Current Research in Infectious Diseases

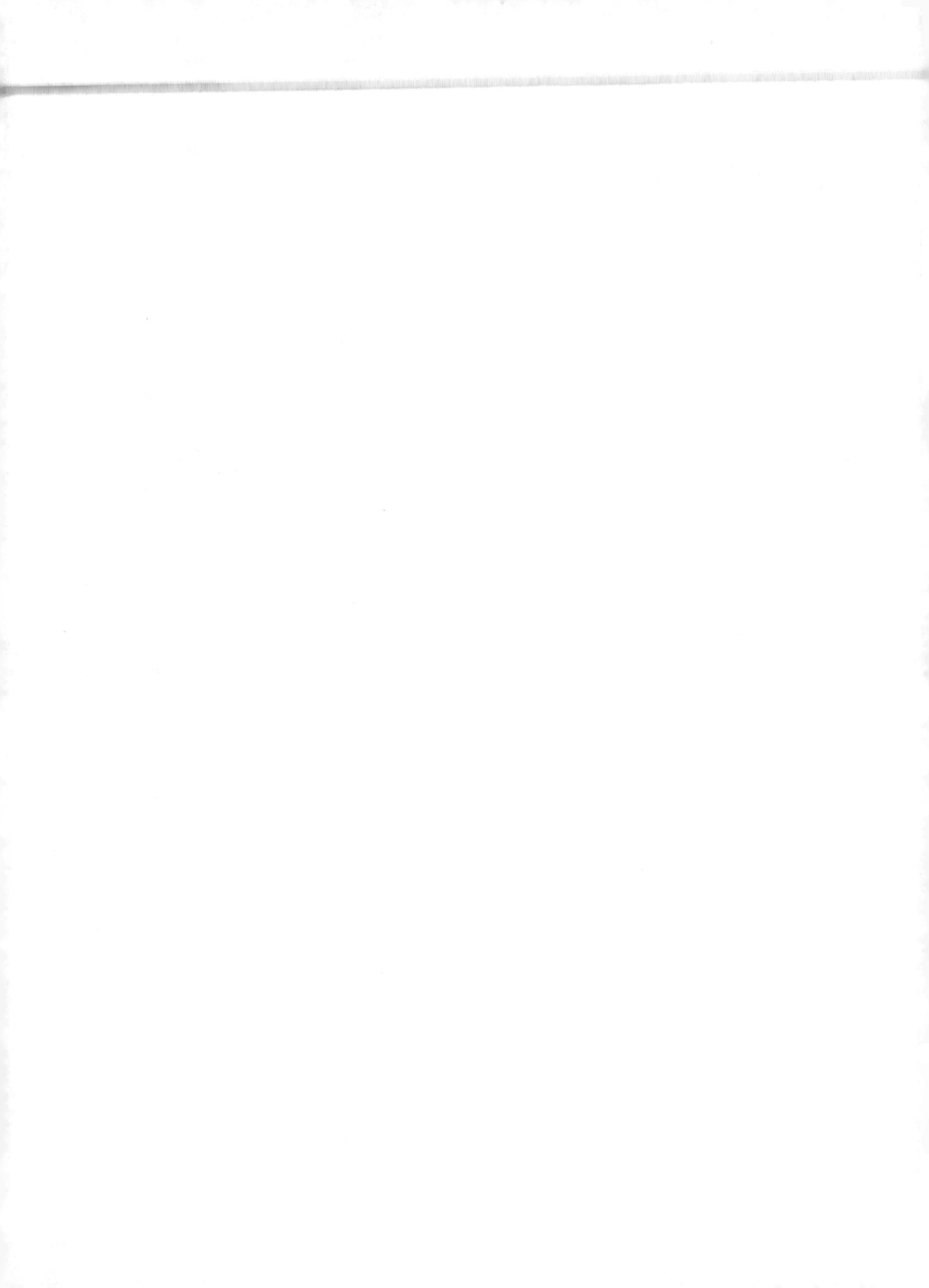

Contents

Current Research in Infectious Diseases

Edited by **Daniel Enger**

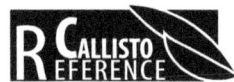

R CALLISTO
REFERENCE

New York

Published by Callisto Reference,
106 Park Avenue, Suite 200,
New York, NY 10016, USA
www.callistoreference.com

Current Research in Infectious Diseases
Edited by Daniel Enger

International Standard Book Number: 978-1-63239-644-0 (Hardback)

Preface

This book aims to highlight the current researches and provides a platform to further the scope of innovations in this area. This book is a product of the combined efforts of many researchers and scientists from different parts of the world. The objective of this book is to provide the readers with the latest information in the field.

Infectious Diseases are an ever growing concern for medical professionals around the globe in today's world. They refer to the disorders caused by the pathogens like bacteria, viruses, germs or fungi. They are acquired by insect bites, consumption of contaminated food or water. These diseases are highly communicable and many of them can be fatal for the living species. Some of the widely known infectious diseases are HIV, Malaria, dengue fever, etc. This book attempts to understand the multiple branches that fall under this discipline and explores the recent researches in the field of infectious diseases. Therefore, this book will help readers in keeping pace with the rapid changes in the world. Coherent flow of topics, student-friendly language and extensive use of examples make this book an invaluable source of knowledge.

I would like to express my sincere thanks to the authors for their dedicated efforts in the completion of this book. I acknowledge the efforts of the publisher for providing constant support. Lastly, I would like to thank my family for their support in all academic endeavors.

Editor

Identifying factors associated with changes in CD4$^+$ count in HIV-infected adults in Saskatoon, Saskatchewan

Kelsey Hunt MSc[1], Prosanta Mondal MSc[2], Stephanie Konrad MSc[1], Stuart Skinner MD MSc[3], Kali Gartner BSc[3], Hyun J Lim PhD[1]

K Hunt, P Mondal, S Konrad, S Skinner, K Gartner, HJ Lim. Identifying factors associated with changes in CD4$^+$ count in HIV-infected adults in Saskatoon, Saskatchewan. Can J Infect Dis Med Microbiol 2015;26(4):207-211.

OBJECTIVE: To assess the impact of clinical and social factors unique to HIV-infected adults in Saskatoon, Saskatchewan, regarding the rate of CD4$^+$ count change, and to identify factors associated with a risk of CD4$^+$ count decline.
METHODS: A retrospective longitudinal cohort study from medical chart reviews at two clinics was conducted in Saskatoon. Univariate and multivariate linear mixed effects models were used to assess the impact of selected factors on CD4$^+$count change.
RESULTS: Four hundred eleven HIV-infected patients were identified from January 1, 2003 to November 30, 2011. Two hundred eighteen (53%) were male, mean (± SD) age was 35.6 ±10.1 years, 257 (70.8%) were First Nations or Métis, 312 (80.2%) were hepatitis C virus (HCV) coinfected and 300 (73.3%) had a history of injection drug use (IDU). In univariate models, age, ethnicity, HCV, IDU, antiretroviral therapy and social assistance were significant. Using ethnicity, HCV and IDU, three multivariate models (models 1, 2, 3) were built due to high correlation. First Nations or Métis ethnicity, HCV coinfection and a history of IDU were associated with significantly lower CD4$^+$ counts in multivariate models. Older age and social assistance were associated with significantly lower CD4$^+$ counts in models 1 and 3. Age was marginally significant in model 2 (P=0.055). Not prescribed antiretroviral therapy was associated with a significantly negative CD4$^+$ count slope in all multivariate models.
CONCLUSION: The unique epidemiology of this HIV-infected population may be contributing to CD4$^+$ count change. Increased attention and resources focused on this high-risk population are needed to prevent disease progression and to improve overall health and quality of life.

Key Words: *CD4$^+$ count; First Nations; HCV; HIV; IDU; Métis; Rapid progression*

Les facteurs d'identification associés aux modifications de la numération de CD4$^+$ chez des adultes infectés par le VIH de Saskatoon, au Canada

OBJECTIF : Évaluer les répercussions des facteurs cliniques et sociaux propres aux adultes infectés par le VIH de Saskatoon, en Saskatchewan, sur le taux de modifications de la numération de CD4$^+$ et déterminer les facteurs associés à un risque de diminution de la numération de CD4$^+$.
MÉTHODOLOGIE : Les chercheurs ont réalisé une étude de cohorte longitudinale rétrospective des dossiers médicaux de deux cliniques de Saskatoon. Ils ont utilisé les modèles linéaires à effets mixtes univariés et multivariés pour évaluer les répercussions de certains facteurs associés aux modifications de la numération de CD4$^+$.
RÉSULTATS : Les chercheurs ont repéré 411 patients infectés par le VIH entre le 1er janvier 2003 et le 30 novembre 2011. Deux cent dix-huit d'entre eux (53 %) étaient de sexe masculin et avaient un âge moyen (± ÉT) de 35,6 ans ±10,1 ans, 257 (70,8 %) étaient Métis ou originaires des Premières nations, 312 (80,2 %) étaient co-infectés par le virus de l'hépatite C (VHC) et 300 (73,3 %) avaient des antécédents de consommation de drogues par injection (CDI). Dans les modèles univariés, l'âge, l'ethnie, le VHC, la CDI, l'antirétrovirothérapie et l'aide sociale étaient déterminants. À l'aide de l'ethnie, du VHC et de la CDI, les chercheurs ont formé trois modèles multivariés (modèles 1, 2, 3) en raison de leur forte corrélation. Le fait d'être Métis ou originaire des Premières nations, d'être co-infecté par le VHC et d'avoir des antécédents de CDI s'associait à des numérations de CD4$^+$ beaucoup plus faibles dans les modèles multivariés. Le fait d'être plus âgé et de recevoir de l'aide sociale s'associait à une numération beaucoup plus faible de CD4$^+$ dans les modèles 1 et 3. L'âge était légèrement significatif dans le modèle 2 (P=0,055). Dans tous les modèles multivariés, l'antirétrovirothérapie ne s'associait jamais à une pente négative de la numération de CD4$^+$.
CONCLUSION : L'épidémiologie unique de cette population infectée par le VIH contribue peut-être à une modification de la numération de CD4+. Il faudra se pencher sur ces patients à haut risque et y injecter plus de ressources pour prévenir l'évolution de leur maladie et améliorer leur santé et leur qualité de vie globales.

The HIV epidemic in Saskatchewan has been growing at an alarming rate since 2003 (1,2). At the present time, the incidence of HIV in Saskatchewan is the highest in Canada (19.6 per 100,000 in 2011), at more than double the national average (7.6 per 100,000) (3). Importantly, the highest recorded incidences have occurred in the most recent years (23.8 per 100,000 in 2009; 20.3 in 2010 and 19.6 in 2011), indicating that the epidemic in this province is not approaching resolution (3).

The epidemiology of HIV in Saskatchewan is unique to Canada in that female sex and/or individuals self-identifying as being of First Nations and Métis ethnicity are over-represented compared with other HIV-infected populations across Canada (4-6). The unfortunate prevalence of low socioeconomic status among First Nations and Métis communities in Canada poses barriers to achieving optimum health.

Such challenges include poverty and the associated housing insecurity and malnutrition, in addition to increased rates of incarceration, injection drug use (IDU) and mental illness. Another unique characteristic of the HIV epidemic in this province is that IDU is the predominant mode of transmission, in contrast to men who have sex with men, which has remained the most commonly reported exposure nationally, since the beginning of the epidemic in Canada (1,2). Given the high prevalence of IDU, this population is also afflicted with high rates of coinfection with hepatitis C virus (HCV), which has been shown to be 10 times more transmissible through IDU than HIV (7-9).

Immune deficiency in AIDS is caused by the virally mediated destruction of CD4$^+$ T cells (10,11). HIV disease progression is characterized by the progressive decline in CD4$^+$ count over time (11-15). The

[1]*Department of Community Health and Epidemiology;* [2]*School of Public Health;* [3]*Department of Medicine, University of Saskatchewan, Saskatoon, Saskatchewan*
Correspondence: Kelsey Hunt, Department of Community Health and Epidemiology, University of Saskatchewan, 107 Wiggins Road, Saskatoon, Saskatchewan S7N 5E5. e-mail keh470@mail.usask.ca

TABLE 1
Baseline and time-dependent patient characteristics according to ethnicity (n=411)

Variables	Total sample (n=411)	First Nations or Métis (n=257, 70.8%)	Others* (n=106, 29.2%)
Follow-up time, months, median (IQR)	27.6 (31.9)	27.6 (29.9)	32.6 (37.7)
Variable at baseline			
Age at enrollment, years, mean ± SD	35.7±10.3	33.7±9.1	41±11.5
Exposure category†			
MSM	21 (6.5)	1 (0.5)	20 (22.0)
MSM/IDU	12 (3.7)	5 (2.3)	6 (6.6)
IDU	244 (75.5)	193 (89.8)	36 (39.5)
Heterosexual contact	46 (14.2)	16 (7.4)	29 (31.9)
Site			
PLP	188 (45.7)	100 (38.9)	80 (75.5)
WSCC	122 (29.7)	84 (32.7)	7 (6.6)
Both	101 (24.6)	73 (28.4)	19 (17.9)
CD4+ count, cells/μL			
n, mean ± SD	300, 379±233	181, 369±218	87, 376±236
Missing, n	111	76	19
CD4+ count, cells/μL			
<200	68 (22.7)	39 (21.6)	21 (24.1)
200–350	88 (29.3)	60 (33.1)	22 (25.3)
>350	144 (48.0)	82 (45.3)	44 (50.6)
Log10 of viral load, copies/mL			
n, mean ± SD	276, 4.3±1.0	167, 4.2±1.0	85, 4.4±1.0
Missing, n	135	90	21
HCV antibody positive	312 (80.2)	227 (92.6)	47 (46.5)
Missing, n	22	12	5
History of IDU	300 (73.3)	222 (87.1)	43 (40.6)
Missing, n	2	2	
STI	134 (32.6)	86 (33.5)	38 (35.8)
Time-dependent variables			
Incarcerated during follow-up	118 (28.7)	89 (34.6)	22 (20.7)
Ever use of social assistance	146 (35.5)	110 (42.8)	25 (23.6)
Ever use of ART	257 (62.5)	167 (65.0)	70 (66.0)
ART naïve	154 (37.5)	90 (35.0)	36 (34.0)
Case management	54 (13.1)	45 (17.5)	4 (3.8)
Clinical AIDS	30 (7.3)	18 (7.0)	12 (11.3)
All-cause mortality	29 (7.1)	20 (7.8)	8 (7.5)

Data presented as n (%) unless otherwise indicated. *48 were missing; †88 were missing. ART Antiretroviral therapy; HCV Hepatitis C virus, IDU Injection drug use; IQR Interquartile range; MSM Men who have sex with men; PLP Positive Living Program; STI Sexually transmitted infection; WSCC Westside Community Clinic

monitoring of CD4+ cell counts over time provides a surrogate measure of HIV disease progression (10). CD4+ cell counts are used by clinicians in determining when to initiate antiretroviral therapy (ART) and other prophylactic therapies in the treatment of opportunistic infections, as well as being commonly used as an end point in clinical studies (10,11,16,17). In the present study, we used CD4+ cell count to evaluate HIV disease progression.

Clinicians in Saskatoon, Saskatchewan caring for HIV-infected individuals have anecdotally reported the observation of a more rapid than expected progression to immunological AIDS (CD4+ count <200 cells/μL) in recent years. The aim of the present study was to examine this phenomenon of rapid progression from HIV infection to immunological AIDS.

The HIV-infected population of Saskatchewan is afflicted with a multitude of health-compromising conditions; this population is understudied and is showing evidence of rapid progression to AIDS. The objectives of the present study were to estimate the rate of CD4+ cell depletion among HIV-infected adults in the city of Saskatoon, and to determine the effects of the following clinical and social factors regarding CD4+cell count changes: age at diagnosis; sex; ethnicity; HCV coinfection; history of IDU; ART; incarceration during follow-up; engagement in case management services; receipt of social assistance; and presence of a sexually transmitted infection (STI).

METHODS
Setting and population
The present study was a retrospective longitudinal cohort anaylsis of HIV-infected patients followed at two clinics in Saskatoon, specializing in the care of this population: the Positive Living Program at Royal University Hospital and the Westside Community Clinic (WSCC).

Data collection
Data were abstracted from patient charts. Inclusion criteria included a new HIV diagnosis of patients ≥18 years of age between January 1, 2003 and November 30, 2011. Patient data abstracted from medical charts included demographics, social history, clinical variables, laboratory data and ART. First CD4+ count and viral load measurement within six months of HIV diagnosis were considered to be baseline measurements.

Data analyses
Patient characteristics at HIV diagnosis (baseline) and during follow-up (time dependent) were summarized using descriptive statistics. A χ^2 test was used to assess associations between categorical variables. Pearson correlation analysis was performed. Independent variables considered included sex, age, ethnicity, HCV seropositivity, coinfection with an STI, IDU, history of incarceration, history of receipt of social assistance, case management (a program of intensive social work at the WSCC) and ART. Before fitting mixed effect models on CD4+ count outcome, the CD4+ count of an individual was summarized in three-month intervals for the first three years and in six-month intervals for the remainder of the study time. If a subject underwent more than one measurement in a given interval, the mean was used. This interval was selected because this is the standard clinical follow-up timeline for patients observed in the two clinics. The interval was increased to six months after the three-year period because there were far fewer patients followed for >3 years compared with patients followed for ≤3 years. CD4+ count was then modelled longitudinally by fitting mixed effects models with random intercept a nd random slope (18). A linear regression of CD4+ count change according to months since diagnosis among 10 randomly selected patients, as well as a linear regression of mean CD4+ count according to months since diagnosis was created to ensure the assumption of a robustly linear change in CD4+ count over time was not violated. Interactions among covariates were examined. Variables were identified as significant using a 0.05 α level. All analyses were performed using SAS version 9.2 (SAS Institute, USA).

The present study was approved by the University of Saskatchewan Ethics Review Board, the Saskatoon Health Region and the WSCC.

RESULTS
A total of 411 patients who had at least one CD4+ recorded met the study inclusion criteria. A total of 2555 CD4+ counts were recorded among all patients (Table 1). One hundred eighty-eight patients were followed at the Positive Living Program, 122 at the WSCC and 101 were followed at both sites. The mean (± SD) age at diagnosis was 35.7±10.3 years and 53% of patients were men. Two hundred fifty-seven (70.8%) patients self-identified as being of First Nations or Métis ethnicity. The most commonly reported exposure category was IDU (75.5%), followed by heterosexual contact (14.2%) and

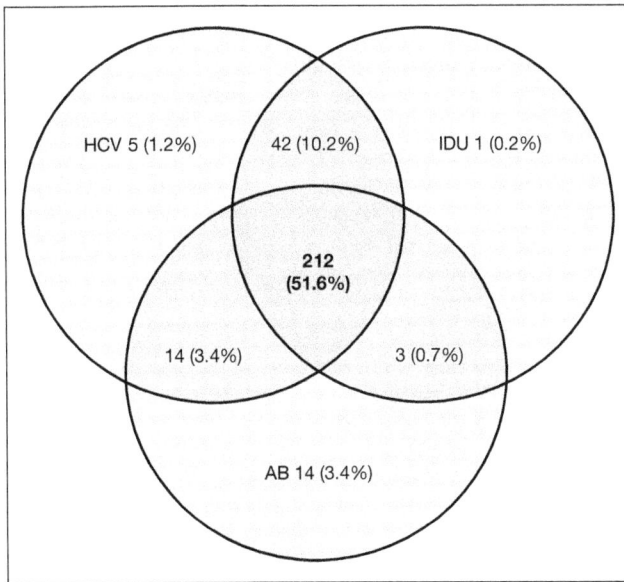

Figure 1) *High correlation among patients coinfected with hepatitis C virus (HCV), injection drug use (IDU) and self-identifying as First Nations or Métis ethnicity (AB). (Note: 53 [12.9%] patients did not possess any of these cofactors and 67 [16.3%] had missing information regarding at least one of these cofactors)*

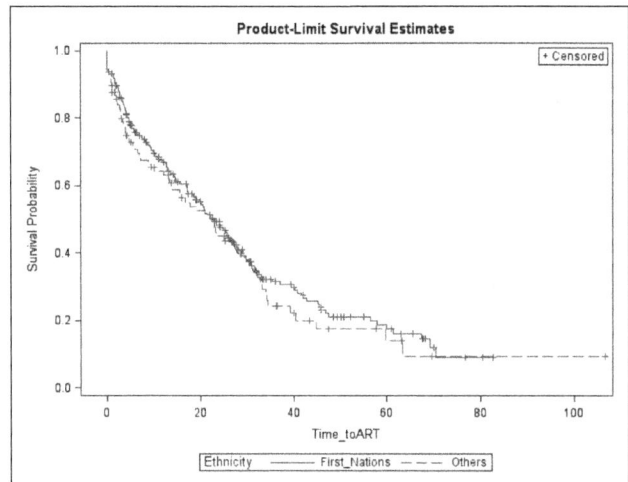

Figure 2) *Time to antiretroviral therapy (ART) initiation among First Nations patients compared with patients of other ethnicities*

men having sex with men (6.5%). Fifty-four (13.1%) patients were case management clients, 146 (35.5%) had a record of receiving social assistance, 134 (32.6%) acquired an STI throughout the course of their care, 312 (80.2%) were HCV seropositive, 300 (73.3%) had a history of IDU, 118 (28.7%) had a history of incarceration and 257 (62.5%) were ever prescribed ART. The mean baseline CD4+count was 379±233 cells/µL and the mean baseline log viral load was 4.3±1 copies/mL. The mean follow-up time for all patients was 32.5 months.

HCV coinfection, First Nations or Métis ethnicity, and IDU were highly correlated (Figure 1). Proportion of HCV coinfection is significantly higher in injection drug users compared with individuals who did not have a history of IDU (98.6% versus 25.8%; P<0.0001). Individuals self-identifying as of First Nations or Métis ethnicity experienced higher odds of having a history of IDU (OR 9.86 [95% CI 5.78 to 16.79]; P<0.0001) and HCV coinfection (OR 14.49 [95% CI 7.80 to 6.91]; P<0.0001). Time to ART initiation was not significantly different between First Nations or Métis and other ethnicity (P=0.43, log-rank test, Figure 2).

In the univariate mixed effects models, ethnicity, social assistance, HCV coinfection, history of IDU and ever use of ART were significant. Sex, age, incarceration, case management and STI coinfection were not significant (results are not shown for the univariate analysis).

All significant covariates from the univariate mixed effects models analysis were included in the multivariate models. Although age was not univariately significant, it was considered to be a potential confounder and added in the multivariate models. Due to the significant correlation among ethnicity, HCV infection and IDU, the following three separate multivariate mixed effects models were built.

Model 1: In the first model incorporating ethnicity (Table 2), the estimated mean regression coefficient of time for the ART-naïve group was −27.18 (95% CI −44.95 to −9.41), suggesting a significant decrease in CD4+ count at a rate of 27.18 cells/µL per year among ART-naïve patients after controlling for other covariates. CD4+ count remained almost unchanged among ART recipients (−27.18+27.94=0.76 cells/µL per year). The rate of CD4+ count change was significantly different between these two groups (27.94 cells/µL per year, P=0.008). First Nations ethnicity (P=0.027), receipt of social assistance (P=0.008) and

higher age at diagnosis (P=0.001) were significant predictors of lower CD4+ count.

Model 2: In the second model incorporating HCV coinfection (Table 3), CD4+ count significantly decreased at a rate of 33.72 cells/µL per year among ART-naive patients (P=0.0001). CD4+ count was not changed among ART-exposed patients (−33.72+37.17=3.45 cells/µL per year). However, the rate of CD4+ count change was significantly different between these two groups (37.17 cells/µL per year, P=0.0003). HCV antibody positivity (P=0.003) and older age at diagnosis (P=0.055) were associated with lower CD4+ counts.

Model 3: In the third model incorporating a history of IDU (Table 4), CD4+ count significantly decreased at a rate of 32.41 cells/µL per year among ART-naive patients after controlling for other covariates (P=0.0002). CD4+ count remained almost unchanged among ART recipients (−32.41+34.08=1.67 cells/µL per year). The rate of CD4+ count change was significantly different between these two groups (34.08 cells/µL per year, P=0.0007). A history of IDU (P=0.042), receipt of social assistance (P=0.042) and increasing age at diagnosis (P=0.026) were significant predictors of lower CD4+ counts.

TABLE 2
Multivariate mixed effects model (model 1) containing First Nations or Métis ethnicity (n=363)

Covariate	β ± SE	95% CI	P
Intercept	618.50±45.63	528.77 to 708.24	<0.0001
Time (in years)	−27.18±9.03	−44.95 to −9.41	0.002
Time*ART (yes)	27.94±10.52	7.31 to 48.57	0.008
First Nations or Métis	−47.20±21.32	−89.03 to −5.37	0.027
Social assistance (yes)	−50.85±19.24	−88.59 to −13.10	0.008
Age at diagnosis	−2.93±0.93	−4.76 to −1.10	0.001

ART Antiretroviral therapy

DISCUSSION

The present study was a retrospective longitudinal cohort analysis of 411 HIV-positive patients diagnosed between January 1, 2003 and November 30, 2011 and followed by physicians at the Positive Living Program and WSCC in Saskatoon, Saskatchewan. We investigated CD4+ changes over time to explore HIV disease progression to immunological AIDS. The objective of the present study was to identify clinical and social factors associated with rates of change in CD4+ counts.

HIV and HCV are both transmitted through IDU (19-22). There is an increased frequency of IDU among incarcerated populations, because patients with more extreme addictions may be at an increased

TABLE 3
Multivariate mixed effects model (model 2) containing hepatitis C virus (HCV) coinfection (n=389)

Covariate	β ± SE	95% CI	P
Intercept	607.17±45.34	518.03 to 696.32	<0.0001
Time (in years)	−33.72±8.69	−50.82 to −16.62	0.0001
Time*ART (yes)	37.17±10.20	17.17 to 57.17	0.0003
HCV (yes)	−67.24±23.28	−112.91 to −21.58	0.003
Social assistance (yes)	−33.57±19.40	−71.63 to 4.49	0.08
Age at diagnosis	−1.72±0.90	−3.49 to 0.04	0.055

ART Antiretroviral therapy

TABLE 4
Multivariate mixed effects model (model 3) containing injection drug use (IDU) (n=409)

Covariate	β±SE	95% CI	P
Intercept	590.62±42.69	506.70 to 674.54	<0.0001
Time (in years)	−32.41±8.47	−49.07 to −15.74	0.0002
Time*ART (yes)	34.08±9.99	14.48 to 53.68	0.0007
IDU (yes)	−42.77±21.02	−84.01 to −1.54	0.042
Social assistance (yes)	−38.92±19.16	−76.51 to −1.33	0.042
Age at diagnosis	−1.97±0.89	−3.70 to −0.23	0.026

ART Antiretroviral therapy

likelihood to incur criminal charges (23,24). IDU and incarceration have been found to be associated with a lower uptake of and adherence to ART (25-29). Additionally, the stress of the prison environment has been found to contribute to a faster rate of decline in CD4$^+$ count (13). The tracking of patients through the prison systems in Saskatchewan has been identified as a barrier to ensuring continuity of care among incarcerated HIV-positive individuals, in particular in ensuring a continual supply of ART. This reduced ability to track a patient's incarceration, duration and release also likely led to an under-representation of the true prevalence of incarceration in the study population. Therefore, the negative impact of incarceration regarding HIV disease progression may be underestimated in the present study.

A longitudinal mixed-effects model found self-identifying as being of First Nations or Métis ethnicity, HCV coinfection, a history of IDU, older age and receipt of social assistance to be associated with significantly lower CD4$^+$ counts in multivariate models. Not being exposed to ART was significantly associated with a negative CD4$^+$ count slope in multivariate mixed effects models.

The mixed effects models have the potential to be developed into clinical tools. These clinical tools may predict the CD4$^+$ counts of patients at follow-up visits and, therefore, potentially be helpful in the identification of patients at risk for rapid progression. By identifying these patients early in the clinical course of HIV disease progression, interventions to mitigate risk factors for rapid progression may be initiated; for example, increased social support to mitigate the effects of low socioeconomic status such as poor nutrition. Such increased social support has recently been introduced at the WSCC in the form of case management service. Associations between engagement in case management services and improvements in overall health among HIV-infected individuals have been previously reported (30-32). Although we did not observe a significant association with increased CD4$^+$ counts and involvement with case management services, this finding was likely due to dataset limitations.

Socioeconomic disadvantages, which are unfortunately prevalent among First Nations and Métis communities, HCV coinfection, a history of IDU, receipt of social assistance and older age at diagnosis were associated with lower CD4$^+$ counts. CD4$^+$ count significantly decreased over time among patients who were never prescribed ART. The present study highlights the urgent need for both clinical, as well as social, interventions to address the HIV epidemic in Saskatchewan.

The findings of the present study may contribute to improvements in clinical care in that these findings may aid clinicians in the identification of HIV-infected patients who may be at risk for rapid progression. The identification of cofactors that can be implicated in contributing to rapid progression to AIDS and/or death has the potential to slow disease progression if the impacts of such cofactors can be mitigated. Earlier and more aggressive ART may be beneficial to patients who can be identified as higher risk for rapid progression to AIDS.

Strengths of the present study include the unique epidemiology of the study population; namely, an over-representation of individuals of First Nations or Métis ethnicity and therefore, an increased prevalence of social and economic disadvantage that unfortunately exists among this population; a high prevalence of HCV coinfection; and a high prevalence of IDU. Another strength is that the follow-up period of the present study

incorporates the course of the emergence of the dramatic increase in incidence of HIV in Saskatchewan.

Limitations of the present study include those of all retrospective data sets, in that we were limited to information that was previously recorded in patient medical records, which may not always have included all of the variables of interest. For example, absolute lymphocyte count, leukocyte count, and information regarding alcohol use and abuse among patients were not available. Alcoholism has known effects on CD4$^+$ counts in HIV-infected patients (33,34). Another limitation of this dataset was an unknown date of seroconversion among many patients, which poses a challenge to an accurate depiction of the entire clinical course of HIV. We were able to arrive at a more accurate depiction of the effects of selected cofactors on the clinical course of HIV through the use of multiple analyses and comparisons of the results of these analyses.

Future studies should include the creation of a prospective cohort database, ideally enrolling at-risk individuals while seronegative, to establish date of seroconversion and, therefore, enable a more accurate and complete depiction of the individual and population-level clinical course of HIV infection. In addition, studies with a longer follow-up period would also allow for a more comprehensive picture of the course of HIV among Saskatchewan patients. Finally, a study examining social factors contributing to the HIV epidemic in Saskatchewan and, in particular, the contribution of social factors to the phenomenon of a rapid progression to AIDS would be of particularly importance to this unique population.

SUMMARY

The HIV-infected population of Saskatoon is characterized according to unique social and clinical factors, which may conspire to contribute to an accelerated progression to AIDS. The variables of HCV coinfection, First Nations or Métis ethnicity and IDU were highly correlated. Ethnicity, receipt of social assistance, older age at diagnosis, HCV coinfection, a history of IDU and ever use of ART were significantly associated with lower CD4$^+$ counts. Patients presenting as HIV positive with one or more of these cofactors can be considered to be at risk for accelerated progression to AIDS. The early identification by clinicians of patients with these risk factors and the implementations of targeted interventions to mitigate the negative health effects of these cofactors may contribute to improved health and quality of life for this HIV-infected population.

ACKNOWLEDGEMENTS: The authors acknowledge the Saskatoon Health Region, the Positive Living Program, the Westside Community Clinic and the thesis committee for their assistance and support of this project.

REFERENCES
1. Saskatchewan Ministry of Health, Population Health Branch. HIV Strategy for Saskatchewan 2010-2013.
2. Public Health Agency of Canada. HIV and AIDS in Canada. Surveillance Report to December 31, 2009. Surveillance and Risk Assessment Division, Centre for Communicable Diseases and Infection Control. 2010.

3. Public Health Agency of Canada. At a Glance – HIV and AIDS in Canada: Surveillance Report to December 31st, 2011. 2012.

4. Disease Prevention Unit, Population Health Branch, Saskatchewan Ministry of Health. HIV and AIDS in Saskatchewan 2010. November 30, 2011.

5. Public Health Agency of Canada. HIV/AIDS Epi Updates – July 2010, Chapter 1: National HIV Prevalence and Incidence Estimates in Canada for 2008. 2011. <www.phac-aspc.gc.ca/aids-sida/publication/epi/2010/1-eng.php#note5> (Accessed March 12, 2012).

6. HIV in Saskatchewan Panel Discussion. February 14, 2011.

7. Montaner JSG, Le T, Hogg R, et al. The changing spectrum of AIDS index diseases in Canada. AIDS 1994;8:693.

8. Des Jarlais DC, Arasteh K, McKnight C, Hagan H, Perlman DC, Semaan S. Associations between herpes simplex virus type 2 and HCV with HIV among injecting drug users in New York City: The current importance of sexual transmission of HIV. Am J Public Health 2011;101:1277.

9. Des Jarlais D, Semaan S. HIV and other sexually transmitted infections in injection drug users and crack cocaine smokers. In: Holmes KK, Spanling PF, Stamm WE, et al (eds). Sexually Transmitted Diseases, 4th edn. New York: McGraw Hill 2008:237-55.

10. Seligmann M, Pinching AJ, Rosen FS, et al. Immunology of human immunodeficiency virus infection and the acquired immunodeficiency syndrome. Ann Intern Med 1987;107:234-42.

11. McCune JM. The dynamics of CD4 T-cell depletion in HIV disease. Nature 2001;410:974-9.

12. Rowland-Jones S, Pinheiro S, Kaul R. New insights into host factors in HIV-1 pathogenesis. Cell 2001;104:473.

13. Griffin MM, Ryan JG, Briscoe VS, Shadle KM. Effects of incarceration on HIV-infected individuals. J Natl Med Assoc 1996;88:639.

14. Anastos K, Gange SJ, Lau B, et al. Association of race and gender with HIV-1 RNA levels and immunologic progression. J Acquir Immune Defic Syndr 2000;24:218.

15. Lyles RH, Muñoz A, Yamashita TE, et al. Natural history of human immunodeficiency virus type 1 viremia after seroconversion and proximal to AIDS in a large cohort of homosexual men. J Infect Dis 2000;181:872.

16. Maini M, Gilson R, Chavda N, et al. Reference ranges and sources of variability of CD4 counts in HIV-seronegative women and men. Genitourin Med 1996;72:27-31.

17. Tsouska C, Bernard N. Markers Predicting progression of human immunodeficiency virus-related disease. Clin Microbiol Rev 1994;7:14-28.

18. Laird NM, Ware JH. Random-effects models for longitudinal data. Biometrics 1982:963-74.

19. Lewden C, Thiébaut R, Boufassa F, et al. Comparison of early CD4 T-cell count in HIV-1 seroconverters in Cote d'Ivoire and France: The ANRS PRIMO-CI and SEROCO cohorts. J Acquir Immune Defic Syndr 2010;53:260.

20. Ledergerber B, Egger M, Erard V, et al. AIDS-related opportunistic illnesses occurring after initiation of potent antiretroviral therapy. JAMA 1999;282:2220-6.

21. Staples JC, Rimland D, Dudas D. Hepatitis C in the HIV (human immunodeficiency virus) Atlanta V.A. (Veterans Affairs Medical Center) Cohort Study (HAVACS): The effect of coinfection on survival. Clin Infect Dis 1999;29:150-4.

22. Dorrucci M, Pezzotii P, Phillips A, Lepri A, Rezza G. Coinfection of hepatitis C virus with human immunodeficiency virus and progression to AIDS. J Infect Dis 1995;172:1503-8.

23. Spaulding A, Stephenson B, Macalino G, Ruby W, Clarke JG, Flanigan TP. Human immunodeficiency virus in correctional facilities: A review. Clin Infect Dis 2002;35:305-12.

24. Freudenberg N. Jail, prisons, and the health of urban populations: A review of the impact of the correctional system on community health. J Urban Health 2001;78:214-35.

25. Jarrin I, Geskus R, Bhaskaran K, et al. Gender differences in HIV progression to AIDS and death in industrialized countries: Slower disease progression following HIV seroconversion in women. Am J Epidemiol 2008;168:532.

26. Pezzotti P, Phillips AN, Dorrucci M, et al. Category of exposure to HIV and age in the progression to AIDS: Longitudinal study of 1199 people with known dates of seroconversion. BMJ 1996;313:583-6.

27. Martin LJ, Houston S, Yasui Y, Wild TC, Saunders LD. All-cause and HIV-related mortality rates among HIV-infected patients after initiating highly active antiretroviral therapy: The impact of Aboriginal ethnicity and injection drug use. Can J Public Health 2011;102:90-6.

28. Palepu A, Tyndall MW, Joy R, et al. Antiretroviral adherence and HIV treatment outcomes among HIV/HCV co-infected injection drug users: The role of methadone maintenance therapy. Drug Alcohol Depend 2006;84:188-94.

29. Mehta S, Moore RD, Graham NMH. Potential factors affecting adherence with HIV therapy. AIDS 1997;11:1665.

30. Gardner LI, Metsch LR, Anderson-Mahoney P, et al. Efficacy of a brief case management intervention to link recently diagnosed HIV-infected persons to care. AIDS 2005;19:423.

31. Katz MH, Cunningham WE, Fleishman JA, et al. Effect of case management on unmet needs and utilization of medical care and medications among HIV-infected persons. Ann Intern Med 2001;135(Part 1):557-65.

32. Fleishman JA, Mor V, Piette J. AIDS case management: The client's perspective. Health Serve Res 1991;26:447.

33. Samet JH, Cheng DM, Libman H, Nunes DP, Alperen JK, Saitz R. Alcohol consumption and HIV disease progression. J Acquir Immune Defic Syndr 2007;46:194-9.

34. Miguez MJ, Shor-Posner G, Morales G, Rodriguez A, Burbano X. HIV treatment in drug abusers: Impact of alcohol use. Addict Biol 2003;8:337.

2

Relapse of visceral leishmaniasis in an HIV-infected patient successfully treated with a combination of miltefosine and amphotericin B

Shauna McQuarrie MD[1], Ken Kasper MD[1,2], Dana C Moffatt MD[2], Daniel Marko MD[3], Yoav Keynan MD PhD[1,2]

S McQuarrie, K Kasper, DC Moffatt, D Marko, Y Keynan. Relapse of visceral leishmaniasis in a HIV-infected patient successfully treated with a combination of miltefosine and amphotericin B. Can J Infect Dis Med Microbiol 2015;26(6):325-329.

The present report documents a 49-year-old HIV-infected man receiving antiretroviral therapy with a suboptimal immune response and a CD4 count of 95 cells/mm^3, despite virological suppression. Investigation of bone marrow was conducted and yielded a diagnosis of visceral leishmaniasis. The clinical course was complicated by gastrointestinal involvment and relapse occurred after amphotericin B therapy. With the addition of miltefosine, the patient no longer presented with bone marrow amastigotes, and displayed an increased CD4 count and negative *Leishmania* polymerase chain reaction results. The present case highlights atypical presentation of visceral leishmaniasis, including poor immune reconstitution and gastrointestinal involvement. The high likelihood of relapse and response to combination therapy are illustrated.

Key Words: *Combination therapy; HIV visceral leishmania coinfection; Miltefosine; Visceral leishmaniasis*

La rechute d'une leishmaniose viscérale chez un patient infecté par le VIH traité au moyen d'une association de miltéfosine et d'amphotéricine B

Le présent rapport rend compte du cas d'un homme de 49 ans atteint du VIH sous antirétroviraux dont la réponse immunitaire était sous-optimale et dont la numération de CD4 était de 95 cellules/mm^3, malgré une suppression virologique. L'examen de la moelle osseuse a confirmé un diagnostic de leishmaniose viscérale. L'évolution clinique de la maladie a été compliquée par une atteinte gastro-intestinale, et le patient a fait une rechute après un traitement à l'amphotéricine B. Après l'ajout de miltéfosine, le patient n'avait plus d'amastigotes de la moelle osseuse, présentait une augmentation de la numération de CD4 et des résultats négatifs de *Leishmania* à la réaction en chaîne par polymérase. Le présent cas fait ressortir la présentation atypique de cette leishmaniose viscérale, y compris la mauvaise reconstitution immunitaire et l'atteinte gastro-intestinale. La forte probabilité de rechute et de réponse à une thérapie combinée est exposée.

A 49-year-old HIV-infected patient receiving antiretroviral therapy who was virologically suppressed, presented with a suboptimal immune response and a CD4 count of 95 cells/mm^3.

The patient was an Ethiopian man who immigrated to Canada. After spending the first two decades of his life in northern Ethiopia near Mekele and Gonder, which are near the Sudanese border, he moved to Addis Ababa and, later, the eastern region of Ogaden. Leaving Kenya in his mid-thirties, he lived in a refugee camp in Kenya for 13 years.

Known to be HIV positive since 2006, he entered care with the Manitoba HIV program on arrival to Canada four years later. His highly active antiretroviral therapy (HAART) regimen, which had been initiated at diagnosis, consisted of twice daily stavudine, lamivudine and nevirapine; he was not receiving any opportunistic infection prophylaxis at the time of his arrival into care in Canada.

Previous medical diagnoses included asthma, gastroesophageal reflux disease and malaria. He had partially completed a course of therapy for malaria shortly before arrival to Canada, and repeat testing was negative. Gastrointestinal symptoms had been present for three years and consisted of retrosternal burning, and intermittent central chest and epigastric pain. This pain radiated to his back, and worsened with eating or with ingesting medications. He experienced two episodes of hematemesis but no melena.

Initial examination revealed a thin man (body mass index 16.1 kg/m^2) with scarring on his chest wall consistent with a past episode of herpes zoster. Abdominal examination revealed a palpable splenic tip. No lymphadenopathy could be discerned, and the remainder of his physical examination was unremarkable.

During the course of his initial assessment, his CD4 count was 95 cells/mm^3, with a discordant CD4 percentage of 17% and a suppressed viral load. Sulfamethoxazole-trimethoprim was subsequently started for *Pneumocystis jirovecii* pneumonia prophylaxis. Due to the patient's symptoms from stavudine and its long-term side effects, his antiretroviral regimen was changed to tenofovir, emtricitabine and nevirapine.

There were other notable abnormalities from his initial laboratory report, including an elevated thyroid stimulating hormone level and pancytopenia (white blood cells [WBCs] 2.67×10^9/L, neutrophils 1.9×10^9, normocytic anemia with a hemoglobin of 81 g/L, platelets initially normal but when repeated were low [121×10^9]). Thyroid replacement was initiated and additional laboratory testing was performed to investigate the etiology of the pancytopenia.

No reticulocytosis was present, rouleaux formation was detected, B$_{12}$ was normal, ferritin was slightly elevated (280 µg/L), and he had low serum iron and total iron-binding capacity. Liver enzyme levels, including lactate dehydrogenase, bilirubin, lipase and creatinine were all within normal limits. There was no evidence of hemolysis. Hemoglobin S screen was positive, and hemoglobin electrophoresis determined no hemoglobin disorders .

Splenomegaly was confirmed using ultrasound (14.3 cm in length, which is considered to be mildly enlarged) and a bone marrow aspirate

[1]*Manitoba HIV Program;* [2]*Department of Internal Medicine, University of Manitoba;* [3]*Diagnostic Services of Manitoba, Winnipeg, Manitoba*
Correspondence: Dr Yoav Keynan, Department of Internal Medicine, Medical Microbiology, Community Health Sciences, University of Manitoba, Winnipeg, Manitoba R3E 0W3. e-mail keynany@yahoo.com

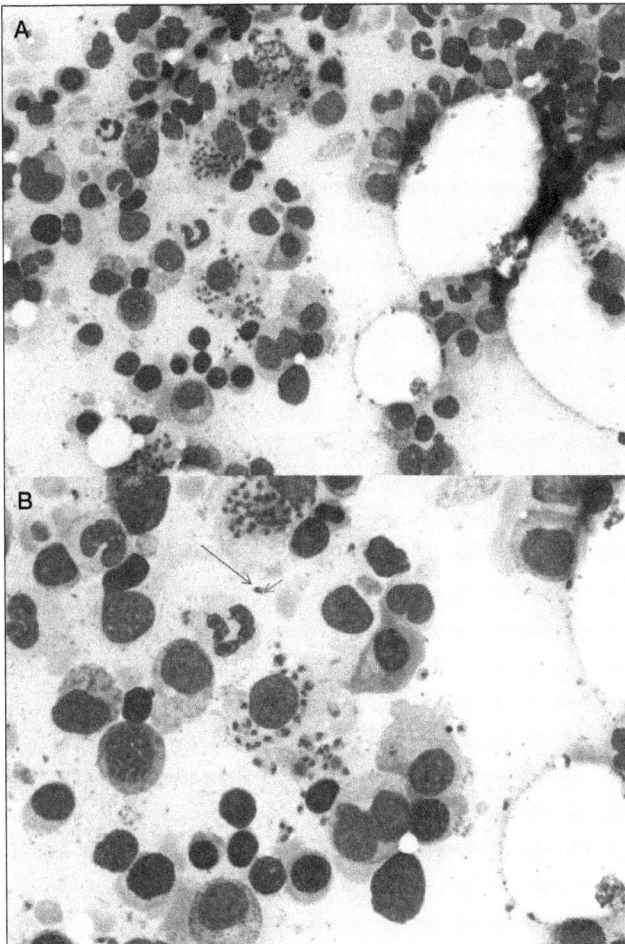

Figure 1) *Giemsa stained bone marrow aspirate demonstrating intra- and extracellular amastigotes (**A**). Nucleus (long arrow) and a kinetoplast (short arrow) are apparent within amastigotes (**B**)*

was proposed to clarify the etiology of his pancytopenia; however, the patient declined to undergo the procedure at that time.

Further laboratory tests performed to investigate his gastrointestinal symptoms revealed positive *Helicobacter pylori* serology for which he was treated with lansoprazole, amoxicillin and clarithromycin. Despite completing the course of therapy, his symptoms persisted and the patient was referred to gastroenterology for further evaluation.

Before being observed, he was hospitalized with bilateral pleural effusions and treated presumptively for tuberculosis (TB) due to his risk factors for TB acquisition and activation (he was from an area where TB is endemic and he was significantly immunocompromised), and the presence of a lymphocytic effusion with a tree-in-bud appearance of his left lower lobe was revealed by computed tomography scan. The pleural fluid was both smear negative and culture negative for TB. He improved clinically after induction therapy with rifampin/isoniazid/pyrazinamide/ethambutol. Ethambutol was switched to moxifloxacin due to ocular symptoms, and induction therapy was followed by isoniazid and rifampin for a subsequent six-month period.

The patient experienced ongoing abdominal pain, fullness, intermittent diarrhea and constipation, as well as nausea and vomiting. A gastroscopy was performed revealing candidal esophagitis and chronic gastritis, including gastric antral and proximal duodenal biopsies illustrating numerous leishmanial parasites. The patient also consented to undergo a bone marrow aspirate to investigate his persistent pancytopenia. Numerous extracellular and intracellular parasites consistent with *Leishmania* amastigotes were observed, and he subsequently underwent treatment with outpatient intravenous (IV)

liposomal amphotericin B 4 mg/kg/day for 10 doses, for a total dose of 40 mg/kg (1).

Initially, his gastrointestinal symptoms improved after treatment. No direct follow-up testing was performed; however, a subsequent ultrasound revealed a reduction of his splenomegaly and his hematological parameters improved (hemoglobin increased from 87 g/L to 101 g/L, WBC count from 2.4×10^9 to 4.3×10^9, neutrophils from 1.48×10^9 to 3.5×10^9 and platelets from 99×10^9 to 187×10^9); however, he had no improvement of his CD4 count.

Unfortunately, over the subsequent nine months, he experienced recurrent gastrointestinal symptoms along with worsening of his hematological parameters.

A repeat bone marrow aspirate performed one year after his initial treatment confirmed the presence of leishmaniasis organisms (Figure 1). His CD4 count at the time was 104 cells/mm^3 (16%) and his HIV viral load was undetectable.

The organism was confirmed to be *Leishmania donovani*, speciated using polymerase chain reaction (PCR).

His antiretroviral regimen was changed to include a protease inhibitor due to its potential for some direct and indirect antileishmanial activity based on in vitro data (2). His new antiretroviral regimen consisted of tenofovir, emtricitabine and darunavir boosted with ritonavir.

Before retreatment of the leishmaniasis, he experienced recurrent epigastric pain and odynophagia and, therefore, endoscopy was repeated. Esophagogastroduodenoscopy revealed candidal esophagitis, and biopsies from both the esophagus and duodenum were positive for leishmaniasis. The esophageal candidiasis was treated with oral fluconazole.

Treatment consisted of IV liposomal amphotericin B (5 mg/kg/dose) for six doses on alternating days (Monday/Wednesday/Friday), along with 28 days of oral miltefosine 100 mg (2.5 mg/kg). He experienced a transient rise in creatinine level, which resolved a few weeks after stopping the amphotericin B.

The patient's epigastric pain improved post-treatment, his splenomegaly resolved and laboratory parameters improved (WBC increased from 2.6×10^9/L to 4.3×10^9/L, neutrophils from 1.8×10^9 to 3.2×10^9, hemoglobin from 82 g/L to 103 g/L and platelets from 68×10^9 to 115×10^9) and his CD4 count rose from 93 cells/mm^3 to 158 cells/mm^3. Splenic aspiration was considered to confirm resolution of the infection; however, with the decrease in splenic size and clearance of infection from the bone marrow after therapy, it was decided that the procedure would not be performed at that time.

A follow-up bone marrow aspirate performed approximately six months post-treatment was free of amastigotes, bone marrow culture was negative for *Leishmania*, as was the aspirate leishmaniasis DNA PCR testing. Serum leishmaniasis DNA PCRs remained negative 15 months after treatment of his relapse, and his most recent CD4 count was 232 cells/mm^3 (20%).

DISCUSSION

Leishmaniasis is a protozoal infection transmitted by the bite of female sandflies, with the majority (90%) of cases being reported from India, Nepal, Bangladesh, Brazil and Sudan. In some regions, up to 30% of the population is asymptomatically infected (3).

Leishmaniasis has three main forms, cutaneous (the most common form), mucocutaneous and visceral (sometimes known as kala-azar). Visceral leishmaniasis (VL) is a disseminated form of the infection caused primarily by the species *Leishmania donovani* and *Leishmania infantum*, and occurs when the organism targets the reticuloendothelial system. Classic features of the disease include chronic fever, weight loss, pancytopenia and organomegaly; however, the majority of individuals with VL are asymptomatic. Our patient lacked the typical symptom of fever, and never developed the expected marked splenomegaly (maximal spleen length was 17.8 cm).

Our patient's diagnosis was made using bone marrow biopsy. Interestingly, because of organism heterogeneity, serological testing for leishmaniasis varies in sensitivity depending on the test used, the individual's region of origin, and is further reduced in HIV coinfection (4).

TABLE 1
Review of published reports of visceral leishmaniasis with gastrointestinal (GI) involvement

Author (reference), year	Symptoms of GI involvement	Patient's country of origin	Site of GI involvement	Treatment	Outcome
McQuarrie et al (present case), 2015					
1	Abdominal pain, nausea, vomiting, diarrhea	Ethiopia, Kenya	Esophagus, gastric antrum and proximal duodenum	Liposomal amphotericin B; relapse treated with liposomal amphotericin B and miltefosine	Responded with negative leishmaniasis antigen titres after second course of treatment
Diro et al (20), 2015					
1		Ethiopia	Oral mucosa (1), rectum (1)	Liposomal amphotericin B	
2	Fever, weight loss, abdominal mass	Ethiopia	Abdominal lymph node	Sodium stibogluconate	Responded
3	Diarrhea, fever, vomiting, oral lesions	Ethiopia	Oral mucosa	Liposomal amphotericin B	Died from septic shock
4	Anal bleeding, fever, weight loss, rectal ulcer	Ethiopia	Rectal mucosa	Sodium stibogluconate	Responded, persistent fecal incontinence
5	Painless nodular skin lesions	Ethiopia	Skin, spleen	Sodium stibogluconate	Responded
Alonso et al (19), 1997					
1	Diarrhea	Spain (travelled to Mexico)	Duodenum	Pentavalent antimonials	Persistent diarrhea and Leishmania seen on follow up duodenal biopsy
2	Diarrhea, fever, abdominal pain, weight loss	Spain	Duodenum	N-methylglutamine antimoniate	Died, renal function deteriorated
Canet et al (21), 2003					
1	Dysphagia	Spain	Midesophageal lesion	Pentavalent antimony and oral allopurinol; sodium stibogluconate every 2 weeks thereafter	Responded
Molaei et al (22), 2007					
1	Fever, abdominal pain, vomiting, diarrhea, weight loss, loss of appetite	Iran	Duodenum	Unknown	Died from sepsis
Hamour et al (23), 1998					
1	Weight loss, polyarthralgia, painless skin lesions	France, Spain	Skin, bone marrow	Amphotericin B, switched to liposomal amphotericin B; relapsed and liposomal amphotericin B triggered renal toxicity; changed to sodium stibogluconate, then IV pentamidine every 2 weeks	Responded, relapsed, responded to second course of treatment
2	Pallor, epigastric tenderness, organomegaly	Fiji/Uganda	Duodenum, bone marrow	Amphotericin B, then pentamidine every 2 weeks	Repeat bone marrow after initial amphotericin B revealed reduction in parasitic load
Jawhar (24), 2011					
1	Abdominal discomfort, diarrhea, vomiting	Yemen	Duodenum, rectum, bone marrow	Sodium stibogluconate	Lost to follow-up

VL is considered to be an opportunistic infection in the context of HIV coinfection. VL increases HIV viral replication and, in turn, is more severe; atypical presentations of VL are more common when patients are coinfected with HIV (5).

We speculate that our patient may have acquired leishmaniasis earlier in life when he lived closer to the Sudanese-Ethiopian border and, subsequently, acquired HIV; however, it is not possible to confirm this hypothesis.

Atypical VL can present variably because of the variety of organ systems that can be involved (eg, the gastrointestinal, respiratory, renal or hepatic systems, among others). In the context of often quite severe immunocompromise due to HIV, the clinician should maintain a high index of suspicion for atypical VL when evaluating symptomatic individuals from areas where leishmaniasis is endemic (6). HIV-positive patients with VL have higher initial leishmaniasis

treatment failure, relapse and mortality rates (7). In our patient, the lack of a rise in CD4 levels, despite suppressive antiretroviral therapy, led to consideration of this diagnosis. A recent study from Spain (8), demonstrated VL to be associated with a high level of immune activation and bacterial translocation (measured by interleukin-6, lipopolysaccharides and, especially, soluble CD14), and poor CD4 rise despite effective HAART.

Treatment of VL
VL can be treated with several agents, such as pentavalent antimonials, amphotericin B, paromomycin and miltefosine; however, the WHO now recommends liposomal amphotericin B as its first preferred regimen in several clinical situations in several geographical regions due to its lower toxicity and excellent clinical efficacy. The markedly increased rates of antimonial toxicity, which HIV-infected individuals

experience when compared with those who are HIV negative limits this medication's use (7,9).

There are other individual agents, such as paromomycin and miltefosine, the latter being the first oral agent. Drawbacks include liver or renal toxicity, cost and varying potential for resistance (2). Miltefosine is well tolerated; however, it has a lower cure rate compared with sodium stibogluconate (an antimonial), and a higher relapse rate (7,10). It is only available in Canada through the Health Canada Special Access program, and the cost for a 28-day course at 100 mg daily is $3,335.48 (personal communication with Manitoba HIV Program pharmacist).

Unfortunately, liposomal amphotericin B is not as widely available as other agents (6,11). It has been shown to be effective in treating HIV/leishmaniasis coinfection, with an initial cure rate of 59.5%; however, less so in HIV-positive leishmaniasis relapse scenarios (38%) (9).

Combination therapy with >1 drug with antileishmanial activity is being considered, given the high failure and relapse rates with monotherapy (9,12-14). All of the above-mentioned drugs are believed to act on different targets (15). A retrospective review of the use of liposomal amphotericin B (30 mg/kg), along with 28 days of miltefosine in an HIV-positive population in Ethiopia, produced an initial cure rate of 87% in HIV-positive leishmaniasis relapse coinfections (7,16). The additive effect of miltefosine may be the result of immunomodulation with boosting of cell-mediated immunity, as illustrated in an experimental model (17).

The hope is that with combination therapy, treatment duration may be shortened, reducing the risk for developing adverse effects, improving compliance and reducing health care costs. Miltefosine, for example, has a very long half-life, and may be well served by being used in combination regimens to prolong and protect its utility (15). More research is needed to determine the best treatment regimen for HIV-coinfected individuals.

Because individuals coinfected with HIV have a higher risk for relapse (up to 60% at one year [5,15]), secondary prophylaxis has been considered. Risk factors for relapse include a very low CD4 count at presentation, past relapse, low body mass index and a CD4 count <200 cells/mm^3 (and especially <100 cells/mm^3) at six months post-treatment (18). Our patient's CD4 count was 71 cells/mm^3 six months after his initial treatment, and 158 cells/mm^3 after the second. An alternative approach is to monitor for serum leishmaniasis DNA PCR, and treat relapses should the PCR become detectable (3).

For individuals diagnosed with leishmaniasis not already receiving HAART, there is no need to delay starting because adverse immune reactions are uncommon and not severe (7). In vitro studies of HIV protease inhibitors have suggested that some may have both direct and indirect antileishmanial effects; however, more research is required to confirm that there is a clinical benefit (2).

Gastrointestinal involvement

Atypical VL is more common in those with HIV coinfection, and can involve systems such as the respiratory, renal, hepatic or gastrointestinal, among others. Gastrointestinal involvement has been extensively reported in the context of *L infantum*, but appears to be relatively common among individuals coinfected with HIV from Ethiopia (6,11). Our client experienced gastrointestinal tract symptoms, which predated his diagnosis by several years, and biopsies confirmed leishmaniasis infection at esophageal, gastric and duodenal sites.

After both treatment courses, his gastrointestinal symptoms resolved and, to date, it appears that the second course of therapy, which combined IV amphotericin B with miltefosine, has been successful. Secondary prophylaxis has not been administered, and the decision was made to follow his leishmaniasis DNA PCR to quickly identify a relapse, should one occur. Fortunately, at last follow-up nine months after he completed treatment, he remained negative.

While the gastrointestinal mucosal appearance may be abnormal, in some situations it may appear unremarkable or suggest an alternate diagnosis. In one article, the diagnosis was made in two individuals based solely on examination of the biopsy material (19), and a negative bone marrow aspirate does not always rule out VL (3). For HIV-positive individuals who are from an area where *Leishmania* is endemic and present with gastrointestinal symptoms, preserving a high index of suspicion for the disease would allow for a greater chance of detection and, therefore, treatment of a potentially curable opportunistic infection.

A review of case reports, which featured gastrointestinal involvement in HIV-positive individuals with VL is summarized in Table 1.

CONCLUSION

Atypical presentations of VL are not uncommon in the HIV-positive population. HIV-coinfected individuals are at risk for atypical site involvement, such as the gastrointestinal tract, and are also at increased risk for relapse after treatment. Gastrointestinal involvement appears to be common among HIV-coinfected individuals from Ethiopia.

Our patient experienced some of the common presenting clinical features of VL (organomegaly and pancytopenia), along with gastrointestinal symptoms but, significantly, without fever. He relapsed after his first course of therapy but, to date, appears to have avoided a relapse after undergoing combination therapy with amphotericin B and miltefosine.

It is important to be aware that leishmaniasis should be included in the differential diagnosis when investigating symptomatic HIV individuals who reside or resided, in leishmaniasis-endemic regions, to ensure that this curable, but otherwise lethal, infection is treated.

While relapse rates are higher than in those who are HIV negative, and there is a need for research to clarify the answers to outstanding questions (such as the role of combination therapy, relapse prevention and appropriate post-treatment monitoring), one of the first challenges is to ensure that individuals with leishmaniasis are diagnosed. This is made more difficult by atypical presentations, such as that observed in our patient, and is why we believed it important to share his experience.

DISCLOSURES: The authors have no financial relationships or conflicts of interest to declare.

REFERENCES

1. AU Russo R, Nigro LC, Minniti S, et al. Visceral leishmaniasis in HIV infected patients: Treatment with high dose liposomal amphotericin B (AmBisome). J Infect 1996;32:133
2. van Griensven J, Diro E, Lopez-Velez R, et al. HIV-1 protease inhibitors for treatment of visceral leishmaniasis in HIV-co-infected individuals. Lancet Infect Dis 2013;13:251-9.
3. van Griensven J, Carrillo E, Lopez-Velez R, Lynen L, Moreno J. Leishmaniasis in immunosuppressed individuals. Clin Microbiol Infect 2014;20:286-99.
4. Abass E, Kang C, Martinkovic F, et al. Heterogeneity of *Leishmania donovani* parasites complicates diagnosis of visceral leishmaniasis: Comparison of different serological tests in three endemic regions. PloS one 2015;10:e0116408
5. van Griensven J, Diro E. Visceral leishmaniasis. Infect Dis Clin North Am 2012;26:309-22.
6. Diro E, van Griensven J, Mohammed R, et al. Atypical manifestations of visceral leishmaniasis in patients with HIV in north Ethiopia: A gap in guidelines for the management of opportunistic infections in resource poor settings. Lancet Infect Dis 2015;15:122-9.
7. Jarvis JN, Lockwood DN. Clinical aspects of visceral leishmaniasis in HIV infection. Curr Opin Infect Dis 2013;26:1-9.
8. Casado J, Abad-Fernandez M, Moreno S, et al. Visceral leishmaniasis as an independent cause of high immune activation, T-cell senescence, and lack of immune recovery in virologically suppressed HIV-1-coinfected patients. HIV Med 2015;16:240-8.
9. Ritmeijer K, ter Horst R, Chane S, et al. Limited effectiveness of high-dose liposomal amphotericin B (AmBisome) for treatment of visceral leishmaniasis in an Ethiopian population with high HIV prevalence. Clin Infect Dis 2011;53:e152-8.

10. Ostyn B, Hasker E, Dorlo TP, et al. Failure of miltefosine treatment for visceral leishmaniasis in children and men in South-East Asia. PLoS One 2014;9:e100220.

11. Diro E, Lynen L, Ritmeijer K, Boelaert M, Hailu A, van Griensven J. Visceral leishmaniasis and HIV coinfection in East Africa. PLoS Negl Trop Dis 2014;8:e2869.

12. Cota GF, de Sousa MR, Fereguetti TO, Rabello A. Efficacy of anti-*Leishmania* therapy in visceral leishmaniasis among HIV infected patients: A systematic review with indirect comparison. PLoS Negl Trop Dis 2013;7:e2195.

13. Sundar S, Chakravarty J. An update on pharmacotherapy for leishmaniasis. Expert Opin Pharmacother 2015;16:237-52.

14. Kumar VD, Verma PR, Singh SK. New insights into the diagnosis and chemotherapy for visceral leishmaniasis. Curr Drug Deliv 2014;11:200-13.

15. van Griensven J, Balasegaram M, Meheus F, Alvar J, Lynen L, Boelaert M. Combination therapy for visceral leishmaniasis. Lancet Infect Dis 2010;10:184-94.

16. van Griensven J, Boelaert M. Combination therapy for visceral leishmaniasis. Lancet 2011;377:443-4.

17. Shivahare R, Vishwakarma P, Parmar N, et al. Combination of liposomal CpG oligodeoxynucleotide 2006 and miltefosine induces strong cell-mediated immunity during experimental visceral leishmaniasis. PLoS One 2014;9:e94596.

18. Cota GF, de Sousa MR, Rabello A. Predictors of visceral leishmaniasis relapse in HIV-infected patients: A systematic review. PLoS Negl Trop Dis 2011;5:e1153.

19. Alonso MJ, Munoz E, Picazo A, et al. Duodenal leishmaniasis diagnosed by biopsy in two HIV-positive patients. Pathol Res Prac 1997;193:43-7.

20. Diro E, Lynen L, Gebregziabiher B, et al. Clinical aspects of paediatric visceral leishmaniasis in north-west Ethiopia. Trop Med Int Health 2015;20:8-16.

21. Canet JJ, Julia J, Martinez-Lacasa J, Garau J. Clinical microbiological case: Esophageal lesion in an AIDS patient. Clin Microbiol Infect 2003;9:421,463-6.

22. Molaei M, Minakari M, Pejhan S, Mashayekhi R, Modaress Fatthi AR, Zali MR. Intestinal leishmaniasis in acquired immunodeficiency syndrome. Iran Red Crescent Med J 2011;13:348-51.

23. Hamour AA, Skelly R, Jowitt SN, et al. Visceral leishmaniasis (Kala-azar) in two patients with HIV-1 infection: Atypical features and response to therapy. J Infect 1998;36:217-20.

24. Jawhar NM. Visceral leishmaniasis with an unusual presentation in an HIV positive patient. SQU Med J 2011;11:269-72.

3

Trichosporon asahii infection after total knee arthroplasty: A case report and review of the literature

Qiang Zuo MSc[1,2]*, Lele Dong BD[2]*, Weidong Mu PhD[1], Lingyun Zhou MSc[3],
Tongping Hu MSc[4], Hua Zhang MSc[5]

Q Zuo, L Dong, W Mu, L Zhou, T Hu, H Zhang. *Trichosporon asahii* infection after total knee arthroplasty: A case report and review of the literature. Can J Infect Dis Med Microbiol 2015;26(1):47-51.

Reports of fungal infection after total knee arthroplasty are extremely rare. In most reports, the infecting organism is a *Candida* species. The present report describes a case involving a 73-year-old immunocompetent woman who underwent total knee arthroplasty and presented one month later with signs of prosthetic infection. She underwent joint debridement and the fluid was sent for culture and sensitivity testing. The culture showed growth of *Trichosporon asahii*. The patient was administered intravenous and intra-articular injections of amphotericin B, followed by antifungal treatment with voriconazole for one year. At 26 months of follow-up, there was no evidence of infection and the patient was ambulating with a walker. To the authors' knowledge, the present case is the first report of *T asahii* infection following knee replacement. Early detection, prompt institution of the appropriate antibiotics and regular follow-up are recommended.

Key Words: *Fungal infection; Periprosthetic; Total knee arthroplasty; Trichosporon asahii*

L'infection à *Trichosporon asahii* après une arthroplastie totale du genou : un rapport de cas et une analyse bibliographique

Les rapports d'infection fongique sont d'une extrême rareté après une arthroplastie totale du genou. Dans la plupart des rapports, l'organisme infectant fait partie des espèces à *Candida*. Le présent rapport décrit le cas d'une femme immunocompétente de 73 ans qui a subi une arthroplastie totale du genou et qui, un mois plus tard, a consulté en raison de signes d'infection prosthétique. Elle a subi un débridement articulaire, et le liquide a été envoyé pour mise en culture et test de sensibilité. La culture a révélé une croissance de *Trichosporon asahii*. La femme a reçu des injections intraveineuses et intra-articulaires d'amphotéricine B, puis un traitement antifongique au voriconazole pendant un an. Après 26 mois de suivi, elle n'avait plus de traces d'infection et pouvait se déplacer avec un déambulateur. En autant que le sache les auteurs, ce cas est le premier rapport d'infection à *T asahii* après une arthroplastie du genou. Ils recommandent le dépistage précoce, l'amorce rapide des antibiotiques pertinents et un suivi régulier.

Incidences of periprosthetic fungal infections following arthroplasty are extremely rare. In the few reported cases, *Candida* species were found to be the primary infecting organisms (1). *Trichosporon asahii* is widely present in the natural environment (2), and *T asahii* infection is more common in patients with immunodeficiency. *T asahii* can infect the lung, skin, hair, lymph nodes or can present as a systemic disseminated infection. The present report describes a case involving primary total knee arthroplasty in a patient without immunodeficiency who presented with a postoperative *T asahii* infection. A review of the literature on the treatment strategy for patients with postoperative fungal infections is also presented.

CASE PRESENTATION

A 73-year-old woman with bilateral osteoarthritis underwent bilateral single-stage total knee replacement. Routine preoperative and preanesthetic investigations were performed. She had a history of hypertension and type 1 diabetes mellitus, and was receiving appropriate medications. Her preoperative fasting blood sugar level was in the range of 6 mmol/L to 10 mmol/L. She did not have a history of intra-articular injections of steroids or any other medications.

The bilateral knee replacement surgery was uneventful. Ceftezole (a first-generation cephalosporin) was administered before the skin incision as a preoperative prophylactic antibiotic. A tourniquet was used bilaterally. A midline skin incision was made and a medial parapatellar approach was used. The surgery lasted for 130 min.

Her postoperative blood sugar levels were regularly monitored, and appropriate medications were administered. The volume of drainage from both knees was larger than usual for the first six days after the procedure. At day 6, the drainage volume was <50 mL and, thus, the drainage tubes were removed. A wound inspection in the right knee revealed that although there was some evidence of superficial poor skin healing, the deep fascia had completely healed. In addition, the patient had a continuous low-grade postoperative fever (37.3°C to 38°C). Laboratory examinations revealed a white blood cell count of $13.6×10^9$/L and a neutrophil percentage of 85.6%. For the first six days, she received a first-generation cephalosporin.

In view of the fever and findings of the wound check, the antibiotic was changed to imipenem/cilastatin sodium, which was given for an additional six days. A wound swab and right knee arthrocentesis culture results were normal at this time. The specimens were inoculated on

Qiang Zuo and Lele Dong contributed equally to this work

[1]*Department of Orthopedics, Provincial Hospital Affiliated to Shandong University, Jinan, Shandong Province;* [2]*Department of Orthopedics, the First Affiliated Hospital of Baotou Medical College, Baotou, Inner Mongolia;* [3]*International Education College, Jiang Xi University of Traditional Chinese Medicine, Nanchang, Jiangxi Province;* [4]*Clinical Laboratory, the First Affiliated Hospital of Baotou Medical College;* [5]*Department of Oncology, the Third Affiliated Hospital of Inner Mongolia Medical College, Baotou, Inner Mongolia, People's Republic of China*

Correspondence: Dr Weidong Mu, Department of Orthopedics, Provincial Hospital Affiliated to Shandong University,
No. 324, Jingwu Road, Jinan 250021, Shandong Province, People's Republic of China. e-mail birchzq@gmail.com

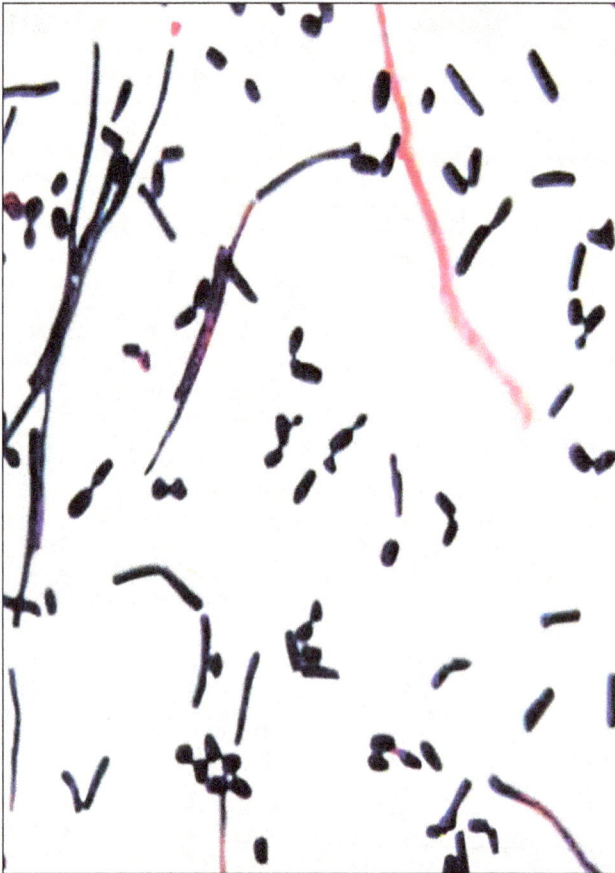

Figure 1) *Colonies of* Trichosporon asahii *after 48 h on Columbia Blood agar at 35°C in ambient air. Morphological features of* T *asahii:* T *asahii is Gram-positive and produces blastoconida of various shapes, well-developed hyphae, pseudohyphae and arthroconida. (Gram stain, magnification ×1000)*

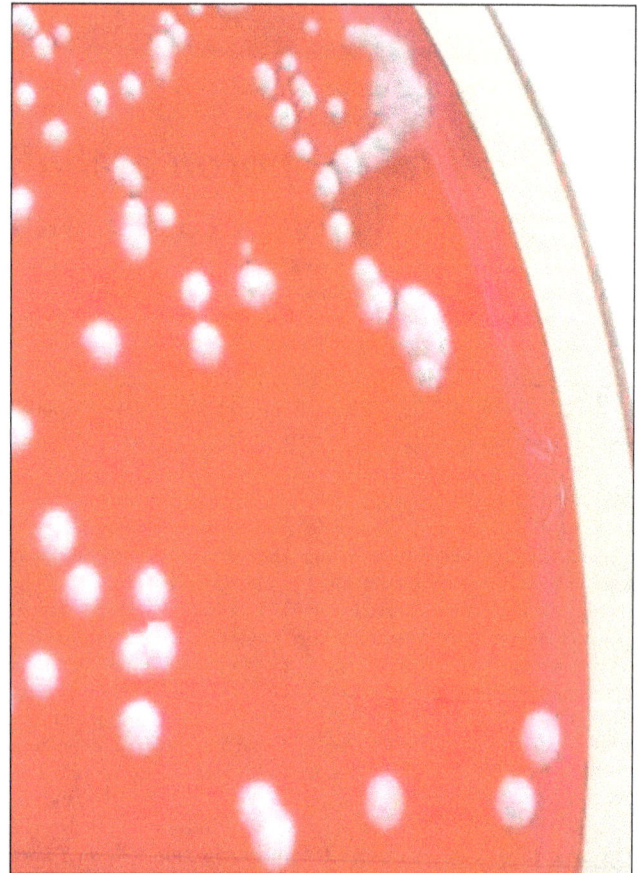

Figure 2) *Colonies of* Trichosporon asahii *after 48 h on Columbia Blood Agar at 35°C in ambient air. Colonies were cream-coloured and smooth. They become dry, moist, shiny, folded, cerebriform and elevated with marginal zones with age*

Columbia Blood agar and China Blue Lactose agar at 35°C in ambient air and cultivated with a Bact/Alert3D Automated Blood Culture System (bioMérieux, France) for three days. Three weeks after surgery, the wound was debrided and resutured due to right knee wound dehiscence. Injectable vancomycin was administered for six days and, subsequently, the wound healed well. One month after the primary surgery, the patient presented with a persistent low-grade fever and recurrent pain on the right side of the left knee joint, which was accompanied by swelling. The temperature of the surrounding skin was also elevated.

Laboratory examinations revealed a normal blood cell count, C-reactive protein level of 27.2 mg/L (normal range 0 mg/L to 5 mg/L) and erythrocyte sedimentation rate of 32 mm/h (normal range 0 mm/h to 15 mm/h). Arthrocentesis revealed that the aspirate from the left knee joint effusion was light yellowish in colour, while aspirate from the right knee effusion was pale, bloody fluid. Both were viscous, not muddy and cultures showed no bacterial growth.

Bilateral joint debridement and lavage was performed. During debridement, pus and necrotic tissue were not present, the synovial fluid was clear and transparent, the surface of the prosthesis was clean and smooth, all of the prosthetic components were stable without any loosening and the bone cement was fixed well. Synovium was completely resected and a pulse lavage system was used to ensure a thorough wash of the joint. In addition, the poly liners were changed. Five days after debridement, intraoperative sampling culture showed no bacterial growth in the right knee; however, the left knee joint fluid culture grew T *asahii* (Figures 1 and 2). The cultures were grown on Columbia Blood agar and China Blue Lactose agar for 24 h to 48 h. The API 20C

identification system (BioMérieux, France) was used to identify T *asahii*, which was sensitive to amphotericin B and voriconazole. Intravenous amphotericin B (1 mg) was administered and increased to 5 mg every subsequent day. However, due to the patient's worsening condition, on the third day, the amphotericin B dose was increased to 25 mg. The patient reported marked improvement in pain three days later. Due to the patient's poor appetite and persistent hypokalemia, the dosage of amphotericin B was not increased to the recommended maximum. Voriconazole alone was started after five weeks, and then after 10 days of intravenous therapy, the dose was changed to 200 mg orally, twice per day. Intra-articular injections of amphotericin B (25 mg once daily) were administered 17 days after surgery. Clinically, the patient continued to improve, her temperature stabilized (with occasional spikes of 37.5°C) and the range of motion of the joint was 0° to 90°.

The patient received oral voriconazole for one year. At the most recent follow-up, which was at 26 months following the primary procedure and 11 months after stopping all antibiotics, including oral voriconazole, the patient's general condition was good, body temperature was normal, function of the right knee had returned to normal, the left knee joint was mildly swollen (Figure 3), there was no joint effusion and the range of motion of the left knee was similar to the preoperative measure. However, there was pain on weight bearing and the patient required a cane for ambulation. Laboratory re-examinations revealed normal C-reactive protein level, erythrocyte sedimentation rate and routine blood tests, as well as liver and kidney function tests. X-rays showed that the prosthesis of the left knee was not loose, there was no evidence of osteolysis, and the prosthesis was well positioned (Figure 4). Laboratory tests and clinical manifestations revealed no drug toxicity and side effects. Left knee arthrocentesis repeatedly showed no growth of T *asahii*.

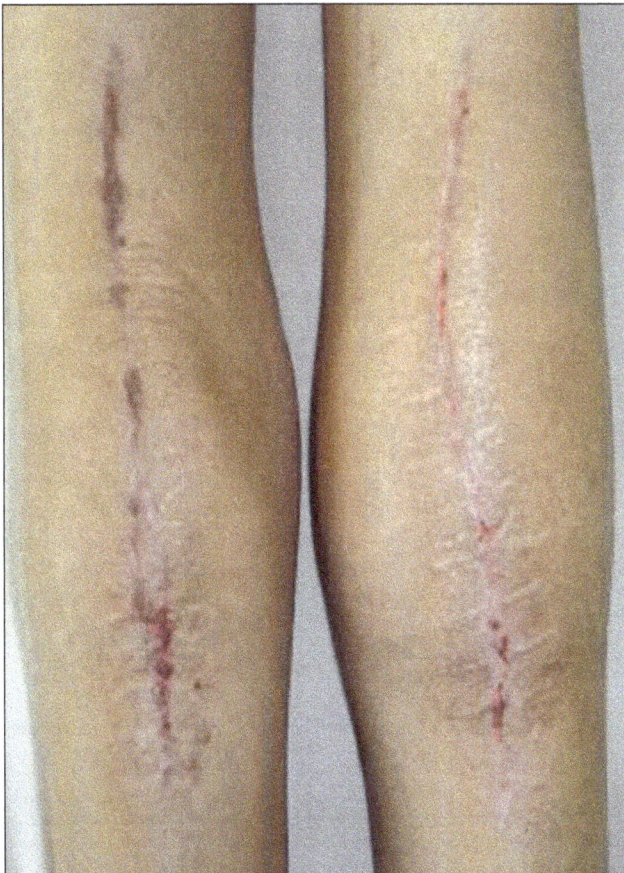

Figure 3) *Gross morphology of the left knee 26 months after surgery. The left knee joint was mildly swollen*

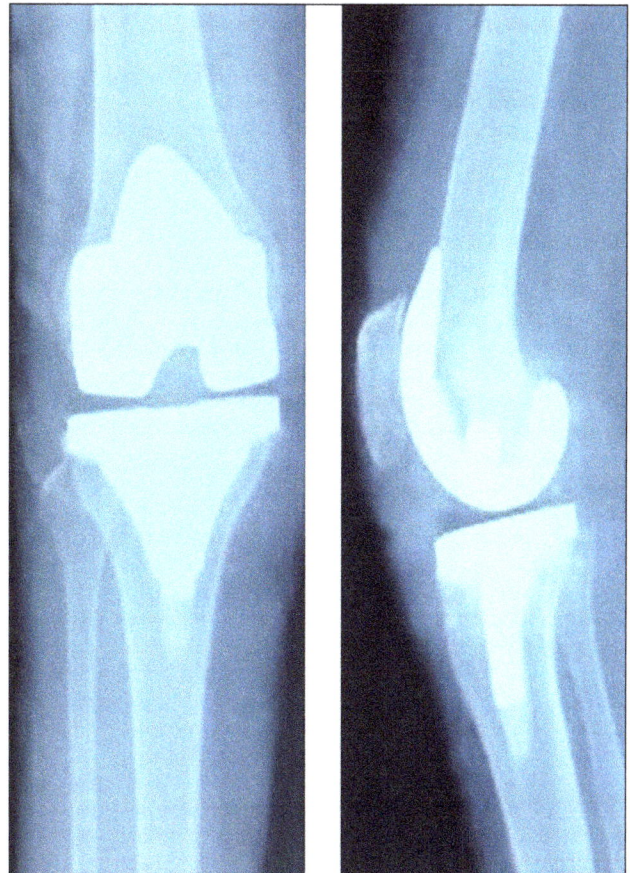

Figure 4) *X-ray of the left knee 26 months after surgery. The prosthesis was not loose and there was no subsidence or migration*

DISCUSSION

Periprosthetic fungal infection cases reported from 1979 to 2012 after artificial joint replacement totaled 57 reports, including 91 cases (3-59). Of these, there were 41 cases of hip replacements, 46 cases of total knee replacements, three cases of shoulder replacement and one case of metacarpophalangeal joint replacement. *Candida albicans* was the most commonly reported pathogen and was cultured in 38 cases. *Candida parapsilosis* was reported in 18 cases, *Candida glabrata* in 10 cases, *Candida tropicalis* in six cases, *Aspergillus fumigatus* in three cases, *Pseudallescheria boydii* in two cases, and one case of each of the following: *Candida guillermondii*, *Aspergillus niger*, *Cryptococcus neoformans*, *Candida lipolytica*, *Phialemonium curvatum*, *Histoplasma capsulatum*, zygomycosis, *Syncephalastrum racemosum*, *Absidia corymbifera*, *Sporotrichum schenckii* and *Rhodotorula minuta*. In addition, there was one case of coinfection by *C parapsilosis* and *C albicans*, and one case of coinfection by *C glabrata* and *C albicans*. The prostheses in 17 of the 91 patients were retained after antifungal therapy, of whom one had persistently painful knee reports during the follow-up, one needed continuous application of fluconazole (63 months), one had sinus tract persistence and three died (the cause of death was not related to joint diseases). Thirty of the 91 patients underwent two-staged reimplantation; swelling and pain during follow-up occurred in four, postoperative bacterial infection occurred in one (antibacterial treatment was successful), and there was one case of secondary infection after surgery (the patient died of heart failure). In addition, 28 of the 91 patients required prosthesis removal, of whom five needed continual treatment with fluconazole and four died. Finally, two of the 91 patients underwent successful single-staged replacement, while arthrodesis was performed in nine of the 91 patients and five of the 91 patients resulted in amputation.

T asahii is widely present in the environment and is present in the normal flora of the human skin, gastrointestinal tract and respiratory tract (60). Formation of biofilms on medical biomaterials in the hospital is very common. Studies have shown the presence of *T asahii* in the wash basins in operating rooms (61). However, the overall incidence of *T asahii* infection is low. As a conditional pathogen, it often causes a systemic disseminated infection in patients with transplantation, blood diseases, malignant tumours, immunodeficiency and leukopenia. The incidence of infection in non-immunodeficient patients is rare, with only one case affecting the central nervous system and lung being reported in an immunocompetent individual (62). There are slightly more than 100 cases of disseminated infection caused by *T asahii* reported worldwide (63). In previous reports, there were no reported cases of prosthesis infection with *T asahii* after arthroplasty. *T asahii* can easily lead to disseminated trichosporosis in particular populations; however, in the present case, blood cultures did not grow *T asahii*, which may be due to the fact that the individual was immunocompetent.

Periprosthetic fungal infections are related to the use of glucocorticosteroids or immunosuppressants, or are observed in patients with malignant tumours. In addition, an increased risk for infection is related to excessive use of antibiotics for a prolonged period, indwelling catheters and patients in the intensive care unit. The patient in the present case underwent multiple surgeries due to postoperative fever and suspicion of bacterial infection. This particular patient may have been at risk for fungal infection due to prolonged use of antibiotics, the presence of indwelling catheters for long periods and multiple instances of recatheterization secondary to multiple surgeries.

Joint infections following arthroplasty are most often bacterial in origin. Because the overall incidence of fungal infection following arthroplasty is very low, microbiology experts and orthopedic surgeons may suspect contamination and incorrectly label the specimen as a false positive. It is difficult to detect fungal infections on pathogenic examination, and arthrocentesis often fails to reveal a positive fungal culture. In the present case, pathogens were not detected even after several synovial fluid cultures before debridement.

In the present case, detection of *T asahii* was successful following debridement and immediate inoculation in blood culture media. Studies have shown that this sampling method can significantly improve the detection rate of specimens (35,51). This method led to a prompt diagnosis, especially given the unexplained signs of infection. The present case report suggests that in cases in which the diagnosis is in doubt due to a confounding clinical picture, such as fever, pain and swelling of unknown origin, a fungal infection must be considered. Such cases warrant an extended culture time, specific culture conditions and a high degree of suspicion for the presence of rare microorganisms.

Common *Candida* infections are sensitive to amphotericin B and triazole drugs (fluconazole, itraconazole, voriconazole and posaconazole). *T asahii* strains are sensitive to amphotericin B and itraconazole (64). In addition, some reports indicate that *T asahii* is highly sensitive to fluconazole and voriconazole in vitro (65); however, fluconazole resistance can occur. In the present case, susceptibility testing of the synovial fluid culture suggested resistance to fluconazole, itraconazole and 5-fluorocytosine; however, the patient was sensitive to amphotericin B and voriconazole. Therefore, it is important to select appropriate drugs and consider the resistance pattern.

Studies have suggested that biofilm formation of *T asahii* is the main factor leading to persistent infection. *T asahii* has a complex three-dimensional structure under electron microscopy. Interestingly, relative to free cells, the resistance of *T asahii* biofilm to voriconazole is 16,000 times greater (66), making it difficult to eradicate with voriconazole alone.

The efficacy of amphotericin B treatment of *Candida* and other fungal infections is well established. However, its renal toxicity can lead to sustained hypokalemia, nausea, vomiting and other side effects. Therefore, the dose is significantly limited in such patients. In the present case, because the application of amphotericin B led to sustained hypokalemia, we administered local intra-articular injections of amphotericin B to increase the local drug concentration. The joint swelling increased after intra-articular injection, but there was no local erythema or rash 24 h after injection. In addition, the patient's skin temperature decreased, the patient reported pain relief and her joint swelling subsided after one week.

As recommended by the Infectious Diseases Society of America, the appropriate time of antifungal treatment for *Candida* arthritis is between six and 12 months (67). In the present case, the patient was treated with antifungal voriconazole for one year. Symptoms did not reappear after withdrawal of the medication, even after 11 months.

Laboratory tests and clinical manifestations indicated no adverse reactions. In comparison, Fabry et al (45) reported a case involving *C albicans* infection of the prosthesis, in which symptoms reappeared two weeks after treatment withdrawal. Thus, there may be a relationship between the duration of the medication and patient recovery after surgery.

Because the patient in the present case refused further surgical treatment, we did not perform a two-stage reimplantation, which was most likely the ideal treatment. In the literature, there are more cases of two-stage reimplantation (30 of 91 cases) and removal of the prosthesis (28 of 91 cases) compared with other surgeries. After the prosthesis is removed, instability and dysfunction may occur and, thus, a two-stage reimplantation is recommended. In two reports by Anagnostakos et al (27) and García-Oltra et al (28), the treatment outcomes were drastically different following two-stage reimplantation. In seven two-stage reimplantation cases, Anagnostakos et al (27) reported only one case that did not accept the reoperation, and treatment of the remaining six cases was successful. In contrast, García-Oltra et al (28) reported that only one case was successful following two-stage replantation after debridement, while the remaining six cases failed. In two-stage replacement surgery, the first step involves the removal of the joint prosthesis and insertion of an antibiotic spacer, as well as long-term application of antifungal treatment. Only two single-staged replacement cases have been successful (6,39). In addition, amputation and arthrodesis are becoming rarer because patients do not accept the outcome. Thus, if revision surgery is not possible or if there are contraindications, long-term use of antifungal therapy with retention of the original prosthesis may be an alternative long-term suppression strategy.

CONCLUSION

Cases of periprosthetic fungal infections after total knee arthoplasty are rare, and the ideal treatment is two-stage revision implantation. However, if the patient's general condition is poor and they are not willing to undergo the revision surgery, long-term treatment with conservative antifungal drugs can be considered on the basis of joint debridement. For immunocompetent patients infected with *T asahii*, the keys to effective treatment are early detection and long-term application of antifungal treatment.

ACKNOWLEDGEMENTS: The authors thank Medjaden Bioscience Limited for assisting in the preparation of the manuscript.

DISCLOSURES: The authors have no conflicts of interest to declare regarding this article.

REFERENCES

1. Azzam K, Parvizi J, Jungkind D, et al. Microbiological, clinical, and surgical features of fungal prosthetic joint infections: A multi-institutional experience. J Bone Joint Surg Am 2009;91:142-9.
2. Sugita T, Nishikawa A, Ichikawa T, et al. Isolation of *Trichosporon asahii* from environmental materials. Med Mycol 2000;38:27-30.
3. Yilmaz M, Mete B, Ozaras R, et al. *Aspergillus fumigatus* infection as a delayed manifestation of prosthetic knee arthroplasty and a review of the literature. Scand J Infect Dis 2011;43:573-8.
4. Langer P, Kassim RA, Macari GS, et al. *Aspergillus* infection after total knee arthroplasty. Am J Orthop 2003;32:402-4.
5. Açikgöz ZC, Sayli U, Avci S, et al. An extremely uncommon infection: *Candida glabrata* arthritis after total knee arthroplasty. Scand J Infect Dis 2002;34:394-6.
6. Baumann PA, Cunningham B, Patel NS, et al. *Aspergillus fumigatus* infection in a mega prosthetic total knee arthroplasty: Salvage by staged reimplantation with 5-year follow-up. J Arthroplasty 2001;16:498-503.
7. Austin KS, Testa NN, Luntz RK, et al. *Aspergillus* infection of total knee arthroplasty presenting as a popliteal cyst. Case report and review of the literature. J Arthroplasty 1992;7:311-4.
8. Graw B, Woolson S, Huddleston JI. *Candida* infection in total knee arthroplasty with successful reimplantation. J Knee Surg 2010;23:169-74.
9. Gaston G, Ogden J. *Candida glabrata* periprosthetic infection: A case report and literature review. J Arthroplasty 2004;19:927-30.
10. Lazzarini L, Manfrin V, De Lalla F. Candidal prosthetic hip infection in a patient with previous candidal septic arthritis. J Arthroplasty 2004;19:248-52.
11. Prenzel KL, Isenberg J, Helling HJ, et al. *Candida* infection in hip allo arthroplasty. Unfallchirurg 2003;106:70-2. German.
12. Ramamohan N, Zeineh N, Grigoris P, et al. *Candida glabrata* infection after total hip arthroplasty. J Infect 2001;42:74-6.
13. Badrul B, Ruslan G. *Candida albicans* infection of a prosthetic knee replacement: A case report. Med J Malaysia 2000;55(Suppl C):93-6.
14. Simonian PT, Brause BD, Wickiewicz TL. *Candida* infection after total knee arthroplasty. Management without resection or amphotericin B. J Arthroplasty 1997;12:825-9.
15. Fukasawa N, Shirakura K. *Candida* arthritis after total knee arthroplasty – a case of successful treatment without prosthesis removal. Acta Orthop Scand 1997;68:306-7.
16. Dunkley AB, Leslie IJ. *Candida* infection of a silicone metacarpophalangeal arthroplasty. J Hand Surg Br 1997;22:423-4.
17. Tunkel AR, Thomas CY, Wispelwey B. *Candida* prosthetic arthritis: Report of a case treated with fluconazole and review of the literature. Am J Med 1993;94:100-3.

18. Koch AE. *Candida albicans* infection of a prosthetic knee replacement: A report and review of the literature. J Rheumatol 1988;15:362-5.
19. Wu MH, Hsu KY. Candidal arthritis in revision knee arthroplasty successfully treated with sequential parenteral-oral fluconazole and amphotericin B-loaded cement spacer. Knee Surg Sports Traumatol Arthrosc 2011;19:273-6.
20. Springer J, Chatterjee S. *Candida albicans* prosthetic shoulder joint infection in a patient with rheumatoid arthritis on multidrug therapy. J Clin Rheumatol 2012;18:52-3.
21. Dutronc H, Dauchy FA, Cazanave C, et al. *Candida* prosthetic infections: Case series and literature review. Scand J Infect Dis 2010;42(11-12):890-5.
22. Kelesidis T, Tsiodras S. *Candida albicans* prosthetic hip infection in elderly patients: Is flucona zole monotherapy an option? Scand J Infect Dis 2010;42:12-21.
23. Merrer J, Dupont B, Nieszkowska A, et al. *Candida albicans* prosthetic arthritis treated with fluconazole alone. J Infect 2001;42:208-9.
24. Lichtman EA. *Candida* infection of a prosthetic shoulder joint. Skeletal Radiol 1983;10:176-7.
25. Phelan DM, Osmon DR, Keating MR, et al. Delayed reimplantation arthroplasty for candidal prosthetic joint infection: A report of 4 cases and review of the literature. Clin Infect Dis 2002;34:930-8.
26. Bruce AS, Kerry RM, Norman P, et al. Fluconazole-impregnated beads in the management of fungal infection of prosthetic joints. J Bone Joint Surg Br 2001;83:183-4.
27. Anagnostakos K, Kelm J, Schmitt E, et al. Fungal periprosthetic hip and knee joint infections clinical experience with a 2-stage treatment protocol. J Arthroplasty 2012;27:293-8.
28. García-Oltra E, García-Ramiro S, Martínez JC, et al. Prosthetic joint infection by *Candida* spp. Rev Esp Quimioter 2011;24:37-41.
29. Johannsson B, Callaghan JJ. Prosthetic hip infection due to *Cryptococcus neoformans*: Case report. Diagn Microbiol Infect Dis 2009;64:76-9.
30. Lerch K, Kalteis T, Schubert T, et al. Prosthetic joint infections with osteomyelitis due to *Candida albicans*. Mycoses 2003;46:462-6.
31. Wada M, Baba H, Imura S. Prosthetic knee *Candida parapsilosis* infection. J Arthroplasty 1998;13:479-82.
32. Fowler VG Jr, Nacinovich FM, Alspaugh JA, et al. Prosthetic joint infection due to *Histoplasma capsulatum*: Case report and review. Clin Infect Dis 1998;26:1017.
33. Darouiche RO, Hamill RJ, Musher DM, et al. Periprosthetic candidal infections following arthroplasty. Rev Infect Dis 1989;11:89-96.
34. Paul J, White SH, Nicholls KM, et al. Prosthetic joint infection due to *Candida parapsilosis* in the UK: Case report and literature review. Eur J Clin Microbiol Infect Dis 1992;11:847-9.
35. Gottesman-Yekutieli T, Shwartz O, Edelman A, et al. *Pseudallescheria boydii* infection of a prosthetic hip joint – an uncommon infection in a rare location. Am J Med Sci 2011;342:250-3.
36. Peel T, Daffy J, Thursky K, et al. Posaconazole as first line treatment for disseminated zygomycosis. Mycoses 2008;51:542-5.
37. Yang SH, Pao JL, Hang YS. Staged reimplantation of total knee arthroplasty after *Candida* infection. J Arthroplasty 2001;16:529-32.
38. Brooks DH, Pupparo F. Successful salvage of a primary total knee arthroplasty infected with *Candida parapsilosis*. J Arthroplasty 1998;13:707-12.
39. Selmon GP, Slater RN, Shepperd JA, et al. Successful 1-stage exchange total knee arthroplasty for fungal infection. J Arthroplasty 1998;13:114-5.
40. Cushing RD, Fulgenzi WR. Synovial fluid levels of fluconazole in a patient with *Candida parapsilosis* prosthetic joint infection who had an excellent clinical response. J Arthroplasty 1997;12:950.
41. Lackner M, De Man FH, Eygendaal D, et al. Severe prosthetic joint infection in an immunocompetent male patient due to a therapy refractory *Pseudallescheria apiosperma*. Mycoses 2011;54 Suppl 3:22-7.
42. Dumaine V, Eyrolle L, Baixench MT, et al. Successful treatment of prosthetic knee *Candida glabrata* infection with caspofungin combined with flucytosine. Int J Antimicrob Agents 2008;31:398-9.
43. Bland CM, Thomas S. Micafungin plus fluconazole in an infected knee with retained hardware due to *Candida albicans*. Ann Pharmacother 2009;43:528-31.
44. Ceffa R, Andreoni S, Borrè S, et al. Mucoraceae infections of antibiotic-loaded cement spacers in the treatment of bacterial infections caused by knee arthroplasty. J Arthroplasty 2002;17:23-8.
45. Fabry K, Verheyden F, Nelen G. Infection of a total knee prosthesis by *Candida glabrata*: A case report. Acta Orthop Belg 2005;71:119-21.
46. Hennessy MJ. Infection of a total knee arthroplasty by *Candida parapsilosis*. A case report of successful treatment by joint reimplantation with a literature review. Am J Knee Surg 1996;9:133-6.
47. Levine M, Rehm SJ, Wilde AH. Infection with *Candida albicans* of a total knee arthroplasty. Case report and review of the literature. Clin Orthop Relat Res 1988;235-9.
48. DeHart DJ. Use of itraconazole for treatment of sporotrichosis involving a knee prosthesis. Clin Infect Dis 1995;21:450.
49. Cutrona AF, Shah M, Himes MS, et al. *Rhodotorula minuta*: An unusual fungal infection in hip-joint prosthesis. Am J Orthop 2002;31:137-40.
50. MacGregor RR, Schimmer BM, Steinberg ME. Results of combined amphotericin B-5-fluorcytosine therapy for prosthetic knee joint infected with Candida parapsilosis. J Rheumatol 1979;6:451-5.
51. Younkin S, Evarts CM, Steigbigel RT. *Candida parapsilosis* infection of a total hip-joint replacement: Successful reimplantation after treatment with amphotericin B and 5-fluorocytosine. A case report. J Bone Joint Surg Am 1984;66:142-3.
52. Lejko-Zupanc T, Mozina E, Vrevc F. Caspofungin as treatment for *Candida glabrata* hip infection. Int J Antimicrob Agents 2005;25:273-4.
53. Nayeri F, Cameron R, Chryssanthou E, et al. *Candida glabrata* prosthesis infection following pyelonephritis and septicaemia. Scand J Infect Dis 1997;29:635-8.
54. Lambertus M, Thordarson D, Goetz MB. Fungal prosthetic arthritis: Presentation of two cases and review of the literature. Rev Infect Dis 1988;10:1038-43.
55. Wyman J, McGough R, Limbird R. Fungal infection of a total knee prosthesis: Successful treatment using articulating cement spacers and staged reimplantation. Orthopedics 2002;25:1391-4.
56. Evans RP, Nelson CL. Staged reimplantation of a total hip prosthesis after infection with *Candida albicans*. A report of two cases. J Bone Joint Surg Am 1990;72:1551-3.
57. Cardinal E, Braunstein EM, Capello WN, et al. *Candida albicans* infection of prosthetic joints. Orthopedics 1996;19:247-51.
58. White A, Goetz MB. *Candida parapsilosis* prosthetic joint infection unresponsive to treatment with fluconazole. Clin Infect Dis 1995;20:1068-9.
59. Lim EV A, Stern PJ. *Candida* infection after implant arthroplasty. A case report. J Bone Joint Surg Am 1986;68:143-5.
60. Walsh TJ, Melcher GP, Lee JW, et al. Infections due to *Trichosporon* species: New concepts in mycology, pathogenesis, diagnosis and treatment. Curr Top Med Mycol 1993;5:79-113.
61. Heslop OD, Nyi Nyi MP, Abbott SP, et al. Disseminated trichosporonosis in a burn patient: Meningitis and cerebral abscess due to *Trichosporon asahii*. J Clin Microbiol 2011;49:4405-8.
62. Rastogi VL, Nirwan PS. Invasive trichosporonosis due to *Trichosporon asahii* in a non-immunocompromised host: A rare case report. Indian J Med Microbiol 2007;25:59-61.
63. Vazquez JA. *Trichosporon* infection Curr Fungal Infect Rep 2010;4:52-8.
64. Badley AD, Van Scoy RE. Long-term follow up of multifocal osteoarticular sporotrichosis treated with itraconazole. Clin Infect Dis 1996;23:394-5.
65. Xia Z, Yang R, Wang W, et al. Genotyping and antifungal drug susceptibility of *Trichosporon asahii* isolated from Chinese patients. Mycopathologia 2012;173:127-33.
66. Di Bonaventura G, Pompilio A, Picciani C, et al. Biofilm formation by the emerging fungal pathogen *Trichosporon asahii*: Development, architecture, and antifungal resistance. Antimicrob Agents Chemother 2006;50:3269-76.
67. Pappas PG, Kauffman CA, Andes D, et al. Infectious Diseases Society of America. Clinical practice guidelines for the management of candidiasis: 2009 update by the Infectious Diseases Society of America. Clin Infect Dis 2009;48:503-35.

4

Public health response to a large-scale endoscopy infection control lapse in a nonhospital clinic

Jacqueline Willmore MPH[1], Edward Ellis MD MPH[2,3], Vera Etches MD MHSc[1,3], Lise Labrecque MHSc BSW[1],
Carla Osiowy PhD[4,5], Anton Andonov MD PhD[4,5], Cameron McDermaid MHSc[1], Anna Majury DVM PhD[6,7],
Camille Achonu MHSc[8], Maurica Maher MD[9], Brenda MacLean RN BScN MEd[1], Isra Levy MD MSc[1]

J Willmore, E Ellis, V Etches, et al. Public health response to a large-scale endoscopy infection control lapse in a nonhospital clinic. Can J Infect Dis Med Microbiol 2015;26(2):77-84.

OBJECTIVE: To determine whether transmission of blood-borne pathogens (BBPs) (hepatitis B virus [HBV], hepatitis C virus [HCV] and HIV) occurred as a result of endoscopy reprocessing failures identified during an inspection of a nonhospital endoscopy clinic in 2011.
METHODS: The present analysis was a retrospective cohort study. Registered notification letters were mailed to 6992 patients who underwent endoscopy from 2002 to 2011 at one Canadian nonhospital endoscopy clinic, informing them of the infection control lapse and offering BBP testing. Multimedia communications and a telephone line supplemented notification. A retrospective study of patients with BBPs was performed with viral genetic testing and risk factor assessment for eligible patients. Risk for infection among patients whose procedure was within seven days of a known positive patient was compared with those whose procedure was performed more than seven days after a known postive patient. The seven-day period was selected as the period most likely to present a risk for transmission based on the documented cleaning procedures at the clinic and the available literature on virus survival.
RESULTS: Ninety-five percent (6628 of 6992) of patients/estates were contacted and 5042 of 6728 (75%) living patients completed BBP testing. Three were newly diagnosed with HBV and 14 with HCV. Twenty-three and 48 tested positive for previously known HBV or HCV, respectively, 367 were immune to HBV due to natural infection and one was immune to HBV due to immunization. None tested positive for HIV. Sequencing did not reveal any relationships among the 46 unique case patients with viral genetic test results available. Ninety-three percent of patients reported alternative risk factors for BBP. An increased risk for infection among those who underwent a procedure within seven days of a known HBV or HCV case was not demonstrated.
CONCLUSIONS: Endoscopy reprocessing failures were not associated with an increased risk for BBP among individuals tested.

Key Words: Endoscopy; Infection control lapse; Public health

La réaction de la santé publique à une vaste défaillance du contrôle des infections en endoscopie dans une clinique non hospitalière

OBJECTIF : Lors de l'inspection d'une clinique d'endoscopie non hospitalière en 2011, déterminer si des pathogènes à diffusion hématogène (PDH; virus de l'hépatite B [VHB], virus de l'hépatite C [VHC] et VIH) sont transmis à cause de la défaillance du retraitement de l'endoscopie.
MÉTHODOLOGIE : Dans la présente étude de cohorte rétrospective, les chercheurs ont posté une lettre recommandée à 6 992 patients qui avaient subi une endoscopie entre 2002 et 2011 dans une clinique canadienne d'endoscopie non hospitalière pour les informer d'une défaillance du contrôle des infections et leur offrir un test de dépistage des PDH. Les communications multimédias et les appels téléphoniques ont complété cet avis. Les chercheurs ont effectué une étude rétrospective des patients ayant des PDH au moyen de tests génétiques viraux et d'une évaluation des facteurs de risque des patients admissibles. Ils ont comparé le risque d'infection entre les patients dont l'intervention avait eu lieu dans les sept jours suivant celle d'un patient positif connu ceux dont l'intervalle dépassait sept jours. Cette période de sept jours était la plus susceptible de constituer un risque de transmission compte tenu des mesures de nettoyage attestées à la clinique et les publications sur la survie des virus.
RÉSULTATS : Les chercheurs ont pris contact avec 95 % (6 628 cas sur 6 692) des patients et des successions, et 5 042 des 6 728 (75 %) patients vivants ont effectué le test de dépistage des PDH. Trois ont obtenu un nouveau diagnostic de VHB et 14, de VHC. De plus, 23 et 48 ont obtenu des résultats positifs à un VHB ou à un VHC déjà connu, respectivement, 367 étaient immuns au VHB en raison d'une infection naturelle et un, grâce à la vaccination. Aucun n'a obtenu de résultat positif au VIH. Le séquençage a révélé l'absence de lien entre les 46 cas uniques de patients pour qui les résultats du test génétique étaient disponibles. Aussi, 93 % des patients ont signalé d'autres facteurs de risques de PDH. Par ailleurs, on n'a pu démontrer d'augmentation du risque d'infection chez les personnes qui avaient subi une intervention dans les sept jours suivant un cas connu de VHB ou de VHC.
CONCLUSIONS : L'échec de retraitement de l'endoscopie ne s'associait pas à une augmentation du risque de PDH chez les personnes qui subissaient un test de dépistage.

More than 1.6 million endoscopic procedures are performed annually in Canada (1). The increasing proportion of colonoscopies and other medical procedures being performed in nonhospital (NH) clinics (2) prompted the College of Physicians and Surgeons of Ontario (CPSO) to launch the Out-of-Hospital Premises Inspection Program in 2010 (3). Before this program was implemented, NH facilities performing procedures such as endoscopies were not inspected. The incidence of infections (primarily bacterial) associated with endoscopy has been reported to be one case per 1.8 million (4). This may underestimate incidence due to a lack of postprocedure surveillance and underreporting. Despite the low estimated incidence of infection, several large-scale endoscopy-related outbreaks and notifications have been reported in the literature (5,6). Few have established transmission of blood-borne pathogens (BBP), such as hepatitis B virus (HBV), hepatitis C virus (HCV) and HIV, as a result of reprocessing errors (7-9). However, HBV and HCV can survive on inanimate surfaces for several

[1]Ottawa Public Health; [2]Public Health and Preventive Medicine Consultant; [3]University of Ottawa, Ottawa, Ontario; [4]National Microbiology Laboratory, Public Health Agency of Canada; [5]University of Manitoba, Winnipeg, Manitoba; [6]Public Health Ontario; [7]Queen's University, Kingston; [8]Public Health Ontario, Toronto; [9]Health Canada, Ottawa, Ontario
Correspondence: Jacqueline Willmore, Ottawa Public Health, 100 Constellation Crescent, 7th Floor West, MC: 26-50, Ottawa, Ontario K2G 6J8.e-mail jacqueline.willmore@ottawa.ca

days depending on conditions (10-14) and infections may go undetected for long periods of time, with serious health consequences (15).

In May 2011, an NH endoscopy clinic in Ottawa, Ontario, was inspected by the CPSO and significant deficiencies in the cleaning and disinfection of the endoscopes since 2002 were identified. Specifically, the inspection found cross-contamination from a dirty endoscope, inadequate decontamination of biopsy forceps, improper use of endoscope processor for high-level disinfection of endoscopes and sterilization of instruments such as biopsy forceps, and no proper cleaning of premises between patients (16). CPSO ordered the clinic physician to cease performing endoscopies at the clinic and notified the Ontario Ministry of Health and Long-Term Care (MOHLTC) about the issue. The MOHLTC notified Ottawa Public Health (OPH), the local public health department. The main objectives of OPH were to assess the risk of transmission of HBV, HCV and HIV to patients and to determine whether a public health response was needed.

METHODS

A decision to notify patients was made by OPH based on assessments of infection risk and ethics considerations, and in consultation with experts in these areas. Due to the large number of affected patients, the clinic could not independently undertake notification and follow-up. An epidemiological investigation, including genetic analysis, was designed to assess whether there was evidence of patient-to-patient transmission of BBP.

Infection risk
The risk for infection with HBV, HCV and HIV was estimated using prevalence estimates (17-19) and the Rutala and Weber methodology (20,21) recommended by the Public Health Agency of Canada. This methodology includes a 14-step protocol for situation management in the event of a possible failure of disinfection or sterilization that could expose patients to an infectious agent. It includes situational evaluation, stakeholder communication, risk evaluation and investigation (20). The risk for infection was estimated to be <1 in 1 million patients for HBV, <1 in 50 million patients for HCV and <1 in 3 billion patients for HIV (22). This process is described in more detail in Appendix 1.

Ethics considerations
Clinical and public health ethics principles and values were considered in deciding whether patient notification was indicated (22). Principles of patient autonomy, the right to know and the professional duty to disclose led to a conclusion that disclosure by the physician and/or public health officials was warranted (23,24). Public health principles of do no harm (nonmaleficence) (25) and protection of the public from harm (26) also supported disclosure, due to the possibility of secondary transmission of BBP to others by infected patients unaware of their infection.

The potential harm of patient distress and anxiety about potential infection with a BBP (however small the risk) that could arise with disclosure was considered (27). However, disclosure is ethical even when the chance of harm is extremely low, although steps must be taken to minimize patient anxiety. Following the principle of transparency, disclosing risk information to patients was determined to be an ethical course of action that would maintain public trust in OPH (23,28).

Patient identification and notification
A 'confirmed patient' underwent an endoscopic procedure in the clinic between April 1, 2002 and June 1, 2011, based on Ontario Health Insurance Plan (OHIP) billing records, clinic records for patients not billed through OHIP, or a plausible history from a self-identified patient lacking billing and clinic records. OPH compiled and managed all patient information related to the response in a secure Microsoft Access database (Microsoft Corporation, USA).

A package was sent by registered mail or personal delivery (to allow for tracking of package receipt or return) to each patient including a letter signed by the Ottawa Medical Officer of Health and the clinic

physician. The letter described the infection control lapse (ICL), stated the estimated numeric risk of BBP infection, offered testing (but did not specifically recommend testing), provided instructions for obtaining free laboratory testing using a prepopulated Public Health Ontario Laboratory requisition (to improve access and facilitate surveillance), conveyed the clinic physician's regret for the incident, and provided a dedicated OPH telephone number and website for further information. Telephone metrics were tracked through Prairie Fyre, a contact management software, and patient satisfaction data were logged electronically by nursing staff who managed the telephones. Local family physicians, infectious disease specialists, gastroenterologists and emergentologists were also notified. Traditional and social media were used to inform patients who could not be reached through postal mail.

Case identification
A 'case patient' had laboratory evidence of an acute, chronic, occult or past HBV infection, an HCV infection or an HIV infection, based on current test results or previously known test results in Ontario's reportable disease database. All assays were performed using a chemiluminescent microparticle immunoassay (Architect i2000SR, Abbott Diagnostics, USA). Assays included qualitative detection of antibody to hepatitis B surface antigen (anti-HBsAg), hepatitis B surface antigen (HBsAg), antibody to hepatitis B core antigen (anti-HBcAg), antibody to HCV (anti-HCV) and HIV p24 antigen and antibodies to HIV type 1 and/or type 2 (HIV-1/HIV-2). Patients acutely or chronically infected with HBV (HBsAg positive), or with evidence of previous or occult infection (HBsAg negative, anti-HBc positive, and anti-HBs ≤100 mIU/mL) were classified as HBV cases. Patients were considered to be immune due to immunization if they were anti-HBsAg positive, HBsAg negative and HBc negative. Patients with positive anti-HCV were classified as HCV cases. HIV-seropositive patients were classified as HIV cases. All samples that tested positive using the initial chemiluminescent microparticle immunoassay were subject to confirmatory testing.

HBV DNA and HCV RNA testing and sequencing
Patients with HBsAg-positive serum samples and those that were potentially occult cases of HBV infection (in the present study, HBsAg negative, anti-HBc positive, and anti-HBs ≤100 mIU/mL) were eligible for HBV DNA testing and eligible samples were sent to the National Microbiology Laboratory, Public Health Agency of Canada for blinded HBV DNA testing. Anti-HCV serology positive patients who had not demonstrated undetectable HCV RNA previously were eligible for HCV RNA testing. Samples were sent to the National Microbiology Laboratory for blinded HCV RNA testing. If nested polymerase chain reactions (PCRs) determined viral nucleic acid positivity (detection limit between 5 IU/mL to 10 IU/mL) in serum samples, HBV DNA and HCV RNA extracted from clinical samples were genotyped and sequenced to assess phylogenetic relatedness of viral samples collected from case patients.

HBV DNA was extracted from 200 µL of sera using silica gel filtration (easyMAG, bioMérieux, Canada) or phenol/chloroform extraction methods to optimize sensitivity (29). Extracted DNA was amplified according to previously published procedures (30,31). Samples that could be amplified by at least two different region-specific primer sets and were HBsAg negative, anti-HBc positive and anti-HBs ≤100 mIU/mL were considered to be occult HBV infection positive (32). A total of 315 base pairs, consistent across all patients, were queried during phylogenetic analysis. The gene sequence evaluated for HBV was the surface/polymerase overlapping sequence. Sanger sequencing provided analysis of the dominant population within the patient quasispecies, which allowed for adequate tracing of transmission events.

HCV RNA was extracted from 250 µL of sera using the automated nucleic acid extraction system NucliSENS easyMag (bioMérieux Inc, USA) and amplified, gel purified, then cycle sequenced with an ABI Prism 3100 Genetic Analyzer (Applied Biosystems, USA) using BigDye v3.1 terminator chemistry. Sequence data obtained were used to determine the HCV genotype of each viral sample and further analysis was performed to determine their phylogenetic relatedness. Genetic distances were estimated by Kimura two-parameter analysis, and a phylogenetic tree was constructed using the maximum likelihood method (33). Significant taxonomic relationships were identified by bootstrap resampling analysis (200 replicates) using the maximum likelihood method. Bootstrap values of ≥70% indicate that the topology of that branch within the phylogenetic tree were considered to be significant or 'related'.

Prevalence, risk factor and OR analysis

To determine whether there was a higher than expected prevalence of any BBP, the prevalence among those tested as a result of the notification was compared with the estimated prevalence in the population of Ottawa (HIV), Ontario (HCV) or Canada (HBV) (as available in the literature), using a Pearson's χ^2 test at $\alpha=0.05$ (17-19).

Public health nurses conducted standardized telephone interviews of case patients regarding any previous test results, HBV immunization and lifetime exposure to recognized risk factors for acute infection (34,35). If the case patient was unavailable and a previous interview record existed, information was abstracted from the provincial reportable disease database. Risk factor responses were collated into mutually exclusive risk factor categories using a previously published hierarchy (35,36).

Odds of infection were calculated using Stata version 12.0 (StataCorp, USA). In this analysis, a case was any confirmed patient who was HBV positive and for whom the HBV status was not known to be positive before their procedure. A control was any confirmed patient who tested negative for HBV. A case or control was considered exposed if they had a clinic visit within seven days after the visit of a known case patient. For the attribution of exposures, confirmed patients who were known to be positive before their endoscopy date were included as transmission exposures: they could act as a source of infection. These confirmed patients were excluded from the analysis because they did not meet case or control definitions. Patients whose laboratory tests indicated they were immune due to immunization were excluded if the vaccination was definitively before their endoscopy procedure. Because some patients had multiple visits, each visit was considered to be an independent case or control visit and the risk analysis was performed on 'patient-visits' rather than individual patients.

The seven-day duration for temporal linking was selected by considering the extent to which endoscope cleaning occurred according to clinic records, although insufficient according to the guidelines (37), and evidence of virus survival in the literature (10-14). Given that HBV and HCV can go undetected for long periods of time (15), all case patients were assumed to be infectious at the time of their clinic visit(s), to consider their infection and transmission risk. Although the seven-day period was believed to present the highest risk to patients, additional exposure periods of 14 days and 28 days were also used as a sensitivity analysis.

RESULTS

Notification results

The notification process resulted in 95% (6628 of 6992) of confirmed patients or estates receiving a package by registered mail or delivery (Table 1). More packages were mailed than confirmed patients due to address changes, and lost or returned packages.

Viral test results

Of 6728 confirmed living patients (96% of 6992 confirmed patients or estates of confirmed patients), 5042 (75%) completed viral testing for at least one BBP as of May 11, 2012. Among living patients, 62% (4173 of 6728) were female and the median age (as of January 1, 2011) was 55.2 years (range 15 to 99 years), older than the 2011 Ontario median age of 40.4 (38). Data regarding sex were missing in 319 cases (4.7%) and age in 171 (2.5%). There were 442 (8.8% of 5042) case patients identified who tested positive for a past or current infection with HBV or HCV, including 12 coinfections (Figure 1). No HIV cases were identified. One

TABLE 1
Patient notification results, as of April 2012

Notification process	n (%)	Total, n
Confirmed patients identified	6992	
Patients confirmed alive at time of notification	6728 (96.2)	6992
Packages sent to patients and estates	7310	
Patients or estates reached by registered mail	6628 (94.8)	6992
Patients who received testing for at least one BBP	5042 (74.9)	6728
Patients tested for HIV	5042 (74.9)	6728
Patients tested for HBV	4703 (69.9)	6728
Patients tested for HCV	4730 (70.3)	6728
Stakeholders notified (eg, physicians, laboratories, hospitals, public health units)	1400	
Calls received by OPH from patients, members of the public	5203	
Calls made by OPH nurses notifying patients of negative laboratory results	4686	
Calls received by OPH from physicians/other health care providers	68	
Patients reached by letter to inform them of option for genetic sequencing	216	

BBP Blood-borne pathogen; HBV Hepatitis B virus; HCV Hepatitis C virus; OPH Ottawa Public Health

case demonstrated immunity to HBV due to vaccination. Forty-eight of 62 HCV cases (77.4%) and 23 of 26 of those with current HBV infection (88.5%) were known from Ontario's reportable disease database. Fifty-six percent (247 of 442) of case patients were female, and the median age was 58.2 years (range 24 to 90 years). Results of initial viral testing in the patients tested as a part of the epidemiological investigation were compared with available general population prevalence estimates for HIV (Ottawa estimate), HCV (Ontario estimate) or HBV (Canadian estimate) (17-19) using Pearson's χ^2 test (Table 2). The prevalence of HBV and HIV was significantly lower than expected, past infection with HBV was within the expected range and the prevalence of HCV was not significantly different than expected.

Ninety-three percent (324 of 350) of HBV or HCV case patients who could be interviewed reported alternate risk factors to endoscopy at the clinic. Patients were assigned to the risk factor with the highest risk (Table 3). Decedents (n=34) and patients who could not be reached and did not have a patient file available (n=31) were excluded.

Statistical analysis did not detect increased odds of HBV or HCV infection among patients potentially exposed to a case patient (Table 4). One case was removed from the analysis because this case was definitively immune before their endoscopy. Sixty-three HBV-positive patients and 50 HCV-positive patients were removed from the risk analysis because they were known to be positive before their procedures. Fourteen- and 28-day periods were also used as periods of exposure, and neither detected increased odds of HBV or HCV infection among exposed patients.

HBV DNA test results

Of HBV cases, 182 were eligible for and were offered DNA testing. A total of 130 HBV DNA tests were performed on 18 HBsAg-positive specimens, 88 HBsAg-negative specimens and 24 specimens in which the HBsAg status was not provided. Twenty specimens were DNA positive according to PCR. Five HBsAg-negative, anti-HBc-positive and anti-HBs-positive (≤100 mIU/mL) specimens, and one specimen in which the HBsAg status was not provided, were considered to be PCR indeterminate because the initial positive PCR result could not be replicated with different primer sets. The 26 sequences were phylogenetically analysed. Three specimens were considered to be occult HBV infection positive (HBsAg negative and PCR positive in different genomic regions). Transmission of HBV related to endoscopy procedures at the clinic was unlikely, as

TABLE 2
Seroprevalence of hepatitis B virus, hepatitis C virus (HCV) and HIV infection for all patients tested as a part of the endoscopy epidemiological investigation

Infection	Patients tested, n	Expected prevalence*, % (n expected)	Observed prevalence, n (%)	Interpretation (Pearson's χ^2 P)	Comparison population
HBsAg positive	4703	2 (94)	26 (0.55)	Lower (P<0.001)	Canada
Anti-HBc positive (past infection)	4703	5–10 (235–470)	366 (7.8)	Within range (NA)	Canada
Anti-HBc positive; HBsAg negative; HBcAg negative (immune)	4703	–	1 (0.02)	–	–
HCV antibody positive	4730	0.94 (44)	62 (1.3)	Not different (P=0.08)	Ontario
HIV antibody positive	5042	0.37 (19)	0 (0)	Lower (P<0.001)	Ottawa

*Data adapted from references 17-19. Anti-HBc Hepatitis B core antibody; HBcAg Hepatitis B core antigen; HBsAg Hepatitis B surface antigen; NA Not applicable

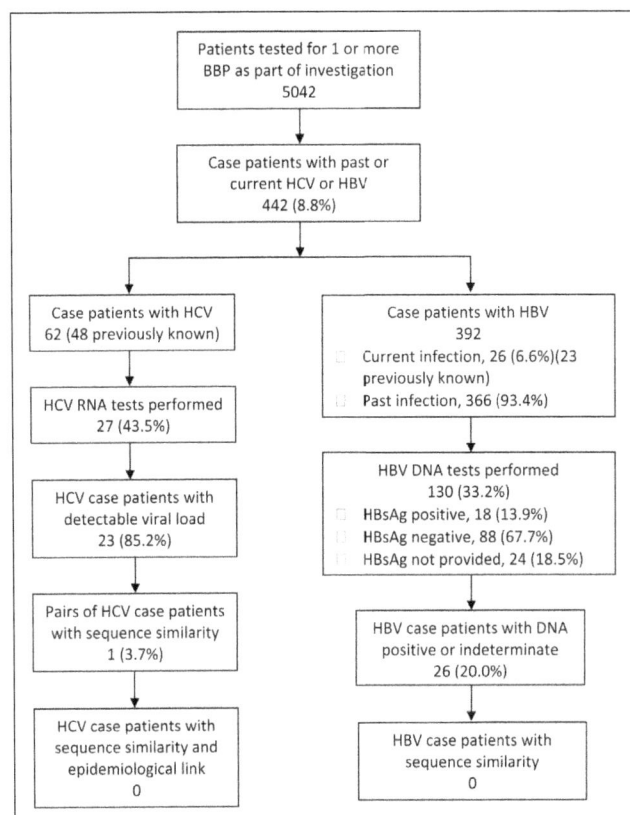

Figure 1) Flow diagram depicting results of testing for hepatitis B virus (HBV) and hepatitis C virus (HCV) among patients tested as part of the epidemiological investigation in Ottawa, Ontario. BBP Blood-borne pathogen; HBsAg Hepatitis B surface antigen

indicated by insufficient sequence similarity based on genotype and placement on the tree (Figure 2C).

HCV RNA test results

Samples from 27 of 55 eligible anti-HCV-positive patients were tested for HCV RNA; of these, 23 were positive with a viral load ranging from 3.57×10^4 IU/mL to 2.46×10^7 IU/mL. Samples from all 23 HCV RNA positive patients were genotyped; subgenotype 1a was the most common (10 cases) followed by subgenotype 1b (six cases). Three cases belonged to subgenotype 3a, three to genotype 4 and one to subgenotype 2a (Figure 2A). One of the three genotype 4 cases belonged to subgenotype 4a, commonly found in Egypt, while the other two were the rarely observed subgenotypes 4v and 4r. A possible transmission event could have occurred only within cases belonging to the same subgenotype.

Analysis of all 1a and 3a cases did not identify clusters of phylogenetically related HCV strains among these patients except for samples H0296/12 and H0501/12; however, these were duplicate samples from the same patient (the laboratory tested all samples in a blind

TABLE 3
Hierarchical, mutually exclusive risk factors* for hepatitis B virus (HBV) or hepatitis C virus (HCV) among interviewed acute cases, chronic carriers and those with evidence of past infection, as of April 2012

Risk factor	HBV Total n=350[†]	HCV Total n=27[†]
Injection drug use	2 (0.6)	10 (37.0)
Non-injection drug use	3 (0.9)	1 (3.7)
Transfusion[‡]	20 (5.7)	2 (7.4)
>2 heterosexual partners	78 (22.3)	2 (7.4)
Men who have sex with men	8 (2.3)	0 (0)
Sex with carrier	7 (2.0)	0 (0)
Tattooing	7 (2.0)	2 (7.4)
Body piercing	64 (18.3)	6 (22.2)
Acupuncture	24 (6.9)	1 (3.7)
Occupational	19 (5.4)	1 (3.7)
HBV/HCV in home	6 (1.7)	0 (0)
Surgery or invasive procedure other than the endoscopy clinic	25 (7.1)	0 (0)
Incarceration	1 (0.3)	0 (0)
Born in a high-prevalence country	60 (17.1)	0 (0)
No disclosed risk	26 (7.4)	2 (7.4)

Data presented as n (%). *Data adapted from references 35 and 36. [†]Decedents (n=34) and patients who could not be reached and did not have a patient file available (n=31) were excluded. [‡]Only transfusions outside Canada anytime (for both HBV and HCV), or transfusions pre-1970 (for HBV) or pre-1990 (for HCV) were included

TABLE 4
Risk analysis of exposure from a clinic visit within seven days of a case patient's visit, as of August 2012*

HBV	Positive	Negative	OR	95% CI
Exposed	340	3893	1.03	(0.84–1.29)
Not exposed	98	1166		

HCV	Positive	Negative	OR	95% CI
Exposed	8	1369	0.87	(0.40–1.87)
Not exposed	28	4148		

*Based on clinic visits because patients could have multiple visits. Excludes patients who were known to be positive before their endoscopy visit. HBV Hepatitis B virus; HCV Hepatitis C virus

manner). Similarly from the six subgenotype 1b cases, sample pairs H0295/12-H0500/12 and H1284/12-H5899/11 carried identical HCV sequences; however, they were also found to be duplicate specimens from the same patients. Interestingly, these two HCV strains were phylogenetically associated (bootstrap value = 87%); however, the epidemiological data did not confirm possible transmission because the visits of these two patients were one year apart. To further investigate the discrepancy between the phylogenetic and epidemiological data, these two HCV strains were analyzed within the NS5B region

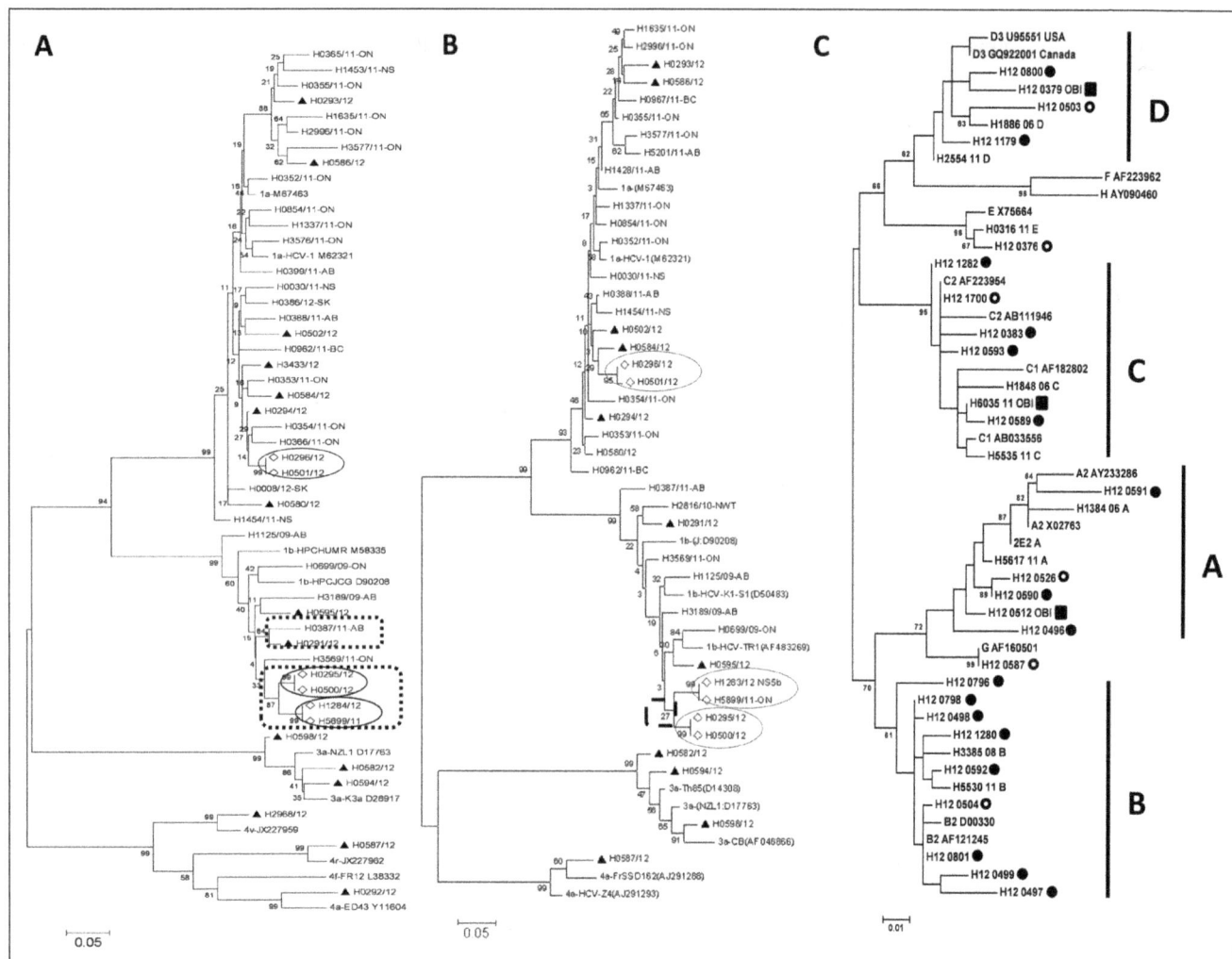

Figure 2) *Results of phylogenetic analysis of hepatitis C virus (**A** and **B**) and hepatitis B virus (HBV) (**C**). **A** Phylogenetic tree based on partial hepatitis C virus E1 genetic region; samples from the Ottawa (Ontario) clinic patients are marked with black triangles. Regional reference clinical cases from Alberta (AB), British Columbia (BC), Ontario (ON) and Saskatchewan (SK), as well as GenBank sequences belonging to different subgenotypes are included for comparison. Investigation cases with identical sequences are marked with open diamonds. Identical or almost identical sequences are encircled. Putative phylogenetic associations are marked with dashed rectangles. **B** Phylogenetic tree based on partial NS5B region: markings as in **A**. Note that the putative phylogenetic association based on partial E1 sequences is not confirmed in NS5B region (samples H1283/12 and 1284/12 belong to the same patient and were collected 10 days apart). **C** Phylogenetic tree of 26 hepatitis B surface antigen (HBsAg)-coding region sequences (315 base pairs; HBV nucleotides 468–782) from 17 HBsAg-positive and nine HBsAg-negative or nonprovided clinic patients. Maximum likelihood analysis was performed using MEGA 5 software and the tree constructed by the Nearest Neighbour Interchange algorithm with 1000 bootstrap replicates (33). Comparative GenBank sequences are designated by the HBV genotype or subgenotype, followed by the accession number. Regional reference and case sequences are designated by a code number preceded by the letter H. The 2E2 A sequence within the genotype A clade denotes the sequence of the positive control used during all polymerase chain reactions (PCRs). Bootstrap confidence values of ≥60% are given. The ruler shows the branch length for a pairwise distance equal to 0.01. Filled circle, HBsAg positive, PCR positive; Open circle, HBsAg negative, PCR indeterminate; Filled square, HBsAg negative, PCR positive*

(Figure 2B) and no support for phylogenetic relatedness was found. These observations highlight the importance of using more than one genetic region for phylogenetic analysis.

DISCUSSION

The public health response to a large-scale ICL in an NH endoscopy clinic included a risk assessment and ethics analysis resulting in a decision to notify almost 7000 patients, and to conduct further epidemiological and genetic investigation of case patients. Our investigation found no evidence for an increased risk of BBP acquisition associated with the endoscopy reprocessing failure. Although three new cases of HBV and 14 new cases of HCV were identified, we did not find any related sequences with an epidemiological link among patients with viral genetic analysis results and most case patients identified alternative risk factors. Additionally, the prevalence of BBP in the patient population that went for testing was not clinically higher than expected,

particularly given that the median age of the patient population was older than the Ontario population and the fact that some patients were undergoing endoscopic procedures because of their HBV or HCV infection. The odds of infection were not significantly higher for patients who underwent a procedure within seven days after a known HBV or HCV case. These data argue against viral transmission during the endoscopic procedure and confirm what others have found with respect to the extremely low risk of transmission of BBP through endoscopy reprocessing failures (7-9).

Successful contact with 95% of patients was within the range (84% to 99%) achieved in similar notification processes in other jurisdictions (7-9,15,39). Factors possibly contributing to the high connection rate included the multipronged communication strategy, as well as repeated attempts to contact patients who did not receive their packages. Patient satisfaction was high on timeliness of services delivered, information provided and staff knowledge, competence and courtesy; the dedicated telephone line was considered to be essential to this outcome and to minimizing patient anxiety. The collaboration between OPH and local, provincial and national laboratories resulted in follow-up of the 75% of patients who chose to get tested. The investigation took almost one year to complete, due to multiple factors including, but not limited to, the lengthy patient identification process, a higher volume of telephone calls from patients than expected, the high number of patients who chose to undergo testing, and the length of time to obtain and report sequential positive and negative results to patients and their physicians. Lack of a predesigned database to manage the large volume of data from various components of the investigation led to data quality and data management problems, which were solved over the course of the investigation.

Limitations to the investigation included the extended risk period (complicating patient follow-up and identification of relevant risk factors among case patients), incomplete clinic patient records, the lack of preprocedure BBP test results for most patients, and having to use general rather than age-specific population prevalence of the BBP to compare with the prevalence found among confirmed patients. Because 25% of patients were not tested, it is possible that associations between case status and exposure may have changed if the status of this group was known. Temporality of case status or viral load and a patient's endoscopy visit could not be determined, in part because negative results for previously known cases are not reported to OPH. Positive patients were considered to be capable of transmitting infection in the OR analysis. The assumption that all positive patients were infectious may influence our outcomes toward the null. Risk factor information was missing for 8% of case patients, and these may be patients at greater risk for transmitting infection. Misclassification of exposures or case status could also affect the results. Because not all eligible patients underwent DNA/RNA testing, a relationship among cases may have been overlooked.

Knowledge gained from this response will be useful for infection control professionals, public health officials and clinicians planning for or managing a potential ICL or other adverse event. While the infection control risk assessment and ethical assessment pointed to the need for a public health response to disclose the ICL to patients, little guidance was available on the most appropriate methods to use. The notification letters to patients and physicians and the dedicated telephone line proved to be vital components of the response. However, we would not recommend the additional cost of registered mail for a patient whose address is likely reliable (such as their OHIP record). Traditional and social media should be used to capture patients who may have recently moved without notifying OHIP. Genetic analysis was essential to complement the epidemiological investigation once new BBP cases were identified.

Given that our findings support the extremely low quantitative risk of infection from an endoscopy-related ICL, unless clear evidence of transmission is found we recommend others follow the Centers for Disease Control and Prevention (Georgia, USA) guidelines for a Category B breach (40). This approach would use a qualitative description of the risk in patient and public communication, explicitly stating that due to the extremely low risk of having been infected, testing for the infections is not generally recommended, but would suggest that patients may call the dedicated telephone line with questions, or speak to their primary health care provider if they would like to discuss testing. Thus, a prepopulated laboratory requisition would not be needed in the package and staff time spent informing patients of negative results by telephone could be avoided. Public health staff would be notified of positive results for reportable BBP as per local protocol and epidemiological investigations of these cases should include questions regarding endoscopies. If new BBP cases among patients with epidemiological links are identified, genetic analyses of these cases and a recommendation for testing of others who share the link (eg, visit on the same day) may then be warranted.

In addition to regular inspections of NH clinics, requirements for reporting of regular training and retraining for NH staff involved in reprocessing could help to prevent future ICLs. A requirement to document

which reusable scope or other instrument is used on which patient could assist in investigations. Because other ICLs had occurred elsewhere in the province, the MOHLTC convened a provincial Task Group on Community Infection Prevention and Control Lapses to make recommendations on how to reduce the number and scale of future lapses, and on consistent public health assessment and management in an ethical and cost-effective manner for ICLs that do occur (41).

ACKNOWLEDGEMENTS: The authors thank members of the Incident Management System and other staff at OPH who contributed to the ICL response, and Epidemiology and Laboratory Services at Public Health Ontario for assistance with laboratory processes and data management.

APPENDIX 1
Estimates for risk of disease transmission
An approach to assessing the risk of disease transmission when there is a failure to follow established infection control procedures has been published by Rutala and Weber (20), and this is the approach is recommended by the Public Health Agency of Canada (21). This method was used to conduct the risk of disease transmission of HIV, HBV and HCV. The following data elements were used to calculate the probability of disease transmission:

- Prevalence of infection (17-19);
- Risk of transmission – risk of transmission for endoscopy alone was calculated using the risk of transmission from mucosal exposure; for endoscopy with biopsy the risk of transmission from percutaneous exposure was used (42,43);
- Likelihood that a nondisinfected instrument was used – various percentages were used to obtain a range of estimates (1%, 10%, 25%, 50%, 75% and 100%);
- Efficacy of cleaning using automated endoscope reprocessor (44);
- Efficacy of disinfection for liquid chemical sterilant (glutaraldehyde).

Endoscope reprocessing involves five steps: precleaning with enzymatic detergent, leak testing, manual cleaning and rinsing, high level disinfection and rinsing, and drying and storing. Automated endoscope reprocessors can be used to perform several functions, but manual cleaning must always be performed before placing the endoscope in a reprocessor.

Data from the manufacturer of the reprocessor used at the facility states that exposure to the disinfectant plus washing in the reprocessor (appropriate length of time and temperature), results in an average $\log_{10}$ reduction in microorganisms (*Mycobacterium terrae*) of 8.2 to 12.2, depending on which endoscope surface was examined. Reprocessor cleaning alone resulted in a 3.4 to 4.6 $\log_{10}$ reduction (this would be approximately 99.99% effective). No information was available concerning reduction in viruses for this reprocessor.

There were uncertainties regarding the effectiveness of the glutaraldehyde used because there was not evidence to show that it was tested for efficacy as required. Given this information and the uncertainties around the effectiveness of the glutaraldehyde used in the facility, risk estimates were calculated using the following two scenarios:

Scenario 1: Assume that the exposure to glutaraldehyde was completely ineffective and that any reduction in bioburden of microorganisms was obtained by washing alone; therefore efficacy of 'cleaning/disinfection' was a 4 $\log_{10}$ reduction (99.99%)

Scenario 2: Assume that the exposure to glutaraldehyde was effective for inactivating viruses and that the reduction in bioburden was 8 $\log_{10}$ (99.999999%).

Estimates for scenario 1
Endoscopy without biopsy:

- HIV 2.25×10^{-11} to 2.25×10^{-10}
- HBV 4.6×10^{-11} to 4.6×10^{-9}
- HCV between risks for HIV and HBV (no transmission risk available for mucosal exposure for HCV to create an estimate, but this approach agrees with the literature [20])

Endoscopy with biopsy:

- HIV 2.7×10^{-11} to 2.7×10^{-10}
- HBV 1.2×10^{-9} to 6×10^{-7}
- HCV 1.7×10^{-9} to 1.7×10^{-8}

Estimates for Scenario 2

Endoscopy without biopsy:

- HIV 2.25×10^{-14} to 2.25×10^{-15}
- HBV 4.6×10^{-13} to 4.6×10^{-11}
- HCV between risks for HIV and HBV (see explanation above)

Endoscopy with biopsy:

- HIV 2.7×10^{-14} to 2.7×10^{-15}
- HBV 1.2×10^{-13} to 6×10^{-11}
- HCV 1.7×10^{-12} to 1.7×10^{-13}

The highest risk estimate was for HBV when a biopsy took place and assumed that the glutaraldehyde being used was ineffective – 6×10^{-7} (6 in 10 million, 0.6 in 1 million).

Limitations

These risk estimates are subject to several limitations. The assessment was based on observations regarding practices noted during one inspection. The efficacy of the enzymatic detergent and the efficacy of manual cleaning were not included in the calculations because the detergent being used was expired. There is scientific literature to suggest that cleaning in reprocessors is equivalent to manual cleaning; however, given the inspector's observations the effect of manual cleaning was not included in these estimates to create a 'worst-case' scenario, which may have resulted in an overestimation of disease transmission risk. There are uncertainties concerning the effectiveness of the glutaraldehyde that was being used and what this would generally be at this facility; there was no additional information provided to refine the estimate. The efficacy of cleaning of viruses by the reprocessor used in the facility was based on extrapolated data from cleaning of bacteria in this reprocessor.

REFERENCES

1. Canadian Association of Gastroenterology. Quality in gastroenterology. Canadian Association of Gastroenterology 2012. <www.cag-acg.org/quality-program-endoscopy> (Accessed December 5, 2012).
2. Alharbi O, Rabeneck L, Paszat LF, et al. Factors associated with colonoscopy performed in nonhospital settings. Can J Gastroenterol 2010;24:419.
3. The College of Physicians and Surgeons of Ontario. Bridging the gap: A patient safety imperative. The Out-of-Hospital Premises Inspection Program Report. The College of Physicians and Surgeons of Ontario, 2012.
4. Schembre DB. Infectious complications associated with gastrointestinal endoscopy. Gastrointest Endosc Clin N Am 2000;10:215.
5. Srinivasan A. Epidemiology and prevention of infections related to endoscopy. Curr Infect Dis Rep 2003;5:467-72.
6. Weber DJ, Rutala WA. The prevention of infection following gastrointestinal endoscopy: The importance of prophylaxis and reprocessing. In: Marino Jr AJ, ed. Gastrointestinal Diseases: An Endoscopic Approach. Thorofare: Slack Inc, 2002:87-106.
7. Holodniy M, Oda G, Schirmer PL, et al. Results from a large-scale epidemiologic look-back investigation of improperly reprocessed endoscopy equipment. Infect Control Hosp Epidemiol 2012;33:649.
8. Bronowicki JP, Venard V, Bott C, et al. Patient-to-patient transmission of hepatitis C virus during colonoscopy. N Engl J Med 1997;337:237-40.
9. Spach DH, Silverstein FE, Stamm WE. Transmission of infection by gastrointestinal endoscopy and bronchoscopy. Ann Intern Med 1993;118:117-28.
10. Bond W, Favero M, Petersen N, Gravelle C, Ebert J, Maynard J. Survival of hepatitis B virus after drying and storage for one week. Lancet 1981;317:550-1.
11. Ciesek S, Friesland M, Steinmann J, et al. How stable is the hepatitis C virus (HCV)? Environmental stability of HCV and its susceptibility to chemical biocides. J Infect Dis 2010;201:1859-66.
12. Doerrbecker J, Friesland M, Ciesek S, et al. Inactivation and survival of hepatitis C virus on inanimate surfaces. J Infect Dis 2011;204:1830-8.
13. Kamili S, Krawczynski K, McCaustland K, Li X, Alter MJ. Infectivity of hepatitis C virus in plasma after drying and storing at room temperature. Infect Control Hosp Epidemiol 2007;28:519-24.
14. Paintsil E, Binka M, Patel A, Lindenbach BD, Heimer R. Hepatitis C virus maintains infectivity for weeks after drying on inanimate surfaces at room temperature: Implications for risks of transmission. J Infect Dis 2014;209:1205-11.
15. Bayoumi A, Strike C, Brandeau M, et al. Report of the Toronto and Ottawa Supervised Consumption Assessment Study. 2012. Toronto, Ontario, St. Michael's Hospital and the Dalla Lana School of Public Health, University of Toronto. <www.catie.ca/sites/default/files/TOSCA%20report%202012.pdf> (Accessed May 1, 2013).
16. The College of Physicians and Surgeons of Ontario. Premises inspection committee report: Dr. C. Farazli MD, FRCP (C) – Level 2. The College of Physicians and Surgeons of Ontario 2011 June 22; <www.cpso.on.ca/CPSO/CMSWebParts/OhpOutcomePdf.aspx?flash=true&pdfid=190586> (Accessed September 1, 2014).
17. Remis RS, Swantee C, Liu J. Report on HIV/AIDS in Ontario 2008. Ontario HIV Epidemiologic Monitoring Unit 2010. <www.ohemu.utoronto.ca/doc/2011/PHERO2008_report_final_rev_Sept2010.pdf> (Accessed December 5, 2012).
18. Remis RS. The epidemiology of hepatitis C infection in Ontario, 2004. Ontario HIV Epidemiologic Monitoring Unit 2007; <www.ohemu.utoronto.ca/doc/EpiHCVOnt.pdf> (Accessed December 5, 2012).
19. Sherman M, Shafran S, Burak K, et al. Management of chronic hepatitis B: Consensus guidelines. Can J Gastroenterol 2007;21(Suppl C):5C.
20. Rutala WA, Weber DJ. How to assess risk of disease transmission to patients when there is a failure to follow recommended disinfection and sterilization guidelines. Infect Control Hosp Epidemiol 2007;28:146-55.
21. Public Health Agency of Canada. Infection Prevention and Control Guideline for Flexible Gastrointestinal Endoscopy and Flexible Bronchoscopy. 2011.
22. Maher M. Issue analysis: Community infection prevention and control breach. Ottawa: Ottawa Public Health; November 17, 2011.
23. Disclosure Working Group. Canadian disclosure guidelines. Edmonton: Canadian Patient Safety Institute, 2008.
24. Canadian Medical Protective Association. Communicating with your patient about harm: Disclosure of adverse events. 2008.
25. Beauchamp TL, Childress JF. Principles of biomedical ethics, 5th edn. Oxford University Press, USA; 2001.
26. University of Toronto Joint Centre for Biothics Pandemic Influenza Working Group. Stand on guard for thee: Ethical considerations in preparedness planning for pandemic influenza. Toronto: University of Toronto, Joint Centre for Bioethics, 2005.
27. Dudzinski DM, Hebert PC, Foglia MB, Gallagher TH. The disclosure dilemma – large-scale adverse events. N Engl J Med 2010;363:978-86.
28. Upshur RE. Principles for the justification of public health intervention. Can J Publ Health 2002;93:101.
29. Osiowy C. Sensitive detection of HBsAg mutants by a gap ligase chain reaction assay. J Clin Microbiol 2002;40:2566-71.
30. Minuk GY, Kowalec K, Caouette S, Larke B, Osiowy C. The prevalence and long term outcome of occult hepatitis B virus infection in community based populations. J Med Virol 2012;84:1369-75.
31. Osiowy C, Andonov A, Borland J, Huynh C, Uhanova J, Minuk G. HBV DNA diagnostic testing: Positivity is in the eye of the beholder (Abstract 1033). Hepatology 2013;58(S1):706A.
32. Raimondo G, Allain J, Brunetto M, et al. Statements from the Taormina expert meeting on occult hepatitis B virus infection. J Hepatol 2008;49:652-7.
33. Tamura K, Peterson D, Peterson N, Stecher G, Nei M, Kumar S. MEGA5: Molecular evolutionary genetics analysis using maximum likelihood, evolutionary distance, and maximum parsimony methods. Mol Biol Evol 2011;28:2731-9.
34. Wu J, Wu HX, Andonov A, et al. Epidemiological profile of newly diagnosed patients with hepatitis C infection in 6 health regions across Canada over an 8-year period. Ann Epidemiol 2007;17:740-1.
35. Boulos D, Goedhuis NJ, Wu J, et al. Enhanced surveillance for acute and likely acute hepatitis B in Canada: 1999 to 2002. Can J Infect Dis Med Microbiol 2005;16:275.

36. Wu HX, Wu J, Wong T, et al. Enhanced surveillance of newly acquired hepatitis C virus infection in Canada, 1998 to 2004. Scand J Infect Dis 2006;38:482-9.

37. Ontario Agency for Health Protection and Promotion (Public Health Ontario). Provincial Infectious Diseases Advisory Committee. Best practices for cleaning, disinfection and sterilization of medical equipment/devices. 3rd edn. May 2013. Toronto: Queen's Printer for Ontario. <www.publichealthontario.ca/en/eRepository/PIDAC_Cleaning_Disinfection_and_Sterilization_2013.pdf> (Accessed November 21, 2014).

38. Statistics Canada. Ontario (Code 35). Census Profile. 2011 Census. Statistics Canada Catalogue no.98-316-XWE . Ottawa: Statistics Canada, 2012.

39. Johnson IL. An outbreak of hepatitis B associated with reusable subdermal electroencephalogram electrodes. CMAJ 2000;162:1127-31.

40. Patel P, Srinivasan A, Perz J. Developing a broader approach to management of infection control breaches in health care settings. Am J Infect Control 2008;36:685-90.

41. Public Health Policy and Programs Branch, Public Health Division, Ministry of Health and Long-Term Care. Report to the Chief Medical Officer of Health from the Community Infection Prevention and Control Lapses Task Group. 2014.

42. Centers for Disease Control and Prevention. 2001. Updates U.S. Public Health Service Guidelines for the Management of Occupational Exposures to HBV, HCV, and HIV and Recommendations for Postexposure Prophylaxis. MMWR 50 (No. RR-11).

43. Morris J, Duckworth GJ, Ridgway GL. Gastrointestinal endoscopy decontamination failure and the risk of transmission of blood-borne viruses: A review. J Hosp Infect 2006;63:1-13.

44. Custom Ultrasonics, 2007. Summary and Overview. Inc. System 83 PlusTM Washer-Disinfector. <www.customultrasonics.com/images/cart_files/83plus2booklet.pdf> (Accessed September 9, 2011).

5

Social network investigation of a syphilis outbreak in Ottawa, Ontario

H D'Angelo-Scott PhD[1], J Cutler MHSc[1], D Friedman PhD[2], A Hendriks MPH[2], AM Jolly PhD[3]

H D'Angelo-Scott, J Cutler, D Friedman, A Hendriks, AM Jolly. Social network investigation of a syphilis outbreak in Ottawa, Ontario. Can J Infect Dis Med Microbiol 2015;26(5):268-272.

BACKGROUND: The incidence of syphilis in Ottawa, Ontario, has risen substantially since 2000 to six cases per 100,000 in 2003, again to nine cases per 100,000 in 2007, and recently rose to 11 cases per 100,000 in 2010. The number of cases reported in the first quarter of 2010 was more than double that in the first quarter of 2009.
OBJECTIVE: In May 2010, the Ontario Ministry of Health and Long Term Care requested the assistance of the Field Epidemiology Program to describe the increase in infectious syphilis rates and to identify social network sources and prevention messages.
METHODS: Syphilis surveillance data were routinely collected from January 1, 2009 to July 15, 2010, and social networks were constructed from an enhanced social network questionnaire. Univariate comparisons between the enhanced surveillance group and the remaining cases from 2009 on non-normally distributed data were conducted using Kruskal-Wallis tests and χ^2 tests.
RESULTS: The outbreak cases were comprised of 89% men. Seventeen of the 19 most recent cases consented to answer the questionnaire, which revealed infrequent use of condoms, multiple sex partners and sex with a same-sex partner. Information regarding social venues where sex partners were met was plotted together with sexual partnerships, linking 18 cases and 40 contacts, representing 37% of the outbreak population and connecting many of the single individuals and dyads.
CONCLUSION: Uncovering the places sex partners met was an effective proxy measure of high-risk activities shared with infected individuals and demonstrates the potential for focusing on interventions at one named bar and one Internet site to reach a high proportion of the population at risk.

Key Words: Canada; Epidemiology; Public health; Sexually transmitted infections; Social network analysis; Syphilis

Une enquête sur les réseaux sociaux d'une éclosion de syphilis à Ottawa, en Ontario

HISTORIQUE : L'incidence de syphilis à Ottawa, en Ontario, a beaucoup augmenté depuis 2000, passant de six cas sur 100 000 habitants en 2003 à neuf cas sur 100 000 habitants en 2007, puis à 11 cas sur 100 000 habitants en 2010. Le nombre de cas signalés pendant le premier trimestre de 2010 a plus que doublé par rapport à celui du premier trimestre de 2009.
OBJECTIF : En mai 2010, le ministère de la Santé et des Soins de longue durée de l'Ontario a demandé l'aide du Programme canadien d'épidémiologie de terrain pour décrire l'augmentation du taux de syphilis infectieuses, en déterminer l'origine dans les réseaux sociaux et établir les messages de prévention.
MÉTHODOLOGIE : Les chercheurs ont colligé systématiquement les données de surveillance sur la syphilis entre le 1er janvier 2009 et le 15 juillet 2010 et en ont établi les réseaux sociaux à partir d'un questionnaire amélioré sur les réseaux sociaux. Au moyen du test de Kruskal-Wallis et des tests du chi carré, ils ont effectué des comparaisons univariées des données non distribuées normalement entre le groupe de surveillance améliorée et les autres cas de 2009.
RÉSULTATS : Les cas d'éclosion se composaient de 89 % d'hommes. Dix-sept des 19 cas les plus récents ont consenti à répondre au questionnaire, qui a révélé un usage peu fréquent du condom, de multiples partenaires sexuels et des relations sexuelles avec des partenaires de même sexe. Les chercheurs ont transcrit sur un graphique l'information relative aux lieux où les partenaires sexuels se sont rencontrés, ce qui a permis de relier 18 cas et 40 contacts, soit 37 % de la population de l'éclosion, et d'associer de nombreux individus uniques et de dyades.
CONCLUSION : La découverte des lieux où les partenaires sexuels se sont rencontrés s'est révélée une mesure indirecte efficace des activités à haut risque partagées avec des personnes infectées et a démontré le potentiel d'intervenir seulement dans un bar précis et un site Internet donné pour joindre une forte proportion de la population à risque.

Since 1987, rates of infectious syphilis have been below 1.6 cases per 100,000 and elimination, defined as <0.5 cases per 100,000, appeared to be a realistic achievement in Canada (1,2). Cases of syphilis then rose from one case per 100,000 in 2000 to 8.85 per 100,000 in 2012 (3).

Ottawa, Ontario, with a population of 812,000 in 2006 (4), experienced a five-fold increase in syphilis since 2001, mostly in men who have sex with men, and a further increase in 2009 (Figure 1). In May 2010, Ottawa Public Health (OPH) requested the assistance of the Canadian Field Epidemiology Program of the Public Health Agency of Canada, through the Ontario Ministry of Health and Long-Term Care. The objectives of the present investigation were to characterize the increase in reported infectious syphilis rates and to identify risk factors and social networks of cases indicative of transmission, which may then be used in interventions. In addition, we aimed to record patients' views and reports regarding sexual-health messaging.

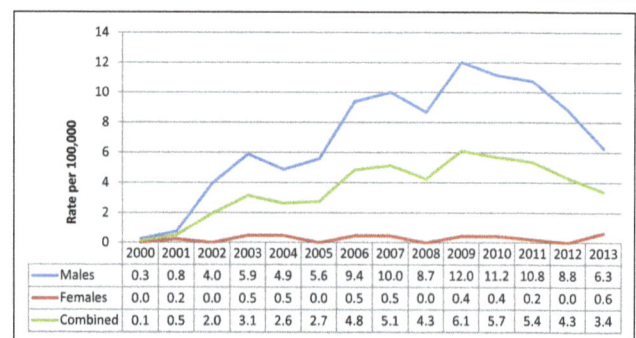

	2000	2001	2002	2003	2004	2005	2006	2007	2008	2009	2010	2011	2012	2013
Males	0.3	0.8	4.0	5.9	4.9	5.6	9.4	10.0	8.7	12.0	11.2	10.8	8.8	6.3
Females	0.0	0.2	0.0	0.5	0.5	0.0	0.5	0.5	0.0	0.4	0.4	0.2	0.0	0.6
Combined	0.1	0.5	2.0	3.1	2.6	2.7	4.8	5.1	4.3	6.1	5.7	5.4	4.3	3.4

Figure 1) *Reported infectious syphilis (primary, secondary and early latent cases only) rate per 100,000 population, males and females, Ottawa, Ontario, 2000 to 2009. Data source: Ontario Ministry of Health and Long-Term Care, integrated Public Health Information System, extracted December 23, 2014.*

[1]Canadian Field Epidemiology Program, Public Health Agency of Canada; [2]City of Ottawa Public Health, Centre for Communicable Disease and Infection Control; [3]University of Ottawa, Ottawa, Ontario
Correspondence: Dr AM Jolly, Epidemiology and Community Medicine, University of Ottawa, Room 3105 Roger Guindon Hall, 451 Smyth Road, Ottawa, Ontario K1H 8M5.e-mail ajolly@uottawa.ca

Sexual networks can be constructed from routinely collected contact-tracing data for bacterial sexually transmitted infections (STIs), by connecting each case and contact point with lines, denoting sexual intercourse. The unusually thorough inquiries, which resulted in a network diagram of the first 44 individuals with HIV and their sex partners in 1984, was one of the first publications demonstrating the unique value of this network approach, clearly revealing the roles of different individuals in transmission (5). However, as was evident in that case, incomplete information regarding sexual contacts, who may be anonymous, often hampers contact tracing. Also evident from that investigation was the importance of self-reported links between men who attended social gatherings in whom AIDS was later diagnosed, and who may also have had sexual, as well as social, contact (5). Requesting information from cases regarding locations where sex partners or friends socialize makes use of 'homophily' in social networks, in which individuals with similar attributes, behaviours and interests cluster together in social groups (6). These social venues were key in defining the outbreak sources, whether as 'pickup joints' for sex partner recruitment or as shared air spaces for tuberculosis transmission (7,8). In a gonorrhea outbreak in northern Alberta, a social network analysis was used to investigate an increase in gonorrhea infections in which cases initially appeared to be disconnected (9). Patronage to a specific bar was found to be the only risk marker in a case-control study. Because almost one-half of the outbreak population of cases and contacts may be accessed by visiting the bar, we decided to use the same approach for this outbreak of infectious syphilis in Ottawa.

METHODS

Residents of Ottawa diagnosed with infectious syphilis, defined according to national case definitions (10) from January 1, 2009 to June 15, 2010, were included in the investigation (n=72). Electronic records were retrieved from the Integrated Public Health Information System, they were then validated and supplementary information was added to each routine surveillance record. For example, contacts known only by an e-mail and sex-partner recruitment venues had not been added into the Integrated Public Health Information System but were added before the analysis, and greatly improved the social network links. An enhanced surveillance questionnaire was developed in consultation with the OPH investigative team and was pilot tested by a case manager. Out of concern for OPH's relationship with the community of men having sex with men, community groups were consulted and approval was obtained from OPH's Research Ethics Board. Twenty syphilis cases from January 2010 to June 2010, which represented 27.7% of all syphilis cases, were contacted up to three times using two different methods (telephone, letter, e-mail, home visits). These 20 cases were the most recent of all 72 cases and, therefore, were more likely to remember details than cases from 2009.

The questionnaire elicited types of sexual partners in the past 12 months including regular, casual and anonymous partners, sex trade clients and group-sex encounters. The questionnaire asked, "What types of partners have you had in the last 12 months before your diagnosis?" Then, there were check boxes for casual, regular and paying partners, without definitions, with a space for participants to indicate how many for each type. Respondents were prompted for visited venues including public venues (including bars), clubs, bath houses, spas, sex clubs, raves, circuit parties, cruising sites or pick-up joints, work, school, prisons, parks, family or friends' homes, Internet sites, adult book and video stores, in Ottawa or in other cities, where they met their sexual partners. Clients were asked whether there had been sexual health messaging at each social venue. Respondents were also asked their opinions regarding actions needed to address the increase in syphilis infections.

Data obtained using enhanced surveillance were combined with demographic data, syphilis staging, HIV coinfection, behavioural risk factors, the names of sexual contacts and incidental free-text fields regarding locations where partners were met were collected as part of a routine case follow-up. Some data regarding exposure and social venues were available through routine surveillance, although

TABLE 1
Characteristics of infectious syphilis cases, Ottawa, Ontario, January 2009 to June 2010*

	2009–2010 cases[†]	Enhanced surveillance cases	Test statistic	P
Total	72	17		
Sex, n (%)				
Male	68 (94.4)	17 (100)		
Female	4 (5.6)	0 (0)	0.73[‡]	1.0
Age, years, mean (% reported)	38.8 (55)	44.0 (17)	1.73[§]	0.81
Contacts, median (interquartile range)	1 (1–1)	1(1–2)	5.63[¶]	0.02
Staging				
Primary	28 (38.9)	2 (11.8)		
Secondary	32 (44.4)	11 (64.7)		
Early latent	11 (15.3)	3 (17.6)		
Infectious neurosyphilis	1 (1.4)	1 (5.9)	5.46[‡]	0.14
HIV coinfection	19 (26.4)	1 (5.9)	6.59[‡]	0.01
Risk exposures/settings				
No condom used	62 (86.1)	14 (82.4)		
Sex with same sex	55 (76.4)	13 (76.5)		
Partner is homosexual	52 (72.2)	13 (76.5)		
New partner in past two months	29 (40.3)	10 (58.8)		
Multiple partners in past six months	18 (25)	4 (23.5)		
Bathhouse	11 (15.3)	1 (5.9)		
Sex with opposite sex	10 (13.9)	3 (17.6%)		
Partner is HIV-positive	9 (12.5)	1 (5.9)		
Met partner through internet	6 (8.3)	0 (0)		
Partner with multiple partners	5 (6.9)	1 (5.9)		
Travel outside province	3 (4.2)	0 (0)		
Judgement impaired by alcohol/drugs	2 (2.8)	0 (0)		
Sex for drugs	1 (1.4)	0 (0)		
Ethnic group				
Caucasian	N/A	14 (82.4)		
Aboriginal		1 (5.9)		
South Asian		1 (5.9)		
West Asian		1 (5.9)		
Named sex partners[†]**				
0	11 (15.3)	2 (11.8)		
1	20 (27.8)	3 (17.6)		
2–5	29 (40.3)	8 (47.1)		
6–10	6 (8.3)	2 (11.8)		
11–20	2 (2.8)	1 (5.9)		
>20	4 (5.6)	1 (5.9)	5.63[¶]	0.02

*Data presented as n (%) unless otherwise indicated. *Includes cases diagnosed up to June 15, 2010 only; [†]Includes only the earliest episode for 4 cases involving 2 episodes each of infectious syphilis in 2009 to 2010; [‡]χ^2 test; [§]t test; [¶]Kruskal-Wallis test; **Totals may differ due to different responses from the same individuals during routine and enhanced surveillance interviews*

they were not consistently collected. It is important to note that the enhanced cases had two opportunities to provide data regarding their sex partners. All unique partners named at both interviews for the 2009 to 2010 period were incorporated into the network diagrams; however, only the data regarding numbers of partners from the first interview were used for statistical tests to avoid ascertainment bias. The incorporation of all routinely available data, together with enhanced data to show clustering around venues for sex partner recruitment, allowed for comparison with previous studies (8,9).

Data analysis

Descriptive and univariate analysis of the data (χ^2, Student's t and Kruskal Wallis tests) were performed using Microsoft Office Excel version 7 (Microsoft Corporation, USA) and Epi Info 6.04 (Centres for Disease Control and Prevention, USA). Where numbers allowed, all cases were compared with the most recent cases for enhanced surveillance to demonstrate that the most recent sample represented the total population of syphilis cases in most respects. Pajek version 1.27 (Pajek, Slovenia) was used to construct and analyze the social networks, where lines represented sexual contact between individuals, who were represented by nodes. A network of all cases and named contacts available from routine data collection was constructed, as well as a network of all cases and contacts who frequented common venues. All of the networks were undirected because the direction of syphilis transmission was unknown. The numbers and sizes of components were counted in which each person was connected to at least one other place or person. The number of links from one person to another immediately adjacent were also counted, which represented the total number of sex partners named by and who named an index case (degree).

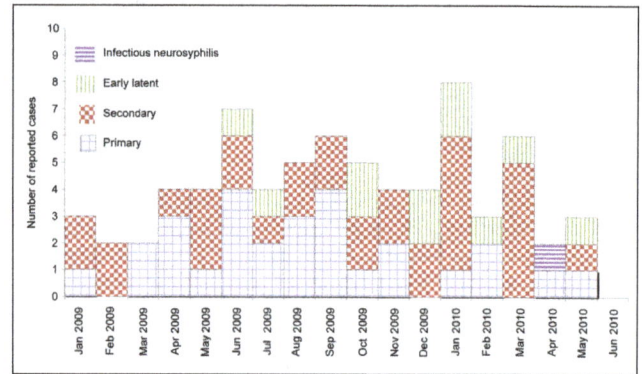

Figure 2) *Reported infectious syphilis cases (primary, secondary and early latent cases only) by month and year of episode, Ottawa, Ontario, January 2009 to June 2010 (includes cases diagnosed up to June 15, 2010 (n=72) [includes only the earliest episode for four cases involving two episodes each of infectious syphilis in 2009 to 2010])*

RESULTS

Routinely collected case data from January 1, 2010 to June 15, 2010

Seventy-two individuals met the infectious syphilis case definition from January 1, 2009 to June 15, 2010 (Table 1). The epidemic curve of infectious syphilis cases during January 1, 2009 to June 15, 2010 was consistent with a propagated outbreak with person-to-person spread (Figure 2). The majority (94.4%) of reported cases were men, ranging from 19 to 63 years of age. Almost one-half of the cases presented with secondary syphilis (44.4%) and 19 (26.4%) were HIV positive. Five of 19 individuals were diagnosed with HIV within one year of their syphilis diagnosis, while 14 cases were diagnosed with HIV more than one year before their diagnosis of syphilis.

Sixty-one (84.7%) cases reported a total of 321 sexual partners ranging from one to 50 partners for each case, of whom only 69 (21.5%) were named. The distribution of the number of named partners (degree) used in the network analysis revealed a highly skewed distribution, known as a 'small world network', in which 90% of respondents who named contacts had one to three partners in the past 12 months, while the remainder had four to 16 named partners. Cases who did not report contact information were similar to those who did, in sex and age (mean of 46.2 and 39.6 years of age, respectively; P=0.14 [Student's t test]).

During routine case follow-up, respondents reported various sex practices including infrequent condom use, sex with a same-sex partner, a homosexual partner, a new partner in the past two months and multiple partners in the past six months (Table 1).

Enhanced surveillance data

Seventeen of 20 (89%) of the most recent cases chosen consented to be reinterviewed, two declined and one was not successfully contacted.

All respondents were men, resembling the majority (94.4%) of routinely reported cases and were of similar ages and syphilis stages compared with the routinely notified group (Table 1). One of the enhanced surveillance respondents (5.9%) was coinfected with HIV, compared with coinfection in 19 (26.4%) of the routine cases (χ^2=6.59; P=0.01). Ethnic background for the 72 reported cases was not collected; however, the majority of the cases who responded to the enhanced surveillance questionnaire were Caucasian (82.4%). The 17 cases contacted for enhanced surveillance reported a total of 81 sexual partners, although only 17 (21.0%) according to name, similar to the routinely reported cases. However, they reported higher numbers of total partners than reported according to routinely notified cases (P=0.02 [Kruskal-Wallis]) (Table 2). Eleven of 17 (64.7%) cases reported having regular sexual partners, 12 (70.6%) reported having casual partners, 11 (64.7%) reported having anonymous partners and four (23.5%) reported having group-sex encounters. There were no cases reporting exchanging sex for money in the past 12 months.

There was no sexual-health messaging reported at informal venues (Table 2). However, there was an awareness of sexual-health messaging in bars and clubs (four of seven responses) and in bathhouses, spas and sex clubs (seven of nine responses) in Ottawa and outside of Ottawa (five of seven responses). The proportion of respondents aware and unaware of sexual-health messaging on Internet sites was evenly split.

Respondents suggested that OPH increase education regarding symptoms, testing and transmission of syphilis, as well as the importance of condom use for oral and anal sex. They suggested targeting specific social venues frequented by the gay population such as bars, Internet sites and bathhouses. The respondents also stressed the need for messaging in other venues, such as public washrooms, to include men who have sex with both women and men. Advertisements directed at the

TABLE 2
Sexual health messaging at social venues reported by infectious syphilis cases through outbreak investigation, Ottawa, Ontario, January 2009 to June 2010 (n=17)

	Sexual health messaging at venue						
	Ottawa			Outside Ottawa			
Social venue	Yes	No	Do not know	Yes	No	Do not know	Total, n
Adult video/bookstore	1 (33.3)	1 (33.3)	1 (33.3)				3
Bar/club	4 (33.3)	1 (8.3)	2 (16.7)	2 (16.7)	1 (8.3)	2 (16.7)	12
Bath house/spas/sex club	7 (50.0)	0 (0)	2 (14.3)	5 (14.3)	1 (7.1)	1 (7.1)	16
Cruising sites	0 (0)	3 (100.0)	0 (0)				3
Family/friends	0 (0)	4 (100.0)	0 (0)				4
Internet	10 (58.8)	7 (41.2)	2(11.8)				19
Private parties	1 (20.0)	1 (8.3)	0 (0)		1 (20.0)	0	3
Other	0 (0)	4 (57.1)	0 (0)	1 (14.3)	2 (28.6)	0	7

Data presented as n (%) unless otherwise indicated

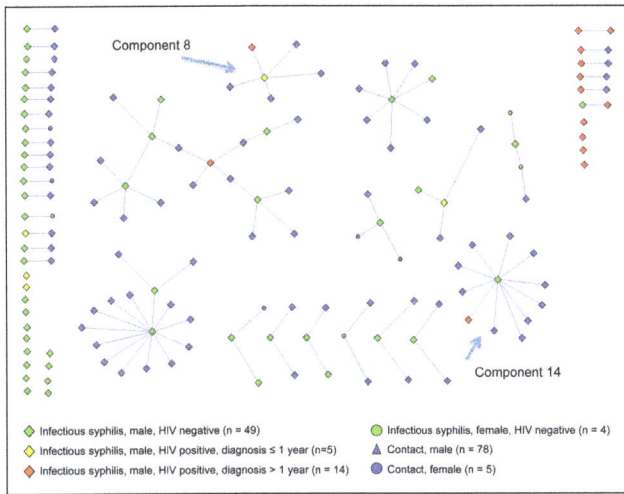

Figure 3) *Sexual network of infectious syphilis cases generated using routinely collected cases and contact data only in a syphilis outbreak, Ottawa, Ontario, January 2009 to June 2010 (n=155). Lines represent sexual contact between individuals*

general public using television, radio and magazines were also suggested to ensure all populations are aware of the messaging. Raising awareness and education of family and emergency room physicians about syphilis was also identified.

Social network data analysis

Including the social venue information collected through routine surveillance, only 155 cases and contacts were linked by sexual intercourse in 55 components consisting of 18 single cases; (11.6% of all cases and contacts) (Figure 3); 23 dyads (only two individuals linked (29.7%), six triads (11.6%), three tetrads (7.7%) and components of six, eight, 12 and 16 each, with the largest being 19 individuals (12%) (Figure 3). Of the 19 infectious syphilis cases coinfected with HIV, 63% were in small components of one or two cases and/or contacts. However, the potential for HIV transmission is illustrated in components eight and 14 (marked by arrows) in which cases who had been diagnosed with HIV were linked to HIV-negative individuals with syphilis or untested contacts.

The 17 enhanced surveillance respondents reported 42 social venues, which included those already noted in the routine surveillance reports; 16 social venues outside of Ottawa and six Internet sites. The most frequently reported social venue was a specific bathhouse in Ottawa, named by six (35%) of the respondents and followed by a popular gay Internet site (29%). Three different bathhouses in Montreal (Quebec) were identified as places to meet partners (24%). In addition, 16 venues in locations >200 km away, such as Florida and Georgia (USA) and Alberta were also named, comprising 38% of all venues.

The above venue data were combined with the networks of 72 routine and enhanced surveillance cases and their 83 named contacts (Figure 4). The network consisted of 45 components ranging in size from one to 95 nodes including 42 social venues. Furthermore, the largest component, previously composed of only 19 nodes (12%), expanded three-fold to contain 18 cases and 40 contacts, representing 37% of the outbreak population (Figure 5). Importantly, a second case with HIV and a female contact who were previously in separate components were now included.

DISCUSSION

Contact tracing of sex partners for individuals with infectious syphilis is universally recommended for the education and treatment of contacts; however, this intervention is limited to known individuals in a sexual relationship. The risk for acquiring an STI is associated with the individual's entire sexual network and not solely with the number of immediate and known sexual partners (9,11,12). In this investigation, the construction of venue-based networks identified previously

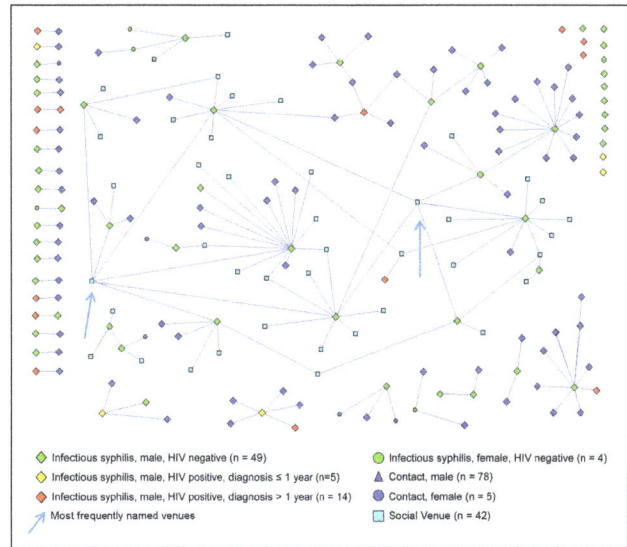

Figure 4) *Social network of infectious syphilis cases, contacts and all venues using data collected from routine and enhanced surveillance cases, according to sex and HIV status, Ottawa, Ontario, January 1, 2009 to June 15, 2010 (n = 197). Squares represent a venue, lines between individuals represent sexual contact while those between individuals and venues represent patronage to that venue*

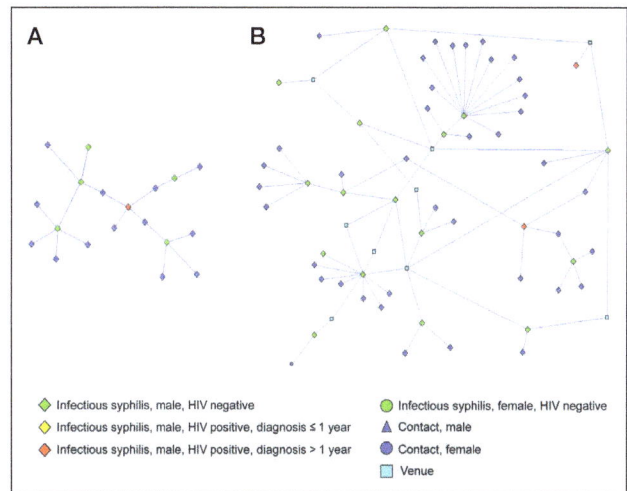

Figure 5) *Largest component of infectious syphilis cases contacts using routinely collected data only (A) and largest component generated from routinely collected data and adding only those venues named by two or more individuals, according to sex and HIV status (B), Ottawa, Ontario, January 1, 2009 to June 15, 2010. Lines between individuals represent sexual contact while those between individuals and venues represent patronage to that venue*

unknown links between a greater number of infectious syphilis cases and their sex partners, and increased connectivity among cases and contacts. This emphasized the concept of HIV and syphilis transmission through an entire sexual network of individuals, rather than as isolated cases for whom the source is unidentified.

We found that more than one-third (37.4%) of the 17 cases within the past six months who answered the enhanced surveillance questions patronized a specific bathhouse in Ottawa and a website. This is a similar proportion to the findings of two previous social network analyses (8,9) in which 49% and 42% of cases and contacts were linked to one local venue. Social network methods are valuable in STI investigation because they include the social context in which sexual intercourse occurs and serve as a proxy measure of homophily, where patronage of places and websites indicates shared, high-risk behaviours. In practice, focusing interventions on a few commonly patronized sites for sexual-health messaging and testing may have the advantage of both precision and efficiency. Conversely, we noted that the men who reported recruiting sex partners >200 km away were significantly more likely to report higher numbers of partners than those who named venues closer to Ottawa (Kruskal-Wallis, P<0.001). This agrees with previous findings that individuals with sex partners recruited from long distances engage in higher risk behaviours than those with local sex partners (13,14).The combination of sex partners locally and far away is ideal in the ability to 'catch' rarer pathogens, such as HIV and syphilis, in a wide net and then transmit them locally (14,15).

HIV transmission is two to five times more likely in couples in whom one has concomitant syphilis (16). Concomitant HIV infection in individuals with syphilis has been reported in several recent outbreaks in Canada (17-21); however, the position in sexual networks of most of the HIV positive men was peripheral, limiting the spread of HIV (22). Futhermore, there were the two HIV-positive men in the large component of the social network from whom HIV may easily spread to the rest.

The present investigation generated several new directions for the public health unit. First, the recording of information regarding venues where cases meet partners was valuable and should continue prospectively so to better serve prevention. Second, thematic analysis of suggestions for interventions identified the need for more sexual-health messaging both at specific, named gay and nongay venues. Finally, an increased need for education of physicians of both gay and heterosexual populations about syphilis symptoms, testing, transmission and the need to use condoms during oral and anal sex, was cited. OPH re-established public health visits to the bathhouses to provide safe-sex practice information and referrals for syphilis testing. OPH also expanded syphilis awareness campaigns, in particular the "Syphilis is Back" campaign, at the 2010 PRIDE events, and educated front line health care providers by hosting a continuing medical education event covering syphilis basics, attended by 200 primary care providers.

There were several limitations associated with the present investigation. First, only 30% of the cases during the time period of interest were followed-up for enhanced surveillance. The cases who completed the enhanced syphilis surveillance questionnaire did not represent the 72 infectious syphilis cases during the investigation period in that they had higher numbers of partners reported, higher numbers of named contacts and lower proportions of coinfection with HIV. An additional limitation was missing sexual partner data, possibly due to poor recall, anonymous partners or unwillingness to identify the partner. However, sex partners who were forgotten have been shown to be similar to those remembered with regard to the proportions subsequently testing positive (23). Finally, verification of the accuracy of the responses regarding the presence of sexual messaging was not possible.

The present investigation demonstrated that inclusion of social venues in network construction increases the connectivity between cases when compared with networks based solely on cases and sexual partners to include previously unknown links. Finally, we found that social network analysis provided a greater understanding of syphilis transmission in the context of the national and international sexual connections, and an opportunity to focus prevention interventions at key locations.

DISCLOSURES: The authors have no financial disclosures or conflicts of interest to declare.

REFERENCES

1. Romanowski B. Proceedings of the National STD Consensus Meeting: Canadian Goals for Syphilis. Canada Commun Dis Rep 1997;23S6:2-9.
2. Scott C. C, Sockett P. Canadian Communicable Disease;1993 Notifiable Disease Annual Summary. Ottawa: Minister of Health, Canada; 1995:5-75.
3. Notifiable Diseases Online. Public Heal Agency Canada. 2012. <http://dsol-smed.phac-aspc.gc.ca/dsol-smed/ndis/charts.php?c=pl> (Accessed August 1, 2015).
4. Canada S. 2006 community profiles. 2010;2011(12/07).
5. Auerbach DM, Darrow WW, Jaffe HW, Curran JW. Cluster of cases of the acquired immune deficiency syndrome; patients linked by sexual contact. Am J Med 1984;76:487-92.
6. Rothenberg R, Narramore J. The relevance of social network concepts to sexually transmitted disease control. Sex Transm Dis 1996;23:24-9.
7. Klovdahl AS, Graviss EA, Yaganehdoost A, et al. Networks and tuberculosis: An undetected community outbreak involving public places. Soc Sci Med 2001;52:681-94.
8. Potterat JJ, Rothenberg RB, Woodhouse DE, Muth JB, Pratts CI, Fogle JS. Gonorrhea as a social disease. Sex Transm Dis 1985;12:25-32.
9. De P, Singh AE, Wong T, Yacoub W, Jolly AM. Sexual network analysis of a gonorrhoea outbreak. Sex Transm Infect 2004;80:280-285.
10. Laboratory Centre for Disease Control HC. Case Definitions for Diseases Under National Surveillance. Canada Commun Dis Rep 2000;26(S3).
11. Ward H. Prevention strategies for sexually transmitted infections: Importance of sexual network structure and epidemic phase. Sex Transm Infect 2007;83:43-9.
12. Klovdahl AS. Social networks and the spread of infectious diseases: The AIDS example. Soc Sci Med 1985;21:1203-16.
13. Calzavara LM, Bullock SL, Myers T, Marshall VW, Cockerill R. Sexual partnering and risk of HIV/STD among Aboriginals. Can J Public Heal 1999;90:186-91.

14. Williams ML, Atkinson J, Klovdahl A, Ross MW, Timpson S. Spatial bridging in a network of drug-using male sex workers. J Urban Health 2005;82s1:135-42.
15. Jolly A, Wylie J. Sexual networks and sexually transmitted infections; The strength of weak (long distance) ties . In: Aral SO, Fenton KA, Lipshutz JA, eds. The New Public Health and STI/HIV prevention. New York: Springer-Verlag; 2013:77-110.
16. Wasserheit JN. Epidemiological synergy. Interrelationships between human immunodeficiency virus infection and other sexually transmitted diseases. Sex Transm Dis 1992;19:61-77.
17. Patrick DM, Rekart ML, Jolly A, et al. Heterosexual outbreak of infectious syphilis: Epidemiological and ethnographic analysis and implications for control. Sex Transm Infect 2002;78:164-9.
18. Rekart ML, Patrick D, Jolly AM, et al. Mass treatment/prophylaxis during an outbreak of infectious syphilis in Vancouver, British Columbia. Canada Commun Dis Rep 2000;26:101-5.
19. Weir E, Fisman D. Syphilis: Have we dropped the ball? CMAJ 2002;167:1267-8.
20. Jayaraman GC, Read RR, Singh AE. Characteristics of individuals with male-to-male and heterosexually acquired infectious syphilis during an outbreak in Calgary, Alberta, Canada. Sex Transm Dis 2003;30:315-9.
21. Leber A, MacPherson P, Lee BC. Epidemiology of infectious syphilis in Ottawa: Recurring themes revisited. Can J Public Health 2008;99:401-5. <www.cpha.ca> (Accessed August 1, 2015).
22. Darrow WW, Potterat JJ, Rothenberg RB, Woodhouse DE, Muth SQ. Using knowledge of social networks to prevent human immunodeficiency virus infections: The Colorado Springs Study. Sociol Focus 1999;32:143-58.
23. Brewer DD, Garrett SB. Evaluation of interviewing techniques to enhance recall of sexual and drug injection partners. Sex Transm Dis 2001;28:666-77.

6

Hepatitis C virus seroconversion among HIV-positive men who have sex with men with no history of injection drug use: Results from a clinical HIV cohort

Ann N Burchell PhD[1,2], Sandra L Gardner PhD[1,2], Tony Mazzulli MD[3,4,5], Michael Manno MSc[1], Janet Raboud PhD[2,6], Vanessa G Allen MD[3], Ahmed M Bayoumi MD MSc[7,8,9], Rupert Kaul MD PhD[9], Frank McGee[10], Peggy Millson MD[2], Robert S Remis MD MPH[2,3], Wendy Wobeser MD MSc[11,12], Curtis Cooper MD[13,14], Sean B Rourke PhD[1,7,15]
on behalf of the Ontario HIV Treatment Network Cohort Study Team*

AN Burchell, SL Gardner, T Mazzulli, et al. Hepatitis C virus seroconversion among HIV-positive men who have sex with men with no history of injection drug use: Results from a clinical HIV cohort. Can J Infect Dis Med Microbiol 2015;26(1):17-22.

BACKGROUND: Internationally, there is a growing recognition that hepatitis C virus (HCV) may be sexually transmitted among HIV-positive men who have sex with men (MSM).
OBJECTIVE: To report the first Canadian estimate of HCV seroincidence in 2000 to 2010 and its risk factors among HIV-positive MSM with no known history of injection drug use.
METHODS: Data from the Ontario HIV Treatment Network Cohort Study, an ongoing cohort of individuals in HIV care in Ontario, were analyzed. Data were obtained from medical charts, interviews and record linkage with the provincial public health laboratories. The analysis was restricted to 1534 MSM who did not report injection drug use and had undergone ≥2 HCV antibody tests, of which the first was negative (median 6.1 person-years [PY] of follow-up; sum 9987 PY).
RESULTS: In 2000 to 2010, 51 HCV seroconversions were observed, an overall incidence of 5.1 per 1000 PY (95% CI 3.9 to 6.7). Annual incidence varied from 1.6 to 8.9 per 1000 PY, with no statistical evidence of a temporal trend. Risk for seroconversion was elevated among men who had ever had syphilis (adjusted HR 2.5 [95% CI 1.1 to 5.5]) and men who had acute syphilis infection in the previous 18 months (adjusted HR 2.8 [95% CI 1.0 to 7.9]). Risk was lower for men who had initiated antiretroviral treatment (adjusted HR 0.49 [95% CI 0.25 to 0.95]). There were no statistically significant effects of age, ethnicity, region, CD4 cell count or HIV viral load.
CONCLUSIONS: These findings suggest that periodic HCV rescreening may be appropriate in Ontario among HIV-positive MSM. Future research should seek evidence whether syphilis is simply a marker for high-risk sexual behaviour or networks, or whether it potentiates sexual HCV transmission among individuals with HIV.

Key Words: *Hepatitis C virus; HIV; Incidence; Men who have sex with men; Syphilis*

La séroconversion au virus de l'hépatite C chez des hommes positifs au VIH qui ont des relations sexuelles avec des hommes sans antécédents de consommation de drogues injectables : les résultats d'une cohorte de VIH clinique

HISTORIQUE : Sur la scène internationale, il apparaît de plus en plus clairement que le virus de l'hépatite C (VHC) peut être transmis sexuellement entre hommes positifs au VIH ayant des relations sexuelles avec des hommes (HARSAH).
OBJECTIF : Rendre compte de la première estimation canadienne de la séro-incidence de VHC entre 2000 et 2010 et de ses facteurs de risque chez les HARSAH positifs au VIH sans antécédents connus de consommation de drogues injectables.
MÉTHODOLOGIE : Les chercheurs ont analysé les données de l'*Ontario HIV Treatment Network Cohort Study*, une cohorte continue de personnes soignées pour le VIH en Ontario. Ils ont tiré les données de dossiers médicaux, d'entrevues et de liens entre les dossiers et les laboratoires provinciaux de santé publique. Ils ont restreint l'analyse à 1 534 HARSAH qui ne déclaraient pas consommer de drogues injectables et qui avaient subi au moins deux tests d'anticorps du VHC, dont le premier était négatif (suivi médian de 6,1 années-personne [AP; somme de 9 987 AP).
RÉSULTATS : De 2000 à 2010, les chercheurs ont observé 51 cas de séroconversion au VHC, pour une incidence globale de 5,1 cas sur 1 000 AP (95 % IC 3,9 à 6,7). L'incidence annuelle variait entre 1,6 et 8,9 cas sur 1 000 AP, sans preuve statistique de tendance temporelle. Le risque de séroconversion était élevé chez les hommes qui n'avaient jamais eu la syphilis (RR rajusté 2,5 [95 % IC 1,1 à 5,5]) et chez les hommes qui avaient eu une infection aiguë par la syphilis dans les 18 mois précédents (RR rajusté 2,8 [95 % IC 1,0 à 7,9]). Le risque était plus faible chez les hommes qui avaient entrepris un traitement antirétroviral (RR rajusté 0,49 [95 % IC 0,25 à 0,95]). L'âge, l'ethnie, la région, la numération des cellules CD4 et la charge virale du VIH n'avaient pas d'effet statistiquement significatif.
CONCLUSIONS : D'après ces observations, il serait judicieux de procéder au dépistage périodique du VHC chez les HARSAH positifs au VIH de l'Ontario. De prochaines recherches devraient viser à établir si la syphilis est un simple marqueur de comportements ou de réseaux sexuels à haut risque ou si elle potentialise la transmission sexuelle du VHC chez les personnes atteintes du VIH.

*Members are listed in the Acknowledgements section
[1]Ontario HIV Treatment Network; [2]Dalla Lana School of Public Health, University of Toronto; [3]Public Health Laboratories, Public Health Ontario; [4]Department of Microbiology, Mount Sinai Hospital; [5]Department of Laboratory Medicine and Pathobiology, University of Toronto; [6]Toronto General Research Institute, University Health Network; [7]Centre for Research on Inner City Health, The Keenan Research Centre in the Li KaShing Knowledge Institute, St Michael's Hospital; [8]Institute of Health Policy, Management and Evaluation, University of Toronto; [9]Department of Medicine, University of Toronto; [10]AIDS Bureau, Ontario Ministry of Health and Long-Term Care; [11]Hotel Dieu Hospital; [12]Queen's University, Kingston; [13]Ottawa Hospital; [14]University of Ottawa, Ottawa; [15]Department of Psychiatry, University of Toronto
Correspondence: Dr Ann N Burchell, Ontario HIV Treatment Network, Suite 600, 1300 Yonge Street, Toronto, Ontario M4T 1X3.
e-mail aburchell@ohtn.on.ca

Outbreaks of hepatitis C virus (HCV) among HIV-positive men who have sex with men (MSM) with no history of injection drug use have been reported from Europe, North America, Australia and Asia (1-6). Although heterosexual HCV transmission is considered to be inefficient (7-9), increasing evidence suggests that sexual transmission occurs among HIV-positive MSM (6). Possible explanations include sexual networks, behavioural factors and biological cofactors, with HCV viral sequence analysis supporting the theory that the HCV epidemic has been driven by changes in sexual behaviour among MSM after 1996, the year of the introduction of combination antiretroviral treatment (ART) (6). Behavioural factors include serosorting (the practice of HIV-positive MSM selectively having unprotected sex with other HIV-positive men); the more common practice of engaging in anal sex because rectal mucosa may be more susceptible than vaginal mucosa; traumatic sexual practices, such as 'fisting', which rupture the skin and cause bleeding; and the use of noninjection recreational drugs (6). Biologically, HIV may increase HCV susceptibility and infectiousness (6). Coinfection with other mucosally disruptive sexually transmitted infections may serve as cofactors (6).

In Canada, the prevalence of HCV in the general population is estimated to be 0.8%, with an annual incidence of 33.7 per 100,000 as of 2009 (10). The majority of infections have been attributed to the sharing of injection drug use equipment, and receipt of blood and blood products before the introduction of HCV screening in 1990. Until recently, sexual transmission was considered to be a theoretically possible but rare mode of transmission in Canada. No HCV acquisition was detected among noninjecting MSM in a large, primarily HIV-negative cohort in Montreal in 1996 to 2001 (11). Anecdotally, Canadian HIV care physicians have not noticed an increase in HCV diagnoses among MSM patients (12). However, ongoing vigilance is important, because if the rate of HCV infection is sufficiently high, occasional screening among HIV-positive MSM would be cost effective (13). Timely diagnosis may prevent further transmission, and may guide treatment and care decisions, because HCV coinfection may complicate HIV therapy (14,15).

We estimated HCV seroincidence among HIV-positive MSM in Ontario with no known history of injection drug use. We hypothesized that syphilis infection would predict HCV seroconversion, because it would be a proxy measure of high-risk sexual behaviour and/or a cofactor for acquisition.

METHODS

The source of the data analyzed in the present study was from the Ontario HIV Treatment Network Cohort Study (OCS) (16). The cohort's source population consists of individuals ≥16 years of age diagnosed with HIV infection who receive medical care at specialty HIV clinics. The 10 participating clinics serve more than three-quarters of HIV patients undergoing viral load testing in the province. Enrollment and ongoing participation in the cohort was voluntary. All participants provided written informed consent. Clinical data obtained as part of participants' routine health care were abstracted from clinic records. From 1995 to 2007, participants self-completed a questionnaire at enrollment. Since 2008, participants have been interviewed annually (16). The study protocol, research instruments and forms received ethical approval from the University of Toronto Human Subjects Review Committee (Toronto, Ontario) and from the individual study sites.

Measurement of coinfection

Testing data were obtained for HIV viral load, HCV and syphilis through record linkage with the provincial Public Health Ontario Laboratories (PHOL). In Ontario, serological screening for hepatitis virus infections can be performed by private laboratories, hospital laboratories or at the PHOL. The PHOL conduct virtually all confirmatory HCV diagnostic serology in Ontario and virtually all HCV-RNA viral load monitoring among the chronically infected. The PHOL is the sole provider of HIV viral load and syphilis serological tests (17).

Analysis

As of December 2011, 5933 participants had enrolled. For the present study, the cohort was limited to 3453 male participants who reported sex with men as their HIV risk factor and/or who self-identified as homosexual or bisexual, did not report injection drug use as their HIV risk factor and did not report drug injection following HIV diagnosis. The cohort was further limited to 2761 men who were under observation in 2000 to 2010 and for whom there was successful record linkage to the HIV viral load database at the PHOL, meaning that any confirmatory or follow-up HCV testing should have been observable. Finally, the cohort was then limited to 1534 men who had at least two linked HCV test records from the PHOL, for which the first was HCV negative; χ^2 and t tests were used to compare the characteristics of the 1227 men who did not meet this criterion with the 1534 men who did. All statistical analyses were conducted using SAS version 9.3 (SAS Institute Inc, USA). All P values were two-sided and statistical significance was determined using the traditional P<0.05.

The incidence density of HCV seroconversion per 1000 person-years (PY) of follow-up was calculated. Person-time was calculated for each subject beginning at the later of the first HCV-antibody negative result, HIV diagnosis date, or January 1, 2000, and ended at the earlier of the last known date of follow-up, date of death (if applicable) or, for cases, the date of the first HCV-antibody positive test. Similarly, the annual incidence density was calculated as the number of new HCV diagnoses during each calendar year per 1000 PY of follow-up in that year. Poisson regression was used for all incidence density calculations and these were reported with 95% CIs.

Risk factors for HCV seroconversion were identified using Cox proportional hazards methods and results are reported as HRs. The effects of the following factors were explored: age; region of residence; ethnicity and time-updated values of CD4 cell count; HIV viral load; whether ART had been initiated; previous reactive syphilis serology and recent diagnosis of acute syphilis infection (defined as a reactive treponemal test and rapid plasma reagin titre ≥1:16, any reactive syphilis test following a previously negative test result, or a fourfold rise in rapid plasma reagin titre for those whose previous syphilis tests were reactive). A multivariable model was first built containing all considered risk factors, then those that were neither associated with HCV seroconversion nor required for adjustment of the remaining risk factors were excluded.

Various sensitivity analyses were conducted. HCV incidence was re-estimated including the additional 746 men who were tested for HCV antibody only once and were nonreactive; it was assumed that these men remained HCV-negative for the duration of follow-up. HR estimates were also recalculated in a Cox model for which the seroconversion event date was reassigned as the midpoint between the last HCV antibody-negative and first HCV antibody-positive test, to account for interval censoring. Finally, the estimates of HCV seroincidence were compared among men who were interviewed in 2008 to 2010 with men who were not interviewed (due to death or loss to follow-up before the introduction of the interview, or participation at one clinic that did not administer interviews). It was hypothesized that injection drug use would be better reported via interview and, thus, that the estimate of HCV seroincidence should be higher among uninterviewed men due to misclassification as noninjectors. The rate of HCV seroincidence among the 174 men who did not report sex with men and 233 women in the cohort who met all other criteria for analysis (except MSM status) was also calculated. Because sexual HCV transmission among individuals with HIV has been primarily reported among MSM (6), it was hypothesized that HCV seroincidence would be lower among heterosexual men and women.

RESULTS

Among the 1534 men who were included in the analysis of HCV seroconversion, men were, on average, 41 years of age, white and living in Toronto at baseline (Table 1). Most had initiated ART. The median HIV viral load was 759 copies/mL and the mean CD4 cell count was 421 cells/mm^3. The included participants were slightly younger, were less likely to live in Ottawa, were more likely to be of nonwhite race, were diagnosed more recently and had higher viral loads compared with the 1227 men who would have been eligible for

TABLE 1
Characteristics of men who have sex with men with no history of injection drug use who were included and excluded from the analysis of hepatitis C virus (HCV) seroincidence, Ontario HIV Treatment Network Cohort Study, 2000 to 2010

Characteristic	Included (n=1534)	Excluded (n=1227)	P[†]
Age at baseline*, years			
<30	150 (9.8)	92 (7.5)	0.14
30–39	541 (35.3)	425 (34.6)	
40–49	584 (38.1)	482 (39.3)	
≥50	259 (16.9)	228 (18.6)	
Mean ± SD	41±9.4	42±9.4	0.009
Region (Ontario)			
Toronto	1142 (74.4)	755 (61.5)	<0.0001
Ottawa	80 (5.2)	205 (16.7)	
Other	312 (20.3)	267 (21.8)	
Race[‡]			
White	1144 (74.6)	971 (79.1)	0.009
Black	72 (4.7)	37 (3.0)	
Aboriginal	121 (7.9)	70 (5.7)	
Other race	194 (12.7)	149 (12.1)	
Year of HIV diagnosis, median (IQR)	1996 (1990–2003)	1993 (1989–1999)	<0.0001
Initiated antiretroviral treatment at baseline*	963 (62.8)	800 (65.2)	0.19
Initiated antiretroviral treatment as of last follow-up	1419 (92.5)	1156 (94.2)	0.07
CD4 cell count/mm^3 at baseline*, mean ± SD	421±260	403±254	0.13
Log$_{10}$ viral load at baseline*, median (IQR)	2.88 (1.69–4.53)	2.42 (1.69–4.14)	0.0005
Ever HCV-positive at last follow-up			
No	1483 (96.7)	1132 (92.3)	<0.0001
Yes	51 (3.3)	95 (7.7)	

*Data presented as n (%) unless otherwise indicated. *Baseline was defined as the later of the first HCV-negative test, the first HIV-positive date, or January 1, 2000; †P values were calculated using χ^2 tests for categorical variables, Wilcoxon signed-rank for medians or Student's t tests for means, as appropriate; ‡Excludes 15 men with unknown race. IQR Interquartile range*

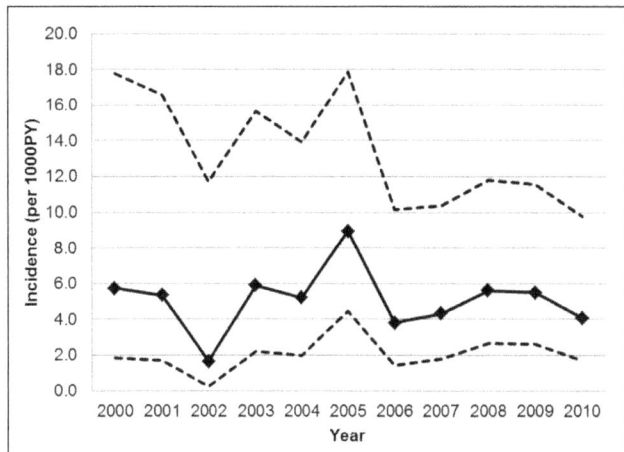

Figure 1) *Hepatitis C virus seroincidence among HIV-positive men who have sex with men in Ontario, 2000 to 2010. Dashed lines represent 95% CIs*

inclusion in the analysis if it were not for the fact that they had not been tested for HCV at least twice with the first test being negative (Table 1). Among these 1227 excluded men, 746 were tested only once and were HCV-negative, 95 tested positive for HCV at their first test and the remainder had no record of ever being tested for HCV.

Men contributed a median of 6.1 PY (interquartile range [IQR] 3.7 to 10.1) of follow-up to the analysis of HCV seroconversion for a total of 9987 PY. The first HCV-negative test occurred a median of 3.6 years after HIV diagnosis (IQR 0.2 to 10.2); all but four patients had their first HCV-negative test post-HIV diagnosis. Men underwent HCV testing a median of two times (75th percentile four times). The median intertest interval was 2.2 years (IQR 1.0 to 4.9) and the median number of HCV tests per year was 0.4 (IQR 0.2 to 0.9).

A total of 51 seroconversions were observed. The first HCV-positive test occurred a median of 9.7 years after HIV diagnosis (IQR 4.5 to 15.0) and 2.7 years after the first HCV-negative test (IQR 0.5 to 5.5). The majority of cases (45 of 51 [89%]) had at least one PHOL record for HCV viral load following the seroconversion date; of these 45, 62% had detectable viral load, 24% had undetectable viral load and for the remainder the result was missing. The overall HCV seroincidence was 5.1 per 1000 PY (95% CI 3.9 to 6.7) with annual rates

that varied from 1.6 to 8.9 per 1000 PY, with no evidence of a temporal trend (Figure 1). In a sensitivity analysis that additionally included person time from the 746 men who tested negative for HCV but who were never tested again, under the assumption that they remained negative, HCV seroincidence was 3.6 per 1000 PY (95% CI 2.7 to 4.7); this estimate provides a plausible lower bound of the underlying true rate.

The strongest risk factor for HCV seroconversion was having ever had reactive syphilis serology (Table 2). An elevation of risk was also observed for men who had evidence of acute syphilis infection within the past 18 months, although the 95% CI included 1.0 (Table 2). Among cases, 20% (10 of 51) had a history of reactive syphilis serology before their first HCV antibody positive test and, among these, 60% had evidence of acute syphilis infection within 36 months of their HCV diagnosis. In a sensitivity analysis using the midpoint date as the event date for cases, the adjusted HRs for ever having syphilis increased from 2.5 (95% CI 1.1 to 5.5) to 2.8 (95% CI 1.2 to 6.4), and the adjusted HR for acute syphilis within the past 18 months declined from 2.8 (95% CI 1.0 to 7.9) to 2.0 (95% CI 0.63 to 6.6).

There was an effect of ART, such that men who had initiated treatment were less likely to experience HCV seroconversion (adjusted HR 0.49 [95% CI 0.25 to 0.95) (Table 2). The magnitude of the HR did not diminish with adjustment for age or time since diagnosis (data not shown), but did diminish to 0.57 (95% CI 0.30 to 1.1) in sensitivity analysis using the midpoint date method. No other examined covariates modified the risk of HCV seroconversion in the primary analysis, in the sensitivity analyses using the midpoint estimate of the seroconversion date or in the analysis that included men who tested HCV negative but who were never tested again (data not shown).

Finally, analyses were conducted in an attempt to quantify the degree of ascertainment bias due to unreported injection drug use (Table 3). Although there was insufficient precision to declare rates statistically significantly different between groups, the incidence was observed to be higher among men who were not interviewed compared with men who were, and the rate among female and heterosexual male participants with no history of injection drug use was one-half the rate of MSM.

DISCUSSION
We analysed data from MSM in HIV care in Ontario from 2000 to 2010 and observed that, among men with no recorded history of injection drug use, the incidence of HCV seroconversion was 5.1 per 1000 PY (95% CI 3.9 to 6.7), which is 15 times higher than that the rate of 0.337 per 1000 observed in the general population in 2009 (10). It is, however, consistent with rates reported among HIV-positive urban MSM internationally, which range from 0 to 12.3 per 1000 PY, and average 6.08 per 1000 PY (95% CI 5.18 to 6.99) (1). At such a rate,

TABLE 2
Risk factors for hepatitis C virus seroconversion among HIV-positive men who have sex with men in Ontario, 2000 to 2010

	Unadjusted HR (95% CI)	Adjusted HR[†] (95% CI)	Adjusted HR[†] (95% CI)
Age, years			
<30	1.00		
30–39	0.83 (0.31–2.2)		
40–49	0.72 (0.27–2.0)		
≥50	1.01 (0.35–3.0)		
Region			
Toronto	1.00	1.00	1.00
Ottawa	1.8 (0.63–5.0)	2.0 (0.69–5.5)	1.9 (0.68–5.4)
Other	1.2 (0.64–2.3)	1.4 (0.73–2.7)	1.4 (0.71–2.6)
Race			
White	1.00		
Black	0.86 (0.21–3.59)		
Aboriginal	1.6 (0.66–3.71)		
Other	0.93 (0.39–2.21)		
CD4 cell count/mm³*			
<200	1.00		
200–499	0.78 (0.36–1.7)		
≥500	0.66 (0.30–1.5)		
HIV viral load*			
Detectable	1.00		
Undetectable	0.90 (0.51–1.6)		
Initiated ART*			
No	1.00	1.00	1.00
Yes	0.49 (0.26–0.95)	0.49 (0.25–0.95)	0.49 (0.25–0.95)
Each additional year since HIV diagnosis*	0.98 (0.94–1.03)		
Ever had reactive syphilis serology*			
No	1.00	1.00	
Yes	2.4 (1.1–5.5)	2.5 (1.1–5.5)	
Acute syphilis within 18 months*			
No	1.00		1.00
Yes	2.9 (1.0–8.0)		2.8 (1.0–7.9)

*Time-varying covariates were updated at each seroconversion event time;
†Multivariate Cox proportional hazards model including all covariates shown.
ART Antiretroviral therapy

TABLE 3
Hepatitis C virus seroincidence among HIV-positive men who have sex with men, by method of ascertainment of injection drug use history, and compared with women and heterosexual men

	Incidence per 1000 person-years (95% CI)
Men who have sex with men with no record of injection drug use	5.1 (3.9–6.7)
Completed one or more interviews	5.0 (3.7–6.7)
Were not interviewed	6.4 (2.6–15.3)
Female participants with no record of injection drug use	2.6 (1.1–6.3)
Male participants who completed one or more interviews and had no record of sex with men or injection drug use	2.1 (0.8–7.9)

cofactor that increases the risk of HIV acquisition several fold (22). There is no evidence that syphilis alters the biological characteristics of HCV; however, this has not been thoroughly studied. An alternative, noncausal explanation for the association between syphilis and HCV may be that a syphilis episode prompts a thorough sexually transmitted infection (STI) work-up, including HCV testing, or vice versa, such that HCV acquisition may precede syphilis infection. We observed that syphilis testing occurred at the time of HCV antibody testing in one-third of diagnosed cases. In sensitivity analysis using the midpoint method to impute event dates, the magnitude of the HR estimate for recent syphilis decreased from 2.8 to 2.0, suggesting that this diagnostic work-up bias may have been present. Our observations require confirmation given our limited precision to quantify risk associated with recent syphilis.

Men who had not yet initiated ART were twice as likely to acquire HCV, a finding that was not due to confounding by age or time since HIV diagnosis. The finding would be consistent with the biological hypothesis that HIV increases susceptibility to HCV, such that suppression of viral load may mitigate this effect (6). However, we observed no direct effect of HIV viral load on HCV risk. Other clinical cohorts in Switzerland (20) and Germany (19) have not observed differences between those receiving and not receiving antiretroviral therapy, suggesting that our finding may be anomalous, unique to our setting or confounded. Further study would be necessary to establish the mechanism for this association, which could be due to behavioural or sexual network factors. Lack of antiretroviral use is associated with behaviours that heighten risk for HCV infection. There is evidence that HCV RNA levels are higher for individuals not on HIV antiretroviral therapy, which would increase risk for onward HCV transmission to partners (23).

The strengths of our analysis included a large sample size, extended follow-up period and use of data from a generally representative cohort of individuals with HIV in Ontario based on characteristics of cumulative HIV diagnoses in Ontario in terms of sex, geographic region, age at diagnosis and HIV exposure category (24). Nevertheless, OCS participants under-represent the recently diagnosed and, compared with nonvolunteer patients at these clinics, participants tend to be older, have been diagnosed for longer and are generally healthier, as measured by CD4 cell count and viral load (25). There was the potential for referral bias given that HCV tests were ordered for clinical care purposes rather than at standardized intervals. MSM participants who did not meet analysis inclusion criteria tended to live in Ottawa, the second-largest city in Ontario, which has experienced high HIV and HCV infection rates among people who inject drugs compared with the remainder of the province (26). As of the last follow-up, HCV coinfection was higher among excluded men (7.7%) than among the men who were included (3.3%); HCV-positive men in the former group were men that tested HCV positive on their first test. All men included in our primary analysis were HCV negative at their first test;

the burden of HCV infection and its sequelae may become considerable. By the end of follow-up, 3.3% of participants were coinfected with HCV. This prevalence is similar to that found in a Canadian venue-based study of MSM, which found that HCV coinfection was present in 4% of HIV-positive MSM who never injected drugs (10).

Men who had ever had syphilis were more than twice as likely to acquire HCV (adjusted HR 2.5 [95% CI 1.1 to 5.5]). We also observed an elevation of risk for men with recent acute syphilis within the past 18 months that approached statistical significance (adjusted HR 2.8 [95% CI 1.0 to 7.9]) but the 95% CI included one, such that we were unable to reject the null hypothesis of no association for recent syphilis. Past syphilis has been noted as a risk factor in univariate analysis of case-control studies in the United Kingdom (18), United States (3) and Germany (19). The Swiss HIV Cohort found a doubling of HCV seroincidence among MSM with past syphilis (adjusted HR 2.1 [95% CI 1.4 to 3.2]) (20). In a Taiwanese analysis of HIV patients, syphilis infection within the past six months was associated with a 7.7-fold increase in odds of HCV seroconversion (21). Syphilis can be considered a proxy measure of high-risk sexual behaviour. It is also possible that syphilitic ulcers potentiate HCV acquisition due to disruption of mucosa (6,20). By analogy, syphilis is an established HIV

however, the fact that HCV retesting was ordered suggests that physicians may have considered these men to be at higher risk for infection, which may have biased our incidence estimates. Such bias due to testing patterns is likely to have diminished with time, because HCV testing has become more frequent in our setting; by 2010, 85% of patients were tested at least once (27). We cannot rule out the possibility that our calculations excluded some undiagnosed seroconversions for men who had not yet been retested for HCV. The rates of HCV seroincidence we observed were consistent with those reported internationally (1), which indicates that bias, if present, was unlikely to be extreme.

We cannot exclude the possibility of HCV acquisition via unreported injection drug use. Compared with MSM who underwent in-depth interviewing, we observed a higher point estimate for HCV seroconversion among men whose assessment of injection drug use history status was based only on a brief, self-completed questionnaire. This suggests that some proportion of HCV cases was likely due to acquisition via unreported sharing of drug use equipment. Nevertheless, the observed association with syphilis infection would be consistent with some sexual transmission.

Our findings have implications for best practices for HCV screening. Current guidelines recommend HCV testing at HIV diagnosis (28,29). Subsequent screening is warranted among HIV-positive MSM who report high-risk sexual behaviour and/or concomitant ulcerative STIs including syphilis (29). Regardless of reported sexual risk behaviour, our observed rate of HCV seroconversion combined with mathematical modelling work by Linas et al (13) suggest that it would be cost effective to conduct rescreening with tests for alanine aminotransferase every six months and HCV antibody annually, as recommended by European AIDS Treatment Network guidelines (30). The higher HCV rate we observed among men who had not yet initiated ART suggests that repeated screening may be especially prudent during this time. Repeated screening for HCV RNA is also warranted for patients who have been successfully treated for HCV infection because reinfection can occur (6,31). Patient education and safer sex counselling to prevent coinfection with STIs remains necessary, especially among men who have only HIV-positive sex partners and may believe that condoms are unnecessary. Finally, future research should seek evidence regarding whether syphilis is simply a marker of high-risk sexual behaviour or networks, or whether it potentiates sexual HCV transmission among individuals with HIV.

ACKNOWLEDGEMENTS: The OHTN Cohort Study Team consists of Dr Sean B Rourke (Principal Investigator, University of Toronto and OHTN), Dr Ann Burchell (Co-Principal Investigator, OHTN), Dr Sandra Gardner (OHTN), Dr Sergio Rueda (OHTN), Dr Ahmed Bayoumi and Dr Kevin Gough, St Michael's Hospital; Dr Jeffrey Cohen, Windsor Regional Hospital; Dr Curtis Cooper, Ottawa General Hospital; Dr Don Kilby, University of Ottawa Health Services; Dr Mona Loutfy and Dr Fred Crouzat, Maple Leaf Medical Clinic; Dr Anita Rachlis and Dr Nicole Mittmann, Sunnybrook Health Sciences Centre; Dr Janet Raboud and Dr Irving Salit, Toronto General Hospital; Dr Edward Ralph, St Joseph's Health Care; Dr Roger Sandre, Sudbury Regional Hospital; Dr Marek Smieja, Hamilton Health Sciences, McMaster University Medical Centre; and Dr Wendy Wobeser, Hotel Dieu Hospital. The authors gratefully acknowledge all of the people living with HIV who volunteered to participate in the OHTN Cohort Study and the work and support of the past and present members of the OCS Governance Committee: Adrian Betts, Anita C Benoit, Les Bowman, Tracey Conway, Patrick Cupido (Chair), Tony Di Pede, Brian Finch, Michael J Hamilton, Brian Huskins, Rick Kennedy, Ken King, Nathan Lachowsky, Joanne Lindsay, Shari Margolese, John McTavish, Colleen Price, Lori Stoltz, Darien Taylor, and Drs Ahmed Bayoumi, Evan Collins, Curtis Cooper, Clemon George, Troy Grennan, Claire Kendall, Greg Robinson and Rosie Thein. The authors thank all of the interviewers, data collectors, research associates and coordinators, nurses and physicians who provide support for data collection and extraction. The authors also thank the OHTN staff and their teams for coordination, data management and administrative support (Kevin Challacombe, Brooke Ellis, Mark Fisher, Ramandip Grewal, Robert Hudder, Veronika Moravan, Nahid Qureshi and Samantha Robinson), and the Public Health Ontario Laboratories for supporting record linkage with the HIV viral load, hepatitis C and syphilis test databases.

DISCLAIMER: The opinions, results and conclusions are those of the authors and no endorsement by the Ontario HIV Treatment Network or Public Health Ontario is intended or should be inferred.

DISCLOSURES AND SOURCES OF FUNDING: The authors have no relevant conflict of interests to declare. This work was supported by Canadian Institutes of Health Research (CIHR) (operating grant 111146 to ANB); a CIHR New Investigator award to ANB; and OHTN Career Scientist awards to JR and CC. The OHTN Cohort Study is funded by the AIDS Bureau, Ontario Ministry of Health and Long-Term Care. This work originated at the Ontario HIV Treatment Network.

REFERENCES

1. Yaphe S, Bozinoff N, Kyle R, et al. Incidence of acute hepatitis C virus infection among men who have sex with men with and without HIV infection: A systematic review. Sex Transm Infect 2012;88:558-64.
2. Van der Helm JJ, Prins M, del Amo J, et al. The hepatitis C epidemic among HIV-positive MSM: Incidence estimates from 1990 to 2007. AIDS Lond Engl 2011;25:1083-91.
3. Fierer DS. Epidemic of sexually transmitted hepatitis c virus infection among HIV-infected men. Curr Infect Dis Rep 2010;12:118-25.
4. Gamage DG, Read TR, Bradshaw CS, et al. Incidence of hepatitis-C among HIV infected men who have sex with men (MSM) attending a sexual health service: A cohort study. BMC Infect Dis 2011;11:39.
5. Van de Laar TJ, Matthews GV, Prins M, et al. Acute hepatitis C in HIV-infected men who have sex with men: An emerging sexually transmitted infection. AIDS Lond Engl 2010;24:1799-812.
6. Bradshaw D, Matthews G, Danta M. Sexually transmitted hepatitis C infection: The new epidemic in MSM? Curr Opin Infect Dis 2013;26:66-72.
7. Vandelli C, Renzo F, Romanò L, et al. Lack of evidence of sexual transmission of hepatitis C among monogamous couples: Results of a 10-year prospective follow-up study. Am J Gastroenterol 2004;99:855-9.
8. Wyld R, Robertson JR, Brettle RP, et al. Absence of hepatitis C virus transmission but frequent transmission of HIV-1 from sexual contact with doubly-infected individuals. J Infect 1997;35:163-6.
9. Terrault NA, Dodge JL, Murphy EL, et al. Sexual transmission of hepatitis C virus among monogamous heterosexual couples: The HCV partners study. Hepatology 2013;57:881-9.
10. Public Health Agency of Canada (PHAC). Hepatitis C in Canada: 2005-2010 Surveillance Report. Ottawa: Centre for Communicable Diseases and Infection Control, PHAC; 2011. <www.catie.ca/sites/default/files/1109-0139-Hep%20C%20Report-EN%20FINAL.pdf> (Accessed May 26, 2014).
11. Alary M, Joly JR, Vincelette J, et al. Lack of evidence of sexual transmission of hepatitis C virus in a prospective cohort study of men who have sex with men. Am J Public Health 2005;95:502-5.
12. CATIE. A Practical Guide to Complementary Therapies for People Living with HIV. Toronto: CATIE; 2004.
13. Linas BP, Wong AY, Schackman BR, et al. Cost-effective screening for acute hepatitis C virus infection in HIV-infected men who have sex with men. Clin Infect Dis 2012;55:279-90.
14. Graham CS, Baden LR, Yu E, et al. Influence of human immunodeficiency virus infection on the course of hepatitis C virus infection: A meta-analysis. Clin Infect Dis 2001;33:562-9.
15. Berenguer J, Alejos B, Hernando V, et al. Trends in mortality according to hepatitis C virus serostatus in the era of combination antiretroviral therapy. AIDS Lond Engl 2012;26:2241-6.
16. Rourke SB, Gardner S, Burchell AN, et al. Cohort profile: The Ontario HIV Treatment Network Cohort Study (OCS). Int J Epidemiol 2012;42:402-11.
17. Mishra S, Boily M-C, Ng V, et al. The laboratory impact of changing syphilis screening from the rapid-plasma reagin to a

treponemal enzyme immunoassay: A case-study from the Greater Toronto Area. Sex Transm Dis 2011;38:190-6.

18. Danta M, Brown D, Bhagani S, et al. Recent epidemic of acute hepatitis C virus in HIV-positive men who have sex with men linked to high-risk sexual behaviours. AIDS Lond Engl 2007;21:983-91.

19. Schmidt AJ, Rockstroh JK, Vogel M, et al. Trouble with bleeding: Risk factors for acute hepatitis C among HIV-positive gay men from Germany – a case-control study. PloS One 2011;6:e17781.

20. Wandeler G, Gsponer T, Bregenzer A, et al. Hepatitis C virus infections in the Swiss HIV Cohort Study: A rapidly evolving epidemic. Clin Infect Dis 2012;55:1408-16.

21. Sun H-Y, Chang S-Y, Yang Z-Y, et al. Recent hepatitis C virus infections in HIV-infected patients in Taiwan: Incidence and risk factors. J Clin Microbiol 2012;50:781-7.

22. Fleming DT, Wasserheit JN. From epidemiological synergy to public health policy and practice: The contribution of other sexually transmitted diseases to sexual transmission of HIV infection. Sex Transm Infect 1999;75:3-17.

23. Cooper CL, Cameron DW. Effect of alcohol use and highly active antiretroviral therapy on plasma levels of hepatitis C virus (HCV) in patients coinfected with HIV and HCV. Clin Infect Dis 2005;(41 Suppl 1):S105-109.

24. Remis RS, Liu J. HIV/AIDS in Ontario: Preliminary Report, 2011. Toronto: University of Toronto; 2013. <www.ohemu.utoronto.ca/doc/PHERO2011_report_preliminary.pdf> (Accessed May 26, 2014).

25. Raboud J, Su D, Burchell AN, et al. Representativeness of an HIV cohort of the sites from which it is recruiting: Results from the Ontario HIV Treatment Network (OHTN) cohort study. BMC Med Res Methodol 2013;13:31.

26. Remis RS, Swantee C, Liu J. Report on HIV/AIDS in Ontario 2009. Toronto: University of Toronto; 2012 <www.ohemu.utoronto.ca/doc/PHERO2009_report_final.pdf> (Accessed April 9, 2013)

27. Gillis J, Smieja M, Cescon A, et al. Risk of cardiovascular disease associated with HCV and HBV co-infection among antiretroviral-treated HIV-infected individuals. Antivir Ther 2014;19:309-17.

28. Public Health Agency of Canada (PHAC). Canadian Guidelines on Sexually Transmitted Infections. Ottawa: Centre for Communicable Diseases and Infection Control, PHAC; 2010.

29. Centers for Disease Control and Prevention (CDC). Sexual transmission of hepatitis C virus among HIV-infected men who have sex with men – New York City, 2005-2010. MMWR Morb Mortal Wkly Rep 2011;60:945-50.

30. European AIDS Treatment Network (NEAT) Acute Hepatitis C Infection Consensus Panel. Acute hepatitis C in HIV-infected individuals: Recommendations from the European AIDS Treatment Network (NEAT) consensus conference. AIDS Lond Engl 2011;25:399-409.

31. Lambers FAE, Prins M, Thomas X, et al. Alarming incidence of hepatitis C virus re-infection after treatment of sexually acquired acute hepatitis C virus infection in HIV-infected MSM. AIDS Lond Engl 2011;25:F21-27.

7

Prevalence of antimicrobial use in a network of Canadian hospitals in 2002 and 2009

Geoffrey Taylor MD[1], Denise Gravel MSc[2], Lynora Saxinger MD[1], Kathryn Bush MSc[3], Kimberley Simmonds MSc[4], Anne Matlow MD[5], Joanne Embree MD[6], Nicole Le Saux MD[7], Lynn Johnston MD[8], Kathryn N Suh MD[9], John Embil MD[6], Elizabeth Henderson PhD[10], Michael John MD[11], Virginia Roth MD[9], Alice Wong MD[12], and the Canadian Nosocomial Infection Surveillance Program

G Taylor, D Gravel, L Saxinger, et al. Prevalence of antimicrobial use in a network of Canadian hospitals in 2002 and 2009. Can J Infect Dis Med Microbiol 2015;26(2):85-89.

BACKGROUND: Increasing antimicrobial resistance has been identified as an important global health threat. Antimicrobial use is a major driver of resistance, especially in the hospital sector. Understanding the extent and type of antimicrobial use in Canadian hospitals will aid in developing national antimicrobial stewardship priorities.

METHODS: In 2002 and 2009, as part of one-day prevalence surveys to quantify hospital-acquired infections in Canadian Nosocomial Infection Surveillance Program hospitals, data were collected on the use of systemic antimicrobial agents in all patients in participating hospitals. Specific agents in use (other than antiviral and antiparasitic agents) on the survey day and patient demographic information were collected.

RESULTS: In 2002, 2460 of 6747 patients (36.5%) in 28 hospitals were receiving antimicrobial therapy. In 2009, 3989 of 9953 (40.1%) patients in 44 hospitals were receiving antimicrobial therapy (P<0.001). Significantly increased use was observed in central Canada (37.4% to 40.8%) and western Canada (36.9% to 41.1%) but not in eastern Canada (32.9% to 34.1%). In 2009, antimicrobial use was most common on solid organ transplant units (71.0% of patients), intensive care units (68.3%) and hematology/oncology units (65.9%). Compared with 2002, there was a significant decrease in use of first- and second-generation cephalosporins, and significant increases in use of carbapenems, antifungal agents and vancomycin in 2009. Piperacillin-tazobactam, as a proportion of all penicillins, increased from 20% in 2002 to 42.8% in 2009 (P<0.001). There was a significant increase in simultaneous use of >1 agent, from 12.0% of patients in 2002 to 37.7% in 2009.

CONCLUSION: From 2002 to 2009, the prevalence of antimicrobial agent use in Canadian Nosocomial Infection Surveillance Program hospitals significantly increased; additionally, increased use of broad-spectrum agents and a marked increase in simultaneous use of multiple agents were observed.

Key Words: *Antimicrobial use; Hospital; Prevalence*

La prévalence d'utilisation d'antimicrobiens dans un réseau d'hôpitaux canadiens en 2002 et 2009

HISTORIQUE : La résistance antimicrobienne croissante est une menace importante pour la santé dans le monde. L'utilisation d'antimicrobiens est un moteur de résistance majeur, particulièrement dans le milieu hospitalier. Il faut comprendre la portée et le type d'utilisation des antimicrobiens dans les hôpitaux canadiens pour établir les priorités nationales en matière de gouvernance antimicrobienne.

MÉTHODOLOGIE : En 2002 et 2009, dans le cadre de sondages de prévalence d'une journée visant à quantifier les infections nosocomiales dans les hôpitaux du Programme canadien de surveillance des infections nosocomiales, les chercheurs ont colligé des données sur l'utilisation des antimicrobiens systémiques par tous les patients des hôpitaux participants. Le jour du sondage, ils ont recueilli les agents précis utilisés (à part les antiviraux et les antiparasitaires) et l'information démographique relative aux patients.

RÉSULTATS : En 2002, 2 460 des 6 747 patients (36,5 %) de 28 hôpitaux recevaient un traitement antimicrobien. En 2009, 3 989 des 9 953 patients (40,1 %) de 44 hôpitaux recevaient un tel traitement (P<0,001). L'utilisation avait beaucoup augmenté au centre du Canada (37,4 % à 40,8 %) et dans l'Ouest canadien (36,9 % à 41,1 %), mais pas dans l'Est canadien (32,9 % à 34,1 %). En 2009, l'utilisation d'antimicrobiens était plus courante dans les unités de transplantation d'organes pleins (71,0 % des patients), les unités de soins intensifs (68,3 %) et les unités d'hématologie-oncologie (65,9 %). Par rapport à 2002, on constatait en 2009 une diminution importante des céphalosporines de première et seconde générations et des augmentations marquées de carbapénèmes, d'antifongiques et de vancomycine. L'utilisation de pipéracilline-tazobactam, en proportion de toutes les pénicillines, est passée de 20 % en 2002 à 42,8 % en 2009 (P<0,001). L'utilisation simultanée de plus d'un agent a également connu une hausse importante, passant de 12,0 % des patients en 2002 à 37,7 % en 2009.

CONCLUSION : De 2002 à 2009, la prévalence d'utilisation d'antimicrobiens dans les hôpitaux du Programme canadien de surveillance des infections nosocomiales a considérablement augmenté. De plus, les chercheurs ont constaté une augmentation marquée d'agents à large spectre et d'utilisation simultanée de multiples agents.

Antimicrobial resistance (AMR) in human bacterial pathogens has been identified as a public health problem of global significance (1-3). Hospitalized patients are at particular risk from antimicrobial-resistant pathogens due to the evolution of AMR after antimicrobial exposure and to the new acquisition of antimicrobial-resistant bacterial strains, such as methicillin-resistant *Staphylococcus aureus* (MRSA), vancomycin-resistant enterococci and *Enterobacteriaceae* such as those with extended-spectrum beta-lactamases or carbapenemases. *Clostridium difficile* infection (CDI) is usually considered to be part of the same public health problem because it shares epidemiological characteristics

[1]*University of Alberta Hospital, Edmonton, Alberta;* [2]*Centre for Communicable Diseases and Infection Control, Public Health Agency of Canada, Ottawa, Ontario;* [3]*Alberta Health Services, Calgary;* [4]*Alberta Health, Edmonton, Alberta;* [5]*The Hospital for Sick Children, Toronto, Ontario;* [6]*Health Sciences Centre, Winnipeg, Manitoba;* [7]*The Children's Hospital of Eastern Ontario, Ottawa, Ontario;* [8]*Queen Elizabeth II Health Sciences Centre, Halifax, Nova Scotia;* [9]*The Ottawa Hospital, Ottawa, Ontario;* [10]*Peter Lougheed Centre, Calgary, Alberta;* [11]*Health Sciences Centre, London, Ontario;* [12]*Royal University Hospital, Saskatoon, Saskatchewan*

Correspondence: Dr Geoffrey Taylor, 2D3.05 WMC, University of Alberta, Edmonton, Alberta T6G 2B7. E-mail geoff.taylor@ualberta.ca

TABLE 1

Antimicrobial use in Canadian Nosocomial Infection Surveillance Program hospitals in 2009: Patient characteristics

Characteristic	Receiving antimicrobial therapy		
	Yes (n=3989)	No (n=5964)	P
Age, years, median (IQR)	62 (43–77)	68 (48–81)	<0.001
Male sex*	2145 (53.8)	2956 (49.9)	<0.001
Infant	213 (5.4)	518 (8.7)	<0.001
Child	329 (8.3)	293 (4.9)	<0.001
Adult	3435 (86.4)	5130 (86.3)	0.89
Type of ward†			
Medicine	1409 (35.3)	2500 (41.9)	<0.001
Surgery	1229 (30.8)	1810 (30.4)	0.62
Intensive care	411 (10.3)	191 (3.2)	<0.001
Neonatal intensive care	131 (3.3)	388 (6.5)	<0.001
Obstetrics/gynecology	49 (1.2)	118 (3.0)	0.004
Hematology/oncology	280 (7.0)	145 (2.4)	<0.001
Solid organ transplant	149 (3.7)	61 (1.0)	<0.001
Trauma/burn	44 (1.1)	48 (0.8)	0.13
Coronary care	41 (1.0)	192 (3.2)	<0.001
Neurosciences/neurosurgery	72 (1.8)	210 (3.5)	<0.001

*Data presented as n (%) unless otherwise indicated. *Data missing from 56 records; †Data missing from 53 records. IQR Interquartile range*

with antimicrobial-resistant pathogens (ie, increasing incidence, association with antimicrobial therapy and primarily affecting hospitalized patients). In the United States, the Centers for Disease Control and Prevention (Georgia) estimates that a minimum of two million infections and 23,000 deaths annually are attributable to AMR, an additional 250,000 illnesses and 14,000 deaths result from CDI, and that most such infections occur in health care settings such as hospitals (2).

Antimicrobial use (AMU) is a major factor driving the occurrence of AMR and CDI. Consequently, antimicrobial stewardship (AS) has recently been established as a new form of clinical quality improvement. It has, as a core part of its mandate, the objective of improving the quality of antimicrobial therapy and, thereby, reducing selection pressures in bacteria favouring the development of AMR (4). AS activity can function at a local, regional/provincial, national or global level.

As in other aspects of public health, surveillance for AMR and AMU provides the information necessary for appropriate action. The Canadian Nosocomial Infection Surveillance Program (CNISP) has performed surveillance for selected antimicrobial-resistant organisms in hospitalized patients since 1994, and has documented the extent and trends over time of MRSA, vancomycin-resistant enterococci, extended-spectrum beta-lactamases, carbapenemase-producing microorganisms and CDI (5-13). In Canada, there are data regarding AMU in ambulatory settings (14-16) but there are little data regarding AMU in Canadian hospitals; this is an important deficiency of information because a considerable proportion of the AMR burden occurs within the hospital sector. In 2002, and again in 2009, CNISP performed one-day prevalence surveys to quantify hospital-acquired infections (HAI) among inpatients in network hospitals on that day (17,18). As part of these surveys, data were also collected on AMU in hospitalized patients. These data represent an important snapshot of information on AMU in hospitals in Canada that may reveal important evolving trends and inform national approaches to AS.

METHODS

Surveillance network
CNISP, a network of 54 acute care hospitals from 10 provinces, is a partnership between the Public Health Agency of Canada (PHAC) and the Canadian Hospital Epidemiology Committee, a group of hospital-based

physician infection prevention specialists. All CNISP hospitals have a university affiliation and provide primary, secondary and tertiary care to adult and/or pediatric patients. Seven hospitals were stand-alone pediatric centres. Surveillance for HAI and AMU in participating hospitals is considered to be within the mandate of hospital infection prevention and control programs and, therefore, does not constitute human research. In most participating hospitals, this surveillance activity does not require institutional review board review.

AMU point prevalence
A point-prevalence survey of all adult and pediatric inpatients was conducted in CNISP hospitals in February 2002 and February 2009, excluding patients on psychiatric units or long-stay units associated with acute care hospitals. Data pertaining to one 24 h period were collected, entered manually into patient data-extraction forms and forwarded to PHAC for data entry and analysis. A unique identifier linked to the patient name was used only to identify patients at the participating hospital and was not transmitted to PHAC. Data elements collected included demographic information, age and sex, information on HAIs, microorganisms isolated, antimicrobials prescribed and use of additional (transmission-based) precautions. Systemic (intravenous or oral) antimicrobial agents in use on the survey day to treat or prevent bacterial, mycobacterial or fungal infections were identified by chart review and classified according to antimicrobial drug class.

Data analysis
The CNISP hospitals were grouped according to region: western (British Columbia, Alberta, Saskatchewan and Manitoba); central (Ontario and Quebec); and eastern (Newfoundland and Labrador, New Brunswick, Prince Edward Island and Nova Scotia).

Each reported antimicrobial agent was grouped into its antimicrobial class using the Anatomical Therapeutic Chemical coding (http://www.whocc.no/atc_ddd_index/). To assess differences among patient populations, continuous variables were expressed using means and medians, and were compared using Student's t tests and Wilcoxon rank-sum tests as appropriate. All tests were two-tailed, and P values of 0.05 were considered to be statistically significant. All analyses were performed using SAS version 9.2 (SAS Inc, USA).

RESULTS
In 2002, 6747 patients in 28 CNISP hospitals were surveyed; 2460 patients (36.5%) were receiving antimicrobial therapy. In 2009, 9953 patients in 44 hospitals were surveyed and 3989 (40.1%; P<0.001) were receiving therapy. According to region, antimicrobial prevalence significantly increased in central Canada (from 37.4% to 40.8%; P<0.01) and in western Canada (from 36.9% to 41.1%; P<0.001), but not in eastern Canada (32.9% to 34.1%; P=0.53). Table 1 describes the characteristics of surveyed patients in 2009, comparing those receiving antimicrobial therapy with those who were not receiving therapy. According to ward type, in 2009, antimicrobial therapy prevalence was highest on solid organ transplant wards (71.0%), hematology/oncology wards (65.9%, an increase from 53.6% in 2002; P<0.001) and intensive care units (68.3%). The prevalence of antimicrobial therapy was lowest on coronary care units (17.6%) and neonatal intensive care units (25.2%). From 2002 to 2009, prevalence increased significantly on surgery wards (34.6% to 40.4%) (Table 2). Table 3 compares the antimicrobial agents in use in 2002 with those in use in 2009 as a proportion of all agents used. Of the agents within the penicillin class, the proportion accounted for by piperacillin-tazobactam increased from 20% in 2002 to 42.8% in 2009 (P<0.001). Figure 1 shows the proportion of patients receiving >1 antimicrobial agent, which significantly increased between 2002 (12.0%) and 2009 (37.7%) (P<0.001). In 2009, among individuals on >1 agent (n=1505), there were 103 cases (7%) in which ≥2 of the same class of antimicrobial agent were in use.

TABLE 2
Antimicrobial prevalence in 2002 and 2009 according to hospital ward type

Ward type	2002	2009	P
Medicine/pediatric medicine	1010 (34.7)	1409 (36.0)	0.044
Surgery	781 (34.6)	1229 (40.4)	<0.001
Intensive care	233 (65.6)	411 (68.3)	0.44
Neonatal intensive care	87 (24.3)	131 (25.2)	0.75
Obstetrics/gynecology	28 (22.8)	49 (29.3)	0.21
Hematology/oncology	158 (53.6)	280 (65.9)	<0.001
Solid organ transplant	71 (68.3)	149 (71.0)	0.62
Trauma/burn	39 (37.5)	44 (47.8)	0.14
Coronary care	50 (29.6)	41 (17.6)	0.53
Other	1 (10.0)	153 (36.3)	0.15
Neurosciences/neurosurgery		72 (25.5)	n/a

Data presented as n (%) unless otherwise indicated

TABLE 3
Comparison of antimicrobial class use in Canadian Nosocomial Infection Surveillance Program hospitals: 2002 and 2009

Antimicrobial class	2002 (2864 patients)	2009 (6048 patients)	P
Penicillins	441 (15.4)	1023 (16.9)	0.07
Cephalosporins			
First generation	347 (12.01)	556 (9.2)	<0.001
Second generation	84 (2.9)	96 (1.6)	<0.001
Third generation	252 (8.8)	446 (7.4)	0.02
Carbapenems	73 (2.6)	238 (3.9)	<0.001
Fluoroquinolones	519 (18.1)	1055 (17.4)	0.43
Aminoglycosides	106 (3.7)	214 (3.5)	0.69
Macrolides	60 (2.1)	144 (2.4)	0.39
Tetracyclines	6 (0.2)	29 (0.5)	0.057
Antifungal agents	124 (4.3)	350 (5.8)	0.004
Antituberculous agents	52 (1.8)	102 (1.7)	0.66
Clindamycin	48 (1.7)	127 (2.1)	0.18
Metronidazole	256 (8.9)	530 (8.8)	0.79
Nitrofurantoin	7 (0.2)	46 (0.8)	0.003
Trimethoprim/ sulfamethoxazole	37 (1.3)	312 (5.2)	<0.001
Vancomycin	123 (4.3)	549 (9.1)	<0.001

Data presented as n (%) unless otherwise indicated

DISCUSSION

Sequential national prevalence surveys have been widely used to assess secular trends in the occurrence of health care-acquired infections and AMU worldwide as a cost-effective approach to obtaining national data to assist in determining priorities for action (19-23). The prevalence data included in the present report represent a useful assessment of AMU in CNISP hospitals at two points in time separated by seven years, from which evolving trends may be recognized. The data suggest that AMU is very high in hospitalized Canadians, and is increasing over time. This rising prevalence in inpatients in CNISP hospitals is in contrast to AMU in ambulatory settings, for which decreased use has been documented over a similar time period (24). These Canadian trends imply that greater national efforts are needed to examine and address the appropriateness of AMU within hospitals in Canada because hospitalized patients are exposed to high-intensity AMU, and antimicrobial-resistant pathogens often arise in hospitals due to antibiotic exposure or are transmitted within hospitals and subsequently selected by antimicrobial exposure.

Within the group of patients receiving antimicrobial therapy, important trends may be developing. Patients surveyed in 2009 were significantly more likely to receive broad-spectrum antimicrobial agents than they were in 2002. Pipercillin-tazobactam, as a proportion of all penicillins, more than doubled in use. Use of carbapenems (imipenem, meropenem, ertapenem), often considered to be the last line of defense against invasive Gram-negative bacteria, remained low in 2009 (3.9% of all agents), but had increased from 2.6% in 2002. In contrast, use of narrower-spectrum agents such as first- and second-generation cephalosporins declined significantly. Furthermore, there was a marked increase in the prevalence of patients simultaneously receiving multiple antimicrobial agents.

Our data are silent regarding the appropriateness of AMU in CNISP hospitals. Having documented the spread of antimicrobial-resistant pathogens in CNISP hospitals, it is possible that increased AMU and increases in use of multiple agents simultaneously is, in part, a consequence as much as a cause of increasing AMR. The twofold increased use of vancomycin between the two surveys is likely a response to an increased prevalence of MRSA and CDI (6,8). In addition, increased use of broad-spectrum agents and antifungal therapy could reflect increasing acuity and complexity of hospital patients. Nevertheless, the data are concerning and point to a need for a better understanding of AMU in Canadian hospitals. More up-to-date information regarding AMU in CNISP hospitals would be an important first step. In addition, there is a need for information on the appropriateness of AMU in hospital clinical practice. Finally, research is required that provides a better understanding of factors driving the AMU trends we have observed, including assessment of forces that influence prescribing in hospitalized patients

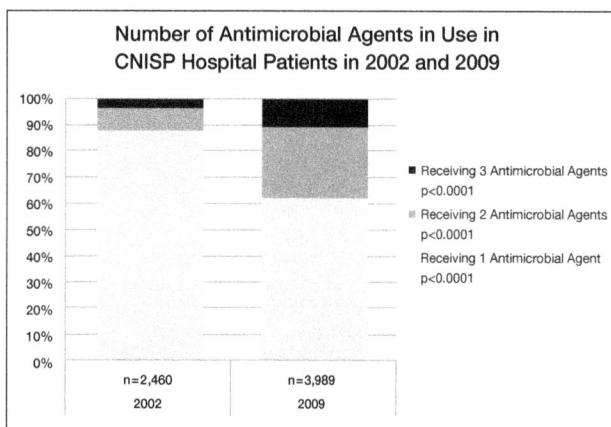

Figure 1) *Number of antimicrobial agents in use in Canadian Nosocomial Infection Surveillance Program (CNISP) hospital patients in 2002 and 2009*

in Canada. This information could then be used to develop appropriate national hospital AS strategies.

Prevalence surveys in other countries have assessed AMU. Our 2009 prevalence (40.1%) appears to be higher than a survey of 172 European hospitals conducted in 2009, which found a prevalence of 29.0% (21), and 32.4% found in three Australian hospitals surveyed in 2012 (22). A report from a 2007 survey in Scotland (25) showed an overall prevalence of AMU at 32.1% of 11,608 patients in acute care hospitals, with 12.6% overall receiving >1 agent. However, direct comparison of prevalence of AMU among countries – and even among hospitals – is hampered by the need to account for differences in survey methods, patient mix, acuity and local microbial ecology. Risk adjustment of AMU is an emerging field, and methods are being developed based on the types of hospital services provided, indexes of patient severity or combinations of both (26).

Our study was subject to limitations. The data reflect only two days of AMU in the same season separated by seven years. Pediatric hospitals were not included in our survey. While large numbers of patients were surveyed, it is possible that the data over- or underestimate true AMU rates in Canadian hospitals. No data are available to fully characterize the trend between 2002 and 2009 – ie, whether a slow persistent increase or a sudden shift in utilization occurred. Similarly, we cannot comment on whether the change in AMU between 2002 and 2009 has continued. CNISP hospitals are primarily large tertiary care teaching institutions; these data may be expected to overestimate prevalence of AMU. While our data reflect some of the only publically available information on AMU in Canadian hospitals, their shortcomings prevent full description of AMU trends in the hospital sector. Ideally, AMU data from a range of Canadian hospitals should be evaluated. As reviewed by Grant et al (27), there are significant gaps in AMR surveillance (particulary in the community sector) in Canada. Only a limited range of target pathogens have been surveyed in subsets of the Canadian hospital sector – primarily performed by our group. AMU surveillance is generally absent and that which occurs is not integrated with AMR surveillance, beyond that occurring within CNISP. Grant et al (26) recommend a range of initiatives, starting with establishment of a coordinated national cross-sectoral AMR and AMU surveillance system. We agree that better data on AMU within the hospital sector are needed.

SUMMARY

Between 2002 and 2009, overall AMU prevalence in major Canadian hospitals significantly increased, and there were substantial shifts in type of agents used. These data can serve as a baseline for future prevalence studies and research into factors influencing the trends we observed.

ACKNOWLEDGEMENT: Members of the CNISP who participated in the Point Prevalence Survey for Healthcare-Acquired Infections: Dr Elizabeth Bryce, Vancouver General Hospital, Vancouver, British Columbia; Dr Gordon Dow, The Moncton Hospital, Moncton, New Brunswick; Dr John Embil, Health Sciences Centre, Winnipeg, Manitoba; Dr Joanne Embree, Health Sciences Centre, Winnipeg, Manitoba; Dr Michael Gardam, University Health Network, Toronto, Ontario; Denise Gravel, Centre for Infectious Disease Prevention and Control, Public Health Agency of Canada; Dr Elizabeth Henderson, Peter Lougheed Centre, Calgary, Alberta; Dr James Hutchinson, Health Sciences Centre, St John's, Newfoundland; Dr Michael John, London Health Sciences Centre, London, Ontario; Dr Lynn Johnston, Queen Elizabeth II Health Sciences Centre, Halifax, Nove Scotia; Dr Pamela Kibsey, Victoria General Hospital, Victoria, British Columbia; Dr Joanne Langley, IWK Health Science Centre, Halifax, NS; Dr Mark Loeb, Hamilton Health Sciences Corporation and St Joseph's Healthcare, Hamilton, Ontario; Dr Anne Matlow, Hospital for Sick Children, Toronto, Ontario; Dr Allison McGeer, Mount Sinai Hospital, Toronto, Ontario; Dr Sophie Michaud, CHUS-Hôpital Fleurimont, Sherbrooke, Quebec; Dr Mark Miller, SMBD–Jewish General Hospital, Montreal, Quebec; Dr Dorothy Moore, Montreal Children's Hospital, Montreal, Quebec; Dr Michael Mulvey, National Microbiology Laboratory, Public Health Agency of Canada; Marianna Ofner, Centre for Infectious Disease Prevention and Control, Public Health Agency of Canada; Ms Shirley Paton, Centre for Infectious Disease Prevention and Control, Public Health Agency of Canada; Dr Virginia Roth, The Ottawa Hospital, Ottawa, Ontario; Jacob Stegenga, Centre for Infectious Disease Prevention and Control, Public Health Agency of Canada; Dr Geoffrey Taylor, University of Alberta Hospital, Edmonton, Alberta; Dr Karl Weiss, Maisonneuve-Rosemont Hospital, Montreal, Quebec; Dr Alice Wong, Royal University Hospital, Saskatoon, Saskatchewan; Dr Dick Zoutman, Kingston General Hospital, Kingston, Ontario.

REFERENCES

1. Public Health Agency of Canada. The chief public health officer's report on the state of public health in Canada, 2013. Infectious Disease the never-ending threat. <http://publichealth.gc.ca/CPHOReport> (Accessed July 2014).
2. Centers for Disease Control and Prevention. Antibiotic resistance threats in the United States, 2013. <www.cdc.gov/drugresistance/threat-report-2013/index.html> (Accessed July 2014).
3. World Health Organization. Antimicrobial resistance: Global report on surveillance 2014. <http://apps.who.int/iris/bitstream/10665/112642/1/9789241564748_eng.pdf> (Accessed July 2014).
4. Dellit T, Owens R, McGowan J, et al. Infectious Diseases Society of America and the Society for Healthcare Epidemiology of America guidelines for developing an institutional program to enhance antimicrobial stewardship. Clin Infect Dis 2007;44:159-77.
5. Simor AE, Ofner-Agostini M, Bryce E, et al. The evolution of methicillin-resistant Staphylococcus aureus in Canadian hospitals: 5 years of national surveillance. CMAJ 2001;165:21-6.
6. Simor AE, Ofner-Agostini M, Gravel D, et al. Surveillance for methicillin-resistant Staphylococcus aureus in Canadian hospital – A report update from the Canadian Nosocomial Infection Surveillance Program. Canada Communicable Disease Report 2005;31:1-7.
7. Ofner-Agostini M, Johnston L, Simor A, et al. Vancomycin resistant enterococci in Canada: Results from the Canadian Nosocomial Infection Surveillance Program, 1999-2005. Infect Control Hosp Epidemiol 2008;29:271-4.
8. Gravel D, Miller M, Simor A, et al. Health care-associated Clostridium difficile infection in adults admitted to acute care hospitals in Canada: A Canadian Nosocomial Infection Surveillance Program study. Clin Infect Dis 2009;48:568-76.
9. Ofner-Agostini M, Simor A, Mulvey M, et al. Risk factors for and outcomes associated with clinical isolates for Escherichia coli and Klebsiella species resistant to extended-spectrum cephalosporins among patients admitted to Canadian hospitals. Can J Infect Dis Med Microbiol 2009;20:e43-e48.
10. Miller M, Gravel D, Mulvey M, et al. Health care associated Clostridium difficile infection in Canada: Patient age and infecting strain type are highly predictive of severe outcome and mortality. Clin Inf Dis 2010;50:194-201.
11. Mataseje LF, Bryce E, Roscoe D, et al. Carbapenem-resistant Gram-negative bacilli in Canada 2009-10: Results from the Canadian Nosocomial Surveillance Project (CNISP). J Antimicrob Chemother 2012;67:1359-67.
12. McCracken M, Wong A, Mitchell R, et al. Molecular epidemiology of vancomycin-resistant enterococcal bacteraemia: Results from the Canadian Nosocomial Infection Surveillance Program, 1999-2009. J Antimicrob Chemother 2013;68:1505-9.
13. Lynch T, Chong P, Zhang J, et al. Characterization of a stable, metronidazole-resistant Clostridium difficile clinical isolate. PLoS One 2013;8;e53757.
14. Glass-Kaastra SK, Finley R, Hutchinson J, Patrick DM, Weiss K, Conly J. Longitudinal surveillance of outpatient beta-lactam antimicrobial use in Canada, 1995 to 2010. Can J Infect Dis Med Microbiol 2014;25:107-12.
15. Glass-Kaastra SK, Finley R, Hutchinson J, Patrick DM, Weiss K, Conly J. Longitudinal surveillance of outpatient quinolone antimicrobial use in Canada. Can J Infect Dis Med Microbiol 2014;25:99-102.
16. Glass-Kaastra SK, Finley R, Hutchinson J, Patrick DM, Weiss K, Conly J. Variation in outpatient oral antimicrobial use patterns among Canadian provinces, 2000 to 2010. Can J Infect Dis Med Microbiol 2014;25:95-8.
17. Gravel D, Taylor G, Ofner M, et al. Point prevalence survey for health-care associated infections within Canadian adult acute care hospitals. J Hosp Infect 2007;66:243-8.
18. Rutledge-Taylor K, Matlow A, Gravel D, et al. A point prevalence survey of health care-associated infections in Canadian pediatric inpatients. Am J Inf Contr 2012;40:491-6.
19. Xie D, Fu X, Wang H, et al. Annual point-prevalence of healthcare-associated infection surveys in a university hospital in China, 2007-2011. J Infect Public Health 2013;6:416-22.
20. Xie D, Xiang L, Li R, Hu Q, Luo Q, Xiong W. A multicenter point-prevalence survey of antibiotic use in 13 Chinese hospitals. J Infect Public Health 2015;8:55-61.

21. Zarb P, Goossens H. European surveillance of antimicrobial consumption (ESAC). Value of a point-prevalence survey of antimicrobial use across Europe. Drugs 2011;71:745-56.
22. Cotta MO, Robertson MS, Upjohn LM, Marshall C, Liew D, Buising KL. Using periodic point-prevalence surveys to assess appropriateness of antimicrobial prescribing in Australian private hospitals. Intern Med J 2014;44:240-6.
23. Llata E, Gaynes R, Fridkin S. Measuring the scope and magnitude of hospital-associated infection in the United States: The value of prevalence surveys. Clin Infect Dis 2009;48:1434-40.
24. Conly J. Antimicrobial resistance programs in Canada 1995-2010: A critical evaluation. Antimicrob Resist Infect Control 2012;1:10.
25. Reilly J, Stewart S, Allardice G, et al. NHS Scotland national HAI prevalence survey. Final Report 2007, Health Protection Scotland (report). <www.documents.hps.scot.nhs.uk/hai/sshaip/publications/national-prevalence-study/report/full-report.pdf> (Accessed March 20, 2015).
26. Ibrahim O, Polk R. Benchmarking antimicrobial drug use in hospitals. Expert Rev Anti Infect Ther 2012;10:445-57.
27. Grant J, Saxinger L, Patrick D. Surveillance of antimicrobial resistance and antimicrobial utilization in Canada. National Collaborating Centre for Infectious Diseases, June 2014.

8

Blastomycosis in northwestern Ontario, 2004 to 2014

Daniel Dalcin MD(c)[1], Syed Zaki Ahmed MD FRCP(C)[1,2]

D Dalcin, Z Ahmed. Blastomycosis in northwestern Ontario, 2004 to 2014. Can J Infect Dis Med Microbiol 2015;26(5):259-262.

Blastomycosis is an invasive fungal disease caused by *Blastomyces dermatitidis* and the recently discovered *Blastomyces gilchristii*. The medical charts of 64 patients with confirmed cases of blastomycosis in northwestern Ontario during a 10-year period (2004 to 2014) were retrospectively reviewed. The number of patients diagnosed with blastomycosis in Ontario was observed to have increased substantially compared with before 1990, when blastomycosis was removed from the list of reportable diseases. Aboriginals were observed to be disproportionately represented in the patient population. Of the patients whose smoking status was known, 71.4% had a history of smoking. 59.4% of patients had underlying comorbidities and a higher comorbidity rate was observed among Aboriginal patients. The case-fatality rate from direct complications of blastomycosis disease was calculated to be 20.3%; this case-fatality rate is the highest ever to be reported in Canada and more than double that of previously published Canadian studies. The clinical characteristics of 64 patients diagnosed with blastomycosis are summarized.

Key Words: *Aboriginal; Blastomycosis; Case-fatality; Clinical characteristics; Northwestern Ontario; Smoking*

La blastomycose au nord-ouest de l'Ontario de 2004 à 2014

La blastomycose est une maladie fongique invasive causée par la *Blastomyces dermatitidis* et le *Blastomyces gilchristii*, récemment découvert. Les chercheurs ont réalisé une analyse rétrospective des dossiers médicaux des 64 patients atteints d'une blastomycose confirmée au nord-ouest de l'Ontario, déclarés sur une période de dix ans (2004 à 2014). Le nombre de patients ayant un diagnostic de blastomycose en Ontario avait considérablement augmenté par rapport à celui d'avant 1990, lorsque la blastomycose a été retirée de la liste de médicaments à déclaration obligatoire. Le nombre d'Autochtones représenté au sein de la population de patients était disproportionné. Chez les patients dont on connaissait le statut de fumeur, 71,4 % avaient des antécédents de tabagisme, 59,4 % présentaient des comorbidités sous-jacentes, et le taux de comorbidités était plus élevé chez les patients autochtones. Le taux de mortalité causé par les complications directes de la blastomycose s'élevait à 20,3 %. C'est le taux le plus élevé jamais déclaré au Canada, soit plus de deux fois celui signalé auparavant dans les études canadiennes. Les caractéristiques cliniques des 64 patients atteints d'une blastomycose diagnostiquée sont résumées.

The Kenora region of northwestern Ontario has the highest reported incidence of blastomycosis in the world (1). Although several published reports have analyzed the epidemiology of blastomycosis in specific regions and time periods of Ontario, a provincial epidemiological understanding of blastomycosis remains unclear since the removal of blastomycosis from the list of reportable diseases in Ontario in 1990 (2). Despite this caveat, the fragmented epidemiological data available suggest that the number of cases of blastomycosis diagnosed per year in northwestern Ontario is increasing (3,4).

Thunder Bay, Ontario is the largest city in northwestern Ontario and provides health services to a large surrounding rural catchment area that contains a substantial Aboriginal population. The Thunder Bay Regional Health Sciences Centre (TBRHSC) is the only academic hospital in northwestern Ontario and is the treatment centre for patients requiring specialized, acute or complex care, in addition to standard local medical services. The objective of the present study was to analyze blastomycosis disease in patients presenting at the TBRHSC.

METHODS

The medical files of 64 patients with confirmed cases of blastomycosis that presented at the TBRHSC from February 1, 2004 to January 31, 2014, were retrospectively reviewed. Similar to Crampton et al (4), confirmed cases of blastomycosis were defined as patients with a clinically compatible illness that was corroborated by a clinical specimen that grew *Blastomyces* species yeast cells in culture or microscopically visualized by a pathologist. The racial status of patients was defined as either Aboriginal or non-Aboriginal. To determine whether the Aboriginal patients in the present study had a statistically significant increased proportion of comorbidities compared with non-Aboriginal patients, a contingency table was used to test for significance using the χ^2 distribution; statistical significance was determined to be $P<0.05$. The Northwest Community Health Integration Network Population Health Profile was used to obtain demographic data on the catchment population of the TBRHSC (5). The present study was approved by the research ethics boards of all involved institutions.

RESULTS

Age and sex
Of the patients with blastomycosis, 65.6% were male. The mean age of patients diagnosed with blastomycosis was 41.2 years (range 12 to 82 years). Patients 20 to 59 years of age accounted for 75% of the patient total (Table 1).

Timing of clinical presentation
Due to incomplete information from patients transferred to the TBRHSC from other facilities, the month and year of diagnosis was available for only 60 patients. Cases of blastomycosis were diagnosed in all months of the year; however, a slightly higher proportion of patients were diagnosed between October and March (60.0% of patients). The number of cases diagnosed per year ranged from two to 11 cases, with a mean of 6.4 cases per year (Figure 1).

Comorbidities
Comorbidities were present in 59.4% of patients; 73.3% of Aboriginal patients were comorbid, compared with 48.5% of the non-Aboriginal patients, and the difference was statistically significant (Tables 2 and 3).

[1]*Northern Ontario School of Medicine;* [2]*Department of Internal Medicine, Thunder Bay Regional Health Sciences Centre, Thunder Bay, Ontario*
Correspondence: Daniel Dalcin, Northern Ontario School of Medicine, 955 Oliver Road, Thunder Bay, Ontario P7B 5E1.
e-mail ddalcin@nosm.ca

TABLE 1
Age, sex, Aboriginal heritage and case-fatality rate among 64 patients with blastomycosis

| Age, years | Age group total | Patients | | | Death count, n | Case fatality, % |
		Male	Female	Aboriginal		
<20	5 (7.8)	4 (80)	1 (20)	3 (60)	0	0.0
20–29	17 (26.6)	9 (52.9)	8 (47.1)	11 (64.7)	3	17.6
30–39	13 (20.3)	10 (76.9)	3 (23.1)	7 (53.8)	3	23.1
40–49	11 (17.2)	8 (72.7)	3 (27.3)	5 (45.4)	2	18.2
50–59	7 (10.9)	3 (42.9)	4 (57.1)	3 (42.9)	3	42.9
60–69	5 (7.8)	4 (80.0)	1 (20.0)	2 (40.0)	1	20.0
70–79	5 (7.8)	2 (40.0)	3 (60.0)	1 (20.0)	1	20.0
>79	1 (1.6)	1 (100.0)	0 (0.0)	0 (0.0)	0	0.0
Total, n	64	41	23	32	13	20.3

Data presented as n (% of age group) unless otherwise indicated

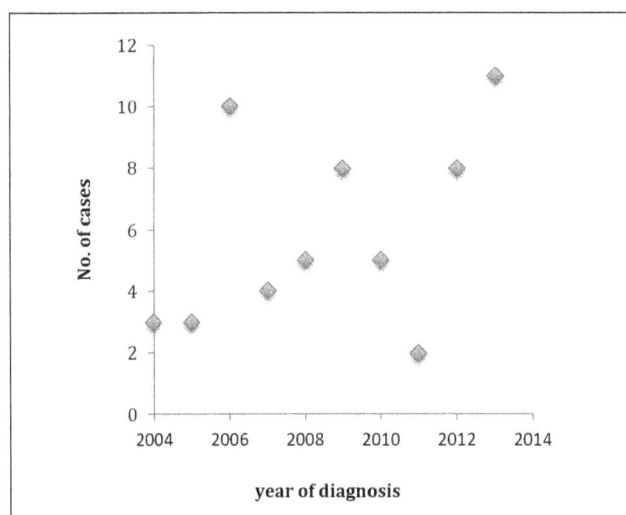

Figure 1) *Number (No) of patients presenting with blastomycosis at the Thunder Bay Regional Health Services Centre (TBRHSC, Thunder Bay, Ontario) according to year of diagnosis from February 1, 2004 to January 31, 2014. The number of cases of blastomycosis diagnosed in Ontario has substantially increased since 1990, when a mean of two cases were diagnosed per year. The mean number of cases diagnosed at the TBRHSC was 6.4 per year*

Aboriginal heritage
Race was specified in 63 (98.4%) of patient medical records. Of the 63 patient medical records that specified Aboriginal status, 30 (47.6%) patients were of Aboriginal heritage.

System involvement
Fifty-five patients (85.9%) had only pulmonary involvement, six patients (9.4%) had central nervous system involvement (three of the six patients with central nervous system involvement also had pulmonary involvement), four patients (6.3%) had skin involvement and one patient (1.6%) had synovial fluid involvement. Two of the 11 patients (18.2%) with extrapulmonary involvement (skin and synovial fluid) were pregnant women.

Smoking status
Smoking status was available for 53 of the 64 patients in the present study. Of these 53 patients, 71.4% had a history of smoking.

Patients who died
Intensive care unit (ICU) care was required for 36 patients. Of these 36 patients, 13 (36.1%) patients died of direct complications of blastomycosis; there were no deaths from patients that did not require ICU care. The overall case-fatality rate observed was 20.3%; this may be the highest case-fatality rate of blastomycosis to be described in Canada.

TABLE 2
Comorbidities of patients diagnosed with blastomycosis according to Aboriginal status

Comorbidity	Patients, n	Aboriginal, n (%)	Non-Aboriginal, n (%)
T1DM	3	2 (66.7)	1 (33.3)
T2DM	14	11 (78.6)	3 (21.4)
Liver failure	1	0 (0)	1 (100)
COPD	4	0 (0)	4 (100)
Renal failure	5	5 (100)	0 (0)
Previous MI	3	1 (33)	2 (66.7)
Tuberculosis	2	1 (50)	1 (50)
Colon cancer	2	0 (0)	2 (100)
Cerebral palsy	2	1 (50)	1 (50)
T2DM and COPD	2	1 (50)	1 (50)
Total	38 (100)	22 (57.9)	16 (42.1)

COPD Chronic obstructive pulmonary disease; MI Myocardial infarction; T1DM Type 1 diabetes mellitus; T2DM Type 2 diabetes mellitus

All patients had a diagnosis of blastomycosis established at the time of death. The age of patients that died ranged from 26 to 73 years (Figure 2). Eleven (84.5%) of the patients that died were between 26 to 55 years of age. Nine (67%) of the patients that died were male.

Smoking status was documented for nine of the 13 patients that died. Eight of the patients that died smoked or had a history of smoking, and one patient identified as a nonsmoker.

Except for one patient, all patients who died had health problems before aquiring blastomycosis. These underlying health problems included: liver failure (n=1), chronic obstructive pulmonary disease (n=2), tuberculosis (n=2), type 1 diabetes mellitus (n=2), type 2 diabetes mellitus (n=1), drug/alcohol abuse (n=1), renal failure (n=1), colorectal cancer (n=1), and both chronic obstructive pulmonary disease and type 2 diabetes mellitus (n=1).

DISCUSSION
Seasonal variation in clinical presentation
Consistent with other reports (1,3,6), 60% of patients were diagnosed between October and March. It has been suggested that the increase in patients diagnosed during the fall and winter months is due to acquisition of *Blastomyces* species conidia during the summer months, followed by a one to six month presymptomatic incubation period (6).

Sex
Similar to the results of other studies (1,4), 65.6% of patients with blastomycosis were male. It is believed that the increase in males affected by blastomycosis is a function of increased environmental exposure (7).

Increased number of cases diagnosed per year post-1990
Based on published epidemiological reports, the number of cases of blastomycosis diagnosed per year in Ontario has increased substantially

TABLE 3
Comparison of comorbid status between Aboriginal and non-Aboriginal patients diagnosed with blastomycosis

Status	Aboriginal	Non-Aboriginal	Total
Comorbid	22	16	38
Non-comorbid	8	17	25
Total	30	33	63

Data presented as n. Of the 64 patients in the present study, race was specified in 63 patients. Of the Aboriginal patients, 73.3% were comorbid, compared with 48.5% of the non-Aboriginal patients, and the difference was statistically significant (Pearson's χ^2=4.054, df=1, P=0.044)

since 1990 (3,8). Leading up to the removal of blastomycosis from the list of reportable diseases in Ontario in 1990, there were only 16 cases of blastomycosis reported in Ontario between 1981 and 1989 (mean of two cases per year) (2,3).

Sixty-four cases of blastomycosis were diagnosed at the TBRHSC during the 10-year period between 2004 and 2014 (mean of 6.4 cases per year), which far exceeds the number of cases diagnosed per year before 1990. This increase in blastomycosis diagnosis is not proportional to the population growth of Ontario. Ontario's population has grown approximately 37% from 1990 to 2014, from an estimated 10 million in 1990 to 13.7 million in 2014 (9). Moreover, the present study only involved patients with blastomycosis presenting to the TBRHSC, suggesting that the actual mean of blastomycosis diagnoses in Ontario is >6.4 cases per year. An epidemiological analysis of blastomycosis in Ontario (1994 to 2003) found 309 cases of blastomycosis were reported in Ontario over a 10-year period (mean of 30.9 cases per year) (3). The same study noted that the number of blastomycosis cases reported per year demonstrated a trend of increasing annual incidence (3).

While Ontario removed blastomycosis from the list of reportable diseases in 1990, Illinois (USA) instated blastomycosis as a mandatory reportable disease in 1994 due to an increased number of diagnosed cases (8). Our results indicate that the number of cases of blastomycosis diagnosed per year has increased substantially since 1990, from a mean of two cases per year in Ontario to a mean of 6.4 cases per year in northwestern Ontario (Figure 1) (3,8).

The reasons for the increase in blastomycosis diagnoses are unclear and require further study. Some possible factors contributing to the increase in blastomycosis diagnoses include increased awareness by clinicians, which may have resulted in a substantial increase in testing rates, or expanding ecological niche of *Blastomyces*. Looking to the future, climate change is projected to create favourable ecological conditions for *Blastomyces* species. The projected drier summers and increased winter precipitation associated with climate change in North America is expected to create optimal conditions for *Blastomyces* species spore dispersal, suggesting that blastomycosis infection may become more prevalent than currently observed (10).

It is clear that the number of blastomycosis diagnoses per year in Ontario has increased considerably compared with the number of cases diagnosed per year before 1990. Given this increase, the possible increase in *Blastomyces* species prevalence associated with climate change, and a significantly high case-fatality rate, it is reasonable to consider reinstating blastomycosis to the list of reportable diseases in Ontario. We, along with other authors, advocate for the reinstatement of blastomycosis to the list of reportable diseases in Ontario (3).

High case fatality
In the present study, 20.3% of patients died from direct complications of blastomycosis, which far exceed the case-fatality rate of the two other Canadian studies that had case-fatality rates of 6.3% and 8%, respectively (4,11). There are several reasons that may account for the high case-fatality rate observed including our patient population and the virulence of *B gilchristii* and *B dermatitidis*.

Because our study evaluated patients at the TBRHSC (a 395-bed hospital) and the other two Canadian studies evaluated patients diagnosed with blastomycosis in hospitals with >150 to 200 beds, our patient

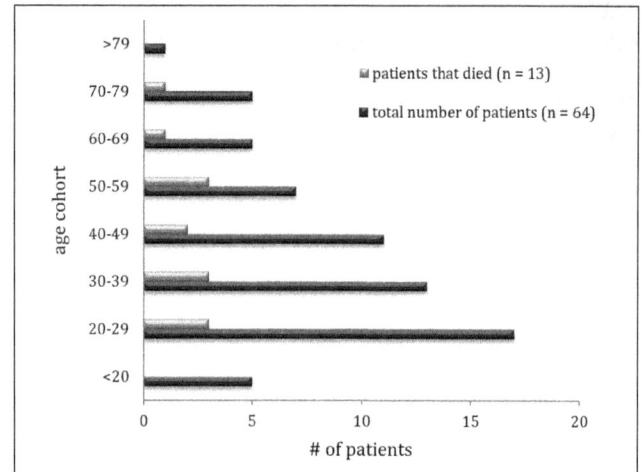

Figure 2) *Age distribution of all patients diagnosed with blastomycosis versus patients diagnosed with blastomycosis who died. Most of the 13 patients who died directly from blastomycosis-related complications at the Thunder Bay Regional Health Services Centre (Thunder Bay, Ontario) were middle-aged. There were no deaths of patients <20 or >79 years of age*

population is selected to be more critically ill and/or comorbid, which would contribute to the higher case-fatality rate observed (4,11). For example, 56.3% of our patients required care in the ICU, compared with the study conducted by Kralt et al (11) where only 10% of patients required ICU care. Although the study conducted by Crampton et al (4) does not discuss what proportion of patients required ICU care, it is clear that our patient population was more seriously ill; 100% of our patients were symptomatic whereas only 91.9% of their patient population was symptomatic. Although the case-fatality rates of these two other studies were also subject to elevation from the underdiagnosis of mild subclinical cases because their analysis only focused on hospitals with >150 to 200 beds, it is clear that our high-case fatality rate is a function of our critically ill patient population.

An additional factor that may have contributed to the high case-fatality rate observed is differences in ecology and virulence among *B dermatitidis* and *B gilchristii* (12). Brown et al (12) analyzed the geographical distribution of *B dermatitidis* versus *B gilchristii* and found that *B gilchristii* clinical isolates were predominantly located in areas where blastomycosis is hyperendemic, such as northwestern Ontario, whereas *B dermatitidis* clinical isolates were broadly distributed across North America. This difference in ecological distribution may be substantiated by differences in virulence between these two fungal species. A preliminary study that compared isolates of *B gilchristii* and *B dermatitidis* found *B gilchristii* to be highly virulent, causing an infection and immunocompetent mice and humans, whereas *B dermatitidis* was described as less virulent and unable to cause illness or death in mice (12). These findings, in the context of our results, provide a framework for further research. Additional analysis is required to determine whether the increased frequency in diagnosis of blastomycosis and associated high case-fatality rate in northwestern Ontario is attributable to the emergence as *B gilchristii* as a more virulent species (12).

Smoking
Of the patients whose smoking status was documented, 71.4% had a history of smoking. Given that 23.2% of the population of Thunder Bay are current or previous smokers and 23.9% of the population of the northwest Local Health Integration Network has a history of smoking, this clearly indicates that smokers are disproportionately affected by blastomycosis (5,13).

The typical course of blastomycosis infection begins with the inhalation of airborne *Blastomyces* species conidia. Under normal physiological conditions, these inhaled conidia are rapidly phagocytized by alveolar macrophages, neutrophils or monocytes (14). However, if phagocytosis is incomplete, the remaining conidia have the potential to transform into a pathogenic yeast form within 24 h to 72 h of inhalation via a temperature-dependent morphological transition. This yeast form of *Blastomyces* species permits infection to persist because the yeast cell is too large to be phagocytized by polymorphonuclear cells (15). Smoking may increase the risk of contracting blastomycosis through several mechanisms that damage the immunocompetency of the respiratory tree, including impaired mucociliary clearance and reduced phagocytic ability of alveolar macrophages (16-20).

Aboriginal status

Because Aboriginals account for only 19.2% of the population of the northwestern Ontario and 47.6% of patients with blastomycosis were identified as Aboriginal, our results indicate that Aboriginals are disproportionately affected by blastomycosis (Table 1) (5). One factor that likely contributed to this observed disparity is comorbidity status. We found that the Aboriginal patients diagnosed with blastomycosis were statistically more likely to be comorbid compared with the non-Aboriginal patients who were diagnosed with blastomycosis (Tables 2 and 3).

In Canada, the smoking rate among Aboriginals is approximately twice as high than that of non-Aboriginals (20). Given this risk factor, it is not surprising that Canadian Aboriginals are disproportionately affected by respiratory disease (21). Although our study did not have statistical power to evaluate this possibility, it is likely that the higher smoking rate among Aboriginals contributed to this disparity.

Limitations

Our study had a small sample size (n=64). Due to the infrequency of disease, it is challenging to obtain a large sample size sufficient to conduct a more robust analysis.

The referral pattern of patients diagnosed with blastomycosis in the Kenora region of northwestern Ontario adds an element of complexity to interpreting our results. Depending on weather, health care resources and patient conditions, patients with blastomycosis in the Kenora area may be transferred to the TBRHSC in Ontario or a hospital in Manitoba.

Our study only examined patients diagnosed, referred or transferred to the TBRHSC. Therefore, mild or subclinical cases of blastomycosis in northwestern Ontario were excluded from the present analysis.

CONCLUSION

Blastomycosis has a wide spectrum of clinical presentation, ranging from subclinical infection to acute respiratory distress syndrome. Nonspecific symptoms, a long incubation period, the lack of a detectable biomarker with high specificity and infrequency of disease contribute to the high rates of late or missed diagnoses (22). Awareness of blastomycosis by clinicians practicing in endemic areas has the potential to reduce the high rate of morbidity and mortality associated with this fungal disease. The present study was the first to evaluate the breadth of blastomycosis disease in the Thunder Bay District of northwestern Ontario. To that end, our results provide valuable clinical information, a framework for further research, and a basis for re-examining the validity of the removal of blastomycosis from the list of reportable diseases in Ontario.

ACKNOWLEDGEMENTS: Daniel Dalcin was funded by a Dean's Medical Student Research Award from the Northern Ontario School of Medicine. The authors are grateful for helpful advice from Dr Eli Nix and Bruce Weaver.

REFERENCES

1. Dwight P, Naus M, Sarsfield P, Limerick B. An outbreak of human blastomycosis: The epidemiology of blastomycosis in the Kenora catchment region of Ontario, Canada. Can Commun Dis Rep 2000;26:82-91.
2. Population and Public Health Branch: Summary of Reportable Diseases 1990. Toronto: Communicable Diseases Control, Ontario Ministry of Health; 1991.
3. Morris S, Brophy J, Richardson S, et al. Blastomycosis in Ontario, 1994–2003. Emerg Infect Dis 2006;12:275-9.
4. Crampton T, Light R, Berg G, et al. Epidemiology and clinical spectrum of blastomycosis diagnosed at Manitoba hospitals. Clin Infect Dis 2002;34:1310-6.
5. Northwest Community Health Integration Network Population Health Profile. <www.northwestlhin.on.ca/resources/~/media/sites/nw/uploadedfiles/Home_Page/Report_and_Publications/Population%20Report%202013%20English.pdf> (Accessed August 12, 2014).
6. Light B, Kralt D, Embil J, et al. Seasonal variations in the clinical presentation of pulmonary and extrapulmonary blastomycosis. Med Mycol 2008;46:835-41.
7. Saccente M, Woods G. Clinical and laboratory update on blastomycosis. Clin Microbiol Rev 2010;23:367-81.
8. Dworkin M, Duckro, Proia N, Semel J, Huhn G. The epidemiology of blastomycosis in Illinois and factors associated with death. Clin Infect Dis 2005;41:107-11.
9. Statistics Canada. Population by year, by province and territory (Number). <www.statcan.gc.ca/tables-tableaux/sum-som/l01/cst01/demo02a-eng.htm> (Accessed on September 15, 2014).
10. Greer A, Ng V, Fisman D. Climate change and infectious diseases in North America: the road ahead. CMAJ 2008;178:715-22.
11. Kralt D, Light B, Cheang M, et al. Clinical characteristics and outcomes in patients with pulmonary blastomycosis. Mycopathologia 2009;167:115-24.
12. Brown E, McTaggart L, Zhang S, et al. Phylogenetic analysis reveals a cryptic species of *Blastomyces gilchristii*, sp. nov. within the human pathogenic fungus *Blastomyces dermatitidis*. PLoS ONE 8:1-13.
13. Statistics Canada 2013 Community Profiles–Health Region. Updated 2008. <www12.statcan.ca/english/census06> (Accessed September 9, 2014).
14. Drutz D, Frey C. Intracellular and extracellular defenses of human phagocytes against *Blastomyces dermatitidis* and yeasts. J Lab Clin Med 1985;105:737-50.
15. Klein B. Immunology of blastomycosis. In: Greenough III, ed. Current Topics in Infectious Diseases. New York: Plenum Publishing Corporation, 1992;133-63.
16. Wanner A, Slathe M, O'Riordan T. Mucociliary clearance in the airways. Am J Resp Crit Care Med 1996;154:1868-1902.
17. Hodge S, Hodge G, Ahern J, Jersmann H, Holmes M, Reynolds P. Smoking alters alveolar macrophage recognition and phagocytic ability: Implications in chronic obstructive pulmonary disease. Am J Respir Mol Biol 2007;37:748-55.
18. Green G, Carolin D. The depressant effect of cigarette smoke on the in vitro antibacterial activity of alveolar macrophages. N Engl J Med 1967;276:421-7.
19. Sethi S, Murphy T. Infection in the pathogenesis and course of chronic obstructive pulmonary disease. N Engl J Med 2008;359:2355-65.
20. Physicians for a Smoke-Free Canada (2013). Factsheets: Smoking among Aboriginal Canadians. <www.smoke-free.ca/factsheets/pdf/cchs/Aboriginal.pdf> (Accessed April 24, 2015).
21. Ospina M, Voaklander D, Senthilselvan A, et al. Incidence and prevalence of chronic obstructive disease among Aboriginal peoples in Alberta, Canada. PLoS One 2015;10:1-13.
22. Chapman W, Dismukes W, Proia, L, et al. Clinical practice guidelines for the management of blastomycosis: 2008 update by the Infectious Diseases Society of America. Clin Infect Dis 2008;46:1801-12.

9

Sepsis due to *Erysipelothrix rhusiopathiae* in a patient with chronic lymphocytic leukemia associated with bronchopneumonia due to *Pseudomonas aeruginosa* and *Escherichia coli*: A case report

Victoria Bîrlutiu MD PhD

V Bîrlutiu. Sepsis due to *Erysipelothrix rhusiopathiae* in a patient with chronic lymphocytic leukemia associated with bronchopneumonia due to *Pseudomonas aeruginosa* and *Escherichia coli*: A case report. Can J Infect Dis Med Microbiol 2015;26(2):108-110.

INTRODUCTION: The present report describes a case of sepsis due to *Erysipelothrix rhusiopathiae* in a patient with B-cell chronic lymphocytic leukemia with no animal exposure, associated with concomitant bronchopneumonia due to *Pseudomonas aeruginosa* and *Escherichia coli*.
CASE PRESENTATION: A 54-year-old Caucasian man presented to an emergency room with a three-day history of chest pain, fever, cough with purulent sputum, chills and dyspnea. The patient had associated erythematous papules on the chest and enlarged axillary, submandibular, pectoral and supraclavicular lymph nodes, which regressed under treatment with penicillin. The patient was found to have sepsis without endocarditis caused by *E rhusiopathiae*, associated with bronchopneumonia that was induced by a double Gram-negative infection.
CONCLUSIONS: The underlying-B cell chronic lymphocytic leukemia may have favoured the development of bacteremia due to *E rhusiopathiae*, which occurred subsequent to glossitis in an immunocompromised host being treated with methylprednisolone and cladribine.

Key Words: Erysipelothrix rhusiopathiae; *Immunocompromised host*; *Sepsis*

Un sepsis causé par un *Erysipelothrix rhusiopathiae* chez un patient atteint d'une leucémie lymphoïde chronique associée à une bronchopneumonie attribuable à un *Pseudomonas aeruginosa* et un *Escherichia coli* : un rapport de cas

INTRODUCTION : Le présent rapport décrit un cas de sepsis causé par un *Erysipelothrix rhusiopathiae* chez un patient atteint d'une leucémie lymphoïde chronique à cellules B sans exposition à des animaux, associée à une bronchopneumonie concomitante attribuable à un *Pseudomonas aeruginosa* et un *Escherichia coli*.
PRÉSENTATION DE CAS : Un homme blanc de 54 ans s'est présenté à l'urgence parce que, depuis trois jours, il avait des douleurs à la poitrine, de la fièvre, une toux accompagnée d'expectorations purulentes, des frissons et une dyspnée. Il avait des papules érythémateuses sur la poitrine et une hypertrophie des ganglions lymphatiques axillaires, submandibulaires, pectoraux et supraclaviculaires, qui ont régressé sous traitement à la pénicilline. Il était atteint d'un sepsis sans endocardite causé par un *E rhusiopathiae*, associé à une bronchopneumonie induite par une double infection Gram négatif.
CONCLUSIONS : La leucémie lymphoïde chronique à cellules B sous-jacente peut avoir favorisé l'apparition d'une bactériémie attribuable à un *E rhusiopathiae*, qui s'est déclarée après une glossite chez un hôte immunodéprimé traité à la méthylprednisolone et à la cladribine.

*E*rysipelothrix rhusiopathiae has been recognized as an etiological agent of infection in animals and humans since 1880 (1), affecting mammals, birds and fish. In humans, infections caused by this agent occur occupationally, especially due to exposures in butchers, farmers and veterinarians, but also builders and fishermen.

The infection occurs after direct manipulation of animals or their products. The manifestations of the infection varies in humans from localized skin infections (erysipeloid) (2) to diffuse skin forms and systemic infections and to sepsis or endocarditis (which may appear after oropharyngeal or gastrointestinal colonization in one-third of patients with skin infection) (3,4).

We report a case of sepsis caused by *E rhusiopathiae* resulting from oropharyngeal colonization and associated with bronchopneumonia induced by a double Gram-negative infection (*Escherichia coli* and *Pseudomonas aeruginosa*) in a patient with chronic leukemia, after a recent course of chemotherapy with methylprednisolone and cladribine.

CASE PRESENTATION

A 54-year-old Caucasian man presented to an emergency department with a three-day history of chest pain, fever, cough with purulent sputum, chills and dyspnea.

The patient had been diagnosed five years previously with B cell chronic lymphocytic leukemia, Binet stage B, and had responded neither to treatment with fludarabine, cyclophosphamide and rituximab regimen, nor a cyclophosphamide, doxorubicin, vincristine and prednisolone regimen.

His current treatment regimen consisted of methylprednisolone 1 g/day, five days/month and cladribine 10 mg/day, three days/month. During these chemotherapy regimens, he had experienced several episodes of soft tissue infections, bacterial pneumonia, disseminated herpes simplex infection and hepatitis B virus infection, and was also undergoing treatment with entecavir.

On physical examination, the patient was observed to have a temperature of 39.6°C, erythematous papules on the chest, a heart rate of

"Lucian Blaga" University Sibiu, Faculty of Medicine Sibiu, Infectious Diseases Clinic, Academic Emergency Hospital Sibiu, Romania
Correspondence: Dr Victoria Bîrlutiu, Alba-Iulia Str. No.79 23/8, Sibiu 550052, Romania. e-mail victoriabirlutiu@yahoo.com

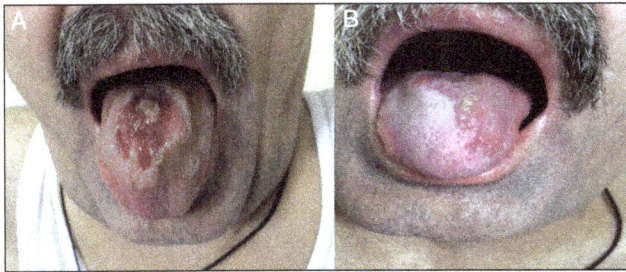

Figure 1) *Ulcerative-necrotic glossitis.* **A** *On admission;* **B** *At discharge*

118 beats/min, blood pressure of 84/50 mmHg, oxygen arterial saturation of 94%, labial herpes, ulcerative-necrotic glossitis (Figure 1) and enlarged axillary, submandibular, pectoral and supraclavicular lymph nodes (Figure 2), with bilateral crackles on chest examination and hepatosplenomegaly. The neurological examination was normal.

Laboratory investigations revealed the following: white blood cell count 3.8×10^9/L (21.6% segmented neutrophils, 54.6% lymphocytes and 19.4% monocytes), hematocrit 35.9%, hemoglobin level 115 g/L, erythrocyte sedimentation rate 82 mm/h, C-reactive protein level 192 mg/L and fibrinogen level 5.44 g/L (15.99 µmol/L). Liver and renal function tests as well as coagulation tests were within normal ranges. Examination of the urine revealed significant pyuria.

An electrocardiogram showed a normal sinus rhythm without conduction abnormalities, and a transesophageal echocardiogram was normal.

Pulmonary radiography showed left perihilar and right infrahilar congestion, and a left pleural effusion. The sputum culture was positive for *P aeruginosa* and *E coli*. The *P aeruginosa* was susceptible to imipenem, meropenem, cefotaxime, ceftazidime, piperacillin, amikacin, netilmicin and fluoroquinolones. The *E coli* was susceptible to amikacin, ceftazidime, gentamicin, imipenem and meropenem. Because the patient had previously developed infections with *P aeruginosa* and *E coli*, empirical treatment with imipenem and gentamicin was initiated. Three days after admission, blood cultures detected the presence of *E rhusiopathiae* (two blood cultures were positive for this bacterium). The laboratory could not test the antibiotic sensitivity of *E rhusiopathiae* in a standardized manner. Therefore, penicillin G 12 million units/day in divided doses was added. During four weeks of treatment with this therapeutic regimen, the patient's symptoms and signs resolved and the patient was discharged in good health. Regression of the enlarged lymph nodes during antibiotic treatment was noted.

DISCUSSION

E rhusiopathiae is a pleomorphic, nonsporulating, nonencapsulated Gram-positive rod-shaped aerobic or facultatively anaerobic organism. *E rhusiopathiae* is recognized as being highly resistant to environmental factors. In the skin, it is capable of producing enzymes, such as hyaluronidase and neuraminidase (5), that facilitate tissue invasion. *E rhusiopathiae* expresses two adhesive surface proteins (6) that bind to collagen types I and IV. In the pathogenesis of infections caused by *E rhusiopathiae*, the following are considered to be important: the neuraminidase, capsule (7) (78.7% of the strains are encapsulated), surface proteins and SpaA antigens (8,9), resistance to phagocytosis and intracellular survival in macrophages.

The role of hyaluronidase in the pathogenesis is controversial because avirulent strains are associated with the loss of the capsule rather than of the hyaluronidase (10). The immunosuppressive conditions in CLL clearly favour the occurrence of *E rhusiopathiae* infections in a suitable host.

The virulence factors cleave the alpha-glycosidic bonds of sialic acid, the mucopolysaccharides present on the surface of mammalian cells, and also play a role in the pathogenesis of arthritis and thrombocytopenia in systemic infection.

CLL is associated with a greater susceptibility to infections due to multiple mechanisms: immunosuppression due to the primary disease,

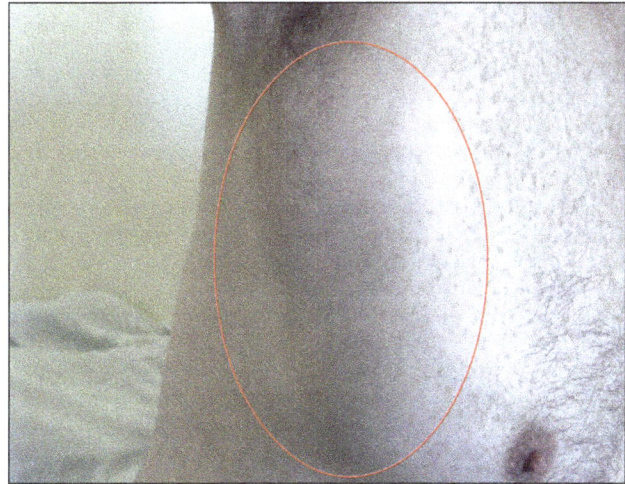

Figure 2) *Axillary lymph nodes*

association with a deficit of cellular-mediated immunity through intrinsic deficiencies or consequent to immunosuppressive therapy (11) (eg, the functional deficit of the T helper cells [12]), an increased activity of T suppressor cells or an inverted CD4/CD8 ratio (13) combined with hypogammaglobulinemia. Deficiency in the complement system also plays an important role in the development of infections due to encapsulated organisms in patients with advanced-stage CLL, along with the decrease in expression of the complement receptors at the level of the B-cell CLL cells (the CR1 and CR2 receptors) and the reduction of the alternative pathway of the complement system (14). The risk for infection in patients with CLL is associated with neutropenia following a progressive bone marrow invasion and immunosuppressive chemotherapy, and also with the decrease in chemotaxis induced by the complement fragment C5a.

In the present case, the patient exhibited relative neutropenia (3.8×10^9/L leukocytes and 21.6% segmented neutrophils), which may have increased the risk for developing a bacterial infection. Facilitating factors associated with the cladribine treatment (15) may have included a decrease in the CD4 level since the beginning of the therapy, which is associated with a greater risk for pneumonia infections and bacterial sepsis (16).

In our case, the patient was undergoing treatment with entecavir due to the reactivation of hepatitis B virus infection, and the last regimen of CLL he was treated with included cladribine and methylprednisolone – all risk factors that favoured the infection. The sputum examination revealed the presence of *P aeruginosa* and *E coli*, sensitive to ciprofloxacin, medication under which the present respiratory manifestations appeared.

E rhusiopathiae infection is described in human pathology as erysipeloid (appearing two to seven days after the skin injury), preceded by local pain or rash, or a purplish plaque at the inoculation site, which is typically very well delimited. Occasionally, there are vesicles with satellite lymphangitis and, rarely, fever, arthralgia or a purpuric rash, appearing as follicular, erythematous papules or a diffuse cutaneous rash with systemic infection – bacteremia and endocarditis (usually aortic valve lesion, sometimes with perivalvular and myocardial abscesses) (17). In immunocompromised hosts, the *E rhusiopathiae* infection may present with bacteremia (18) or endocarditis after oropharyngeal or gastrointestinal tract colonization. *E rhusiopathiae* has been associated with acute leukemia in a child (19) and in neonatal sepsis (20) but has not, to our knowledge, been associated with double Gram-negative infection in B-cell CLL in an adult patient. Some authors have described an association with lupus (21), oropharyngeal cancer (17), perforation of the sigmoid colon (22) and HIV infection. A variety of infections have been reported including acute meningitis (23), chronic meningitis, cerebral abscesses, peritonitis associated with peritoneal dialysis, pleural effusion, septic arthritis (24) and septic shock (25). Recently, a case of pneumonia caused by *E rhusiopathiae* was described in an immunocompetent patient (26). To date, >90 cases of bacteremia have been described, most with endocarditis affecting native valves, especially the aortic valve, with an associated 38% mortality, as compared with 20% for other etiologies. The treatment of choice is penicillin; however, *E rhusiopathiae* is also sensitive to cephalosporins, quinolones, clindamycin, erythromycin and imipenem, but resistant to vancomycin, chloramphenicol, daptomycin and tetracycline. We postulate that our patient acquired *E rhusiopathiae* by ingestion of undercooked fish and became bacteremic, consequent to glossitis occuring in an immunocompromised setting induced by treatment with methylprednisolone and cladribine.

Bacteremia was suspected in the present case because the patient was found to have *P aeruginosa* and *E coli* in the sputum; three days after admission, *E rhusiopathiae* was isolated in blood cultures. The patient had associated erythematous papules on his chest and axillary, supraclavicular and pectoral lymphadenopathy was present, which

regressed under treatment with penicillin. The clinical improvement was not observed after starting the imipenem treatment, but the patient became afebrile with the addition of the penicillin to the treatment regimen. The present case highlights the importance of complete bacteriological identification of isolates in the immunocompromised patient who is at risk for developing multi-etiological infections.

CONSENT: Written informed consent was obtained from the patient for publication of this case report and any accompanying images. The study was accepted by the Ethics Committee of the hospital, which encouraged publication of the article.

ACKNOWLEDGEMENTS: The author expresses special thanks to Alexandru George Bratu for language assistance and Rares-Mircea Birlutiu for drafting the manuscript.

REFERENCES

1. Brooke CJ, Riley T. *Erysipelothrix rhusiopathiae*: Bacteriology, epidemiology and clinical manifestations of an occupational pathogen. J Med Microbiol 1999;48:789-99.
2. Reboli AC, Farrar WE. *Erysipelothrix rhusiopathiae*: An occupational pathogen. Clin Microbiol Rev 1989;2:354-9.
3. Bille J, Racourt J, Swaminathan B. Listeria, erysipelothrix and kurthia. In: Baron E, Ptaller M, Tenover F, Yolken R, Murray P, eds. Manual of Clinical Microbiology. Washington, DC: American Society for Microbiology Press, 1999:346-56.
4. Gorby GL Jr, Peacock JE. *Erysipelothrix rhusiopathiae* endocarditis: Microbiologic, epidemiologic, and clinical features of an occupational disease. Rev Infect Dis 1988;10:317-25.
5. Wang Q, Chang BJ, Mee BJ, Riley TV. Neuraminidase production by *Erysipelothrix rhusiopathiae*. Vet Microbiol 2005;107:265-72.
6. Shimoji Y, Ogawa Y, Osaki M. Adhesive surface proteins of *Erysipelothrix rhusiopathiae* bind to polystyrene, fibronectin, and type I and IV collagens. J Bacteriol 2003;9:2739-48.
7. Lachmann PG, Deicher H. Solubilization and characterization of surface antigenic components of *Erysipelothrix rhusiopathiae* T28. Infect Immun 1986;52:818-22.
8. Galan JE, Timoney JF. Cloning and expression in *Escherichia coli* of a protective antigen of *Erysipelothrix rhusiopathiae*. Infect Immun 1990;58:3116-21.
9. Makino SI, Yamamoto K, Murakami S, et al. Properties of repeat domain found in a novel protective antigen, SpaA, of *Erysipelothrix rhusiopathiae*. Microb Pathog 1998;25:101-9.
10. Tsiodras S, Samonis G, Keating MJ, Kontoyiannis DP. Infection and immunity in chronic lymphocytic leukemia. Mayo Clin Proc 2000;75:1039-54.
11. Chiorazzi N, Fu SM, Montazeri G, Kunkel HG, Rai K, Gee T. T cell helper defect in patients with chronic lymphocytic leukemia. J Immunol 1979;122:1087-90.
12. Platsoucas CD, Galinski M, Kempin S, Reich L, Clarkson B, Good RA. Abnormal T lymphocyte subpopulations in patients with B cell chronic lymphocytic leukemia: An analysis by monoclonal antibodies. J Immunol 1982;129:2305-12.
13. Schlesinger M, Broman I, Lugassy G. The complement system is defective in chronic lymphatic leukemia patients and in their healthy relatives. Leukemia 1996;10:1509-13.
14. Marquart HV, Gronbaek K, Christensen BE, Svehag SE, Leslie RG. Complement activation by malignant B cells from patients with

chronic lymphocytic leukaemia (CLL). Clin Exp Immunol 1995;102:575-81.
15. O'Brien S, Kantarjian H, Estey E, et al. Lack of effect of 2-chlorodeoxyadenosine therapy in patients with chronic lymphocytic leukemia refractory to fludarabine therapy. N Engl J Med 1994;330:319-322.
16. Schlesinger M, Broman I, Lugassy G. The complement system is defective in chronic lymphatic leukemia patients and in their healthy relatives. Leukemia 1996;10:1509-13.
17. Campbell D, Cowan M. Septicemia and aortic valve endocarditis due to *Erysipelothrix rhusiopathiae* in a homeless man. Case Rep Infect Dis 2013;2013:4 pages.
18. Sheng WH1, Hsueh PR, Hung CC, Fang CT, Chang SC, Luh K. Fatal outcome of *Erysipelothrix rhusiopathiae* bacteremia in a patient with oropharyngeal cancer. J Formos Med Assoc 2000;99:431-4.
19. Coman G, Miron I, Pânzaru C, Cârlan M, Petraru E. *Erysipelothrix rhusiopathiae* bacteremia in a child with acute leukemia. Revista medico-chirurgicala a Societatii de Medici si Naturalisti din Iasi 1997;101:218-22.
20. Jones N, Khoosal M. *Erysipelothrix rhusiopathiae* septicemia in a neonate. Clin Infect Dis 1997;24:511.
21. Thomas N, Jesudason M, Mukundan U, John TJ, Seshadri MS, Cherian AM. Infective endocarditis caused by *Erysipelothrix rhusiopathiae* in a patient with systemic lupus erythematosus. J Assoc Physicians India 1996;44:223.
22. Callon RA Jr, Brady PG. Toothpick perforation of the sigmoid colon: An unusual case associated with *Erysipelothrix rhusiopathiae* septicemia. Gastrointest Endosc 1990;36:141-3.
23. Joo EJ, Kang CI, Kim WS, et al. Acute meningitis as an initial manifestation of *Erysipelothrix rhusiopathiae* endocarditis. J Infect Chemother 2011;17:703-5.
24. Vallianatos PG, Tilentzoglou AC, Koutsoukou AD. Septic arthritis caused by *Erysipelothrix rhusiopathiae* infection after arthroscopically assisted anterior cruciate ligament reconstruction. Arthroscopy 2003;19:E26.
25. Ognibene, FP, Cunnion RE, Gill V, Ambrus J, Fauci AS, Parrillo JE. *Erysipelothrix rhusiopathiae* bacteremia presenting as septic shock. Am J Med 1985;78:861-4.
26. Meric M, Ozcan SK. *Erysipelothrix rhusipathiae* pneumonia in an immunocompetent patient. J Med Microbiol 2012;61:450-1.

10

Edwardsiella tarda bacteremia. A rare but fatal water- and foodborne infection: Review of the literature and clinical cases from a single centre

Yuji Hirai MD PhD[1,2], Sayaka Asahata-Tago MD[1], Yusuke Ainoda MD PhD[1],
Takahiro Fujita MD PhD[1], Ken Kikuchi MD PhD[1]

Y Hirai, S Asahata-Tago, Y Ainoda, T Fujita, K Kikuchi.
Edwardsiella tarda bacteremia. A rare but fatal water- and
foodborne infection: Review of the literature and clinical cases
from a single centre. Can J Infect Dis Med Microbiol
2015;26(6):313-318.

BACKGROUND: *Edwardsiella tarda* bacteremia (ETB) can be a fatal
disease in humans.
OBJECTIVES: To determine the significant risk factors associated
with death caused by ETB, and to examine the geographical, seasonal,
environmental and dietary factors of the disease.
METHODS: A retrospective, observational, case control study was
performed. The PubMed MEDLINE and Japanese Medical Abstract
Society (www.jamas.or.jp) databases were searched for ETB case
reports and meeting abstracts. In additon, retrospective chart reviews
of patients with ETB at the Tokyo Women's Medical University
Hospital (Tokyo, Japan) were conducted to evaluate the risk factors
associated with death using multivariate analyses.
RESULTS: The literature search yielded 46 publications, comprising 72
cases from the English (n=30), French (n=1), Spanish (n=1) and
Japanese (n=14) literature. Five cases at the Tokyo Women's Medical
University Hospital were also included. Of the included 77 cases, the
mean age was 61 years and 39% of patients were female; 77.2% of the
cases occurred between June and November, and 45.5% were reported in
Japan. Dietary factors (raw fish/meat exposure) were reported for 10.4% of
patients and 12.9% reported environmental (ie, brackish water) exposure.
The overall mortality rate was 44.6%; however, this rate increased to
61.1% for ETB patients with soft tissue infections. Liver cirrhosis was
determined to be an independent risk factor associated with death (OR
12.0 [95% CI 2.46 to 58.6]; P=0.00213) using multivariate analyses.
DISCUSSION: To our knowledge, the present analysis was the first
and largest multi-language review of ETB. Clinical characteristics of
ETB resemble those of *Aeromonas*, typhoid fever and *Vibrio vulnificus*
infections, in addition to sharing similar risk factors.
CONCLUSION: ETB should be categorized as a severe food- and
waterborne infection, which results in high mortality for patients with
liver cirrhosis.

Key Words: *Bacteremia; Edwardsiella tarda; Foodborne infection; Food
habits; Liver cirrhosis; Risk factors; Waterborne infection*

La bactériémie à *Edwardsiella tarda*. Une infection
d'origine hydrique et alimentaire, mais fatale :
analyse bibliographique et cas cliniques dans un
seul centre

HISTORIQUE : Chez les humains, la bactériémie à *Edwardsiella tarda*
(BET) peut être mortelle.
OBJECTIFS : Déterminer les facteurs de risque importants liés aux
décès causés par la BET et examiner les facteurs géographiques, saison-
niers, environnementaux et diététiques de la maladie.
MÉTHODOLOGIE : Les chercheurs ont effectué une étude cas-
témoins d'observation rétrospective. Ils ont fait des recherches dans les
bases de données MEDLINE de PubMed et de la Société japonaise de
communications médicales (www.jamas.or.jp) pour trouver les comptes
rendus de BET et les communications de cas lors de colloques et con-
grès. Ils ont également procédé à une analyse rétrospective des dossiers
de patients atteints d'une BET à l'hôpital universitaire de Tokyo pour
femmes, au Japon, pour évaluer les facteurs de risque liés aux décès à
l'aide d'analyses multivariées.
RÉSULTATS : L'analyse bibliographique a permis d'extraire 46 publications, soit 72 cas tirés de publications anglophones (n=30), francophones
(n=1), espagnoles (n=1) et japonaises (n=14). Cinq cas de l'hôpital
universitaire de Tokyo pour femmes étaient également inclus. Les 77 cas
avaient un âge moyen de 61 ans, et 39 % étaient de sexe féminin, 77,2 %
s'étaient déclarés entre les mois de juin et novembre et 45,5 % provenaient du Japon. Chez 10,4 % des patients, des facteurs diététiques (poisson cru, exposition à la viande) étaient en cause, tandis que 12,9 %
présentaient une exposition environnementale (eau saumâtre). Le taux
de mortalité globale s'élevait à 44,6 %, mais passait à 61,1 % chez les
patients atteints d'une BET et d'infections des tissus mous. D'après les
analyses multivariées, la cirrhose était un facteur de risque indépendant
de décès (RC 12,0 [95 % IC 2,46 à 58,6]; P=0,00213).
EXPOSÉ : En autant que nous le sachions, il s'agissait de la plus vaste
analyse sur la BET et de la première à être multilingue. Les caractéristiques cliniques de la BET ressemblent à celles des infections à
Aeromonas et à *Vibrio vulnificus* et de la typhoïde en plus de partager
des facteurs de risque similaires.
CONCLUSION : La BET devrait être classée parmi les graves infections d'origine hydrique et alimentaire qui entraînent des taux de
mortalité élevés chez les patients atteints d'une cirrhose.

E dwardsiella tarda is a motile, facultatively anaerobic, Gram-
negative rod that is categorized as a member of the family
Enterobacteriaceae. The genus *Edwardsiella* was first recognized by
Trabulsi et al (1) in 1962, followed by a description of *E tarda* in
the mid-1960s. These organisms have successively been named the
"Bartholomew group" by King and Adler (2), the "Asakusa group" by
Sakazaki (3) and "*Edwardsiella*" by Ewing et al (4).

E tarda is typically isolated from fresh or brackish water environ-
ments such as river mouths. It has also been isolated from the intestines
of humans (after eating fresh water food sources such as catfish [5] or
eels [6]) and from animals, including reptiles and freshwater fish.

E tarda rarely causes infections in humans. The colonization rate in
humans ranges from 0.0073% in the Japanese (7) to 1% in Panamanians
(8). Approximately 80% of *E tarda* infections in humans are characterized

---

[1]*Department of Infectious Diseases, Tokyo Women's Medical University;* [2]*Department of General Medicine, Faculty of Medicine, Juntendo
University, Toyko, Japan*
*Correspondence: Dr Yuji Hirai, Department of Infectious Diseases, Tokyo Women's Medical University, 8-1 Kawada-cho, Shinjuku,
Tokyo 162-8666, Japan.e-mail: hirai.yuji@twmu.ac.jp*

TABLE 1

Clinical characteristics of 77 patients with *Edwardsiella tarda* bacteremia (ETB)

	Overall n (%)	Survived, n	Died, n	Univariate analysis P	Multivariate analysis OR (95% CI)	P
Cases, n	77	44	33			
Age, years, mean (range) OR mean ± SD	61 (2 days – 101 years)	54.02±26.2	55.9±24.4	0.75		
>65 years of age	31 (40.3)	17	14	0.818		
<1 year of age	6 (7.8)	3	3	1		
Female sex	30 (39.0)	20	10	0.166		
Underlying diseases						
Cancer	29 (37.7)	13	16	1		
Hepatobiliary cancer	17 (22.1)	6	11	0.0531	3.2 (0.76 – 13.4)	0.111
Gastric/colon cancer	5 (6.5)	3	2	1		
Noncancer						
Liver cirrhosis	13 (16.9)	2	11	0.000567	12.0 (2.46 – 58.6)	0.00213
Galbladder stone, chorecystitis	21 (27.3)	16	5	0.0434	0.351 (0.104 – 1.19)	0.093
Diabetes	7 (9.1)	2	5	0.131		
Complication of ETB						
Meningitis	4 (5.2)	1	3	0.308		
Liver abscesss	10 (13.0)	7	3	0.502		
Diarrhea	19 (24.7)	13	6	0.295		
Soft tissue infection	18 (23.4)	7	11	0.103		
Intrauterine infection	3 (3.9)	3	0	0.3498		
No complication	35 (45.5)	21	14	0.817		
Antimicrobial agents						
Penicillins	19 (24.7)	12	7	0.398		
Cepharosporins	26 (33.8)	15	11	0.781		
Carbapebens	8 (10.4)	4	4	1		
Others (eg, aminoglycosides)	16 (20.8)	10	6	0.104		
Behavior/dietary risk factors						
Alcoholism	5 (6.5)	3	2	1		
Exposure						
To raw food	8 (10.4)	6	2	0.454		
To fresh or marine water, animal feces	10 (13.0)	6	4	1		
Geographical area						
Japan	35 (45.5)	19	16	0.653		
United States (US)	12 (15.6)	9	3	0.216		
States around the Gulf of Mexico	5 (6.5)	4	1	1		
Republic of China (Taiwan)	10 (13.0)	6	4	1		
Other region (Not Japan, US, Taiwan)	19 (24.7)	9	10	0.104		
Season of onset (northern hemisphere)						
Summer (June to November)	18 (23.4)	13	5	0.117		
Period of time from onset to patient dying	20 h – 61 days (median 8 days)					

as gastroenteritis and *E tarda* is primarily isolated from stool samples. Extraintestinal infections, such as endocarditis, empyema, hepatobiliary infections, peritonitis, intra-abdominal abscesses, osteomyelitis, wound infections and meningitis, have been reported less frequently. While *E tarda* bacteremia (ETB) occurs relatively rarely (<5%), it can be fatal in humans (9). However, little is known about the clinical epidemiology of ETB. Therefore, we aimed to document the clinical epidemiology of ETB, including independent risk factors associated with death, the geographical and seasonal distributions, as well as environmental and dietary risks, based on previous reports and recent clinical cases of ETB at our institution (Tokyo Women's Medical Univeristy [TWMU] Hospital [Tokyo, Japan]).

METHODS

A retrospective, observational, case control study was performed. The present analysis comprised literature and retrospective chart reviews. A search was conducted for case reports and case series involving ETB, published between January 1968 and December 2013, with

the PubMed MEDLINE and Japanese Medical Abstracts Society ICHUSHI (www.jamas.or.jp) databases using the following keywords: "*Edwardsiella tarda*", "*E tarda*" and "infection". An episode of ETB was defined as ≥1 positive blood cultures yielding *E tarda* from the same patient. Results meeting the following criteria were included: published case reports or abstracts from scientific meetings; patients of any age; and articles published in any language including English, French, Spanish and Japanese. Exclusion criteria included: negative blood culture; no description of *E tarda* infection; animal cases; experimental studies; and review articles.

In addition, the medical records of patients, regardless of age, with ETB admitted to the TWMU (a 1423-bed university hospital in Tokyo, Japan) between April 2000 and December 2013, were included in the retrospective chart review.

The following data were obtained from both published and TWMU-admitted cases that fulfilled the inclusion criteria: age; sex; underlying disease; antibiotic treatment; complications related to the ETB; geographical area; month of ETB onset; history of exposure to

TABLE 2

Antimicrobial susceptibility of *Edwardsiella tarda* isolated from blood culture; five cases from Tokyo Women's Medical University (TWMU; Tokyo, Japan) and eight cases from the literature

| Age, years/sex | Underlying disease(s) | Complication | Exposure/ dietary risk | Minimum inhibitory concentration (MIC), mg/L | | | | | | | | TWMU case or reference | Country | Year |
				ABPC	CEZ	CTX	IPM/CS	GM	LVFX	TMP-SMX	Colistin			
88/female	GBS	Cholecystitis	ND	<2	<2	<8	<1	<1	<0.5	<2	16 (R)	TWMU-1	Japan	2004
80/male	LC,HCC	EC	ND	<2	<2	<8	<1	<1	<0.5	<2	24 (R)	TWMU-2	Japan	2004
84/male	BCa	Cholecystitis	ND	<4	<4	<8	<1	<1	<2	<2	32 (R)	TWMU-3	Japan	2010
80/female	PCa	Liver abscess	ND	<4	<4	<8	<1	<1	<2	<2	0.125 (S)	TWMU-4	Japan	2013
46/female	Ce-Ca	EC	Sushi	<4	<4	<8	<1	<1	<2	<2	32 (R)	TWMU-5	Japan	2013
14/female	none	Liver abscess	Immigrant	S	ND	ND	ND	ND	ND	ND	R	13	Thailand	1969
46/male	none	EC	Travel to Mexico	0.25	1 (cefalothin)	ND	ND	0.25	ND	ND	R	18	United States	1980
39/male	Alcoholism	EP, DC	ND	S	S	S	S	S	S	S	ND	41	Japan	1988
67/male	HCC,LC	NF	ND	S	S	S	S	S	S	S	ND	42	Japan	1996
76/male	DM,HCC	Liver abscess	Sushi	ND	<8	<8 (CAZ)	<1 (MEPM)	<16 (AMK)	<2	ND	ND	51	Japan	2011
21/female	SCA	None	ND	<2	<4	<0.5	<1	2	<0.25	<2	ND	39	Columbia	2008
46/female	SLE	PID	ND	<2	<4	<1	<1	<1	<0.12	ND	ND	53	Japan	2012
67/female	NHL	NF	ND	<4	<4	<8	<1	<1	<1	<2	ND	52	Japan	2012

ABPC Ampicillin; AMK Amoxicillin; BCa Bile duct cancer; CAZ Ceftazidime; Ce-Ca Cervical cancer; CEZ Cefazolin; CTX Cefotaxime; DC Discitis; DM Diabetes mellitus; EC Endstage cancer; EP Endophthalmitis; GBS Gallbladder stone; GM Gentamicin; HCC Hepatocellular carcinoma; IPM/CS Imipenem cilastatin; LC Liver cirrhosis; LVFX Levofloxacin; MEPM Meropenem; ND Not described; NF Neurofibromatosis; NHL Non-Hodgkin lymphoma; PCa Pancreatic cancer; PID Pelvic inflammatory disease; R Resistant (MIC not described); S Susceptible (MIC not described); SCA Sickle cell anemia; SLE Systemic lupus erythematosus; TMP-SMX Trimethoprim/sulfamethoxazole

environmental risk factors; dietary history to include dietary risk factors; and crude mortality after ETB within 90 days. The case definition for survival required a report of whether the patient survived, or no report of death, in published articles or medical records from cases at TWMU. During the study period, 112,796 blood samples were obtained under sterile conditions and were processed using BACTEC 9240 (Becton Dickinson Diagnostic Instrument Systems, USA) until March 11, 2011, and BacT/ALERT 3D (bioMérieux, France) from April 2011 onward. Strains of *E tarda* were identified using MicroScan WalkAway 96si (Siemens, Germany). The five cases of ETB identified were included in the present study. The species identification of *E tarda* was also confirmed using matrix-assisted laser desorption ionization–time of flight mass spectrometry (Microflex LT with MALDI-Biotyper version 3.1, Bruker Daltonik, Germany). Susceptibility of *E tarda* isolated from blood cultures was tested retrospectively in accordance with the standards of the Clinical and Laboratory Standards Institute using E-test (bioMérieux, France).

Continuous data were compared using a *t* test and categorical data were compared using Fisher's exact tests; P<0.05 was considered to be statistically significant. Multivariate analyses were used to determine the independent risk factors associated with mortality using forward stepwise logistic regression. All variables with P<0.1 in univariate analyses were entered into the multivariate model. Statistical analyses were performed using R version 3.0.3 (www.r-project.org).

The study protocol was approved by the TWMU Hospital Medical Ethics Committee (No. 3052).

RESULTS

The literature search resulted in 234 articles from the PubMed MEDLINE database and 68 articles from the ICHUSHI database, published between January 1968 and December 2013. Of these, 202 and 54 publications were excluded, according to inclusion criteria, from the PubMed MEDLINE and ICHUSHI databases, respectively. The resulting 46 publications, published between 1968 and 2013, were retrieved from the English (n=30) (8-37), French (n=1) (38), Spanish (n=1) (39) and Japanese (n=14) literature (40-53). A total of 72 cases were described in the retrieved publications and five cases diagnosed at the TWMU were also included, resulting in 77 cases for analysis.

The mean age of the patients was 61 years (range two days to 101 years) and 30 cases (30 of 77 [39%]) involved women. Underlying diseases included cancer (29 of 77 [37.6%]); hepatobiliary cancer (17 of 77 [20.8%]) and liver cirrhosis (13 of 77 [16.8%]). Six (6.5%) cases involved neonatal patients. Thirteen (16.9%) cases occurred in healthy individuals without any underlying disease and there were 35 (45.5%) cases of uncomplicated ETB. Eighteen (23.4%) cases involved soft tissue infections, 24.7% involved diarrhea, 13.0% involved liver abscess and 3.9% involved meningitis. Despite appropriate antimicrobial therapy, the overall mortality rate was 44.6% (33 of 74, no mortality data available for three cases [14,46,49]); however, this rate increased to 61.1% (11 of 18) for patients with soft tissue infections.

Treatment using the following antimicrobial agents was described in 51 cases (66.2%): cephalosporin (n=26), penicillin (n=19) and carbapenems (n=8). Although no significant differences were found with respect to age, sex, complications of ETB, geographical area or season of onset among cases in which the patient died compared with cases in which the patient survived, liver cirrhosis (OR 12.0 [95% CI 2.46 to 58.6]; P=0.00213) was considered to be an independent risk factor associated with death in multivariate analyses (Table 1). Antibiotic susceptibility of the *E tarda* strains that were isolated from the blood cultures is summarized in Table 2. Six cases in the literature reported susceptibility to ampicillin, cefazolin, imipenem, levofloxacin and gentamicin, in cases in which each drug minimum inhibitory concentrations were measured (13,18,39,41,42,51-53). Reduced susceptibility to colistin was found in four of five strains (80%) at the TWMU and two of two strains (13,18) in the literature. Reported environmental risks included direct exposure to fresh or brackish water (lacerated forearm after a fall into brackish water [28] and fishing [28,36]), soil (farming [8] and gardening [12]) and animal feces (working in a zoo [20]). The parents of two neonatal cases were exposed to fresh water; the father from one case was a dock maintenance worker at a lake and his wife participated in a baptism involving immersion in a lake while pregnant, and a mother from another case washed clothes in a river resulting in confirmed maternal colonization (29,50). Reported dietary risks included exposure to raw fish/sushi (48,50,51) (TWMU-5 in Table 2), raw meat (27), ceviche during a trip to

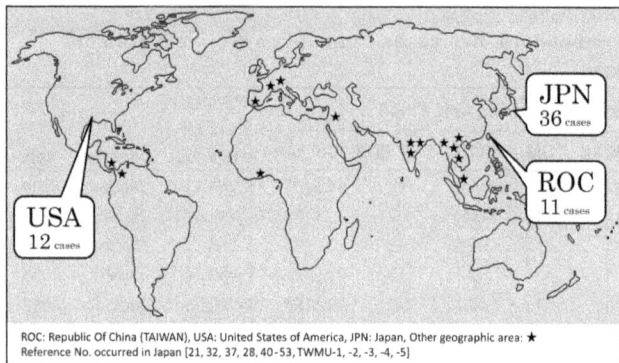

ROC: Republic Of China (TAIWAN), USA: United States of America, JPN: Japan, Other geographic area: ★
Reference No. occurred in Japan [21, 32, 37, 28, 40-53, TWMU-1, -2, -3, -4, -5]

Figure 1) *Number (No) of* Edwardsiella tarda *bacteremia cases according to location on the world map. TWMU Tokyo Women's Medical University, Tokyo, Japan*

Ecuador (45) and unpasteurized goat's milk (46). The geographical distribution of ETB is shown in Figure 1. The most frequently reported geographical area of ETB cases was Japan (35 of 77 [45.5%]) (21,32,37,40-53) (TWMU-1, -2, -3, -4, -5 in Table 2), followed by the United States (US) (12 of 77 [15.6%]) and the Republic of China (Taiwan) (10 of 77 [13.0%]). Five of 12 (41.6%) cases from the US occurred in states located around the Gulf of Mexico (Louisiana, n=2 [12,32]; Florida, n=1 [15]; Texas, n=1 [18]; and Mississippi, n=1 [24]). Of the cases from the US, 66.7% (eight of 12) occurred in states by the ocean (five cases near the Gulf of Mexico (12,15,18,24,32); New York, n=2 [22,33]; and California, n=1 [13]). No reports of ETB cases in the southern hemisphere were found in the present review. The seasonal distribution of ETB is shown in Figure 2. The majority of the cases that provided a description of the time of onset (18 of 22 [81.8%]) (10,12,13,15,16,18,21,25,28,33,38,40-42,45,50,51) (TWMU-1, -2, -3, -4, -5 in Table 2) occurred during the northern hemisphere summer and autumn months (June to November).

DISCUSSION

To our knowledge, the present study was the first and largest multi-language review of ETB. The results indicate that the overall mortality related to ETB is 44.6%, and ETB may be more likely to occur in the humid and subtropical climates of Eastern Asia and near the Gulf of Mexico in the US, particularly during summer and autumn months. Furthermore, environmental and dietary risk factors, such as exposure to brackish water and raw food consumption, may play a role in ETB.

ETB occurs infrequently (<5%) (9), and the risk factors are not well established. Investigating similarities with other species may provide some clues regarding the mechanisms related to ETB. Previous case series suggest that up to 50% of ETB patients also had hepatobiliary diseases, including alcoholic cirrhosis (9). Interestingly, the authors indicated that conditions resulting in iron overload, such as cirrhosis, sickle cell anemia, leukemia and the neonatal state, are also considered to be risk factors for ETB (9). In the present analysis, 66.2% of the cases involved hepatobiliary diseases, including cancer. Twenty-one (27.3%) of these cases involved gallbladder stones with recurrent episodes of cholecystitis. The rate of underlying diseases may be higher in ETB than in other *E tarda* infections; this may indicate that the presence of underlying disease increases the risk for developing ETB. However, the results of our multivariate analyses suggest, for the first time, that liver cirrhosis is an independent risk factor associated with death in ETB. Cholecystitis with gallbladder stones may increase the risk for ETB in a way similar to that of human typhoid fever. Moreover, the overall rate of underlying diseases in ETB may be higher than in other *E tarda* infections, potentially indicating that the presence of underlying disease increases the risk for ETB and subsequent high mortality from ETB.

In addition, reservoir-related *Aeromonas* species are similar to *E tarda*. Both can cause a wide spectrum of diseases among warm- and

cold-blooded animals, including fish, reptiles, amphibians, mammals and humans. Population sizes of both species can grow quite large, generally peaking in the warmer temperatures of the summer months in temperate freshwater lakes and chlorinated drinking water, and have been associated with contact wtih reptiles, including those kept as pets (54). *Vibrio vulnificus* can also cause severe disseminated infection associated with exposure to seawater and brackish water. Severe *V vulnificus* infections in humans are also responsible for liver cirrhosis. Therefore, clinical characteristics of *E tarda* infections in humans resemble those of *Aeromonas*, typhoid fever and *V vulnificus* infections, and share similar environmental risks. It is well known that necrotizing fasciitis type 3, which is known as a marine infection and can be fatal within 48 h, is caused by *Vibrio* or *Aeromonas* species. Therefore, it should be recognized that *E tarda* can also result in necrotizing fasciitis type 3. In addition, previous reports indicate that the mortality rate of ETB is nearly 50%, which is similar to that of *V vulnificus* (55) or severe infections caused by *Aeromonas* species (56,57).

E tarda infections, including ETB, are considered to be foodborne. Despite this, dietary risk factors for ETB have not been well established or documented. In addition, most of the cases of ETB are suspected to occur endogenously through primary colonization and infection in the human intestinal tract. However, documented *E tarda* infections in humans have resulted from the consumption of infected or contaminated food such as fish (58). According to the Food and Agriculture Organization of the United Nations Statisitcs Division (FAOSTAT) Food Balance Sheet 2006 (http://faostat.fao.org/), Japan has one of the world's highest per capita seafood consumption rates. *E tarda* has been isolated from raw flounder in Japanese fish farms (58). Interestingly, *E tarda* has been reported to result in a 60% to 90% mortality rate among Japanese eels (59), and a traditional custom in Japan, dating from the 18th century, is to eat cooked eel at the end of July. Furthermore, 71% of the eels from the eel farms in Korea (60) have been reported to carry *E tarda*.

Toward the end of the 1960s in the US, *E tarda* was linked to catfish, mainly in the waters of Arkansas, Mississippi, Texas and Louisiana (61). Despite the small number of cases in the current study, approximately one-half of the cases occurred around the Gulf of Mexico, which receives a supply of nutrient-rich water from several rivers. Individuals residing in these areas may be exposed to high concentrations of *E tarda* through the water or contaminated food. According to data from the National Fisheries Institute, tilapia, pangasius and catfish are consumed in the US. They are farmed in fresh water and 79% of already-dressed catfish in the US carry *E tarda* (62). Given the collective findings of the available literature, we suspect that dietary exposures also affect the risk for ETB.

Little is known about the recent prevalence of *E tarda* colonization in healthy individuals; no recent data are available from large-scale studies in any country. A study conducted in the 1970s (7), is one of the few to report that only 26 of 353,600 Japanese individuals were healthy carriers of *E tarda*. We suspect that the rate of colonization in stool appears to be high among individuals in areas with a high consumption of raw fish contaminated with *E tarda*. The colonization rate in humans may be affected by changes in dietary habits and increased travel, and the use of novel techniques, such as matrix-assisted laser desorption ionization–time of flight mass spectrometry, may improve identification of *E tarda*, which was previously underestimated.

Trimethoprim/sulfamethoxazole-resistant *E tarda* has been clinically isolated in a pediatric patient with X-linked chronic granulomatous disease and osteomyelitis in Japan (63). No multidrug-resistant strains of *E tarda* were found in the current study. There are several studies showing at least 90% of *E tarda* strains to be colistin resistant. Natural resistance of *E tarda* to colistin or polymyxin B has been suggested, but its mechanism was unelucidated (64). Feedstuffs for domesticated animals are exposed to colisin in Japan (65) and some European countries. Antibiotic resistance in *E tarda* may emerge as an issue related to environmental antibiotic exposure in food production. Geographical differences among the Republic of China (Taiwan)

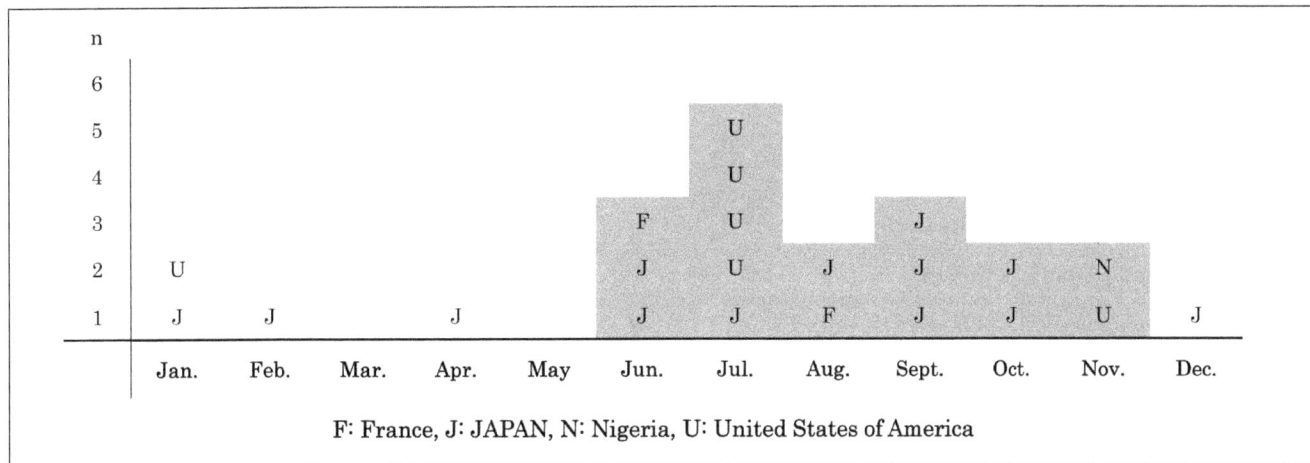

Figure 2) *The seasonal distribution of 22* Edwardsiella tarda *bacteremia cases. Apr April; Aug August; Dec December; Feb February; Jan January; Jul July; Jun June; Mar March; Oct October; Sept September; Nov November*

and the US in the antimicrobial susceptibility of *E tarda*, isolated from food-producing animals, have been previously described (66). Seasonal distribution of human *E tarda* gastroenteritis has not been previously demonstrated (9). In addition, information has not been available regarding the time of year for extraintestinal *E tarda* infections in previously reported cases. The results of the current review suggest that there may, in fact, be a seasonal distribution of ETB, and exposure to higher concentrations of *E tarda* in the warmer temperatures of the summer months may increase the risk for ETB (61). For example, Eastern Asia, which includes Japan and the Republic of China (Taiwan), and the states of the US near the Gulf of Mexico, reported the highest rates of ETB and belong to climates that are similar – humid and subtropical.

In addition, dietary customs vary according to geographical region. Therefore, dietary factors may play a role in the geographical or seasonal distributions of ETB.

Taking all of this into account, we propose two reasons for the high prevalence of ETB in Japan. The first is that Japan is geographically rich in brackish water areas and rivers. Second, the Japanese consume a relatively large amount of raw seafood, which may be contaminated with *E tarda*.

The present review had limitations. One was the retrospective nature of the data, including the use of previously reported literature and only five recent cases from our institute. Fourteen of 72 cases from the literature were described only in the Japanese language. Therefore, publication and resource bias may have affected our results. The second limitation is that we focused on the results of blood cultures; however, sensitivity of blood cultures may vary during a long study period.

CONCLUSIONS

ETB may be categorized as a severe food- and waterborne infection similar to *Aeromonas*, *Vibrio* and *Salmonella* (typhoid fever) infections, which result in high mortality in patients with severe underlying diseases such as liver cirrhosis. Geographical and seasonal distributions may characterize ETB. The clinical epidemiology, including dietary risk factors and the current incidence of ETB should be further established.

DISCLOSURES: The authors have no financial relationships or conflicts of interest to declare.

ACKNOWLEDGEMENTS: Results from this study were presented, in part, as a poster (Presentation number 1263) at ID Week 2013, San Francisco, October 2 to 6, 2013.

REFERENCES

1. Trabulsi LR, Ewing WH. Sodium acetate medium for the differentiation of Shigella and Escherichia cultures. Public Health Lab 1962;20:137-40.
2. King BM, Adler DL. A previously undescribed group of Enterobacteriaceae. Am J Clin Pathol 1964;41:230-2.
3. Sakazaki R. A proposed group of the family Enterobacteriaceae, the Asakusa group. Int Bull Bacteriol Nomencl Taxon 1965;15:45-7.
4. Ewing WH, McWhorter AC, Escobar MR, Lubin AH. *Edwardsiella*, a new genus of Enterobacteriaceae, based on a new species, *E.tarda*. Int Bull Bacteriol Nomencl Taxon 1965;15:33-8.
5. Wyatt LE, Nickelson R, Vanderzant C. *Edwardsiella tarda* in freshwater catfish and their environment. Appl Environ Microbiol 1979;38:710-4.
6. Joh SJ, KIM MJ, Kwon HM, Ahn EH, Jang H, Kwon JH. Characterization of *Edwardsiella tarda* isolated from farm-cultured eels, *Anguilla japonica*, in the Republic of Korea. J Vet Med Sci 2011;73:7-11.
7. Onogawa T, Terayama T, Zenyoji H. Distribution of *Edwardsiella tarda* and hydrogen sulfide-producing *Escherichia coli* in healthy persons. J Jpn Assoc for Infect Dis (Kansenshogaku Zasshi) 1976;50:10-7.
8. Kournay M. Vasquez MA, Saenz R. Edwardsiellosis in man and animals in Panama: Clinical and epidemiological characteristics. Am J Trop Med Hyg 1977;26:1183-90.
9. Janada JM, Sharon LA. Infections associated with the genus *Edwardsiella*: The role of *Edwardsiella tarda* in human diseases. Clin Infect Dis 1993;17:742-8.
10. Okubadejo OA, Alausa KO. Neonatal meningitis caused by *Edwardsiella tarda*. Br Med J 1968;3:357-8.
11. Sonnenwirth AC, Kallus BA. Meningitis due to *Edwardsiella tarda*. First report of meningitis caused by *E.tarda*. Am J Clin Pathol 1968;49:92-5.
12. Pankey GA, Seshul MB. Septicemia caused by *Edwardsiella tarda*. J La State Med Soc 1969;121:41-3.
13. Jordan GW, Hadley WK. Human infection with *Edwardsiella tarda*. Ann Intern Med 1969;70:283-8.
14. Bockemühl J, Pan-Urai R, Burkhardt F. *Edwardsiella tarda* associated with human disease. Pathol Microbiol 1971;37:393-401.
15. Sachs JM, Pacin M, Counts GW. Sickle hemoglobinopathy and *Edwardsiella tarda* meningitis. Am J Dis Child 1974;128:387-8.
16. Le Frock JL, Klainer AS, Zuckerman K. *Edwardsiella tarda* bacteremia. South Med J 1976;60:188-90.
17. Koshi G, Lalitha MK. *Edwardsiella tarda* in a variety of human infections. Indian J Med Res 1976;64:1753-9.
18. Clarridge JE, Musher DM, Fainstein V, Wallace RJ Jr. Extraintestinal human infection caused by *Edwardsiella tarda*. J Clin Microbiol 1980;11:511-4.

19. Ovartlarnporn B, Chayakul P, Suma S. *Edwardsiella tarda* infection in Hat Yai Hospital. J Med Assoc Thai 1986;69:599-603.

20. Marínez ML, Lázaro ME, Albillos A, et al. *Edwardsiella tarda* bacteremia. Eur J Clin Microbiol Infect Dis 1987;6:599-600.

21. Funada H, Kameoka J, Machi T, Matsuda T. *Edwardsiella tarda* septicemia complicating acute leukemia. Jpn J Med 1987;27;325-8.

22. Vohra K, Torrijos E, Jhaveri R, Gordon H. Neonatal sepsis and meningitis caused by *Edwardsiella tarda*. Pediatr Infect Dis J 1988;7;814-15.

23. Wilson JP, Waterer RR, Wofford JD, Chapman SW. Serious infections with *Edwardsiella tarda*. A case report and review of the literature. Arch Intern Med 1989;149:208-10.

24. Jaruratanasirikul S, Kalnauwakul S. *Edwardsiella tarda*: A causative agent in human infections. Southeast Asian J Trop Med Public Health 1991;22:30-4.

25. Fournier S, Pialoux G, Feuillie V, Fleury J, Dupont B. *Edwardsiella tarda* septicemia with cellulitis in a patient with AIDS. Eur J Clin Microbiol Infect Dis 1997;16:551-3.

26. Osiri M, Tantawichien T, Deesomchock U. *Edwardsiella tarda* bacteremia and septic arthritis in a patient with diabetes mellitus. Southeast Asian J Trop Med Public Health 1997;28:669-72.

27. Yang CH, Wang CK. *Edwardsiella tarda* bacteraemia-complicated by acute pancreatitis and pyomyoma. J Infect 1999;38:124-6.

28. Slaven EM, Lopez FA, Hart SM, Sanders CV. Myonecrosis caused by *Edwardsiella tarda*: A case report and case series of extraintestinal E.tarda infections. Clin Infect Dis 2001;32:1430-3.

29. Mowbray EE, Buck G, Humbaugh KE, Marshall GS. Maternal colonization and neonatal sepsis caused by *Edwardsiella tarda*. Pediatrics 2003;111:e296-8.

30. Wang IK, Kuo HL, Chen YM, et al. Extraintestinal manifestations of *Edwardsiella tarda* infection. Int J Clin Pract 2005;59:917-21.

31. Yousuf RM, How SH, Amran M, Hla KT, Shah A, Francis A. *Edwardsiella tarda* septicemia with underlying multiple liver abscesses. Malays J Pathol 2006;28:49-53.

32. Tamada T, Koganemaru H, Matsumoto K, Hitomi S. Urosepsis caused by *Edwardsiella tarda*. J Infect Chemother 2009;15:191-4.

33. Golub V, Kim AC, Krol V. Surgical wound infection, tuboovarian abscess, and sepsis caused by *Edwardsiella tarda*: Case reports and literature review. Infection 2010;38:487-9.

34. Kadam SD. *Edwardsiella tarda* – a case report. Indian J Pediatr 2013;80:63-4.

35. Hashavya S, Averbuch D, Berger I, et al. Neonatal sepsis following maternal amnionitis by *Edwardsiella tarda*: A case report and a review of the literature. Eur J Pediatr 2011;170:111-3.

36. John AM, Prakash JA, Simon EG, Thomas N. *Edwardsiella tarda* sepsis with multiple liver abscesses in a patient with Cushing's syndrome. Indian J Med Microbiol 2012;30:352-4.

37. Ohara Y, Kikuchi O, Goto T, et al. Successful treatment of a patient with sepsis and liver abscess caused by *Edwardsiella tarda*. Intern Med 2012;51:2813-7.

38. Peyrade F, Bondiau P, Taillan B, Boscagli A, Roa M, Dujardin P. *Edwardsellia tarda* septicemia in chronic lymphoid leukemia. Rev Med Interne 1997;18:233-4.

39. Perez RDA, Ramirez AG. Sepsis por Edwardsiella tarda y asociación con anemia falciforme: Reporte de caso y revision de la literatura. Medicina & Laboratorio 2008;14:43-8.

40. Mori K, Yamazaki A, Kishikawa E, Sugizaki N, Kume H. A case of sepsis caused by *Edwardsiella tarda*. J Jpn Assoc Infect Dis (Kansenshogaku Zasshi) 1983;57:273-9.

41. Harada M, Yoshida H, Oomagari K, Sakai T, Abe H, Tanikawa K. A case of sepsis caused by *Edwardsiella tarda* complicated panophthalmitis and pyogenic spondylitis. J Jpn Assoc Infect Dis (Kansenshogaku zasshi) 1990;64:620-4.

42. Matsushima S, Yajima S, Taguchi T, et al. A fulminating case of *Edwardsiella tarda* septicemia with necrotizing fasciitis. J Jpn Assoc Infect Dis (Kansenshogaku zassshi) 1996;70:631-6.

43. Tohira H, Yokota J. *Edwardsiella tarda*. Nihon rinsho 2001;(Suppl 1):235-8.

44. Maruge S, Mizuguchi M, Yasuda T, et al. A case of necrotizing fasciitis with septic shock due to *Edwadsiella tarda*. J Jpn Assoc Infect Dis (Kansenshogaku Zasshi) 2005;79(Suppl 1):228.

45. Fujimoto M, Nakao K, Fujikawa K, et al. A case of rapidly progressive fatal septic shock following necrotizing fasciitis due to *Edwardsiella tarda* with hepatitis C virus related liver cirrhosis complicated hepatocellarcarcinoma Kanzo 2006;47:273-4.

46. Nishiyama H, Tarumoto K, Fujikawa K. A case of necrotizing fasciitis due to *Edwardsiella tarda*. J Jpn Soc Clin Microbiol 2007;17(Suppl 1):130.

47. Takahashi K, Ikeda M, Matsubayashi H, et al. Intrauterine infection caused by *Edwardsiella tarda*. Kanto Journal of Obstetrics and Gynecology 2007;44:73-6.

48. Tamura T, Ito K, Tsuchiya R, et al. A case of septic shock with necrotizing fasciitis caused by *Edwardsiella tarda*. J Jpn Soc Care Med 2009;16:207-8.

49. Fujii M, Ooki T, Yoshiko M. A case of necrotizing fasciculitis caused by *E.tarda* in a patient with peritoneal dialysis. J Jpn Soc Dial Ther 2009; (Suppl 42):739.

50. Hara K, Ouchi H, Kitahara M, Shibano K, Miyauchi T, Ishiguro H. A case of fasciitis localized in the calf muscles associated with *Edwardsiella tarda* sepsis. Clin Neurol (Rinsho Shinkeigaku) 2011;51:694-8.

51. Tokunaga S, Tanino T, Koda M, et al. A case of sepsis due to *Edwardsiella tarda* with alcoholic liver cirrhosis complicated by hepatocellular carcinoma and lung cancer. Kanzo 2011;52:120-5.

52. Sato M, Satomura H, Odaka I. Septic shock caused by *Edwardsiella tarda*. Journal of Chiba Association of Medical Technologists 2012;115:56-9.

53. Tanaka C, Nishikawa N, Mushika M, et al. Intrauterine infection which caused sepsis by *Edwardsiella tarda*. Tokai J Obstet Gynecol 2013;49:285-9.

54. Nagel P, Serritella A, Layden TJ. *Edwardsiella tarda* gastroenteritis associated with a pet turtle. Gastroenterology 1982;82:1436-7.

55. Matsumoto K, Ohshige K, Fujita N, et al. Clinical features of *Vibrio vulnificus* infections in the coastal areas of the Ariake Sea, Japan. J Infect Chemother 2010;16:272-9.

56. Wang JH, Wang CY, Chi CY, Ho MW, Ho CM, Lin PC. Clinical presentations, prognostic factors, and mortality in patients with *Aeromonas sobria* complex bacteremia in a teaching hospital: A 5-year experience. J Microbiol Immunol Infect 2009;42:510-5.

57. Dryden M, Munro R. Aeromonas septicaemia: Relationship of species and clinical features. Pathology 1989;21:111-4.

58. Rashid MM, Honda K, Nakai T, Muroga K. An ecological study on *Edwardsiella tarda* in flounder farms. Fish Pathology 1994;29:221-7.

59. Kim KI, Kang JK, Park JY, Joh SJ, Lee HS, Kwon YK. Phenotypic traits, virulence-associated gene profile and genetic relatedness of *Edwardsiella tarda* isolates from Japanese eel *Anguilla japonica* in Korea. Lett Appl Microbiol 2014;58:168-76.

60. Joh SJ, Ahn EH, Lee HJ, Shin GW, Kwon JH, Park CG. Bacterial pathogens and flora isolated from farm-cultured eels (*Anguilla japonica*) and their environmental waters in Korean eel farms. Vet Microbiol 2013;163:190-5.

61. Meyer FP, Bullock GL. Edwardsiella tarda, a new pathogen of channel catfish (*Ictalurus punctatus*). Appl Microbiol 1973;25:155-6.

62. Wyatt LE, Ranzell N, Vanderzant C. *Edwardsiella tarda* in freshwater catfish and their environment. Appl Environ Microbiol 1979;38:710-4.

63. Kawai T, Kusakabe H, Seki A, Kobayashi S, Onodera M. Osteomyelitis due to trimethoprim/sulfamethoxazole-resistant *Edwardsiella tarda* infection in a patient with X-linked chronic granulomatous disease. Infection 2011;39:171-3.

64. Muyembe T, Vandepitte J, Desmyter J. Natural colistin resistance in *Edwardsiella tarda*. Antimicrob Ag Chemother 1973;4:521-4.

65. Marshall BM, Levy SB. Food animals and antimicrobials: Impacts on human health. Clin Microbiol Rev 2011;24:718-33.

66. Waltman WD, Shotts EB. Antimicrobial susceptibilities of *Edwardsiella tarda* from the United States and Taiwan. Vet Microbiol 1986;12;277-82.

11

Canada's National Advisory Committee on Immunization: Celebrating 50 years

Shalini Desai MD MHSc FRCP(C)[1], Shainoor J Ismail MD MSc FRCP(C)[2],
Robert Lerch RN BScN MSc[3], Bryna F Warshawsky MD CCFP[4], Ian Gemmill MD CCFP[?]

S Desai, SJ Ismail, R Lerch, BF Warshawsky, I Gemmill. Canada's National Advisory Committee on Immunization: Celebrating 50 years. Can J Infect Dis Med Microbiol 2015;26(3):126-128.

Vaccines have saved more lives than any other innovation in modern medicine. National immunization committees play a vital role in the development of evidence-based recommendations for the use of vaccines. The present article describes the evolution and work of the National Advisory Committee on Immunization in Canada as the group marks its 50th anniversary. The article also provides insight into the future challenges that the committee is likely to face.

Key Words: *Advisory committee; Canada; Decision making; Immunization programs*

Le Comité consultatif national de l'immunisation du Canada : 50 ans à célébrer

Les vaccins ont sauvé plus de vies que n'importe quelle autre innovation de la médecine moderne. Les comités nationaux d'immunisation jouent un rôle essentiel dans la préparation de recommandations fondées sur des données probantes relatives à l'utilisation des vaccins. Le présent article décrit l'évolution et le travail du Comité consultatif national de l'immunisation du Canada, qui célèbre son cinquantième anniversaire. Il contient également un aperçu des prochains défis que le comité devra probablement relever.

Often referred to as a modern miracle, vaccines are one of the most important public health measures (1), having saved more lives than any other innovation in modern medicine (2). Vaccine knowledge and development have advanced significantly since the first inoculation against smallpox in 1796. With rapid advances in vaccine development in the 1960s (including polio, measles, mumps and rubella vaccines [3]) came the creation of the National Advisory Committee on Immunizing Agents in Canada in the fall of 1964. This event marked the beginning of a long history of coordinated, expert advice on vaccines in this country. In honour of the 50th anniversary of the creation of what is now referred to as the National Advisory Committee on Immunization (NACI), the present article highlights the history and successes of this highly regarded committee, and discusses future challenges.

THE HISTORY OF NACI

The National Advisory Committee on Immunizing Agents was initially established in 1964 with a mandate to provide advice on immunizing agents to the Department of National Health and Welfare, and to make recommendations on immunizing agents that appeared to warrant special consideration to the Dominion Council of Health. In 1975, the mandate was revised to focus on advice related to the introduction of new vaccines in Canada and to assist in the development of immunization programs. In 1978, the name of the committee was changed to the National Advisory Committee on Immunization, reflecting the revised mandate for consideration of procedures related to immunization and immunization coverage.

Over the years, NACI has evolved from providing advice on only a few vaccines to now providing technical guidance for >50 different authorized vaccine products to prevent 24 different diseases (4). NACI is a highly regarded scientific advisory committee that has been recognized globally as one of 15 "well-established National Immunization Technical Advisory Groups" (5) that can be regarded as a resource in establishing similar groups in other countries to enhance the use of evidence-based decision-making processes in the development of immunization programs and policies. In Canada, the National Advisor on Healthy Children and Youth has recognized the importance of the work of NACI, and recommended that "the federal government continue to support the work of the National Advisory (Committee) on Immunization (NACI) in getting valuable information to health care providers and parents" (6).

THE PEOPLE AND THE PROCESS

The current mandate of NACI is to provide the Public Health Agency of Canada (PHAC) with ongoing and timely medical, scientific and public health advice related to vaccines and certain immunoglobulins for both adult and pediatric populations (7). This is accomplished through the efforts of appointed expert members, liaison representatives from organizations with an interest in immunizations and vaccines, as well as ex officio representatives from relevant areas of the federal government, and secretariat support through the Centre for Immunization and Respiratory Infectious Diseases (8). The vaccine industry provides valuable information to the committee related to products in development and ongoing clinical trials, but they do not participate in NACI's funding, its deliberations or in the development of its recommendations. Members are expected to express their personal opinions as informed by their professional expertise, experience and relevant evidence. Members are asked to submit conflict of interest declarations annually and provide updates as they arise. These declarations are assessed for impact on NACI deliberations and recommendations, with potential management strategies including limited participation on specific agenda items. The intent of the committee is

[1]*Public Health Agency of Canada, Toronto, Ontario;* [2]*Public Health Agency of Canada, Edmonton, Alberta;* [3]*Public Health Agency of Canada, Ottawa;* [4]*Public Health Ontario, Toronto, Ontario*
Correspondence: Dr Shalini Desai, Public Health Agency of Canada, 180 Queen Street West, Toronto, Ontario M5G 1V2.
e-mail shalini.desai@phac-aspc.gc.ca

to ensure that unbiased expert advice, based on best practices and evidence, is provided to assist PHAC in informing the Canadian public health community and frontline providers.

As the committee has evolved, a scientific methodology and more transparent process have been embraced for making recommendations. A search of relevant published data, along with grey literature, is conducted to understand the currently available information regarding vaccine efficacy, effectiveness, immunogenicity and safety. Cost and cost-effectiveness is not currently considered in NACI deliberations. The literature review is generally guided by a working group chairperson to ensure that all relevant data are reviewed. These data are then synthesized, along with a ranking of the level and quality of evidence. Canadian epidemiology, using a variety of published and unpublished sources, is used to understand the burden of disease and the potential for improving health at a population level for a particular disease. The committee then 'puts it all together' by reviewing the benefits and risks, following which the evidence is translated into scientifically grounded recommendations (9).

KNOWLEDGE TRANSLATION

Once NACI has made its recommendations, several products are developed to ensure that they are available to a variety of stakeholders. NACI's recommendations can be found in the Canadian Immunization Guide (4) (the Guide), in advisory committee statements and in detailed literature reviews (7). These materials are made available on PHAC's website (www.phac-aspc.gc.ca/naci-ccni/index-eng.php#rec).

The Guide is intended to support the front-line immunizer in providing the right vaccine at the right time to the right person via the right route and at the right dose. It also assists health care professionals in responding to questions from potential vaccine recipients or their caregivers, including providing current knowledge regarding vaccine safety. In 2014, the Guide has been moved from its traditional book format to an Internet-based 'ever-green' format. This change allows for timely updating of information and improvements in providers' ability to obtain the most accurate information.

Advisory committee statements provide details of the Canadian epidemiology related to the disease under consideration, an overview of the efficacy, effectiveness, immunogenicity and safety of a particular vaccine, and a summary of NACI's recommendations for the use of that vaccine. More details regarding the literature review that was conducted to support the development of the statement and its recommendations are often published separately. The literature review, the advisory statement or both contain detailed tables summarizing and assessing each individual study that was considered.

The number of advisory committee statements written annually has increased over the years, reflecting the increase in the number, complexity and specific indications for use of vaccine products. For example, NACI issues an annual influenza statement. Each year, this statement provides an overview of the epidemiology from the previous year's influenza season and a summary of the vaccines available in Canada for the upcoming influenza season, along with

their recommended usage. Recent updates to the influenza statement have included a change in the recommended pediatric dose for those six to 36 months of age from 0.25 mL to 0.5 mL (10), a preferential recommendation of live attenuated intranasal influenza vaccine for children two to six years of age (11), a recommendation for vaccination of egg-allergic individuals when this had previously been a contraindication (10) and the progressive expansion of the age indications for routine influenza vaccination, which is now recommended for everyone ≥6 months of age (12,13). Current issues being considered include the use of quadrivalent vaccines that provide protection against both lineages of influenza B and the possible preferential use of more efficacious vaccines in certain age groups. As new products, evidence and indications evolve, NACI revisits its recommendations to keep them up to date, relevant, and based on the best and most current evidence.

FUTURE CHALLENGES

Vaccine innovation and development is continuing at an impressive pace. Vaccine development pipelines contain candidate vaccines targeted not only against infectious diseases, but also to prevent chronic diseases. Vaccine technologies are also expanding, with the potential to prevent a range of diseases that have proved to be challenging to address with current technologies. As these new products come to market, there will be an increasing demand for rigorous, unbiased guidance to understand how they can be used to improve the health of Canadians.

NACI currently focuses on the epidemiology and the scientific aspects of a vaccine product. As the vaccine landscape becomes more complex, it may be necessary to expand this mandate to include other elements in the analysis and recommendations; for example, the feasibility and acceptability of a new vaccine, as well as the cost effectiveness and societal impact. Additional attention must also be devoted to vaccine program considerations including vaccine uptake, vaccine hesitancy, and surveillance systems to monitor vaccination programs and vaccine safety. Given this possible expanded mandate, it may be necessary to employ a different model of creating vaccine guidance and recommendations; however, it will continue to be essential to ensure that the processes used by NACI are systematic, rigorous, transparent, timely and unbiased.

SUMMARY

Over the past 50 years, NACI has contributed to the practice of immunization by providing thoughtful, practical and evidence-based guidance to individual vaccine providers, as well as to provinces and territories for their publically funded programs. NACI and PHAC, which supports NACI's work, recognize the importance of this work and are committed to continuing to provide this advice within the rapidly changing landscape of vaccine development and a possible evolving mandate of the committee. As it has been in the past 50 years, the advice of NACI will continue to be vital to supporting the future delivery and uptake of the modern miracle of vaccines.

REFERENCES

1. Ehreth J. The global value of vaccination. Vaccine 2003;21:596-600.
2. How vaccination saves lives. United Kingdom: National Health Service, 2014 (updated April 4 2014). <www.nhs.uk/conditions/vaccinations/pages/vaccination-saves-lives.aspx> (Accessed October 14, 2014).
3. Taking shots: The modern miracle of vaccines. Medscape Pediatrics, 2004 (updated June 24, 2004). <www.medscape.com/viewarticle/481059> (Accessed October 14, 2014).
4. Canadian immunization guide. Ottawa: Public Health Agency of Canada; 2014 (updated April 23, 2014). <www.phac-aspc.gc.ca/publicat/cig-gci/index-eng.php>(Accessed October 14, 2014).
5. Gessener B, Duclos P, DeRoeck D, Nelson E. Informing decision makers: Experience and process of 15 national immunization technical advisory groups. Vaccine 2010;28(S1):1-5.
6. Leitch K. Reaching for the top: A report by the advisor on healthy children and youth. Ottawa: Health Canada, 2007. Report No.:978-0-662-46456-3.

7. National Advisory Committee on Immunization. Ottawa: Public Health Agency of Canada, 2014 (updated May 16, 2014). <www.phac-aspc.gc.ca/naci-ccni/index-eng.php>(Accessed October 14, 2014).
8. Ismail S, Langley J, Harris T, Warshawsky B, Desai S, FarhangMehr M. Canada's National Advisory Committee on Immunization (NACI): Evidence-based decision-making on vaccines and immunization. Vaccine 2010;28(Suppl 1):58-63.
9. National Advisory Committee on Immunization. Evidence-based recommendations for immunization: Methods of the national advisory committee on immunization. CCDR 2009;35(ACS-1). <www.phac-aspc.gc.ca/publicat/ccdr-rmtc/09vol35/acs-1/index-eng.php> (Accessed October 14, 2014).
10. National Advisory Committee on Immunization. Statement on seasonal influenza vaccine 2011-2012. CCDR 2011;38(ACS-5). <www.phac-aspc.gc.ca/publicat/ccdr-rmtc/11vol37/acs-dcc-5/index-eng.php> (Accessed October 14, 2014).

11. National Advisory Committee on Immunization. Revised wording to the National Advisory Committee on Immunization (NACI) recommendation for live attenuated influenza vaccine (LAIV) in healthy children and adolescents 2-17 years of age. CCDR 2013;39(ACS-4). <www.phac-aspc.gc.ca/publicat/ccdr-rmtc/13vol39/acs-dcc-4/index-eng.php> (Accessed October 14, 2014).

12. National Advisory Committee on Immunization. Statement on seasonal influenza vaccine for 2012-2013. CCDR. 2012;38(ACS-2).

<www.phac-aspc.gc.ca/publicat/ccdr-rmtc/12vol38/acs-dcc-2/index-eng.php> (Accessed October 14, 2014).

13. Statement on seasonal influenza vaccine 2014-2015. Ottawa: Public Health Agency of Canada, 2014 (updated September 19, 2014). <www.phac-aspc.gc.ca/naci-ccni/flu-grippe-eng.php> (Accessed October 14, 2014).

12

Improving health care efficiency through the integration of a physician assistant into an infectious diseases consult service at a large urban community hospital

Melissa Decloe MSc CCPA[1,2], Janine McCready MD FRCPC[1,3],
James Downey MD FRCPC PhD[1,3], Jeff Powis MD FRCPC MSc[1,3]

M Decloe, J McCready, J Downey, J Powis. Improving health care efficiency through the integration of a physician assistant into an infectious diseases consult service at a large urban community hospital. Can J Infect Dis Med Microbiol 2015;26(3):130-132.

BACKGROUND: Physician assistants (PAs) have recently been introduced into the Canadian health care system in some provinces; however, there are little data demonstrating their impact.
METHODS: A retrospective case-control study was conducted between January 2010 and December 2013. Length of stay (LOS) and mortality were examined in the infectious diseases consult service (IDCS) compared with hospital-wide controls. The two-year period before the introduction of the PA to the IDCS of a large urban community hospital in Canada (2010 to 2011) was compared with the two-year period following the introduction of the PA (2012 to 2013).
RESULTS: Following the introduction of a PA to the IDCS, there was a decrease in time to consultation from 21.4 h to 14.3 h (P<0.0001). LOS was significantly decreased among IDCS patients by 3.6 days more than that seen in matched hospital-wide controls (P=0.0001). Mortality did not significantly change after PA introduction in either cases or controls.
DISCUSSION/CONCLUSION: PAs can improve health efficiencies in the Canadian health care setting, leading to reduction in LOS.

Key Words: *Length of stay; Mortality; Physician assistant*

Améliorer l'efficacité des soins de santé par l'intégration d'un auxiliaire médical au service de consultations infectieuses d'un grand hôpital général en milieu urbain

HISTORIQUE : Les auxiliaires médicaux (AM) ont récemment été intégrés au système de santé de certaines provinces canadiennes, mais on possède peu de données pour en évaluer les répercussions.
MÉTHODOLOGIE : Les chercheurs ont réalisé une étude rétrospective cas-témoins entre janvier 2010 et décembre 2013. Ils ont comparé la durée de séjour (DdS) et la mortalité au service de consultation en infectiologie (SCI) à celles de sujets témoins de tout l'hôpital. Ils ont comparé la période de deux ans avant l'arrivée des AM au SCI d'un grand hôpital général urbain du Canada (2010 et 2011) à la période de deux ans suivant leur arrivée (2012 et 2013).
RÉSULTATS : Après l'arrivée des AM au SCI, les chercheurs ont constaté une diminution du délai avant la consultation, qui est passé de 21,4 h à 14,3 h (P<0,0001). La DdS a régressé d'au moins 3,6 jours chez les patients du SCI par rapport à celle des sujets témoins de l'ensemble de l'hôpital (P=0,0001). La mortalité ne changeait pas de manière significative après l'arrivée des AM, que ce soit pour les cas ou les sujets-témoins.
INTERPRÉTATION : Les AM peuvent améliorer l'efficacité du milieu canadien de la santé et réduire la DdS.

Physician assistants (PAs) are academically trained, dependent health care providers who work in various clinical settings to support the clinical duties of the supervising physician (1). They have been practicing in Canada since the 1960s in the armed forces and have recently been introduced into civilian practice in some provinces (2). Manitoba and Ontario have established PA training programs (2) and Alberta has recently introduced a pilot project to implement PAs (3). The impact of PAs in other jurisdictions, particularly in the United States, has been well studied and extrapolated to inform the introduction of PAs in Canada. The generalizability of the United States literature is limited by the substantial differences between health care systems; specifically, the significant differences in health care funding. Given that the profession remains in its infancy in Canada, research has only begun to emerge examining the integration of PAs in Canadian practice (4). To date, the majority of Canadian studies have aimed to describe the role of PAs in Canada (5-8) as well as physician and patient attitudes toward PAs (9-12). Three studies were identified that aimed to evaluate outcomes relating to implementing a PA into Canadian practice; however, all were limited by their lack of a control group (13-15). To date, no study has evaluated the impact of integrating a PA into a hospital-based medicine subspeciality in Canada. Therefore, we aimed to evaluate the impact of integrating a PA into a medicine subspeciality on health care efficiency and patient outcomes.

METHODS

Starting in November 2011, the Infectious Diseases Consult Service (IDCS) at Toronto East General Hospital (Toronto, Ontario), a 515-bed urban community hospital, introduced a PA with assistance from a Career Start Grant for Physician Assistant Graduates through Health Force Ontario (16). The PA was a Canadian Certified Physician Assistant and had completed a Canadian training program in 2011. Infectious diseases (ID)-specific training consisted of two weeks in the offsite microbiology laboratory as well as ongoing one-on-one mentorship with the ID specialists during daily case reviews.

A retrospective case-control study was conducted between January 2010 and December 2013. The two-year period before the introduction

[1]*Division of Infectious Diseases, Department of Medicine, Toronto East General Hospital, Toronto;* [2]*Physician Assistant Education Program, McMaster University, Hamilton;* [3]*Department of Medicine, University of Toronto, Toronto, Ontario*
Correspondence: Dr Jeff Powis, Division of Infectious Diseases, Department of Medicine, Toronto East General Hospital, Toronto, Ontario. e-mail jpowi@tegh.on.ca

TABLE 1

Baseline characteristics of the infectious diseases cohort (cases) and hospital-wide cohort (controls)

Variable	Cases (n=3386)	Controls (n=13,493)
Age, years, mean ± SD	65.9±18.4	65.9±18.3
Sex		
Male	1735 (51.2)	6899 (51.1)
Female	1651 (48.8)	6594 (48.9)
Medical diagnosis partition	2677 (79.1)	10,685 (79.2)
Study period		
Before physician assistant	1547 (45.7)	6160 (45.7)
After physician assistant	1839 (54.3)	7333 (54.3)

Data presented as n (%) unless otherwise indicated

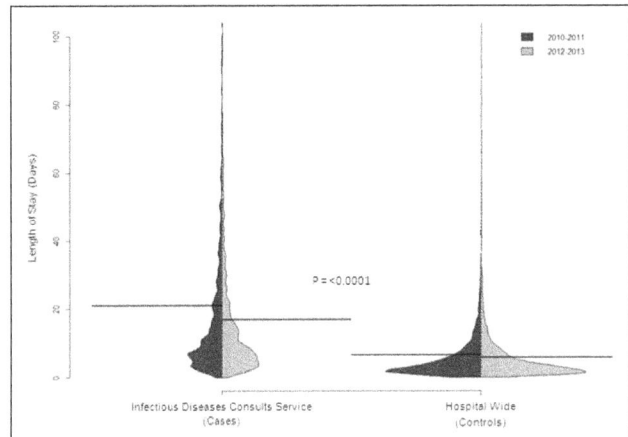

Figure 1) *Violin plot illustrating the distribution of length of stay (LOS) in the infectious diseases consult service cohort (cases and the hospital-wide cohort [controls]) pre and post introduction of the infectious diseases physician assistant. The average LOS in each group is illustrated with the bold black line. The differential change in LOS in the cases and the controls is statistically significant (P<0.0001)*

of the PA (2010 to 2011) was compared with the two-year period following the introduction of the PA (2012 to 2013). The primary objective of the present study was to evaluate the impact of PA introduction on inpatient length of stay (LOS) and mortality among IDCS patients, compared with a matched hospital-wide control group. The inclusion of a control group was critical to determine the independent impact of PA introduction to the IDCS from other hospital-wide quality improvement interventions that may have impacted LOS or mortality.

Patients were included if they were seen by the IDCS during their inpatient stay during the workweek when the PA was working. Patients from the complex continuing care unit, day surgery, mental health and those who were seen in the emergency department but not admitted to hospital were excluded. LOS, mortality and time to consult data were obtained from the hospital electronic medical record. In the LOS and mortality data set, LOS and mortality data were retained for each patient on each unique hospital encounter. The hospital-wide data for the control cohort were obtained from the electronic medical records through hospital decision support. Controls were determined from a hospital-wide data set and were matched to cases according to sex (exact), admission date (±15 days), age (±5 years) and diagnosis partition (medical or surgical). The diagnosis partition is part of the Canadian Institute for Health Information's Case Mix Groups methodology, which assigns patients into more homogenous groups for determination of complexity and estimated resource use (17). The aim was to match cases to controls with a 1:4 ratio (18,19). Age and diagnosis partition were weighted at two times admission date. Duplicate consults were removed from the time to consultation analysis but were retained if requested >24 h after the initial consult.

Time to ID consult in the period before the introduction of the ID PA (preintervention) was compared with the period following the introduction of the ID PA (postintervention) with the Mann-Whitney U test. A matched case-control analysis was conducted for the LOS and the mortality variables. Of the 3386 patient encounters in the case cohort, 3347 were matched to four controls, 30 were matched to three controls, seven were matched to two controls, one was matched to one control and only one case was not matched to any controls. The unmatched case was a 94-year-old male medical patient.

To estimate differences in means and proportions in LOS and mortality between the cases and controls in the preintervention period to the postintervention period, a generalized estimating equation (GEE) was used. For LOS, a linear GEE model was used to account for the continuous nature of the LOS variable. For the mortality analysis, a logistic GEE model was used for the binary nature of the mortality variable. The project was approved by the local research ethics board.

RESULTS

Following the introduction of the PA to the IDCS, the average time to consult decreased from 21.4 h to 14.3 h (P<0.0001). Characteristics of cases and controls are shown in Table 1.

Among patients seen by the IDCS, there was 21.0% reduction in LOS, with the average LOS decreasing from 20.5 days to 16.2 days following the introduction of the PA. In the hospital-wide matched cohort, there was a 10.6% reduction in LOS, with the average LOS decreasing from 6.8 days to 6.1 days from the pre- to postintervention period. There is a statistically significant decrease in the differential change of LOS among patients seen by the IDCS compared with the hospital-wide matches of 3.6 days (95% CI 1.8 to 5.5 days; P=0.0001) (Figure 1).

The proportion of deaths among ID-consulted patients decreased from 0.26 to 0.22 from the pre- to postintervention period; in the hospital-wide cohort, the proportion of deaths decreased from 0.055 to 0.051 during the study period. There was no statistically significant difference in the differential change in the proportion of deaths in the two cohorts (P=0.14).

INTERPRETATION

Following the introduction of the PA to the IDCS at Toronto East General Hospital, decreases in both time to consultation and LOS were observed. When LOS in the IDCS cohort was compared with the hospital-wide control cohort, a statistically significant difference in the rate of change of 3.6 days was seen. This suggests that the observed decrease in LOS after introduction of the PA was unique to the IDCS and, therefore, cannot be attributed to any other hospital-wide interventions. Although a trend toward decreasing mortality was observed among the IDCS cohort after introduction of the PA, this did not reach statistical significance.

The significant change in LOS among the ID-consulted cohort in the post-ID PA time periods is likely related to the more rapid time to consultation as well as the fact that the ID PA's primary job responsibility was to the ID consult service. Dedicated ID PA availability likely translated into more frequent follow-up assessments, improved accessibility and facilitated communication to other care providers. Although we did not measure which factors led to the observed reductions in LOS, the PA likely served as a conduit for immediate knowledge translation to consulting services.

Although advancements in the management of ID through new antimicrobials or delivery of current treatments may have been introduced during the study period, none would be anticipated to have such a considerable impact on LOS.

No previous studies have examined LOS in admitted patients in which PAs have been involved in patient care; one previous study examined LOS in the emergency department when PAs were on duty and demonstrated similar findings. Ducharme et al (14) examined LOS in the emergency department in a 14-day study period before the introduction of PAs compared with a 14-day study period following the introduction of the PA, and a 30.3% decrease in LOS in the emergency department was observed when PAs were on duty (95% CI 21.6% to 39.0%; P<0.01). The findings of this study, however, are limited by the lack of a control group. We are unaware of any literature that evaluated outcomes associated with the introduction of a PA to inpatients, including medicine subspecialities, in the Canadian health care system.

Two studies were identified that conducted cost analyses of using PAs in Canada. Sigurdson (15) conducted a business case analysis that examined PAs employed on a plastic surgery team in Halifax, Nova Scotia and found that a PA could be cost efficient when a double operating room model was used for surgical services. Bohm et al (13) demonstrated similar findings in their study examining a PA employed as a surgical assist in an arthroplasty program in Winnipeg (Manitoba). In their study, PAs were cost neutral with general practitioner surgical assistants, but decreased surgical wait times from 44 weeks in the pre-intervention time period to 30 weeks postintroduction of the PA (13). Our study did not undertake a financial analysis associated with the decreased LOS in hospital in patients because it was beyond the scope of the current project. However, a decrease in LOS by 3.6 days per patient would undoubtedly be associated with significant cost savings when the cost per day of hospital admission is considered and could form the basis of a business plan to justify employing a PA.

The present study used a matched case-control methodology to examine two years of data in the period before the introduction of the PA and two years of data following the introduction of the PA. This resulted in a large sample size and allowed for the examination of trends over a four-year period, serving to reduce the chance that seasonal variations in patient volumes or other initiatives impacted the findings. One of the largest limitations of our study is that no measure of patient severity or complexity was available for matching. The mortality rate and the average LOS were higher in the IDCS cohort compared with the hospital-wide cohort, demonstrating that the IDCS cohort and the hospital-wide cohort are likely systematically different from one another. More information may have been gained from the mortality analysis if we were able to match cases based on patient complexity or severity. It should be reiterated, however, that the inclusion of the hospital-wide cohort was not for direct comparison of these two very different groups, but rather to provide context for our IDCS analysis. The present study was also limited by its retrospective design; thus, there may be unmeasured confounders biasing our results that were differentially affecting the IDCS patients. Finally, only a subset of the IDCS patients were included in the analysis because only patients seen by the ID PA during the work week were included; therefore, these results cannot be generalized to the ID service as a whole.

The present study demonstrates that a PA can be successfully integrated into a specialty service with a complex patient population. This is a unique role for a PA in Canada and, therefore, it is unclear whether these results can be generalized to other inpatient medicine subspecialities employing PAs. Further studies that aim to evaluate PA-related outcomes in health care efficiencies would be of significant benefit to the Canadian PA literature.

The present study demonstrated that with the addition of a PA to the IDCS, health care efficiency improved, as measured by time to consult and LOS. These findings also support the objective that the introduction of PAs in Canada would provide greater access to care and potential cost savings through efficiencies achieved in the delivery of care (2).

REFERENCES

1. Canadian Association of Physician Assistants – About Physician Assistants. <https://capa-acam.ca/about-pas/> (Accessed May 6, 2014).
2. HFO. Ontario's Physician Assistant Initiative: An Overview. 2009 <www.healthforceontario.ca/UserFiles/file/AHP/Inside/PA-overview-may-2009-en.pdf> (Accessed April 7, 2014).
3. Alberta Health Services – Physician Assistants. 2014. <www.albertahealthservices.ca/8754.asp> (Accessed April 7, 2014).
4. Hamilton GM, Decloe MD. Reviewing the Evidence for Canada's Physician Assistant Initiative. University of Toronto Medical Journal 2011;88:88-90.
5. Jones IW. Where the Canadian physician assistants are in 2012. JAAPA 2012;25:54.
6. Jones IW, Seo B, Chauhan TS, Buske L. The results of the first Canadian national physician assistant survey. JAAPA 2011;24:63.
7. Jones IW, St-Pierre N. Physician assistants in Canada. JAAPA 2014;27:11-3.
8. Doan Q, Sabhaney V, Kissoon N et al. The role of physician assistants in a pediatric emergency department: A center review and survey. Pediatr Emerg Care 2012;28:783-8.
9. Doan Q, Hooker RS, Wong H, et al. Canadians' willingness to receive care from physician assistants. Cana Fam Physician 2012;58:e459-64.
10. Doan Q, Piteau S, Sheps S, et al. The role of physician assistants in pediatric emergency medicine: The physician's view. CJEM 2013;15:321-9.
11. Taylor MT, Wayne Taylor D, Burrows K, Cunnington J, Lombardi A, Liou M. Qualitative study of employment of physician assistants by physicians: Benefits and barriers in the Ontario health care system. Can Fam Physician 2013;59:e507-13.
12. Busse JW, Riva JJ, Nash JV, et al. Surgeon attitudes toward nonphysician screening of low back or low back-related leg pain patients referred for surgical assessment: A survey of Canadian spine surgeons. Spine 2013;38:E402-8.
13. Bohm ER, Dunbar M, Pitman D, Rhule C, Araneta J. Experience with physician assistants in a Canadian arthroplasty program. Can J Surg 2010;53:103-8.
14. Ducharme J, Alder RJ, Pelletier C, Murray D, Tepper J. The impact on patient flow after the integration of nurse practitioners and physician assistants in 6 Ontario emergency departments. CJEM 2009;11:455-61.
15. Sigurdson L. Meeting challenges in the delivery of surgical care. [Abstract]. Winnipeg, September 27 to 29, 2007: The Royal College of Physicians and Surgeons of Canada 2007 Annual Conference. Clin Invest Med 2007;30:S35-S6.
16. Health Force Ontario – Career Start Grant for Physician Assistant Graduates (2013). 2013. <www.healthforceontario.ca/UserFiles/file/Floating/Program/PA/pa-career-start-info-package-2013-en.pdf> (Accessed April 7, 2014).
17. Canadian Institute of Health Information. DAD resource intensity weights and expected length of stay. Ottawa: Canadian Institute of Health Information, 2004.
18. Rosenbaum PR. Optimal matching for observational studies. J Am Stat Assoc 1989;84:1024-32.
19. Bergstralh EJ, Kosanke JL. Computerized Matching of Controls. Rochester: Section of Biostatistics, Mayo Foundation 1995.

13

Lyme disease: Knowledge and practices of family practitioners in southern Quebec

Cécile Ferrouillet DMV MPH[1,2], François Milord MD MSc[2,3], Louise Lambert MD MSc[3],
Anne Vibien MD FRCP[4], André Ravel DMV PhD[1,5]

C Ferrouillet, F Milord, L Lambert, A Vibien, A Ravel. Lyme disease: Knowledge and practices of family practitioners in southern Quebec. Can J Infect Dis Med Microbiol 2015;26(3):151-156.

BACKGROUND: Public health authorities in Quebec have responded to the progressive emergence of Lyme disease (LD) with surveillance activities and education for family physicians (FPs) who are key actors in both vigilance and case management.

OBJECTIVES: To describe FPs' clinical experience with LD, their degree of knowledge, and their practices in two areas, one with known infected tick populations (Montérégie) and one without (regions nearby Montérégie).

METHODS: In the present descriptive cross-sectional study, FPs were recruited during educational sessions. They were asked to complete a questionnaire assessing their clinical experience with Lyme disease, their knowledge of signs and symptoms of LD, and their familiarity with accepted guidelines for diagnosing and treating LD in two clinical scenarios (tick bite and erythema migrans).

RESULTS: A total of 201 FPs participated, mostly from Montérégie (n=151). Overall, results revealed a moderate lack of knowledge and suboptimal practices rather than systematically insufficient knowledge or inadequate practices. A majority of participants agreed to more education on LD. As expected, FPs from Montérégie had a higher clinical experience with tick bites (57% versus 25%), better knowledge of LD endemic areas in Canada and erythema migrans characteristics, and better management of erythema migrans (72% versus 50%).

CONCLUSION: The present study documented the inappropriate intention to order serology tests for tick bites and the unjustified intention to use tick analysis for diagnostic purposes. Such practices should be discouraged because they are unnecessary and overuse collective laboratory and medical resources. In addition, public health authorities must pursue their education efforts regarding FPs to optimize case management.

Key Words: *Lyme disease; Health knowledge, attitudes, practice; Quebec*

La maladie de Lyme : Les connaissances et les pratiques des médecins de famille du sud du Québec

HISTORIQUE : Les autorités en santé publique du Québec ont répondu à l'émergence progressive de la maladie de Lyme (ML) par des activités de surveillance et des formations pour les médecins de famille (MF), qui sont des acteurs majeurs en matière de vigilance et de prise en charge.

OBJECTIFS : Décrire l'expérience clinique des MF à l'égard de la ML, leur degré de connaissances et leurs pratiques dans deux régions, l'une comptant des populations connues de tiques infectées (Montérégie) et l'autre n'en comptant pas (régions à proximité de la Montérégie).

MÉTHODOLOGIE : Dans la présente étude transversale descriptive, les MF ont été recrutés pendant des séances de formation. Ils ont été invités à remplir un questionnaire visant à évaluer leur expérience clinique de la ML, leurs connaissances des signes et symptômes de cette maladie et leurs connaissances des directives acceptées pour diagnostiquer et traiter la ML pour deux scénarios cliniques (piqûre de tique et érythème migrant).

RÉSULTATS : Au total, 201 MF ont participé, la plupart provenant de la Montérégie (n=151). Dans l'ensemble, les résultats ont révélé un manque modéré de connaissances et des pratiques sous-optimales plutôt que des connaissances systématiquement insuffisantes ou des pratiques inadéquates. La majorité des participants ont convenu avoir besoin de plus de formation sur la ML. Comme prévu, les MF de la Montérégie avaient une plus grande expérience clinique des piqûres de tique (57 % par rapport à 25 %), connaissaient mieux les régions endémiques de la ML au Canada et les caractéristiques de l'érythème migrant et prenaient mieux en charge l'érythème migrant (72 % par rapport à 50 %).

CONCLUSION : La présente étude a permis de constater l'intention inappropriée de demander des tests sérologiques après une piqûre de tique et d'analyser les tiques pour corroborer le diagnostic de ML. Il faut décourager ces pratiques, car elles sont inutiles et favorisent la surutilisation collective des laboratoires et des ressources médicales. Par ailleurs, les autorités en santé publique doivent poursuivre leurs efforts de formation auprès des MF pour optimiser la prise en charge des cas.

Lyme disease is a vector-borne zoonotic disease caused by the bacterium *Borrelia burgdorferi* and is transmitted by the tick *Ixodes scapularis* in the northeastern region of the United States bordering Canada (1), where this illness is endemic. It is the first tick-borne disease that has emerged in southwestern Quebec, more specifically in the region of Montérégie (2-4) (Figure 1). In 2008, a predictive model mapped high-risk regions for *I scapularis* establishment in the southern area of Quebec (5). Five areas were further confirmed by active surveillance in south-central Montérégie and along the Saint Lawrence River in Montérégie (3). None have been confirmed in the region of Estrie. The Lanaudière

region was not sampled at that time because it was further away from the high-risk areas for tick establishment identified by the model. From 2010 to 2012, southern Quebec regional public health authorities conducted an awareness campaign of Lyme disease for family physicians and informed them about the areas with established tick populations in Montérégie. Since then, surveillance activities support that ticks have become established in high-risk areas further north and east of Montérégie (6). Lyme disease has been a reportable disease in Quebec since November 2003. Between 2004 and 2012 inclusively, 138 cases have been reported, with 101 of the cases contracted outside the

[1]*Groupe de recherche en épidémiologie des zoonoses et santé publique, Faculté de médecine vétérinaire, Université de Montréal, St Hyacinthe;* [2]*Direction des risques biologiques et de la santé au travail, Institut national de santé publique du Québec, Montréal;* [3]*Direction de santé publique, Agence de la santé et des services sociaux de la Montérégie, Longueuil;* [4]*Service de microbiologie-infectiologie, CSSS Richelieu-Yamaska;* [5]*Département de pathologie et microbiologie, Faculté de médecine vétérinaire, Université de Montréal, St Hyacinthe, Québec*
Correspondence: Dr Cécile Ferrouillet, 3200 rue Sicotte, CP 5000, St-Hyacinthe, Quebec J2S 7C6 e-mail cecile.ferrouillet@umontreal.ca

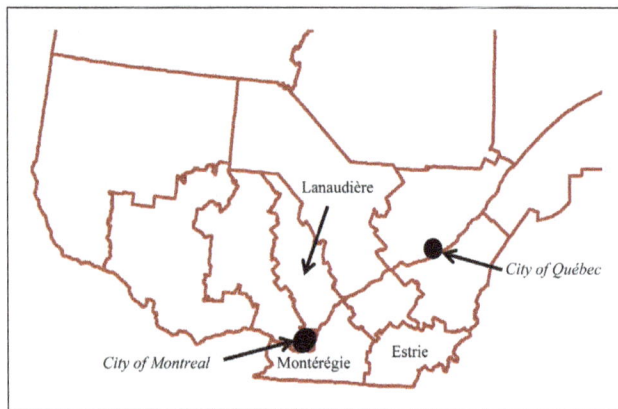

Figure 1) *Regions of Quebec included in the present study*

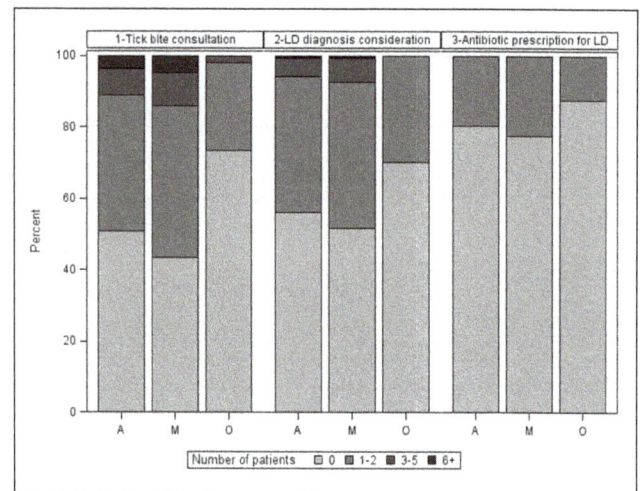

Figure 2) *Number of different patients seen in 2011 by family physicians in three clinical situations (tick bite consultation, Lyme disease [LD] diagnosis consideration, antibiotic prescription for LD) and according to region. A All; M Montérégie; O Other*

province, 31 contracted indigenously and six unknown. Most of the indigenous cases occurred after exposure to the Montérégie region (27 of 31) (7). Despite the low number of reported cases, the average number of serologies for Lyme disease processed by the public health laboratory increased from 1380 in 2004 to 2600 in 2012 (B Serhir, *Laboratoire national de santé publique du Quebec*, personal communication, 2012). The annual number of positive serologies for new patients corresponds grossly to the number of declared cases of Lyme disease. Twenty-five patients with a positive serology were identified in 2011 and 43 were identified in 2012.

Because of its emergence in southern Quebec, it is important to ensure that front-line practitioners know how best to manage these cases. A descriptive study of Quebec family physicians was performed to describe their clinical experience related to Lyme disease, their knowledge of the disease, and their familiarity with practices regarding the diagnosis and management of cases to validate whether these practices are compliant with the most recent guidelines (8). The value of such a study is to improve general practitioners' knowledge and practices concerning this emerging disease and, if necessary, to optimize the management of individual patients and the use of collective resources.

METHODS

The present study was cross-sectional, descriptive and exploratory in nature. The target population was all family physicians whose principal place of practice was within Montérégie or within Estrie and Lanaudière, which are both border regions in southern Quebec. Family physicians were recruited during continuing medical education activities. Of the 15 professional associations contacted, 11 were interested in participating and seven allowed the authors to contact their members during the study period from May to September 2012. The study was briefly explained to the family physicians by one of the authors and they were invited to participate. Those who accepted provided the data for the study on site immediately. The study was approved by the Research Ethics Board of the Faculty of Medicine of the Université de Montréal (Montreal, Quebec; certificate 12-063-CERES-D) as well as by the ethics committees of relevant groups.

The measuring instrument used for data collection was a self-administered, anonymous two-page questionnaire featuring 19 questions: six questions on their profile; one question on their clinical experience with Lyme disease during the past year; five questions regarding their clinical practice; five questions regarding their knowledge; and two questions regarding their need for information. 'Clinical experience with Lyme disease' refers to whether a physician has encountered a patient who presents at least one feature of potential exposure to Lyme disease or has signs of exposure such as a tick on the body, tick bites, erythema migrans, etc. The questionnaire used was modelled after those used by Magri et al (9) and Henry et al (10) for the assessment of knowledge, beliefs and practices regarding Lyme disease. The authors merged and translated the questionnaires, and modified the questions

regarding practice to take into account the frequent use of serological diagnosis in Quebec and the low number of cases actually diagnosed. To adapt to a region in which Lyme disease is emerging, clinical vignette answers included 'don't know' and 'need information' as well as an answer combining the simultaneous prescription of serology and antibiotics. The resulting questionnaire was then reviewed by five experts in the field and pretested using a convenience sample of 10 family physicians before minor changes were made to obtain the final version (Supplementary Figure 1; go to www.pulsus.com).

Descriptive analyses were performed by dividing the respondents into two regions (Montérégie and outside Montérégie), taking into account that known populations of ticks carrying the Lyme disease agent were established only in Montérégie at the time. Proportions between the regions were compared using a Fisher's exact test computed in SAS version 9.4 (SAS Institute, USA) with the significance level set at 0.05, and the 95% CIs around the proportions were calculated with an approximation of normal distribution. In addition, multiple correspondence analysis (MCA) was used to probe the existence of general practitioner subgroups within the data by finding similar answer profiles. MCA is a descriptive statistical technique designed to explore and visualize the relationships between ≥3 categorical variables (11). Beyond the intensive mathematical computation, the most interesting output of MCA is the representation of the several categorical variables on a two-dimensional map that minimizes deformation and underscores the relationships between categories of the variables included in the analysis. Each category is plotted on the map and interpreted based exclusively on their location. The two axes and the distances between points have no straightforward interpretation. Points in the middle of the figure, close to the axis origin, reveal categories that have no remarkable association with any other categories. On the other hand, points located away from the origin and found in approximately the same direction highlight some notable associations between the categories they represent. The analyzed variables were the management of a tick bite case, the identification and analysis of a tick for the diagnosis of Lyme disease, the recognition of erythema migrans, the management of erythema migrans, fever and erythema migrans as symptoms of the first stages of Lyme disease, as well as clinical experience with potential cases of Lyme disease. MCA was conducted using XLStat 2007.5 software (Addinsoft, France).

RESULTS

Participants were recruited during the course of 10 continuing medical education events between May and September 2012, three of which

TABLE 1
Demographic characteristics of survey respondents and comparison with regional and provincial data

	Present study, Montérégie	Present study, other regions	Province of Québec (13)	Province of Québec (14)	Montérégie (14)
n	151	50	1525	7719	1427
Women*, %	53 (45–61)†	68 (52–81)	47	NA	55
Average number of years in practice	24.2 (22.3–26.0)	23.1 (19.2–27.0)	NA	19	19.2
First-line practice exclusively, %	60 (51–68)	68 (52–81)	NA	38 (37–39)	NA
Second-line practice exclusively, %	7 (3–12)	7 (2–18)	NA	21 (20–22)	NA
Average number of patients seen per week	78 (71–85)	83 (69–97)	81 (78–83)	NA	NA

*Data presented as mean (95% CI) unless otherwise indicated; *Of the 201 respondents overall, 14 from Montérégie and nine from the other regions did not specify sex; NA Not applicable*

TABLE 2
Respondents' practice regarding Lyme disease according to region

Scenario	Montérégie (n=151)	Other regions (n=50)	Total (n=201)
You have a patient with a known tick bite, no symptoms, and normal findings on examination. What do you do or what would you do? (one choice only)			
Serology for Lyme disease	26 (17)	5 (10)	31 (16)
Antibiotic treatment for Lyme disease	8 (5)	0 (0)	8 (4)
Serology and antibiotic treatment for Lyme disease	34 (23)	7 (14)	41 (21)
No serology, no antibiotics, educate patient, follow up as needed	41 (27)	10 (20)	51 (26)
I need more information to manage this patient	34 (23)	26 (53)	60 (30)
Other action or treatment*	7 (5)	1 (2)	8 (4)
Knowing that a patient's tick bite occurred in an endemic area (an area with numerous ticks infected with *Borrelia burgdorferi*), does your patient management differ?†			
No	54 (47)	9 (39)	63 (45)
Yes (action added to their initial answer)	21 (18)	8 (35)	29 (21)
Add serology and/or antibiotic	18	8	26
Tick analysis	1	0	1
No serology, no antibiotics, educate patient, follow up as needed	1	0	1
No serology, antibiotics only	1	0	1
Do not know, no answer, information needed	41 (35)	6 (26)	47 (34)
You diagnose erythema migrans (erythematous skin lesion typical of Lyme disease) in a patient. What do you do or what would you do? (one choice only)			
Serology for Lyme disease	11 (7)	5 (10)	16 (8)
Antibiotic treatment for Lyme disease	8 (5)	3 (6)	11 (5)
Serology and antibiotic treatment for Lyme disease	101 (67)	22 (44)	123 (61)
No serology, no antibiotics, educate patient, follow up as needed	0 (0)	0 (0)	0 (0)
I need more information to manage this patient	31 (21)	20 (40)	51 (25)
Other action or treatment	0 (0)	0 (0)	0 (0)

*Data presented as n (%) or n. Number of respondents per vignette may differ from the total number of respondents because of a few missing answers *Action or treatment proposed: seven respondents mentioned an action related to ticks (tick identification and/or tick testing for B burgdorferi) and one respondent mentioned antibioprophylaxis; †Respondents needing information to manage a patient with a tick bite were removed from data.*

included a presentation on Lyme disease, among other topics. Physicians working in private practice, in hospitals and in local community service centers were reached. In total, 201 general practitioners answered the questionnaire, for a participation rate of 59% (ranging from 28% to 100%). Of the 201 participants, 151 (75%) practised in Montérégie and represented 11% of the general practitioners in this region (ranging from 3% to 19%) according to subregion. Compared with provincial statistics, the respondents had, on average, a higher number of years of practice (four or five additional years), and were more often in front-line practice exclusively, thus less so in hospitals (Table 1). This sample can be considered representative for the objectives of the present study.

Answers regarding clinical experience with Lyme disease are presented in Figure 2. Fifty-one percent of the respondents had never experienced a tick bite consultation, 56% had never considered a diagnosis of Lyme disease and 80% had never prescribed antibiotics for Lyme disease. Most of the respondents with clinical experience were exposed to one or

two cases. The proportion of respondents who had been consulted at least once for a tick bite was higher in Montérégie than in the others regions (57% [95% CI 48% to 65%] versus 27% [95% CI 15% to 41%]). The answers regarding management of cases are presented in Table 2. In the case of a consultation for a tick bite without any symptoms or other conditions, respondents were divided between the suggested answers – 30% of them needed information to manage the case and 26% chose the right answer (absence of serology and antibiotics, education of the patient and follow-up as needed). Four percent of the respondents decided to treat patients with antibiotics, which is not a routine procedure but may be offered for prevention of Lyme disease after a recognized tick bite in an area with a prevalence of ticks infected with B burgdorferi >20%. Twenty-one percent of physicians said that they would have managed the case differently if the same patient had been bitten in a known endemic area, while 34% had no opinion. Faced with erythema migrans, 66% correctly chose to prescribe antibiotics (with or without serology),

TABLE 3
Respondents' beliefs and knowledge regarding Lyme disease (LD)

	Yes	No	Don't know
Believed a patient could contract LD in his practice region			
Montérégie	113 (78)	10 (7)	21 (15)
Other regions	25 (53)	13 (28)	9 (19)
Total	138 (72)	23 (12)	30 (16)
Knew LD-endemic areas in the United States	129 (66)	47 (24)	18 (9)
Knew LD-endemic areas in Canada	101 (52)	64 (33)	31 (16)
Knew LD-endemic areas in Europe	18 (10)	109 (59)	57 (31)
Recognized characteristics that define erythema migrans (bull's-eye lesion, expanding lesion [≥5 cm], occurs in 60% to 80% of cases, no pain)	80 (40)	67 (34)	52 (26)
Believed that tick identification and tick testing for *Borrelia burgdorferi* is a decision tool for LD diagnosis	133 (69)	28 (14)*	33 (17)
Believed that tick identification and tick testing for *B burgdorferi* is used to identify LD risk zones in Quebec	173 (88)*	3 (2)	21 (11)
Recognized early signs and symptoms related to early stage LD			
Fever	131 (75)*	21 (12)	22 (13)
Erythema migrans	169 (91)*	7 (4)	10 (5)
Myalgia and arthralgia	126 (71)*	31 (18)	20 (11)
Auriculoventricular heart block	7 (5)*	75 (50)	69 (46)
Cranial neuritis	21 (14)*	68 (44)	64 (42)
Recognized early signs and symptoms not related to early stage LD			
Diarrhea	55 (36)*	18 (12)	80 (52)

Data presented as n (%). *Correct answer

while 25% needed more information to manage the case. Respondents from Montérégie and others regions differed with regard to their answers to the tick bite and erythema migrans questions. Compared with physicians from other regions, a lower proportion of respondents from Montérégie needed information to manage the patient and a higher proportion chose an appropriate management of erythema migrans by prescribing antibiotics (with or without serology) (72% [95% CI 64% to 79%] versus 50% [95% CI 38% to 63%]).

Participants' knowledge of Lyme disease and the expression of their need for information on the subject are presented in Table 3. Asked about the existence of Lyme disease in their practice region, 78% (95% CI 71% to 84%) of participants from Montérégie responded affirmatively (which is true according to the known population of ticks established in 2011-2012 in this region) compared with 53% (95% CI [39% to 67%]) for those from the other regions (where there was no known population of ticks established in 2011-2012, but where passerine birds could drop off infected ticks). Asked about their knowledge of endemic areas, 52% of all respondents declared knowing those in Canada, 66% in the United States and 10% in Europe. The proportions of those who did not answer were 16%, 9% and 31%, respectively. There appears to be a higher proportion of respondents who did not know the endemic areas in Canada in regions other than Montérégie (49% [95% CI 35% to 63%] versus 27% [95% CI 20% to 34%]). Regarding the characteristic that did not correspond to erythema migrans, 40% answered correctly among the four options suggested, while 26% indicated not knowing. There appears to be a higher proportion of respondents from Montérégie than from the other regions who knew characteristics of erythema migrans (46% [95% CI 38% to 54%] versus 24% [95% CI 12% to 36%]). Sending a tick taken from a patient to the laboratory for identification and searching for *B burgdorferi* was considered to be useful for the diagnosis of Lyme disease (which is false) by 69% of respondents and useful for identifying the areas at risk in the province of Quebec (which is true) by 88%. Regarding the symptoms associated with Lyme disease, a majority (≥75%) answered accurately for erythema migrans, fever, myalgia and arthralgia, while a minority (≤36%) answered accurately for atrioventricular block, cranial neuritis and diarrhea (the latter is not a symptom of Lyme disease). For these three symptoms, 42% to 52% of respondents indicated not knowing. A

majority of respondents (≥84%) expressed a need for information for each of the three topics suggested: recognizing erythema migrans, laboratory tests and treatment. For providing this information, continuing medical education activity was chosen by 73% of respondents, medical literature by 63% and website by 48%. Physicians reported using various information sources on Lyme disease during the study period, with a preference for their public health newsletter (51%), a website (46%) or another professional (colleague, infectious disease specialist or public health physician) (26%). Eleven percent said they did not have any source of information at the time (7% in Montérégie and 22% in the other regions).

The MCA map shows four most striking features (Figure 3). Correct answers are not highly clustered, which means that physicians providing correct answers to all questions were uncommon. The answers indicating lack of knowledge ('don't know' and 'need more information' combined) are clustered on the right side of the map, indicating a tendency of a lack of knowledge for several questions for some physicians. The bubbles showing the numbers of patients with possible Lyme disease seen in 2011 are distributed from the right to the left of the map and in the opposite direction of the answers, indicating a lack of knowledge and suggesting a positive relationship between the numbers of potential Lyme disease cases seen by physicians and their knowledge (whether accurate or not) about the disease. Finally, incorrect answers or those indicating a lack of knowledge are spread all over the map, indicating an absence of pattern for incorrect answers to several questions. This shows a moderate lack of knowledge among physicians rather than systematic insufficient knowledge or practices and shows that this gap tends to decrease with clinical experience.

DISCUSSION
In the present study, general practitioners' clinical experience with Lyme disease in 2011 was relatively rare. In 2011, 49% of family physicians participating in the present study were consulted at least once for a tick bite and 44% considered a Lyme disease diagnosis at least once. Our study does not reveal any unsafe practices for the patient; however, it reveals some doctor misconceptions such as the intention to prescribe serology or antibiotherapy for a tick bite without any other symptoms and the intention to use tick analysis for human diagnostic

Eryt: no

Fever: no

Lesion: sero

Tick for Dx: no

Not eryt: freq

Eryt: dk

Bite: educ

Bite: AB

Not eryt: pain

LD-Dx: 3-5

Lesion: AB

Fever: dk

Bite: sero

LD-Dx: 1-2

Not eryt: dk

Lesion: info

LD-Dx: 6-10

LD-Dx: 0

Eryt: yes

Lesion: sero+AB

Tick for Dx: dk

Bite: info

Byte: sero+AB

Fever: yes

Tick for Dx: yes

Not eryt: large

Not eryt: small

Bite: other

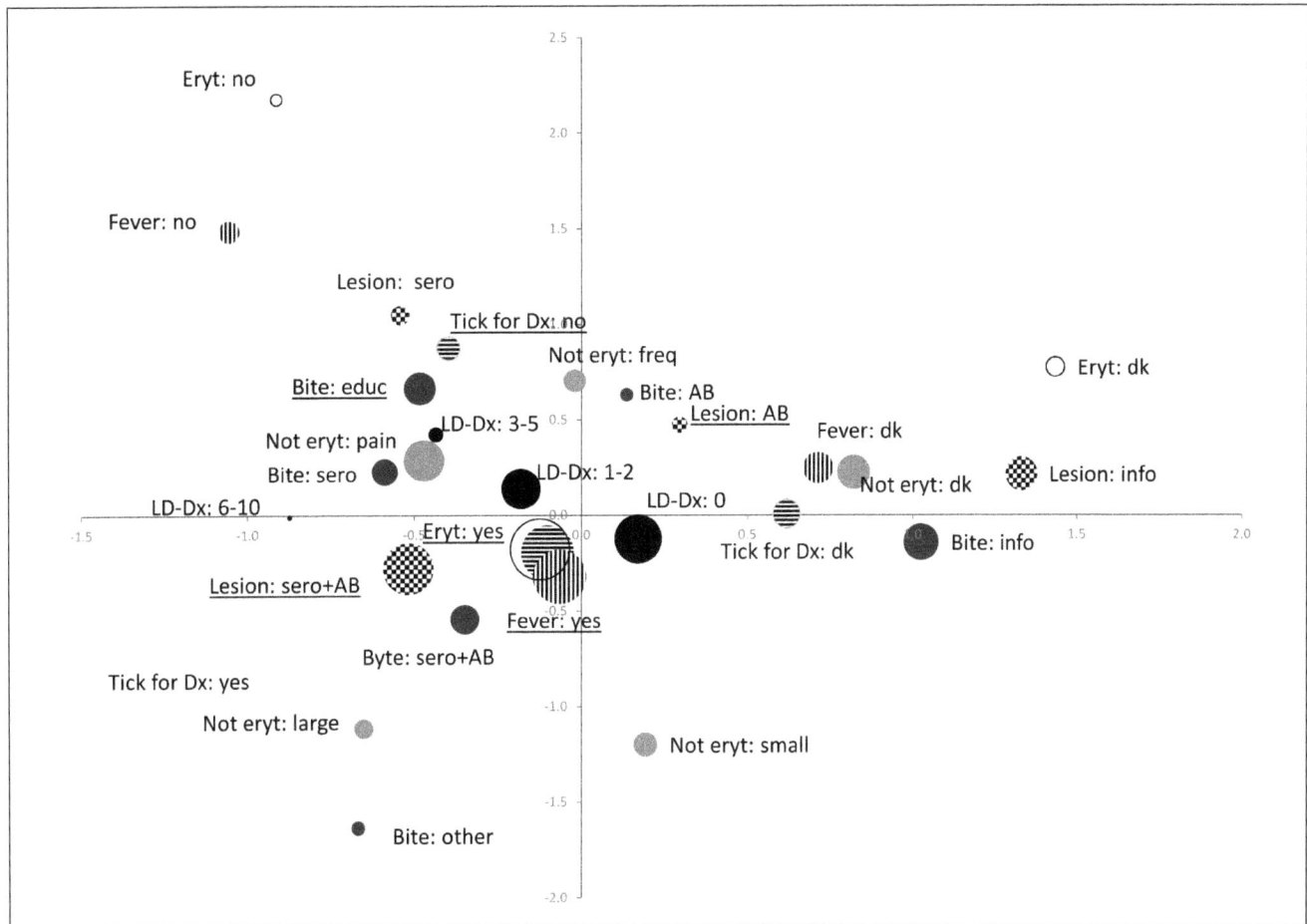

Figure 3) *Map resulting from the multiple correspondence analysis of 151 general practitioners' answers to six questions. The bubbles represent the relative location of each possible answer given for every question on the two-dimensional plan that shows most of the variability in the answers. The size of the bubbles is proportional to the number of respondents for the variable it represents. The questions were the following. 1) 'When faced with a patient with a known tick bite but no symptoms and normal findings on examination, what do you do or what would you do?' (dark gray bubble). The choices were 'serology for Lyme disease' (Bite: sero), 'antibiotic treatment for Lyme disease' (Bite: AB), 'serology and antibiotic treatment for Lyme disease' (Bite: sero+AB) , 'no serology, no antibiotics, educate patient, follow up as needed' (Bite: educ), 'I need more information to manage this patient' (Bite: info), 'other action or treatment' (Bite: other). 2) 'When faced with a patient with erythema migrans (erythematous skin lesion typical of Lyme disease), what do you do or what would you do?' (checked bubble). The choices were 'serology for Lyme disease' (Lesion: sero), 'antibiotic treatment for Lyme disease' (Lesion: AB), 'serology and anti- biotic treatment for Lyme disease' (Lesion: sero+AB), 'no serology, no antibiotics, educate patient, follow up as needed' (Lesion: educ), 'I need more informa- tion to manage this patient' (Lesion: info), 'other action or treatment' (Lesion: other). 3) 'A patient brings you a tick that bit him/her. You send the tick to the laboratory for identification and to test for B burgdorferi. According to you, are the lab results useful for the diagnosis of Lyme disease?' (horizontally striped bubble). Answer choices were 'yes' (Tick for Dx: yes), 'no' (Tick for Dx: no), and 'don't know' (Tick for Dx: dk). 4) 'What is the only characteristic that does not comply with the classical definition of erythema migrans?' (light gray bubble). The choices were 'bull's-eye lesion' (Not eryt: small), 'expanding lesion larger than or equal to 5 cm' (Not eryt: large), 'lesion occurs in 60% to 80% of cases' (Not eryt: freq), 'painful lesion' (Not eryt: pain), 'don't know' (Not eryt: dk). 5) 'In the case of fever, do you think the patient is in an acute phase of Lyme disease?' (vertically striped bubble). The choices were 'yes' (Fever: yes), 'no' (Fever: no), or 'don't know' (Fever: dk). 6) In a case of erythema migrans, do you think the patient is in an acute phase of Lyme disease?' (white bubble). Choices were 'yes' (Eryt: yes), 'no' (Eryt: no), or 'don't know' (Eryt: dk). Correct answers to the six questions are underlined on the map. Finally, the dark bubbles show the number of patients for whom the physician thought Lyme disease was a potential diagnosis during the year 2011 (LM-Dx: 0 patients, LM-Dx: 1-2 patients, LM-Dx: 3-5 patients and LM-Dx: 6-10 patients). See the figure highlights in the text.*

purposes. Treatment of patients with antibiotics (doxycycline) is not a routine procedure but may be offered for prevention of Lyme disease after a recognized tick bite to adult patients and to children ≥8 years of age when all of the following circumstances exist: the attached tick can be reliably identified as an adult or nymphal *I scapularis* tick that is estimated to have been attached for ≥36 h on the basis of the tick's degree of engorgement with blood or when there is certainty about the time of exposure to the tick; prophylaxis can be started within 72 h of the time that the tick was removed; ecological information indicates that the local prevalence of infection of these ticks with *B burgdorferi* is ≥20%; and doxycycline treatment is not contraindicated (8). In fact,

antibiotic use for prevention of Lyme disease after a recognized tick bite is not recommended in Quebec because the prevalence of ticks infected with *B burgdorferi* is between 10% and 15%.

Family physicians' knowledge should be improved both on a clinical level (symptoms of Lyme disease and characteristics of ery- thema migrans) and on an epidemiological level (areas at risk). Multiple correspondence analysis shows a lack of general knowledge rather than inaccurate knowledge or practice. Physicians recognize their need for training on several aspects of diagnosis and treatment of this disease. Family physicians from Montérégie distinguish them- selves from those of the other regions because more of them were consulted for a tick bite, knew characteristics of erythema migrans and Lyme disease endemic zones in Canada, and chose an appropriate management of erythema migrans by prescribing antibiotics (with or without serology).

Differences in practice observed between family physicians from Montérégie and those of the other regions may be due to their clinical experience with tick bites or potential cases of Lyme disease as well as to the work of local public health authorities to develop awareness. In Montérégie, the public health newsletter provided physicians in 2010 and 2012 with critical information on epidemiology and clinical management of Lyme disease and their website made available various tools and reference documents. Since 2011-2012 in Estrie, the information on Lyme disease for professionals was updated on their website while no specific communication was made in Lanaudière. There is a small difference between the number of physicians who prescribed antibiotics for Lyme disease (n=38, one to two patients each) and the number of cases reported to public health authorities for the same period (n=32 in 2011). This difference may be due to a biased estimate during the study or to the underreporting of cases. There may be under-reporting of cases in Quebec; however, this is limited because physicians were encouraged to declare erythema migrans with compatible exposure, and the majority of physicians prescribe a serology in the presence of erythema migrans and a positive result is automatically reported to public health by the laboratory. Among physicians who did not need information to manage a patient with a tick bite, the proportion of physicians with an accurate answer (absence of serology and antibiotics, education of the patient and second consultation if needed) is lower than in similar studies conducted in low endemic areas (10) or moderately endemic areas (9,12), the proportion of physicians using only antibiotics (prophylactic antibiotic therapy) is equal to similar studies, and the proportion of physicians requesting a serology (with or without antibiotics) is higher. Among the physicians not needing information to manage a patient with erythema migrans, the proportion of physicians who prescribe antibiotics is similar to the other study conducted in a low endemic area (10).

One study limitation is the possible selection bias in terms of recruiting physicians with an interest in Lyme disease. Some physicians (n=47) were surveyed before training on Lyme disease; however, they have the same practices and knowledge as the other respondents. Recall bias exists for questions related to the number of cases in the past 12 months. The questionnaire was fine-scaled and there were very few answers in the higher categories. An overestimation for these questions is unlikely; an underestimation is possible, but is likely limited because a patient with suspected Lyme disease is noteworthy. The answers to the clinical vignettes may reflect what is medically expected rather than what would be done in reality. The options 'don't know' and 'need information was added to the questionnaire to limit this. Finally, some questions used a specific terminology, such as clinical manifestations in the *early stages* of Lyme disease, which may have been misinterpreted by some respondents.

CONCLUSION

The present study documents the inappropriate intention to order serology tests for tick bites and the unjustified intention to use tick analysis for diagnostic purposes, two practices that overuse the collective laboratory and medical resources. Public health authorities must provide more information to general practitioners to improve their knowledge and optimize management of cases. They must also communicate the usefulness of looking for ticks with B *burgdorferi* to keep our knowledge of risk areas current.

An increase in locally acquired cases was observed in Montérégie in 2013 and 2014, supporting the need to better inform family physicians. A follow-up study may be conducted to verify the impact of continuing information campaigns to raise awareness and improve practice. Research investigating the best methods for family physicians to acquire knowledge on slowly emerging diseases that do not manifest themselves as outbreaks would also be useful.

SOURCE OF FUNDING: This study was funded by the *Fonds vert dans le cadre de l'Action 21 du Plan d'action 2006-2012 sur les changements climatiques du gouvernement du Quebec.*

REFERENCES

1. Bacon RM, Kiersten JK, Mead PS. Surveillance for Lyme disease-United States, 1992-2006. MMWR 2008;57(SS10):1-9.
2. Nguon S, Milord F, Ogden NH, Trudel L, Lindsay LR, Bouchard C. Étude épidémiologique sur les zoonoses transmises par les tiques dans le sud-ouest du Québec-Rapport de l'année 2007. Québec: Institut national de la santé publique du Québec, 2008. <www.inspq.qc.ca/pdf/publications/1139_EtudeZooonoses2007.pdf> (Accessed May 4, 2014).
3. Nguon S, Milord F, Trudel L, et al. Étude épidémiologique sur les zoonoses transmises par les tiques dans le sud-ouest du Québec – rapport de l'année 2008. Québec, QC: Institut national de la santé publique du Québec, 2009. <www.inspq.qc.ca/pdf/publications/1140_EtudesZoonoses2008.pdf> (Accessed May 4, 2014).
4. Ogden NH, Bouchard C, Kurtenbach K, et al. Active and passive surveillance and phylogenetic analysis of Borrelia burgdorferi elucidate the process of Lyme disease risk emergence in Canada. Environ Health Perspect 2010;118:909-14.
5. Ogden N, St-Onge L, Barker I, et al. Risk maps for range expansion of the Lyme disease vector, Ixodes scapularis, in Canada now and with climate change. Int J Health Geogr 2008;7:24.
6. Ferrouillet C, Fortin A, Milord F, et al. Proposition d'un programme de surveillance intégré pour la maladie de Lyme et les autres maladies transmises par la tique Ixodes scapularis au Québec. Québec, QC: Institut national de la santé publique du Québec, 2014. <www.inspq.qc.ca/pdf/publications/1819_Programme_Maladie_Lyme.pdf> (Accessed February 12, 2015).
7. Milord F, Leblanc M-A, Markowski F, Rousseau M, Lévesque S, Dion R. Flash Vigie: Surveillance de la maladie de Lyme au Québec – Bilan 2004-

2012. Québec, QC: Ministère de la Santé et des Services sociaux, 2013. <http://publications.msss.gouv.qc.ca/acrobat/f/documentation/2006/06-271-02W-vol8_no5.pdf> (Accessed May 4, 2014).
8. Wormser G, Dattwyler R, Shapiro E, et al. The clinical assessment, treatment, and prevention of Lyme disease, human granulocytic anaplasmosis, and babesiosis: Clinical practice guidelines by the Infectious Diseases Society of America. Clin Infect Dis 2006;43:1089-134.
9. Magri JM, Johnson MT, Herring TA, Greenblatt JF. Lyme disease knowledge, beliefs, and practices of New Hampshire primary care physicians. J Am Board Fam Pract 2002;15:277-84.
10. Henry B, Crabtree A, Roth D, Blackman D, Morshed M. Lyme disease: Knowledge, beliefs, and practices of physicians in a low-endemic area. Can Fam Physician 2012;58:e289-e95.
11. Greenacre MJ. Theory and applications of correspondence analysis. London: Academic Press; 1984.
12. Murray T, Feder HM, Jr. Management of tick bites and early Lyme disease: A survey of Connecticut physicians. Pediatrics 2001;108:1367-70.
13. Anonymous. National Physician Survey 2010. <http://nationalphysiciansurvey.ca/> (Accessed May 27, 2014).
14. Paré I, Ricard J. Le profil de pratique des médecins omnipraticiens québécois 2006-2007. 2e version. Fédération des médecins omnipraticiens du Québec, Québec, 2008. Bibliothèque et Archives nationales du Québec – ISBN 978-2-921361-51-4. <www.fmoq.org/fr/organization/clinical/resources/Lists/Billets/Post.aspx?ID=1> (Accessed May 4, 2014).

14

Antimicrobial use over a four-year period using days of therapy measurement at a Canadian pediatric acute care hospital

Bruce R Dalton BScPhm PharmD[1,2], Sandra J MacTavish MSc[1,3], Lauren C Bresee BScPharm ACPR MSc PhD[1,3,4], Nipunie Rajapakse MD[5,6,7], Otto Vanderkooi MD[5,6,7], Joseph Vayalumkal MD[5,6,7], John Conly MD[7,8,9,10]

BR Dalton, SJ MacTavish, LC Bresee, et al. Antimicrobial use over a four-year period using days of therapy measurement at a Canadian pediatric acute care hospital. Can J Infect Dis Med Microbiol 2015;26(5):253-258.

BACKGROUND: Antimicrobial resistance is a concern that is challenging the ability to treat common infections. Surveillance of antimicrobial use in pediatric acute care institutions is complicated because the common metric unit, the defined daily dose, is problematic for this population.

OBJECTIVE: During a four-year period in which no specific antimicrobial stewardship initiatives were conducted, pediatric antimicrobial use was quantified using days of therapy (DOT) per 100 patient days (PD) (DOT/100 PD) at the Alberta Children's Hospital (Calgary, Alberta) for benchmarking purposes.

METHODS: Drug use data for systemic antimicrobials administered on wards at the Alberta Children's Hospital were collected from electronic medication administration records. DOT were calculated and rates were determined using 100 PD as the denominator. Changes over the surveillance period and subgroup proportions were represented graphically and assessed using linear regression.

RESULTS: Total antimicrobial use decreased from 93.6 DOT/100 PD to 75.7 DOT/100 PD (19.1%) over the 2010/2011 through to the 2013/2014 fiscal years. During this period, a 20.0% increase in PD and an essentially stable absolute count of DOT (2.9% decrease) were observed. Overall, antimicrobial use was highest in the pediatric intensive care and oncology units.

DISCUSSION: The exact changes in prescribing patterns that led to the observed reduction in DOT/100 PD with associated increased PD are unclear, but may be a topic for future investigations.

CONCLUSION: Antimicrobial use data from a Canadian acute care pediatric hospital reported in DOT/100 PD were compiled for a four-year time period. These data may be useful for benchmarking purposes.

Key Words: *Antimicrobial stewardship; Antimicrobial use; Days of therapy; Pediatric; Surveillance*

L'utilisation d'antimicrobiens sur une période de quatre ans mesurée d'après les jours de traitement dans un hôpital pédiatrique canadien de soins aigus

HISTORIQUE : La résistance aux antimicrobiens nuit à la capacité de traiter les infections courantes. Il est difficile de surveiller l'utilisation d'antimicrobiens dans les établissements de soins aigus en pédiatrie, parce qu'il est difficile d'établir l'unité métrique habituelle, qui est la dose quotidienne définie, au sein de cette population.

OBJECTIF : Après quatre ans sans initiative de gérance des antimicrobiens précise, les chercheurs ont quantifié l'utilisation des antimicrobiens pédiatriques au moyen des jours de traitement (JdT) par 100 jours-patients (JP) (JdT/100 JP) à l'*Alberta Children's Hospital* de Calgary en vue d'une analyse comparative.

MÉTHODOLOGIE : À partir des dossiers électroniques sur l'administration des médicaments, les chercheurs ont colligé les données sur l'utilisation des antimicrobiens systémiques administrés dans les services de l'*Alberta Children's Hospital*. Ils ont calculé les JdT et déterminé les taux à l'aide du dénominateur 100 JP. Ils ont représenté graphiquement les changements pendant la période de surveillance et les proportions des sous-groupes et les ont évalués à l'aide de la régression linéaire.

RÉSULTATS : L'utilisation totale d'antimicrobiens a reculé de 93,6 JdT/100 JP à 75,7 JdT/100 JP (19,1 %) entre les exercices 2010-2011 et 2013-2014. Pendant cette période, les chercheurs ont observé une augmentation de 20,0 % des JP et une numération absolue de JdT pratiquement stable (diminution de 2,9 %). Dans l'ensemble, l'utilisation d'antimicrobiens était plus élevée dans les unités pédiatriques de soins intensifs et d'oncologie.

EXPOSÉ : On ne sait pas exactement quels changements aux profils de prescription ont donné lieu à la réduction observée de JdT/100 JP et à l'augmentation connexe de JP, mais cette question pourrait faire l'objet de prochaines recherches.

CONCLUSION : Pendant quatre ans, les chercheurs ont compilé les données sur l'utilisation d'antimicrobiens en JdT/100 JP dans un hôpital pédiatrique canadien de soins aigus. Ces données peuvent être utiles dans une analyse comparative.

A ntimicrobial resistance is a global public health threat that increasingly challenges our ability to prevent and treat infections (1-4). Infections with multiple drug-resistant organisms have been shown to result in increased mortality, morbidity and reduced quality of life (1,2). The lack of development of new antimicrobials to replace the older ineffective agents has made antimicrobial resistance an urgent situation (2). To assess antimicrobial stewardship initiatives, baseline measurement of antimicrobial use is required. Defined daily doses are commonly used to assess antimicrobial use in adult medicine but is based on adult dosing and, therefore, is problematic for assessment in pediatric

[1]*Department of Pharmacy Services, Alberta Health Services, Calgary;* [2]*O'Brien Institute of Public Health, Cumming School of Medicine, University of Calgary, Calgary, Alberta;* [3]*School of Pharmacy, University of Waterloo, Waterloo, Ontario;* [4]*Department of Community Health Sciences, Cumming School of Medicine;* [5]*Department of Pediatrics, Section of Infectious Diseases;* [6]*Department of Medicine, Cumming School of Medicine, University of Calgary;* [7]*Alberta Children's Hospital Research Institute, Alberta Health Services;* [8]*Department of Pathology and Laboratory Medicine, Cumming School of Medicine;* [9]*Synder Institute for Chronic Diseases;* [10]*Department of Microbiology, Immunology and Infectious Diseases, Cumming School of Medicine, University of Calgary, Calgary, Alberta*
Correspondence: Dr Bruce R Dalton, Department of Pharmacy Services, Foothills Medical Centre, 1403-29th Street Northwest, Calgary, Alberta T2N 2T9. e-mail bruce.dalton@albertahealthservices.ca

populations (5). The WHO International Working Group for Drug Statistics Methodology do not recommend that defined daily doses be used in assessment of antimicrobial use in pediatrics (6,7). In children, the days of therapy (DOT) measurement is preferred for measuring antibiotic use because it is independent of age- and weight-related differences in doses (6). The DOT unit of measure is defined as one day in which a patient is given a drug, regardless of dose (6). The ability to quantify pediatric antimicrobial use through DOT measurements provides a value that is numerically comparable with adult antibiotic use, more applicable to a variety of populations and is less likely to be affected by different dosing schemes (6,8).

The objectives of the present study were to initiate antimicrobial surveillance at the Alberta Children's Hospital (ACH; Calgary, Alberta) over a four-year period, to quantify pediatric antimicrobial use and to provide a basic descriptive epidemiological analysis of our data. There are few published data available regarding Canadian antimicrobial use in pediatric acute care settings. The present study provides an overview of systemic antibacterial (J01) and antifungal (J02) use according to ward at the ACH, covering fiscal years (April through March) from April 2010 to March 2014.

METHODS
Setting
The ACH is an acute care tertiary pediatric centre located in Calgary, Alberta. A new structure opened in 2007 that included units for oncology/hematology/bone marrow transplants, pediatric intensive care, neonatal intensive care, day surgery and mental health, as well as three general medicine/surgery units. The present investigation quantified antimicrobial use over a 51-month period from January 2010 to March 2014. During the study period, the total number of inpatient beds available were 125 in January 2010 and 141 in March 2014. Wards increasing their capacity included general medicine/surgery (increased by two beds), neonatal intensive care (increased by six beds) and pediatric intensive care (increased by eight beds). Sunrise Clinical Manager version 5.8 (Eclipsys Corporation, USA) was introduced for use in 2009, featuring electronic prescribing, patient care management, laboratory and diagnostic imaging results, and electronic medication administration records (eMAR), for all patients admitted to the ACH. Tools for antimicrobial stewardship, such as pediatric antimicrobial reference cards, were provided to prescribers and other health care professionals, but no specific interventional initiatives had been conducted in recent years. There were no notable formulary changes in high-use agents during the study period.

Data collection
Drug use data for all provincial inpatient formulary systemic antibacterial and systemic antifungal medications administered on wards at the ACH were collected from the Sunrise Clinical Manager eMAR system, which was used by nursing staff to record the details of administration of each dose of medication. Patient days (PD) data were collected from the Data Integration Measurement and Reporting unit of Alberta Health Services, who collects and provides health care statistics for Alberta Health Services facilities. Preoperative antimicrobial prophylaxis given in the operating room may not be captured electronically and, therefore, was excluded from analysis. Antibiotics given in the emergency department and ambulatory clinics were also excluded from the present study.

Drug classification
Drugs were classified based on the WHO anatomical therapeutic chemical classifications, and systemic antibacterial and antifungal agents were included and reported as the sum of those two groups and separately. Agents were grouped into clinically relevant drug categories, derived by consensus of the Calgary Zone Antimicrobial Stewardship Committee (CASC) as follows: broad-spectrum Gram-negative active agents (BGNA) that included piperacillin/tazobactam, carbapenems and ticarcillin/clavulanate; Gram-positive antimicrobial-resistant organism

active agents that included vancomycin, linezolid, tigecycline and daptomycin; narrow-spectrum agents that included first-generation cephalosporins, ampicillin, amoxicillin, penicillin G, penicillin V, cloxacillin and aminoglycosides; and second- to fifth-generation cephalosporins. Agents not included in any of the above categories were included as 'unclassified' antibacterial agents.

Units of measure
Antimicrobial use was measured in DOT for antimicrobials signed off on eMAR, consistent with methods previously described (5,6,8). If a single patient received two different antimicrobial agents within one day, it counted as two DOT (5). The rate of antimicrobial use was expressed as DOT/100 PD, consistent with Canadian recommendations for expressing antimicrobial use (9). DOT were assigned to a ward based on the location of the patient at the time of the first administration of the antimicrobial during each 24 h period. Centrality and dispersion of reported means and standard deviations for site-level use were determined using Microsoft Excel 2010 (Microsoft Corporation, USA). Percentage changes were expressed in terms of use rate relative to the baseline (2011 fiscal year) for all agents and wards. Hospital-level use was analyzed in terms of measures for total antimicrobials (DOT and DOT/100 PD) and the hospital capacity measure PD against time (fiscal period) using ordinary least squares regression for the period of April 2010 to March 2014 and reported Pearson correlation. P<0.05 was considered to be statistically significant. Three months of data were excluded to capture seasonal variations equitably. SPSS version 19 (IBM Corporation, USA) was used for calculation of correlation coefficients. Proportion of each drug class measured was expressed as percentage of total.

Ethical considerations
The A pRoject Ethics Community Consensus Initiative (ARECCI) ethics screening tool (10) was completed to assess the ethical risk to study participants and whether a review through a research ethics board was necessary. The assessment tool included consideration of the positions of the individuals processing the data (in the present case, a staff member and a summer student). The present project was deemed to be a quality improvement project with 'minimal risk' to participants and, as a result, ethics approval was deemed to be unnecessary. The ARECCI ethics guidelines for quality improvement and evaluation projects were used to guide the present project.

RESULTS
Data from ACH eMARs showed a steady decrease in antimicrobial use at the ACH over the 2011 to 2014 fiscal years (Figure 1A.) Total antimicrobial use decreased from 93.6 DOT/100 PD to 75.7 DOT/100 PD (19.1% decrease over the four years [Table 1]). This decrease was reciprocally associated with a change in PDs (increase by 20.0%, Figure 1B.), but change in absolute number of DOT was minor (−2.9%) (Figure 1C). In terms of administration, the majority of antimicrobials were given parenterally (73.6% to 75.3%). Oral antimicrobial use accounted for 23.1% to 25.0% of total antimicrobial use each year and inhaled antimicrobials represented <1% of DOT for all years.

The percent change in individual antimicrobial use at the ACH over the four-year period was determined and reported along with antimicrobial use for each fiscal year (Table 1). A decline in the use of most individual agents was observed during the study period, with a few notable exceptions. These exceptions included oral amoxicillin/clavulanate (35.5% increase), amoxicillin (29.8% increase), parenteral ceftriaxone (66.9% increase), as well as several other agents of which use did not exceed 1 DOT/100 PD (Table 1). Agents from each of the CASC-derived categories decreased in use from 2011 to 2014 and were numerically dominated by one or two agents. Specifically, the BGNA group decreased by 24.1% and piperacillin/tazobactam accounted for 68.6% of the use. Vancomycin was dominant in the Gram-positive antimicrobial-resistant active agents group, accounting for 95.1% of the group, and the use of this group decreased by 35.7%.

The use of narrow-spectrum agents decreased by 16.4% and ampicillin and cefazolin made up 55.0% of the category. Cefotaxime and ceftriaxone accounted for 77.9% of the second- to fifth-generation cephalosprins group, which declined by 26.8% over four years. Fluconazole was the antifungal with the highest mean use of 4.17 DOT/100 PD, accounting for 74.9% of antifungal use (Table 1). The decrease in use of systemic antibacterials unclassified in the system was 18.2% and systemic antifungal agents fell from 5.9 DOT/100 PD to 4.8 DOT/100 PD from 2011 to 2013, but increased again in 2014 to 6.0 DOT/100 PD (Table 1).

Individual ward use summaries for 2014, 2011 to 2014 change and proportion of each CASC-derived drug category are presented in Table 2. Different patterns of both types and amounts of anti-infectives used on various wards were observed. The pediatric intensive care unit had the highest antimicrobial mean (± SD) use of 129.9±6.1 DOT/100 PD, of which narrow-spectrum agents were the largest portion. In addition, relative to medical/surgical units, there was a higher portion of BGNA (17.3% versus 4.2% to 6.1%) and Gram-positive antimicrobial-resistant active agents (16.1% versus 3.6% to 8.8%) use on the pediatric intensive care unit. The oncology ward also experienced a very high use of total antibacterial and antifungal drugs (mean 120.7±13.5 DOT/100 PD), which decreased by 17.4% over the four years of surveillance and was notable for high use of antifungal agents (27.9%).

DISCUSSION

A 19.1% decrease in the rate of DOT/100 PD over a four-year period was observed. Awareness of the directions of trends is valuable for those initiating new antimicrobial stewardship initiatives because evaluations of these programs should consider trends that are already occurring. We observed an associated increase in PDs by 20% with little change in absolute DOT count (Figures 1B and 1C, Table 2). However, the knowledge that the denominator of the rate of antimicrobial use changed while the numerator was static does not provide extensive insight into prescribing patterns, the quality of antimicrobial use or the infectious acuity of the patients. Investigations to determine whether changes in the number of admissions receiving antimicrobials or whether the length of therapy on antimicrobials occurred are potential areas of further inquiry.

Internally, in our institution, a categorization scheme of antimicrobial agents that groups agents that may have common therapeutic use together (eg, broad-spectrum Gram-negative activity) was developed because traditional classification schemes heavily rely on the chemical structure, which may have less relevance for antimicrobial use surveillance. It is recognized that there are agents that are used to a significant degree that have not been added into a category; however, it was believed that these would be better left unclassified, as opposed to being included in a category that would, therefore, become less specific. For example, had amoxicillin/clavulanate been added to the BGNA group, this would broaden the therapeutic indications that the group covers. In all four CASC-derived antibacterial drug categories, there was a decrease in rate of antimicrobial use by 16.5% to 35.7% from the 2011 to 2014 fiscal years (Table 1). Among individual agents, there were a few increases in rate of use, such as with ceftriaxone, (2.68 DOT/100 PD to 4.48 DOT/100 PD, 66.9%) (Table 1). We are unclear on the reasons for these observed rate increases; however, in the case of ceftriaxone, most of the increase in use rate occurred during the 2010/2011 fiscal year (2.68 DOT/100 PD to 4.12 DOT/100 PD; 51.8%). The change observed may reflect a shift from the use of cefotaxime to ceftriaxone because both are third-generation cephalosporins with similar spectrum of activity. Over the period of observation, the total rate of the two agents decreased by 15.4% (11.00 DOT/100 PD to 9.26 DOT/100 PD).

The data revealed that the highest antibacterial and antifungal use took place in the pediatric intensive care unit, where the four-year mean value was 129.9 DOT/100 PD. The hematology-oncology

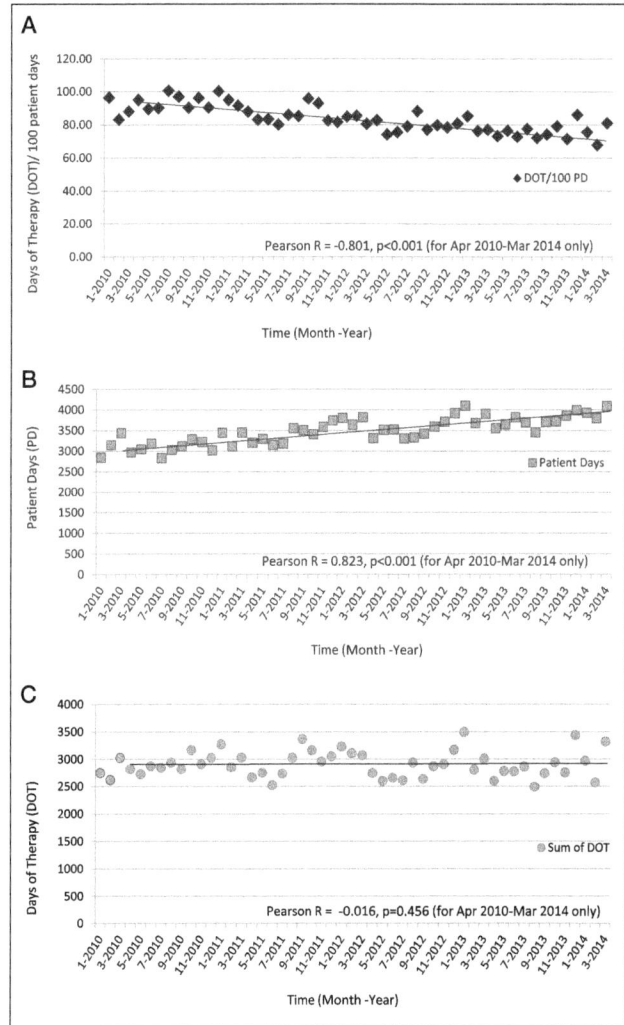

Figure 1) *Alberta Children's Hospital (ACH, Calgary, Alberta) systemic antibacterial and antifungal use according to year and month, mean (± SD) (83.49±8.14 days of therapy [DOT]/100 patient days [PD]) (**A**); ACH PD (denominator of the data in Figure 1A), mean 3502.27±315.92 PD (**B**); ACH systemic antibacterial and antifungal use according to year and month (numerator of the data in Figure 1A), mean 2908.33±240.49 DOT (**C**); Period from from January 2010 to April 2014; Regression line and descriptive statistics calculated from April 2010 to March 2014 (see text for explanation)*

ward had lower overall use than the pediatric intensive care unit and a greater use of antifungals. This high use of anti-infectives is not surprising because bacterial and fungal infections are common in these two patient populations (11,12).

It is difficult to compare antimicrobial use at one institution with another because of differences in patient populations and because there are limited published data. Five relevant recent studies using DOT to quantify antimicrobial use in pediatric acute care centres (13-16) or the pediatric patient population in acute care general hospitals (6) were identified. Study population, specific antimicrobials reported and changes over time of the reports are detailed in Table 3, along with results of our surveillance (on systemic antimicrobials) for comparison. Cited references reported DOT/1000 PD; therefore, we converted their results to DOT/100 PD to ease comparison. Others have noted reductions in overall antimicrobial use assessed by DOT/100 PD (15), but have not reported on the change in either absolute count of DOT or PDs, which may be useful dimensions for assessment of the success of antimicrobial stewardship initiatives.

TABLE 1
Antimicrobial use according to days of therapy per 100 patient days and fiscal year (month of year end)

	Anatomical therapeutic chemical code	Year				2011–2014 change in use, %	Proportion of agent in group (all years), %
		2011	2012	2013	2014		
All systemic antibacterials (J01) and antifungals (J02)		93.56	85.10	79.54	75.71	−19.1	
Broad-spectrum Gram-negative agents*		9.97	8.70	8.35	7.57	−24.1	–
Ertapenem	J01DH03	0.14	0.17	0.24	0.11	−16.7	1.9
Meropenem	J01DH02	3.41	2.38	2.64	1.76	−48.5	29.5
Piperacillin/tazobactam	J01CR05	6.41	6.16	5.46	5.68	−11.5	68.6
Gram-positive antimicrobial-resistant organism active agents*		8.69	7.96	6.82	5.59	−35.7	–
Linezolid	J01XX08	0.21	0.25	0.67	0.25	17.7	4.8
Vancomycin	A07AA09 (O) J01XA01 (P)	8.48	7.71	6.10	5.34	−37.0	95.1
Narrow-spectrum agents*		29.37	26.17	25.57	24.54	−16.4	–
Amoxicillin	J01CA04	2.00	1.67	2.48	2.60	29.8	8.3
Ampicillin	J01CA01	6.67	5.60	5.53	5.88	−11.9	22.4
Cefazolin	J01DB04	8.67	8.70	8.51	8.57	−1.2	32.6
Cephalexin	J01DB01	1.16	1.50	1.36	1.08	−6.7	4.8
Cloxacillin	J01CF02	1.25	0.72	0.62	0.48	−61.5	2.9
Gentamicin	J01GB03	5.74	5.05	3.81	3.56	−38.0	17.2
Penicillin G sodium	J01CE01	0.71	0.66	0.59	0.37	−48.3	2.2
Penicillin V potassium	J01CE02	0.51	0.30	0.60	0.32	−37.0	1.6
Tobramycin	J01GB01	2.58	1.96	2.04	1.56	−39.5	7.7
Second- to fifth-generation cephalosporins*		16.04	14.06	12.74	11.73	−26.8	–
Cefepime	J01DE01	0.02	0.02	0.10	0.67	3519.0	1.5
Cefixime	J01DD00	0.28	0.32	0.18	0.21	−23.7	1.8
Cefotaxime	J01DD01	9.32	6.78	6.33	4.78	−48.8	49.9
Cefprozil	J01DC10	0.91	0.70	0.28	0.19	−79.7	3.8
Ceftazidime	J01DD02	1.54	1.28	1.15	1.16	−24.8	9.4
Ceftriaxone	J01DD04	2.68	4.12	4.01	4.48	66.9	28.0
Cefuroxime	J01DC02	1.24	0.79	0.65	0.23	−81.7	5.3
Other systemic antibacterials		21.64	21.31	19.14	17.70	−18.2	–
Amoxicillin/clavulanate	J01CR02	1.35	1.40	1.65	1.83	35.5	7.8
Ciprofloxacin	J01MA02	2.22	2.53	1.91	1.71	−23.1	10.5
Clarithromycin	J01FA09	0.77	0.64	0.31	0.20	−74.2	2.4
Clindamycin	J01FF01	2.89	2.77	2.38	2.01	−30.4	12.6
Colistin	J01XB01	0.12	0.10	0.01	0.03	−75.2	0.3
Erythromycin	J01FA01	0.62	0.20	0.06	0.23	−63.4	1.4
Levofloxacin	J01MA12	0.68	0.46	0.48	0.61	−10.5	2.8
Metronidazole	J01XD01	7.90	8.53	7.63	7.12	−10.0	39.1
Nitrofurantoin	J01XE01	0.50	0.45	0.42	0.34	−31.9	2.1
Piperacillin	J01CA12	0.05	0.00	0.01	0.00	−100.0	0.1
Sulfamethoxazole/trimethoprim	J01EE01	4.18	3.89	3.78	3.47	−17.0	19.2
Tetracycline	J01AA07	0.05	0.00	0.04	0.00	−100.0	0.1
Trimethoprim	J01EA01	0.30	0.32	0.46	0.15	−49.4	1.5
Systemic antifungals		5.95	5.38	4.80	6.02	1.3	–
Amphotericin B	J02AA01	0.03	0.00	0.05	0.08	143.6	0.8
Amphotericin B liposomal	J02AA01-lipid	0.23	0.15	0.69	0.24	2.5	5.9
Caspofungin	J02AX04	0.16	0.00	0.01	0.00	−100.0	0.8
Fluconazole	J02AC01	4.99	4.39	3.06	4.17	−16.5	74.9
Itraconazole	J02AC02	0.03	0.00	0.00	0.24	592.3	1.2
Micafungin	J02AX05	0.03	0.22	0.61	0.46	1330.6	6.0
Posaconazole	J02AC04	0.00	0.01	0.00	0.00	NA	0.1
Voriconazole	J02AC03	0.47	0.61	0.39	0.84	79.5	10.4

*No daptomycin, fifth-generation cephalosporin, imipenem/cilastatin, ticarcillin/clavulanate, penicillin G benzathine or posaconazole use occurred during the study period; Cefoxitin had 0.1 days of therapy per 100 patient days in 2012; Tigecycline and amikacin each had 0.1 days of therapy per 100 patient days in 2013; Streptomycin had 0.1 days of therapy per 100 patient days in 2014. J01 Systemic antimicrobial agents-WHO anatomical therapeutic chemical classification; J02 Systemic antifungal agents-WHO anatomical therapeutic chemical classification. Refer to methods section for further explanation. NA Not available; O Oral, P parenteral

TABLE 2
Antimicrobial use according to ward type

| | 2011–2014 | | Proportion of ward or hospital total in fiscal year 2014, % | | | | | |
Ward	2014 total DOT/100 PD (all J01 & J02 agents)	change in use (%)	BGNA	GPAA	NSA	SFGC	Other J01	J02
Whole hospital	71.1	−20.2	10.4	7.3	32.1	14.6	27.2	8.5
Medical/surgical units 1–3	70.0	−21.8	5.0	6.3	38.6	17.1	30.2	2.7
Oncology/bone marrow transplant	112.2	−17.4	22.5	4.0	10.2	6.3	26.6	30.5
Pediatric intensive care unit	129.8	−5.4	17.3	16.1	24.0	19.4	19.4	3.9
Neonatal intensive care unit	62.1	−11.2*	13.3	13.3	43.1	12.5	12.7	5.0
Mental health	3.1	32.2	0.0	0.0	13.3	0.0	86.7	0.0
Day surgery	60.4	11.3	0.8	0.3	73.4	2.0	23.5	0.0

Neonatal intensive care unit change in rate from 2012 (first complete fiscal year) to 2014; Year designation refers to fiscal year (April–March) year-end month. BGNA Broad-spectrum Gram-negative active agents; DOT/100 PD Days of therapy per 100 patient days; ICU Intensive care unit; J01 Systemic antimicrobial agents-WHO anatomical therapeutic chemical classification; J02 Systemic antifungal agents-WHO anatomical therapeutic chemical classification; GPAA Gram-positive antimicrobial-resistant organism active agents; NSA Narrow-spectrum agents; SFGC Second- to fifth-generation cephalosporins. Refer to methods section for further explanation

TABLE 3
Other studies reporting inpatient pediatric antimicrobial use

Reference	Years of surveillance	Patient population	Antibiotics reported	Range reported (DOT/100 PD)*	Change over years
6	2002–2007	Pediatric population in general acute care centres in the United States	J01	53.7–56.0	None
13	2007–2010	One acute pediatric centre in the United States located within a larger adult hospital	J01, J02 and J05	72.9–81.5	Increase in broad-spectrum agents; decrease in narrow-spectrum agents
14	2010	Specific high-use disease groups including cystic fibrosis, other patients with pneumonia, skin and soft tissue infections, or an appendectomy in a network of freestanding children's hospitals in the United States	J01	69.8	NA
15,16	2004–2014	Network of freestanding children's hospitals in the United States	J01	60.0-83	Decrease
Present study	2011–2014	One freestanding pediatric hospital in Canada	J01	67.1–85.7	Decrease

Range reported: antimicrobial total use from each reference was converted into days of therapy per 100 patient days (DOT/100 PD) to compare with the Alberta Children's Hospital data. J01 Systemic antibacterial agents-WHO anatomical therapeutic chemical classification; J02 Systemic antifungal agents-WHO anatomical therapeutic chemical classification; J05 Systemic antiviral agents-WHO anatomical therapeutic chemical classification; NA Not available

The present report established a baseline of antimicrobial use at the ACH for future reference and may be useful to other pediatric institutions in Canada. We acknowledge that the present study has limitations. We did not evaluate the use of agents in terms of appropriateness of the therapy or their use as treatment versus prophylaxis. Antimicrobial use intensity may drive the development of resistance, regardless of the appropriateness of the therapy for an individual patient and, therefore, is an accepted metric for antimicrobial resistance surveillance purposes (17,18). Some data were excluded because the location at the time of administration of the antimicrobial was missing; however, these were few and unlikely to significantly alter our results. Perioperative doses are commonly given in the operating theatre, where it is uncommon practice to record their administration on the eMAR. Depending on the procedure, surgical patients may also receive doses of the same prophylactic agent postoperatively outside of the operating theatre on the same day and a DOT would be assigned to the patients; therefore, we believe this limitation to be minor. There is occasional nonformulary antimicrobial use at ACH that was not captured in the eMAR data, but the provincial inpatient formulary is mostly inclusive of systemic antibacterials and systemic antifungals because of the diverse populations the formulary serves. The possibility exists that some doses signed off by nurses were subsequently not administered to the patient, but equally, there is the possibility of doses having

been given but not signed off. We do not have data to assess these possibilities at this time but believe that if such events occur they are infrequent and would not change our findings to a clinically relevant degree. We believe that the eMAR is a better source of data than pharmacy dispensing systems, and have previously observed a 20% greater antimicrobial drug use with pharmacy dispensing system data versus eMAR data using the same metric units (19). In addition, a simple linear regression of the monthly data points of total antimicrobial use without adjustment for seasonality was performed. So that one season was not over-represented, we only used the latter entire four-year period of the total 51 months of observation in calculation of regression coefficient and summary statistics and excluded data for three months. Without a seasonal variable fitted to our model, prediction of use in a specific future month(s) may not be accurate; however, we do not intend that this model be used for that purpose. Despite these limitations, the strengths of the present report include the use of DOT as a primary metric, which is more appropriate for pediatric patients than the WHO-recommended anatomical therapeutic chemical per defined daily dose system, which uses a standardized adult dose that is not applicable given the weight-based dosing regimens used in children.

In conclusion, we believe surveillance of antimicrobial use is an integral part of antimicrobial stewardship. In the pediatric acute care setting, there have been only a few published surveillance projects using utilization metrics appropriate for this population but the need for such information in this unique patient population is as important as in the adult population. Our results contribute to this literature and demonstrate the importance of ongoing antimicrobial use surveillance in a pediatric population.

ACKNOWLEDGEMENTS: The authors gratefully acknowledge the contribution of Kevin Lonergan, who extracted data from the Sunrise Clinical Manager eMAR system for analysis.

REFERENCES

1. World Health Organization. Antimicrobial resistance fact sheet N° 194. <www.who.int/mediacentre/factsheets/fs194/en/> (Accessed June 3, 2014).
2. World Health Organization. Antimicrobial resistance global report on surveillance. <http://apps.who.int/iris/bitstream/10665/112642/1/9789241564748_eng.pdf?ua=1> (Accessed June 25, 2014).
3. Centers for Disease Control and Prevention. Antibiotic resistance threats in the United States, 2013. <www.cdc.gov/drugresistance/threat-report-2013/pdf/ar-threats-2013-508.pdf> (Accessed December 15, 2014).
4. Public Health Agency of Canada. Antimicrobial resistance and use in Canada: A federal framework for action. <http://healthycanadians.gc.ca/alt/pdf/drugs-products-medicaments-produits/antibiotic-resistance-antibiotique/antimicrobial-framework-cadre-antimicrobiens-eng.pdf> (Accessed December 15, 2014).
5. Polk RE, Fox C, Mahoney A, Letcavage J, MacDougall C. Measurement of adult antibacterial drug use in 130 US hospitals: Comparison of defined daily dose and days of therapy. Clin Infect Dis 2007;44:664-70.
6. Pakyz AL, Gurgle HE, Ibrahim OM, Oinonen MJ, Polk RE. Trends in antibacterial use in hospitalized pediatric patients in United States academic health centers. Infect Control Hosp Epidemiol 2009;30:600-3.
7. WHO Collaborating Centre for Drug Statistics Methodology. Guidelines for ATC classification and DDD assignment 2014. <www.whocc.no/filearchive/publications/2014_guidelines.pdf> (Accessed June 25, 2014).
8. Kubin CJ, Jia H, Alba LR, Yoko Furuya E. Lack of significant variability among different methods for calculating antimicrobial days of therapy. Infect Control Hosp Epidemiol 2012;33:421-3.
9. Hutchinson JM, Patrick DM, Marra F, et al. Measurement of antibiotic consumption: A practical guide to the use of the anatomical therapeutic chemical classification and defined daily dose system methodology in Canada. Can J Infect Dis Med Microbiol 2004;15:29-35.
10. Alberta Innovates Health Solutions. ARECCI Tool. <www.aihealthsolutions.ca/arecci/screening/55035/af524cd22bdf1743ecbd0fdd5f43766f> (Accessed December 4, 2014).
11. Arnold C. Decreasing antibiotic overuse in neonatal intensive care units: Quality improvement research. Proc (Bayl Univ Med Cent) 2005;18:280-4.
12. Cecinati V, Principi N, Brescia L, Esposito S. Antibiotic prophylaxis in children with cancer or who have undergone hematopoietic cell transplantation. Eur J Clin Microbiol Infect Dis 2014;33:1-6.
13. Levy ER, Swami S, Dubois SG, Wendt R, Banerjee R. Rates and appropriateness of antimicrobial prescribing at an academic children's hospital, 2007-2010. Infect Control Hosp Epidemiol 2012;33:346-53.
14. Gerber JS, Kronman MP, Ross RK, et al. Identifying targets for antimicrobial stewardship in children's hospitals. Infect Control Hosp Epidemiol 2013;34:1252-8.
15. Hersh AL, De Lurgio SA, Thurm C, et al. Antimicrobial stewardship programs in freestanding children's hospitals. Pediatrics 2015;135:33-9.
16. Hersh AL, Beekmann SE, Polgreen PM, Zaoutis TE, Newland JG. Antimicrobial stewardship programs in pediatrics. Infect Control Hops Epidemiol 2009;30:1211-17.
17. Dellit TH, Owens RC, McGowan JE Jr, et al. Infectious Diseases Society of America and the Society for Healthcare Epidemiology of America. Guidelines for developing an institutional program to enhance antimicrobial stewardship. Clin Infect Dis 2007;44:159-77.
18. Ganguly NK, Arora NK, Chandy SJ, et al. Rationalizing antibiotic use to limit antibiotic resistance in India. Indian J Med Res 2011;134:281-94.
19. Dalton BR, Sabuda DM, Bresee LC, Conly JM. Assessment of antimicrobial metrics; days of therapy versus defined daily doses and pharmacy dispensing records versus nursing administration data. Infect Control Hosp Epidemiol 2015;36:688-94.

15

Antimicrobial susceptibility of Canadian isolates of *Helicobacter pylori* in Northeastern Ontario

Nelson F Eng PhD[1], Gustavo Ybazeta PhD[1], Katrina Chapman BSc[1], Nya L Fraleigh MSc[1], Rebecca Letto MSc[1],
Eleonora Altman PhD[2], Francisco Diaz-Mitoma MD PhD[1]

NF Eng, G Ybazeta, K Chapman, et al. Antimicrobial susceptibility of Canadian isolates of *Helicobacter pylori* in Northeastern Ontario. Can J Infect Dis Med Microbiol 2015;26(3):137-144.

BACKGROUND: *Helicobacter pylori* plays a significant role in gastritis and ulcers. It is a carcinogen as defined by the WHO, and infection can result in adenocarcinomas and mucosa-associated lymphoid tissue lymphomas. In Canada, rates of antimicrobial resistance are relatively unknown, with very few studies conducted in the past 15 years.
OBJECTIVE: To examine rates of resistance in Sudbury, Ontario, compare antimicrobial susceptibility methods and attempt to determine the molecular basis of antibiotic resistance.
METHODS: Patients attending scheduled visits at Health Sciences North (Sudbury, Ontario) provided gastric biopsy samples on a volunteer basis. In total, 20 *H pylori* isolates were collected, and antimicrobial susceptibility testing (on amoxicillin, tetracycline, metronidazole, ciprofloxacin, levofloxacin and clarithromycin) was conducted using disk diffusion and E-test methods. Subsequently, genomic DNA from these isolates was sequenced to detect mutations associated with antimicrobial resistance.
RESULTS: Sixty-five percent of the isolates were found to be resistant to at least one of the listed antibiotics according to E-test. Three isolates were found to be resistant to ≥3 of the above-mentioned antibiotics. Notably, 25% of the isolates were found to be resistant to both metronidazole and clarithromycin, two antibiotics that are normally prescribed as part of first-line regimens in the treatment of *H pylori* infections in Canada and most of the world. Among the resistant strains, the sequences of 23S ribosomal RNA and *gyrA*, which are linked to clarithromycin and ciprofloxacin/levofloxacin resistance, respectively, revealed the presence of known point mutations associated with antimicrobial resistance.
CONCLUSIONS: In general, resistance to metronidazole, ciprofloxacin/levofloxacin and clarithromycin has increased since the studies in the early 2000s. These results suggest that surveillance programs of *H pylori* antibiotic resistance may need to be revisited or improved to prevent antimicrobial therapy failure.

Key Words: *Antimicrobial susceptibility*; Helicobacter pylori; *Northern Ontario; Resistance*

La susceptibilité antimicrobienne d'isolats canadiens d'*Helicobacter pylori* au nord-est de l'Ontario

HISTORIQUE : L'*Helicobacter pylori* contribue énormément à la gastrite et aux ulcères. L'OMS le définit comme un cancérigène, et l'infection peut provoquer l'apparition d'adénocarcinomes et de lymphomes de tissus lymphoïdes associés aux muqueuses. Au Canada, on connaît relativement peu les taux de résistance antimicrobienne, car très peu d'études ont été réalisées sur le sujet depuis 15 ans.
OBJECTIF : Examiner les taux de résistance à Sudbury, en Ontario, comparer les méthodes de susceptibilité antimicrobienne et tenter de déterminer le fondement biologique de la résistance antibiotique.
MÉTHODOLOGIE : Les patients qui allaient à un rendez-vous prévu au *Health Sciences North* de Sudbury ont remis les résultats de biopsies gastriques sur une base volontaire. Au total, 20 isolats de *H pylori* ont été recueillis, et les tests de susceptibilité antimicrobienne (à l'amoxicilline, à la tétracycline, au métronidazole, à la ciprofloxacine, à la lévofloxacine et à la clarithromycine) ont été effectués au moyen de la diffusion sur disque et de l'essai E. L'ADN génomique de ces isolats a ensuite été séquencé pour déceler les mutations associées à la résistance antimicrobienne.
RÉSULTATS : Selon l'essai E, 65 % des isolats étaient résistants à au moins un des antibiotiques énumérés. Notamment, 25 % des isolats étaient résistants à la fois au métronidazole et à la clarithromycine, tous deux normalement prescrits en première ligne pour traiter les infections à *H pylori* au Canada et dans la plupart des régions du monde. Parmi les souches résistantes, les séquences d'ARN ribosomique 23S et de *gyrA*, qui sont liées à la résistance à la clarithromycine et à la ciprofloxacine-lévofloxacine, respectivement, révélaient la présence de mutations de points connus associés à une résistance antimicrobienne.
CONCLUSIONS : En général, la résistance au métronidazole, à la ciprofloxacine-lévofloxacine et à la clarithromycine a augmenté depuis les études réalisées au début des années 2000. D'après ces résultats, il faudra peut-être revoir ou améliorer les programmes de surveillance de l'antibiorésistance au *H pylori* pour prévenir l'échec du traitement antimicrobien.

*H*elicobacter pylori is a bacterial human pathogen that preferentially colonizes the stomach and is found in 50% of the world's population, causing dyspepsia, gastritis and peptic ulcers (1). The WHO has classified this organism as a class I carcinogen that can cause stomach cancers, which, after diagnosis, has only a 27% survival rate (2-4). In Canada, the prevalence of *H pylori* is approximately 20% to 30% (5,6). However, in developing countries, rates can be as high as 80% (7). As of 2007, the incidence in the province of Ontario was approximately 23%, with men twice as likely to be infected as women (29.4% versus 14.9%) (5). Infection is strongly correlated with crowding, smoking, diet and poor sanitation (8-11). Unfortunately, such conditions exist within the most vulnerable populations in Canada; specifically, some First Nations communities have demonstrated rates as high as 95% (12).

[1]*Advanced Medical Research Institute of Canada, Sudbury;* [2]*National Research Council of Canada, Ottawa, Ontario*
Correspondence: Dr Francisco Diaz-Mitoma, Advanced Medical Research Institute of Canada, 41 Ramsey Lake Road, Sudbury, Ontario P3E 5J1.
e-mail fdiazmitoma@amric.ca

Eradication of *H pylori* is dependent on successful treatment with a proton pump inhibitor (PPI), such as omeprazole, lansoprazole and rabeprazole, and at least two antibiotics among clarithromycin (CLR), metronidazole (MTZ), amoxicillin (AMX) and tetracycline (TET) (13-16). In Canada, one of the standard recommended first-line regimens is a triple therapy consisting of a PPI, CLR, and either AMX or MTZ for up to 14 days (17). Alternatively, a quadruple regimen including a PPI, bismuth, MTZ and TET for up to 14 days may be required (18). Initially, both regimens had eradication rates >90% in 2000 (19), but this had dropped to 70% 10 years later (20), well below the recommended 80% outlined by Maastricht IV guidelines (21). A major contributor to the decline in efficacy is the increasing prevalence of antimicrobial resistance through selection, mutation and the development of emerging efflux pumps. This compels the necessity of susceptibility testing to manage the infection effectively (13). In one study, nearly 50% of patients in Germany were unable to eradicate *H pylori* because of resistance to both CLR and MTZ (22). In another study, nitroimidazole resistance was a contributing factor of eradication rates dropping by 15% to 50% (23). A recent study evaluated whether a new regimen of AMX plus a high dose of lansoprazole can achieve ≥90% eradication of *H pylori* (24). It was believed that the high PPI dose could affect the stomach environment and increase antimicrobial susceptibility; however, the desired eradication rate was not achieved. With mounting evidence that antimicrobial resistance affects clinical outcomes, there is a need to place more emphasis on a surveillance program to monitor resistance to guide the treatment of *H pylori* infections.

One of the mechanisms by which *H pylori* acquires resistance to antibiotics is through vertical transmission of mutations. For example, it is well documented that CLR resistance is linked to point mutations at nucleotide A2142 and A2143 in the 23S ribosomal (r)RNA gene (*rrn*) (25,26). Resistance to TETs were observed when all three nucleotides at positions 926 to 928 of the 16S rRNA gene were mutated (27,28). However, determining whether newly discovered mutations are responsible for antimicrobial resistance is a challenging task. Care must be taken because several mutations can appear in any given gene, and only through methodical evaluation (eg, site-directed mutagenesis of a susceptible wild-type *H pylori* strain) can a proper conclusion be made about a particular mutation leading to resistance.

Recent reporting of *H pylori* in Canada has been sporadic, with the most recent comprehensive epidemiological analyses on prevalence and antimicrobial resistance in Canada as a whole being published in 2000 (29) and 2004 (30). More recently, a study in the Arctic region of Canada has examined rates of antimicrobial resistance in an Aboriginal community in Aklavik, Northwest Territories (31). Additionally, there was a report in 2007 about the prevalence of *H pylori* in Ontario (5), and in a First Nations community in Sioux Lookout in Northwestern Ontario (32). In 1998, studies in Alberta showed that MTZ resistance was 14%, while CLR resistance was 3% (33). While it is currently unknown how *H pylori* has progressed in prevalence or whether antimicrobial resistance has increased across Canada, *H pylori* resistance to CLR across Europe doubled from 9% to 18% between 1998 and 2008, suggesting that antimicrobial resistance has increased globally (21).

The present pilot study provides a small glimpse into *H pylori* antimicrobial susceptibility in Northeastern Ontario by examining rates of antibiotic resistance for patients who attended Health Sciences North (HSN) in Sudbury, Ontario, for care. Different methods to determine antimicrobial resistance are compared and molecular detection of mutations known to be associated with antibiotic resistance are examined. Our introductory findings show increased local rates of antimicrobial resistance. As such, the extent of rising antimicrobial resistance rates of *H pylori* should be examined nationally and internationally as a means to prevent further treatment failure.

METHODS

Gastric biopsy collection, processing and culturing of *H pylori*
The HSN Research Ethics Board in Sudbury, Ontario, approved the research protocol. Patients who were scheduled for gastroscopies as part of their regular health care were asked for informed consent to collect blood and additional biopsy samples for the present study. In total, 301 patients were recruited to the study (117 men and 184 women); 127 participants were ≥60 years of age. Demographically, 280 identified themselves as Caucasian, 18 as First Nations, two as of African descent and one as of Indian descent. At HSN, gastric biopsies are typically sent for histology to identify *Helicobacter*-like organisms using Giemsa staining. Presence of these organisms would then prompt physicians to prescribe standard levels of treatment with a follow-up later. Physicians in the endoscopy unit who participated in the present study extracted additional biopsies and placed them into tubes containing transport medium consisting of thioglycollate medium (Oxoid, Canada), as per the manufacturer's instructions. To increase the likelihood of recovering *H pylori*, the biopsies were processed within 20 min of biopsy collection (E Altman, National Research Council of Canada, personal communication).

Briefly, biopsies were ground between two glass slides to break up the tissue and then plated on Columbia blood agar (BD Difco, USA) supplemented with a final concentration of 7% defibrinated horse blood (Quelab, Canada) and antibiotics (Sigma-Aldrich, Canada) as previously described (34). The plates were then placed into the Invivo$_2$ 500 Hypoxia Workstation (Ruskinn Technology Ltd, United Kingdom) at 37°C under microaerophilic conditions (5% O$_2$, 10% CO$_2$, 85% N$_2$) for a minimum of 48 h to two weeks to facilitate the culture of *H pylori*. Colonies were streaked for isolation on fresh media and subsequently cultured under the same conditions for 48 h to 72 h. When sufficient growth had occurred, samples were prepared for storage in Brain Heart Infusion broth (BD Difco) supplemented with 20% glycerol (Fisher Scientific, Canada) at −80°C. Enough bacteria were resuspended to cause turbidity in the freezing media. *H pylori* isolates were minimally cultured (two to five times due to varying rates of growth) to prevent the introduction of mutations under selective pressure.

Biochemical and polymerase chain reaction identification of *H pylori*
A KOH test was performed to rapidly determine whether isolated bacteria were Gram negative (35). A small amount of bacteria on a loop was added to a drop of 3% KOH (Sigma-Aldrich, Canada) on a microscope slide. A positive reaction (ie, Gram negative) was indicated if the mixture became viscous within 30 s and a string of the mixture was observed by raising the loop approximately 1 cm from the slide.

H pylori colonies were identified by positive catalase, urease and oxidase tests as previously described (36). Catalase was determined to be present if a drop of 3% H$_2$O$_2$ (Sigma-Aldrich) on a slide with bacteria led to effervescence. A urease test was considered to be positive if bacteria introduced in a solution of Brucella broth (BD Difco), urea (Sigma-Aldrich) and phenol red (Sigma-Aldrich) at pH 6.8 to 7.0 (yellow colour) turned pink or red within 24 h. Finally, a positive reaction for oxidase was indicated when bacteria smeared on filter paper dampened with N,N,N,N-tetramethyl-p-phenylenediamine dihydrochloride (Kovacs reagent, Sigma) left a purple colour on the filter paper.

The identity of *H pylori* was confirmed and further characterized by amplifying 16S rRNA, *cagA*, *ureC* and *ureA*, with primers listed in Table 1 using the Multiplex PCR Kit (Qiagen, Canada) as per the manufacturer's instructions in the VapoProtect gradient thermocycler (Eppendorf, Canada). Expected size amplicon lengths of 522, 294, 400 and 411 base pairs, respectively, were resolved on a 2% agarose gel using the PowerPac HC (BioRad, Canada).

Antimicrobial susceptibility
Antimicrobial susceptibility testing was conducted using two methods (disk diffusion and E-test). Colonies from two- to three-day-old pure culture of *H pylori*, grown on nonselective Mueller-Hinton (MH) agar (BD Difco) plates and supplemented with 5% defibrinated horse blood (Quelab), were resuspended in phosphate-buffered saline to a McFarland standard of 2 (approximately 6×10^8 cfu/mL) for the disk

diffusion testing, and a standard of 3 (approximately 1.0×10^9 cfu/mL) for the E-test. *H pylori* 26695 was used as a negative control because the strain is susceptible to all of the antibiotics tested in the present study (37,38).

The disk diffusion test followed the guidelines as set out by the European Committee on Antimicrobial Susceptibility Testing (EUCAST), April 2013, for microaerophilic bacteria (39). Bacterial suspensions were applied to the MH blood agar plates using a sterile cotton swab within 30 min, and the antibiotic disks were applied within 15 min on three separate occasions and averaged. The plates were incubated in the microaerophilic chamber at 37°C for three days, at which time the zones of inhibition were measured in millimetres. The disks (Oxoid) used were AMX (10 µg/disk), CLR (15 µg/disk), TET (30 µg/disk), MTZ (5 µg/disk), ciprofloxacin (CIP; 5 µg/disk), and levofloxacin (LVX; 5 µg/disk) as suggested by EUCAST and the Clinical and Laboratory Standards Institute standards for antibiotic content. Resistance was determined when zones of inhibition were ≤25 mm for AMX, ≤30 mm for CLR and TET, ≤16 mm for MTZ (39), and ≤30 mm for CIP (40) and LVX (41).

For the E-test, the same inoculation procedure was applied except with the use of a 3 McFarland standard. Each E-test strip (BioMérieux, Canada) of the same antibiotics as above was applied onto the MH blood agar plates, incubated similarly as with the disk diffusion test, and readings were taken after three days, according to the manufacturer's instructions. The breakpoints used to classify strains as susceptible or resistant are as follows, according the latest EUCAST recommendations as of January 2014 (42): ≤0.12 µg/mL susceptible, >0.12 µg/mL resistant for AMX; ≤1 µg/mL susceptible, >1 µg/mL resistant for CIP, LVX and TET; ≤0.25 µg/mL susceptible, >0.5 µg/mL resistant for CLR; and ≤8 µg/mL susceptible, >8 µg/mL resistant for MTZ. The E-test evaluation was conducted in duplicate on two different occasions.

Genomic DNA extraction

H pylori was grown in Columbia broth (Quelab) supplemented with 10% fetal bovine serum with shaking at 100 rpm using a MaxQ 6000 incubated shaker (Thermo Scientific, USA) under microaerophilic conditions at 37°C for 48 h to 72 h. Subsequently, the broth culture was centrifuged at 1700 × *g* for 20 min. The supernatant was removed, and the pellet was resuspended in phosphate-buffered saline and then centrifuged again. Following removal of the supernatant, resuspension buffer (50 mM Tris-HCl, pH 7.5 [BioShop, Canada], 10 mM EDTA [BioShop], 100 mg/mL RNase A [Fermentas, Canada]) was added with an equal volume of a mixture of a 25:24:1 ratio of phenol (Fisher), chloroform (BioShop) and isoamyl alcohol (BioShop), respectively (PCI). The mixture was shaken for 2 min to 3 min and then centrifuged at 15000 × *g* in the Sorvall Legend Micro 17 centrifuge (Fisher) for 10 min. Twice, the supernatant was carefully retrieved and then another equal volume of PCI was added, mixed and centrifuged as previously described. RNase A/T1 (Fermentas) was then added to the supernatant and allowed to incubate in a 37°C water bath for 1 h. PCI was once more added to remove the RNase. Approximately 2.5 to 3 times the volume of an ethanol mix (0.16 M of sodium acetate in 500 mL absolute ethanol) was added to initiate DNA precipitation. After incubation at –20°C overnight, the solution was centrifuged again at 15000 × *g* to pellet the precipitated DNA. The pellet was then washed with 70% ethanol and dried using a Hetovac VR-1 vacuum centrifuge (Heto Lab Equipment, Denmark). DNase- and RNase-free water was used to solubilize the DNA. The purity and concentration of the DNA was verified using agarose gel electrophoresis and a Nanodrop 2000c Spectrophotometer (Fisher), respectively.

Sequencing of *H pylori* genome

All genome sequences generated at the Advanced Medical Research Institute of Canada and HSN were produced using an Ion Torrent PGM (Life Technologies, Canada) sequencing technology.

TABLE 1
Primers used for polymerase chain reaction

Gene	Primer sequence (5′ → 3′)	Reference
16S rRNA	GCTAAGAGATCAGCCTATGTCC	71
	TGGCAATCAGCGTCAGGTAATG	
cagA	AATACACCAACGCCTCCAAG	72
	TTGTTGCCGCTTTTGCTCTC	
ureC	AAGCTTTTAGGGGTGTTAGGGGTTT	73
	AAGCTTACTTTCTAACACTAACGC	
ureA	GCCAATGGTAAATTAGTT	74
	CTCCTTAATTGTTTTTAC	

rRNA Ribosomal RNA

The following gene sequences, obtained from GenBank, are involved with antimicrobial resistance and were used to query the entire genomes (43): 16S rRNA (TET) GI: 6626253, 23S rRNA (CLR) GI: 881379, gyrase A (*gyrA*, CIP/LVX) GI: 12057207, penicillin-binding protein 1A (*pbp1A*, AMX) GI: 6626253 and oxygen-insensitive NADPH nitroreductase (*rdxA*, MTZ) GI: 308035684. BLAST v2.2.29+ (44) searches were performed with each gene sequence against each *H pylori* genome. Genome contigs were manually inspected to check for artifacts in the extracted gene sequences using Gap5 v1.2.14-r (45). Extracted genes were saved in FASTA format and visualized in Seaview v4.5.0 (46). Gene alignments were performed using MUSCLE v3.8.31 (47). Each alignment was inspected for stop codons, insertions/deletions and frame shifts. The final alignments for the coding sequences were performed following their codon structure.

RESULTS

Patient recruitment, collection and identification of *H pylori*

Between October 2012 and November 2013, 301 patients volunteered to participate in the present study to provide gastric biopsy samples. Twenty of these participants (13 male, seven female) tested positive for *H pylori*. Biochemical testing on the isolated bacteria indicated positive reactions for urease, catalase and oxidase. In addition, polymerase chain reaction (PCR) was conducted on the bacterial isolates and 19 of 20 were found to have fragments of *ureA*, *ureC* and 16S rRNA. While the latter two amplicons were detected from the isolate from participant 60, *ureA* was only detected upon sequencing. Only seven of 20 indicated the presence of *cagA* according to PCR. According to the pathology reports, nearly all the patients had gastritis, while four of these patients also had metaplasia or hyperplasia (Table 2). One pathology report was not available. At the time of biopsy, 90% (18 of 20) of the positively identified patients were ≥50 years of age.

Disk diffusion assay

The antimicrobial resistance of the 20 *H pylori* isolates to AMX, TET, MTZ, CIP, LVX and CLR is listed in Table 3 as the average zone of inhibition, measured in millimetres. Results are also listed in Table 4 as being susceptible or resistant. Of 20 isolates, eight were resistant for MTZ (40%), six were resistant for CIP and LVX (30%), and eight were resistant for CLR (40%). None of the isolates were resistant to AMX or TET. Multiple resistances, outside of CIP and LVX (fluoroquinolones), were also observed. Two of 20 isolates (10%) were resistant to both MTZ and to the fluoroquinolones, three (15%) were resistant to CLR and the fluoroquinolones, five (25%) were resistant to MTZ and CLR, while two (10%) were resistant to MTZ, CLR and to the fluoroquinolones.

Minimum inhibitory concentration determination using E-test

The disk diffusion method alone is not sufficient to evaluate *H pylori* antimicrobial resistance because it is not yet standardized. As such, the E-test, following the manufacturer's instructions, was performed in addition to determine minimum inhibitory concentration (MIC) as recommended by EUCAST. Table 4 shows the resulting MIC determination

TABLE 2
Resistance profile of 20 *Helicobacter pylori* isolates according to disk diffusion and E-test methods

Isolate number	Pathology	AMX 10 µg*	AMX MIC[†]	TET 30 µg*	TET MIC[†]	MTZ 5 µg*	MTZ MIC[†]	CIP 5 µg*	CIP MIC[†]	LVX 5 µg*	LVX MIC[†]	CLR 15 µg*	CLR MIC[†]
45	No pathology performed	S	<0.016	S	<0.023	S	<0.75	R	>32	R	<8	R	>256
60	Chronic gastritis, metaplasia	S	<0.023	S	<0.094	R	>256	S	<0.064	S	<0.094	S	<0.19
63	Chronic gastritis	S	<0.016	S	<0.032	R	<0.75	S	<0.125	S	<0.125	S	<0.064
66	Chronic gastritis, hyperplasia	S	<0.016	S	<0.25	R	>256	R	>32	R	>32	R	>256
103	Chronic gastritis	S	<0.023	S	<0.019	S	<0.75	S	<0.38	S	<0.25	S	<0.047
104	Gastritis	S	<0.032	S	<0.032	R	<64	S	<0.19	S	<0.19	R	>256
163	Chronic gastritis	S	<0.023	S	<0.125	R	>256	S	<0.75	S	<0.5	R	>256
170	Chronic gastritis	S	<0.016	S	<0.047	S	<0.5	S	<0.019	S	<0.019	R	>256
173	Acute and chronic gastritis	S	<0.016	S	<0.047	S	<0.38	S	<0.25	S	<0.25	S	<0.064
181	Chronic gastritis	S	<0.016	S	<0.125	S	<0.5	S	<0.125	S	<0.125	S	<0.047
195	Chronic gastritis	S	<0.016	S	<0.032	R	>256	S	<0.125	S	<0.094	R	>256
207	Chronic gastritis	S	<0.032	S	<0.023	S	<0.094	S	<0.064	S	<0.125	S	<0.094
209	Chronic gastritis	S	<0.016	S	<0.032	S	<0.125	R	>32	R	>32	S	<0.047
227	Chronic gastritis	S	<0.016	S	<0.094	S	<0.047	R	>32	R	<6	S	<0.023
236	Chronic gastritis	S	<0.016	S	<0.023	S	<0.38	S	<0.19	S	<0.25	S	<0.032
239	Chronic gastritis	S	<0.064	S	<0.125	R	<48	R	>32	R	>32	R	<96
243	Chronic gastritis, metaplasia	S	<0.032	S	<0.25	R	>256	S	<0.38	S	<0.38	S	<0.094
263	Chronic gastritis, metaplasia	S	<0.064	S	<0.047	S	<0.75	S	<0.25	S	<0.19	R	>256
283	Chronic gastritis	S	<0.032	S	<0.25	S	<1	R	>32	R	>32	S	<0.023
288	Chronic gastritis	S	<0.016	S	<0.023	S	<0.5	S	<0.094	S	<0.125	S	<0.023

Per disk; [†]µg/mL. AMX Amoxicillin; CIP Ciprofloxacin; CLR Clarithromycin; LVX Levofloxacin; MIC Minimum inhibitory concentratio; MTZ Metronidazole; R Resistant; S Susceptible; TET Tetracycline

TABLE 3
Average zone diameters (in mm) of inhibition according to disk diffusion

Isolate number	AMX	TET	MTZ	CIP	LVX	CLR
45	58.0	54.0	20.7	6.0	14.7	6.0
60	53.3	55.7	9.3	46.0	44.7	54.3
63	62.0	60.3	14.0	47.7	46.7	50.7
66	59.3	50.0	6.0	6.0	6.0	7.7
103	54.7	52.0	19.0	39.7	38.7	52.7
104	53.7	56.7	7.0	43.0	39.7	7.3
163	44.3	58.0	6.0	36.3	34.7	6.0
170	56.7	57.7	16.5	39.3	38.0	6.0
173	56.0	51.7	30.0	39.3	37.7	46.3
181	52.0	40.0	26.3	40.3	44.0	55.0
195	54.7	61.3	6.0	47.3	46.0	6.0
207	60.3	66.7	47.7	49.3	49.0	60.7
209	59.7	57.0	26.7	6.0	6.0	48.3
227	56.7	50.3	16.7	6.0	18.0	48.3
236	56.7	61.7	35.7	44.7	41.0	52.7
239	49.7	52.0	6.0	6.0	15.0	6.0
243	65.0	53.7	6.0	39.0	40.7	54.0
263	51.3	64.0	32.3	44.7	44.0	6.0
283	54.7	52.7	22.3	6.0	6.0	59.7
288	60.3	63.3	23.3	45.3	45.3	57.3

AMX Amoxicillin; CIP Ciprofloxacin; CLR Clarithromycin; LVX Levofloxacin; MTZ Metronidazole; TET Tetracycline

using E-test strips. In evaluating AMX, the MIC was 0.064 µg/mL in two isolates, 0.032 µg/mL in four isolates, 0.023 µg/mL in three isolates and 0.016 µg/mL in 11 isolates. Because the breakpoint for AMX is 0.12 µg/mL, all of the isolates were deemed to be susceptible to AMX. All of the isolates were also susceptible to TET; the breakpoint is 1 µg/mL and the MIC values for all of the isolates were ≤0.25 µg/mL. Of the 20 isolates, seven were found to be resistant to MTZ (35%) because their MIC values were ≥48 µg/mL, which is higher than the breakpoint value of 8 µg/mL.

Quinolone resistance was observed in six isolates (30%), which had MIC values much greater (>6 µg/mL) than the 1 µg/mL breakpoint. Finally, CLR testing showed that seven isolates had the maximum MIC values that were listed on the E-test strip (256 µg/mL), while one was 96 µg/mL, giving rise to a total of eight resistant isolates (40%) that were well above the 0.5 µg/mL breakpoint. There was excellent correspondence between disk diffusion and E-test; however, the isolate from participant 63 was not resistant to MTZ according to E-test, while disk diffusion results suggested resistance. Patterns of multiple resistances were nearly identical to those found by disk diffusion except for those related to isolate 63. There was at least one antibiotic resistance found in 13 of the isolates (65%).

Detection of mutations in *H pylori* genes associated with antimicrobial resistance

To corroborate these data on antimicrobial susceptibility, five *H pylori* genes, which have been documented to be associated with antimicrobial resistance when mutated, were examined. These genes (AMX – *pbp1a*; TET – 16S rRNA; MTZ – *rdxA*; CIP/LVX – *gyrA*; CLR – 23S rRNA) were compared with the sequences from the isolates in the present study (Table 5). The genomes collected were originally for another project at the authors' laboratory; therefore, only the five genes were extracted for analysis.

Seven of the eight strains that were found to be resistant to CLR showed a point mutation, A2143G, in the 23S rRNA sequence, while the other strain from participant 263 revealed an A2142G mutation (Table 5). These mutations were not detected among the strains susceptible to CLR. Six strains that were resistant to CIP and LVX were also found to have mutations. Five had the G271A point mutation in the *gyrA* gene, while one isolate had an A272G mutation. The susceptible strains did not possess these mutations. Interestingly, while many strains were found to be resistant to MTZ, only two showed unique mutations to the *rdxA* gene, which has not been previously documented. One showed a C16T point mutation that led to a stop codon, and an insert at nucleotide 121 with the sequence GAAATCGCC, which kept the remainder of the sequence in frame. No other mutations that have been documented to be involved with resistance were detected in the other resistant strains. There were amino acid mutations detected in the *pbp1a* gene that

TABLE 4
Comparison of antimicrobial susceptibility according to disk diffusion and E-test

	Disk diffusion			E-test	
	Isolates, n (%)			Isolates, n (%)	
Antimicrobial agent	Susceptible	Resistant	Range, µg/mL	Susceptible	Resistant
Amoxicillin	20 (100)	0 (0)	0.016–256	20 (100)	0 (0)
Tetracycline	20 (100)	0 (0)	0.016–256	20 (100)	0 (0)
Metronidazole	12 (60)	8 (40)	0.016–256	13 (65)	7 (35)
Ciprofloxacin	14 (70)	6 (30)	0.002–32	14 (70)	6 (30)
Levofloxacin	14 (70)	6 (30)	0.002–32	14 (70)	6 (30)
Clarithromycin	12 (60)	8 (40)	0.016–256	12 (60)	8 (40)

TABLE 5
Molecular detection of *Helicobacter pylori* mutations that may be linked to antimicrobial resistance

Isolate number	23S rRNA		gyrA		rdxA		pbp1A	
	CLR S/R	Mutation	CIP/LVX S/R	Mutation	MTZ S/R	Mutation	AMX S/R	Mutation
45	R	A2143G (26)	R	G271A (57)	S		S	V45I (64), V16I (64), S543R (66)
60	S		S		R	nd	S	V16I, S543R
63	S		S		R	nd	S	
66	R	A2143G	R	G271A	R	nd	S	
103	S		S		S		S	S543T (present study)
104	R	A2143G	S		R	nd	S	V16I, S543R
163	R	A2143G	S		R	nd	S	S543N (present study)
170	R	A2143G	S		S		S	S543R
173	S		S		S		S	
181	S		S		S		S	S543R
195	R	A2143G	S		R	C16T (stop) (present study)	S	V16I, S543R
207	S		S		S		S	S543N
209	S		R	G271A	S		S	S543R
227	S		R	A272G (57)	S		S	V16I, S543R
236	S		S		S		S	
239	R	A2143G	R	G271A	R	nd	S	S543R
243	S		S		R	ins121GAAATC-GCC (present study)	S	V16I, S543R
263	R	A2142G (26)	S		S		S	T556S (65), S543R
283	S		R	G271A	S		S	S543R
288	S		S		S		S	

AMX Amoxicillin; CIP Ciprofloxacin; CLR Clarithromycin; LVX Levofloxacin; MTZ Metronidazole; nd Did not detect any mutations that have been previously linked to antimicrobial resistance; R Resistant; rRNA Ribosomal RNA; S Susceptible; TET Tetracycline

have been associated with AMX resistance; however, all of the isolates were susceptible to the antibiotic and, thus, the mutations may not be involved in resistance. They include individual and combinations of V16I, V45I, T556S, A599T, S543R and G595S mutations. Interestingly, some of the isolates have newly found mutations for S543 to asparagine or threonine, or insertions at G595, but whether they appear as single or multiple mutations, they do not appear to be sufficient to confer resistance. No known mutations of 16S rRNA that are responsible for TET resistance were found, which was consistent with the present findings that all of the isolates were susceptible to TET.

DISCUSSION

Monitoring emerging antimicrobial-resistant strains of H pylori is paramount for therapeutic treatment to be successful. While Canada has a lower prevalence rate than the global average, increased international travel and immigration from countries that have high endemic rates of H pylori should be a signal that surveillance should not only continue in Canada and the world, but also perhaps increase.

The present study was the first to examine antimicrobial susceptibility in Northern Ontario. It is surprising that a relatively high percentage of

resistance to certain antibiotics was found by E-test, namely MTZ (35%), CLR (40%) and CIP/LVX (30%), despite the small number of H pylori isolates in the study. To compare, in 2000, Fallone (29) determined that MTZ resistance in Canada was between 11% and 48%, while resistance to CLR was 0% to 12%. The variation in data evaluated by Fallone reflected the difficulty in discerning primary and secondary resistance when results were reported. For CIP/LVX, it was estimated that resistance in Canada was <10% in 2004 (30). It is possible that the data we obtained could be attributed to region-specific demographics, and that a broader and larger sample size would be a better reflection of antimicrobial resistance in Ontario. However, the fact remains that a large percentage of antibiotic resistance was found. The data suggest that not only will physicians need to identify H pylori quickly, but also that susceptibility testing should be part of the clinical evaluation so that treatment can be tailored to combat the infection more effectively, rather than relying on consensus guidelines, and to prevent or slow the development of antimicrobial resistance.

In Canada, the incidence of AMX resistance was <2% as of 1997 (48), while there has yet to be any public information on resistance rates, if any, of TET since 2000 (29). Our work is consistent with previous data in that AMX and TET resistance have yet to become more prevalent in Canada and that, for the time being, they remain effective in H pylori eradication.

There was 100% agreement in results determining susceptibility or resistance of H pylori between the use of antimicrobial disks and the E-test for five of the six antibiotics tested. For MTZ, 19 of 20 isolates were consistent with one another. This is in relative agreement with previous studies that used conditions closely resembling our methodology, in which there was a 7% discrepancy when evaluating MTZ resistance (49).

While 100% agreement between the E-test and disk diffusion assay was not observed with MTZ, the small percentage of discrepancy should be an indication that outside of MTZ, disk diffusion may be able to provide rapid and cost-effective insight into antimicrobial resistance. The greatest challenge in using it to evaluate MTZ resistance is that a standard zone diameter does not exist and that several other factors complicate a proper evaluation (50). The Clinical and Laboratory Standards Institute, EUCAST and the British Society for Antimicrobial Chemotherapy do not recommend the use of antibiotic disks for clinical studies because the stability of the antibiotics on the disk may be compromised after 48 h to 72 h of growth, which is normally required for testing H pylori. Regardless, many laboratories still use this approach as a cost-effective measure to monitor emerging resistant H pylori strains. The agar dilution method is considered to be the gold standard and is effective in large batch studies to provide accurate MICs, but is technically too demanding to be a viable test for everyday practice (51,52). The E-test method generally has a more consistent antibiotic release, is able to tolerate prolonged incubation and can provide MICs (53). However, an E-test strip costs approximately 100 times more than an antimicrobial disk, which can be prohibitive in terms of cost and access in developing countries where they try to establish surveillance programs, especially because incidence rates of H pylori are often higher in some developing nations (7). As such, laboratories in countries such as India, Iran and Turkey continue to use disk diffusion to determine susceptible and resistant H pylori strains, while efficiently selecting for more effective therapies (39,54-56). If the cost and the ease of evaluation are prohibitive factors in screening for H pylori antimicrobial resistance, disk diffusion, with the possible exception of MTZ, should be an acceptable approach through the development of standardized zones of inhibition.

The mutations detected in the 23S rRNA gene that led to CLR resistance in the present study were consistent with the same mutations that have been described previously (26). The A2142 and A2143 nucleotides are located in the peptidyl transferase loop of the secondary structure of the gene and, as such, the mutations to guanine cause a conformational change in the loop, leading to decreased binding of CLR (26). Similarly, mutations in the gyrA gene (G271A, A272G, which correspond to amino acid changes D91N and D91G) that led to resistance to CIP and LVX are also well known in a previous study (57). These mutations have been very consistent in literature as mutations that confer resistance, and served as a validation for our antimicrobial susceptibility results. Recently, it has been suggested that an efflux pathway may also be involved in CLR resistance (13).

In contrast to CLR and the quinolones tested, the mechanism behind MTZ resistance is significantly more complicated. All seven isolates resistant to MTZ, as determined by E-test, did not possess any mutations that are known to cause H pylori to be resistant to the drug (37,58). In fact, it has not been possible to clearly identify a set of rdxA mutations that consistently accounted for resistance (59,60). However, two of the strains, those from patient 195 (C16T mutation leading to a stop codon) and patient 243 (an insert of nine nucleotides), did show new mutations that may lead to resistance. These mutations would need to be investigated individually using a control strain to determine whether they are involved with MTZ susceptibility. Studies have shown that other genes, such as frxA, may also be involved with MTZ resistance when mutated (61). It has also been shown that MTZ resistance can occur without any mutations to the rdxA or frxA genes,

suggesting that another mechanism may be involved (62), such as the Fur protein that, when mutated, may be able to eliminate the drug (63). Clearly, the complex mechanism behind MTZ resistance will need to be evaluated in future studies.

In our study, every isolate was susceptible to AMX; however, several mutations that were previously described as being linked to resistance were discovered to be present in our isolates. Amino acid mutations such as V45I and V16I, found in six of our isolates, confirmed previous studies in which they were determined to have no effect on antimicrobial susceptibility (64). The mutations G595S and A599T have also been described previously, although it is unknown what their contribution is to resistance because they were part of a series of mutations that led to drug resistance (64). In the present study, we found amino acid insertions at position 595, yet no resistance was found. Another mutation (T556S) was found to be singly capable of conferring resistance in one study (65); however, this was not the case in the present study. Mutations at serine 543 have also been linked to resistance, although not necessarily as a single mutation (66). Fifteen of the 20 isolates had mutations at this amino acid, but no resistance was conferred. H pylori from participant 263 had both T556S and S543R mutations, yet this strain was still susceptible to AMX. This suggests that multiple mutations to pbp1A may be required to confer resistance. High-level resistance to AMX may also involve mutations to porin proteins, notably HopB (AlpB), HopC (AlpA) and HopD (65,67).

While we report relatively high resistance rates against CLR, MTZ and CIP/LVX, it should be noted that we were unable to determine whether these were primary or secondary resistances. When treatment with an antibiotic fails, it would normally result in a higher probability of a selection of an isolate that is resistant, particularly with MTZ and CIP and, thus, we cannot preclude the possibility that patients may have been previously treated with antibiotics (68,69). It is then possible that there is horizontal transfer of resistance to susceptible strains in individuals who are infected with more than one strain (70).

H pylori is pathogenic and potentially carcinogenic. The present pilot study provides a small, yet important, glimpse into the prevalence of H pylori in Northeastern Ontario, in addition to the frequency and molecular mechanisms of antimicrobial-resistant strains. While the present study examined cases of H pylori from one institution within a relatively small geographical area, the high proportion of antimicrobial resistance relative to previous reports is alarming. With the presence of strains in the present study that are resistant to multiple antibiotics, particularly MTZ and CLR, which are most frequently used under current treatment guidelines, carefully devised regimens examining antimicrobial susceptibility of H pylori strains and consideration of past use of antibiotics, rather than adherence to consensus guidelines, may be preferable. The Maastricht IV guidelines do allow for appropriate changes in treatment if it is not effective due to high prevalence of antibiotic resistance. However, this information needs to be available before changes can be initiated. Routine antimicrobial susceptibility testing would be a good place to start. Future studies to determine whether our results are found in other jurisdictions will need to be conducted to determine whether increased antimicrobial resistance of H pylori is widespread.

Despite emerging studies of other mechanisms of antibiotic resistance, chromosomal mutations in H pylori remain the primary source. If other mechanisms are involved, whole genome sequencing provides an opportunity to examine mutations during disease progression or selection, which may lead to a tailored treatment that would facilitate H pylori eradication instead of resistance selection.

ACKNOWLEDGEMENTS: This work was funded by the Northern Ontario Academic Medicine Association awarded to FDM. The authors thank Drs Kim Stephen Tilbe, Heather Boudreau, Jagan Reddy and Robert Smith for volunteering their services in the endoscopy unit at HSN and extracting gastric biopsies.

DISCLOSURES: The authors have no conflicts of interest to declare.

REFERENCES

1. Cheung J, Goodman K, Munday R, et al. *Helicobacter pylori* infection in Canada's arctic: Searching for the solutions. CanJGastroenterol 2008;22:912-6.
2. Survival rates for stomach cancer by stage. Am Cancer Soc 2013. <www.cancer.org/cancer/stomachcancer/detailedguide/stomach-cancer-survival-rates> (Accessed July 15, 2014).
3. McColl KE. Clinical practice. *Helicobacter pylori* infection. N Engl J Med 2010;362:1597-604.
4. Schistosomes, liver flukes and *Helicobacter pylori*. IARC Working Group on the Evaluation of Carcinogenic Risks to Humans. Lyon, 7-14 June 1994. IARC Monogr Eval Carcinog Risks Hum 1994;61:1-241.
5. Naja F, Kreiger N, Sullivan T. *Helicobacter pylori* infection in Ontario: Prevalence and risk factors. Can J Gastroenterol 2007;21:501-6.
6. Thomson AB, Barkun AN, Armstrong D, et al. The prevalence of clinically significant endoscopic findings in primary care patients with uninvestigated dyspepsia: The Canadian Adult Dyspepsia Empiric Treatment – Prompt Endoscopy (CADET-PE) study. Aliment Pharmacol Ther 2003;17:1481-91.
7. Graham DY, Adam E, Reddy GT, et al. Seroepidemiology of *Helicobacter pylori* infection in India. Comparison of developing and developed countries. Dig Dis Sci 1991;36:1084-8.
8. Graham DY, Malaty HM, Evans DG, Evans DJ Jr, Klein PD, Adam E. Epidemiology of *Helicobacter pylori* in an asymptomatic population in the United States. Effect of age, race, and socioeconomic status. Gastroenterology 1991;100:1495-501.
9. Moayyedi P, Axon AT, Feltbower R, et al. Relation of adult lifestyle and socioeconomic factors to the prevalence of *Helicobacter pylori* infection. Int J Epidemiol 2002;31:624-31.
10. Woodward M, Morrison C, McColl K. An investigation into factors associated with *Helicobacter pylori* infection. J Clin Epidemiol 2000;53:175-81.
11. Olafsson S, Berstad A. Changes in food tolerance and lifestyle after eradication of *Helicobacter pylori*. Scand J Gastroenterol 2003;38:268-76.
12. Bernstein CN, McKeown I, Embil JM, et al. Seroprevalence of *Helicobacter pylori*, incidence of gastric cancer, and peptic ulcer-associated hospitalizations in a Canadian Indian population. Dig Dis Sci 1999;44:668-74.
13. Vakil N, Vaira D. Treatment for *H. pylori* infection: New challenges with antimicrobial resistance. J Clin Gastroenterol 2013;47:383-8.
14. Delaney BC, Qume M, Moayyedi P, et al. *Helicobacter pylori* test and treat versus proton pump inhibitor in initial management of dyspepsia in primary care: Multicentre randomised controlled trial (MRC-CUBE trial). BMJ 2008;336:651-4.
15. Sharma VK, Howden CW. A national survey of primary care physicians' perceptions and practices related to *Helicobacter pylori* infection. J Clin Gastroenterol 2004;38:326-31.
16. Megraud F, Lehours P. *Helicobacter pylori* detection and antimicrobial susceptibility testing. Clin Microbiol Rev 2007;20:280-322.
17. Bourke B, Ceponis P, Chiba N, et al. Canadian Helicobacter Study Group Consensus Conference: Update on the approach to Helicobacter pylori infection in children and adolescents – an evidence-based evaluation. Can J Gastroenterol 2005;19:399-408.
18. Hunt R, Fallone C, Veldhuyzan van Zanten S, et al. Canadian Helicobacter Study Group Consensus Conference: Update on the management of *Helicobacter pylori*--an evidence-based evaluation of six topics relevant to clinical outcomes in patients evaluated for *H pylori* infection. Can J Gastroenterol 2004;18:547-54.
19. Cuadrado-Lavin A, Salcines-Caviedes JR, Carrascosa MF, et al. Antimicrobial susceptibility of *Helicobacter pylori* to six antibiotics currently used in Spain. J Antimicrob Chemother 2012;67:170-3.
20. Graham DY, Fischbach L. *Helicobacter pylori* treatment in the era of increasing antibiotic resistance. Gut 2010;59:1143-53.
21. Malfertheiner P, Megraud F, O'Morain CA, et al. Management of *Helicobacter pylori* infection – the Maastricht IV/Florence Consensus Report. Gut 2012;61:646-64.
22. Heep M, Kist M, Strobel S, Beck D, Lehn N. Secondary resistance among 554 isolates of *Helicobacter pylori* after failure of therapy. Eur J Clin Microbiol Infect Dis 2000;19:538-41.
23. Sycuro LK, Pincus Z, Gutierrez KD, et al. Peptidoglycan crosslinking relaxation promotes *Helicobacter pylori*'s helical shape and stomach colonization. Cell 2010;141:822-33.
24. Attumi TA, Graham DY. High-dose extended-release lansoprazole (dexlansoprazole) and amoxicillin dual therapy for *Helicobacter pylori* infections. Helicobacter 2014;19:319-22.
25. Occhialini A, Urdaci M, Doucet-Populaire F, Bébéar CM, Lamouliatte H, Mégraud F. Macrolide resistance in *Helicobacter pylori*: Rapid detection of point mutations and assays of macrolide binding to ribosomes. Antimicrob Agents Chemother 1997;41:2724-8.
26. Versalovic J, Shortridge D, Kibler K, et al. Mutations in 23S rRNA are associated with clarithromycin resistance in *Helicobacter pylori*. Antimicrob Agents Chemother 1996;40:477-80.
27. Gerrits MM, de Zoete MR, Arents NLA, Kuipers EJ, Kusters JG. 16S rRNA mutation-mediated tetracycline resistance in *Helicobacter pylori*. Antimicrob Agents Chemother 2002;46:2996-3000.
28. Trieber CA, Taylor DE. Mutations in the 16S rRNA genes of *Helicobacter pylori* mediate resistance to tetracycline. J Bacteriol 2002;184:2131-40.
29. Fallone CA. Epidemiology of the antibiotic resistance of *Helicobacter pylori* in Canada. Can J Gastroenterol 2000;14:879-82.
30. Best L, Haldane DJ, Veldhuyzen Van Zanten S. *Helicobacter pylori* antibiotic resistance in Canadian populations. Gastroenterology 2004;126:S1293.
31. Cheung J, Morse AL, Goodman KJ, et al. Prevalence of *Helicobacter pylori* and antibiotic resistance in an Aboriginal population in Canada's Arctic: Preliminary results from the Aklavik *H. pylori* Project. Gastroenterology 2009;136:A341.
32. Sethi A, Chaudhuri M, Kelly L, Hopman W. Prevalence of *Helicobacter pylori* in a First Nations population in northwestern Ontario. Can Fam Physician 2013;59:e182-7.
33. Taylor DE, Jiang Q, Fedorak RN. Antibiotic susceptibilities of *Helicobacter pylori* strains isolated in the Province of Alberta. Can J Gastroenterol 1998;12:295-8.
34. Hiratsuka K, Logan SM, Conlan JW, et al. Identification of a D-glycero-D-manno-heptosyltransferase gene from *Helicobacter pylori*. J Bacteriol 2005;187:5156-65.
35. Halebian S, Harris B, Finegold SM, Rolfe RD. Rapid method that aids in distinguishing Gram-positive from Gram-negative anaerobic bacteria. J Clin Microbiol 1981;13:444-8.
36. Garcia LS, ed. Clinical Microbiology Procedures Handbook, 3rd edn. Washington, DC: ASM Press, 2007.
37. Wang G, Wilson TJ, Jiang Q, Taylor DE. Spontaneous mutations that confer antibiotic resistance in *Helicobacter pylori*. Antimicrob Agents Chemother 2001;45:727-33.
38. Toledo H, López-Solís R. Tetracycline resistance in Chilean clinical isolates of *Helicobacter pylori*. J Antimicrob Chemother 2010;65:470-3.
39. EUCAST. Antimicrobial susceptibility testing. EUCAST disk diffusion method. <www.eucast.org/fileadmin/src/media/PDFs/EUCAST_files/Disk_test_documents/Manual_v_3.0_EUCAST_Disk_Test.pdf> (Accessed April 2013).
40. Boyanova L, Stancheva I, Spassova Z, Katzarov N, Mitov I, Koumanova R. Primary and combined resistance to four antimicrobial agents in *Helicobacter pylori* in Sofia, Bulgaria. J Med Microbiol 2000;49:415-8.
41. Lee CC, Lee VWY, Chan FKL, Ling TKW. Levofloxacin-resistant *Helicobacter pylori* in Hong Kong. Chemotherapy 2008;54:50-3.
42. The European Committee on Antimicrobial Susceptibility Testing. Breakpoint tables for interpretation of MICs and zone diameters. Version 4.0, 2014.
43. Mégraud F. *H pylori* antibiotic resistance: Prevalence, importance, and advances in testing. Gut 2004;53:1374-84.
44. Camacho C, Coulouris G, Avagyan V, et al. BLAST+: architecture and applications. BMC Bioinformatics 2009;10:421.
45. Bonfield JK, Whitwham A. Gap5 – editing the billion fragment sequence assembly. Bioinformatics 2010;26:1699-703.
46. Gouy M, Guindon S, Gascuel O. SeaView version 4: A multiplatform graphical user interface for sequence alignment and phylogenetic tree building. Mol Biol Evol 2010;27:221-4.
47. Edgar RC. MUSCLE: Multiple sequence alignment with high accuracy and high throughput. Nucleic Acids Res 2004;32:1792-7.
48. Fedorak R, Archambault A, Flamm R, Osato M, Stamler D. Antimicrobial susceptibility of *H. pylori* in Canada to three key antibiotics: Metronidazole, clarithromycin and amoxicillin. Gastroenterology 1997;112:A115.
49. Smith C, Perkins J, Tompkins DS. Comparison of Etest and disc diffusion for detection of antibiotic resistance in *Helicobacter pylori*. PHLS Microbiol Dig 1997;14:21-3.

50. Weiss K, Laverdière M, Restieri C. Comparison of activity of 10 antibiotics against clinical strains of *Helicobacter pylori* by three different techniques. Can J Gastroenterol 1998;12:181-5.

51. Osato MS. Antimicrobial susceptibility testing for *Helicobacter pylori*: Sensitivity test results and their clinical relevance. Curr Pharm Des 2000;6:1545-55.

52. DeCross AJ, Marshall BJ, McCallum RW, Hoffman SR, Barrett LJ, Guerrant RL. Metronidazole susceptibility testing for *Helicobacter pylori*: Comparison of disk, broth, and agar dilution methods and their clinical relevance. J Clin Microbiol 1993;31:1971-4.

53. Cederbrant G, Kahlmeter G, Ljungh A. The E test for antimicrobial susceptibility testing of *Helicobacter pylori*. J Antimicrob Chemother 1993;31:65-71.

54. Mishra KK, Srivastava S, Garg A, Ayyagari A. Antibiotic susceptibility of *Helicobacter pylori* clinical isolates: Comparative evaluation of disk-diffusion and E-test methods. Curr Microbiol 2006;53:329-34.

55. Falsafi T, Mobasheri F, Nariman F, Najafi M. Susceptibilities to different antibiotics of *Helicobacter pylori* strains isolated from patients at the pediatric medical center of Tehran, Iran. J Clin Microbiol 2004;42:387-9.

56. Ozbey G, Bahcecioglu IH, Acik MN. Resistance rates to various antimicrobial agents of *Helicobacter pylori* isolates in Eastern Turkey. Int J Mol Clin Microbiol 2012;2:148-52.

57. Moore RA, Beckthold B, Wong S, Kureishi A, Bryan LE. Nucleotide sequence of the gyrA gene and characterization of ciprofloxacin-resistant mutants of *Helicobacter pylori*. Antimicrob Agents Chemother 1995;39:107-11.

58. Paul R, Postius S, Melchers K, Schäfer KP. Mutations of the *Helicobacter pylori* genes rdxA and pbp1 cause resistance against metronidazole and amoxicillin. Antimicrob Agents Chemother 2001;45:962-5.

59. Mendz GL, Mégraud F. Is the molecular basis of metronidazole resistance in microaerophilic organisms understood? Trends Microbiol 2002;10:370-5.

60. Chisholm SA, Owen RJ. Mutations in *Helicobacter pylori* rdxA gene sequences may not contribute to metronidazole resistance. J Antimicrob Chemother 2003;51:995-9.

61. Marais A, Bilardi C, Cantet F, Mendz GL, Mégraud F. Characterization of the genes rdxA and frxA involved in metronidazole resistance in *Helicobacter pylori*. Res Microbiol 2003;154:137-44.

62. Bereswill S, Krainick C, Stähler F, Herrmann L, Kist M. Analysis of the rdxA gene in high-level metronidazole-resistant clinical isolates confirms a limited use of rdxA mutations as a marker for prediction of metronidazole resistance in *Helicobacter pylori*. FEMS Immunol Med Microbiol 2003;36:193-8.

63. Choi SS, Chivers PT, Berg DE. Point mutations in *Helicobacter pylori*'s fur regulatory gene that alter resistance to metronidazole, a prodrug activated by chemical reduction. PLoS One 2011;6:e18236.

64. Kim BJ, Kim JG. Substitutions in penicillin-binding protein 1 in amoxicillin-resistant *Helicobacter pylori* strains isolated from Korean patients. Gut Liver 2013;7:655-60.

65. Matteo MJ, Granados G, Olmos M, Wonaga A, Catalano M. *Helicobacter pylori* amoxicillin heteroresistance due to point mutations in PBP-1A in isogenic isolates. J Antimicrob Chemother 2008;61:474-7.

66. Kwon DH, Dore MP, Kim JJ, et al. High-level β-lactam resistance associated with acquired multidrug resistance in *Helicobacter pylori*. Antimicrob Agents Chemother 2003;47:2169-78.

67. Co E-MA, Schiller NL. Resistance mechanisms in an in vitro-selected amoxicillin-resistant strain of *Helicobacter pylori*. Antimicrob Agents Chemother 2006;50:4174-6.

68. Goodwin CS, Marshall BJ, Blincow ED, Wilson DH, Blackbourn S, Phillips M. Prevention of nitroimidazole resistance in *Campylobacter pylori* by coadministration of colloidal bismuth subcitrate: Clinical and in vitro studies. J Clin Pathol 1988;41:207-10.

69. Tompkins DS, Perkin J, Smith C. Failed treatment of *Helicobacter pylori* infection associated with resistance to clarithromycin. Helicobacter 1997;2:185-7.

70. Fantry GT, Zheng QX, Darwin PE, Rosenstein AH, James SP. Mixed infection with cagA-positive and cagA-negative strains of *Helicobacter pylori*. Helicobacter 1996;1:98-106.

71. Engstrand L, Nguyen AM, Graham DY, el-Zaatari FA. Reverse transcription and polymerase chain reaction amplification of rRNA for detection of *Helicobacter* species. J Clin Microbiol 1992;30:2295-301.

72. Tummuru MK, Cover TL, Blaser MJ. Cloning and expression of a high-molecular-mass major antigen of *Helicobacter pylori*: Evidence of linkage to cytotoxin production. Infect Immun 1993;61:1799-809.

73. Labigne A, Cussac V, Courcoux P. Shuttle cloning and nucleotide sequences of *Helicobacter pylori* genes responsible for urease activity. J Bacteriol 1991;173:1920-31.

74. Clayton C, Kleanthous K, Tabaqchali S. Detection and identification of *Helicobacter pylori* by the polymerase chain reaction. J Clin Pathol 1991;44:515-6.

16

Development and validation of a *Pneumocystis jirovecii* real-time polymerase chain reaction assay for diagnosis of *Pneumocystis* pneumonia

Deirdre L Church MD PhD[1,2,3], Anshula Ambasta MD[3], Amanda Wilmer MD[4], Holly Williscroft MLT[1], Gordon Ritchie PhD[4,5], Dylan R Pillai MD[1,2,3], Sylvie Champagne MD[4,5], Daniel G Gregson MD[1,2,3]

DL Church, A Ambasta, A Wilmer, et al. Development and validation of a *Pneumocystis jirovecii* real-time polyermase chain reaction assay for diagnosis of *Pneumocystis* pneumonia. Can J Infect Dis Med Microbiol 2015;26(5):263-267.

BACKGROUND: *Pneumocystis jirovecii* (PJ), a pathogenic fungus, causes severe interstitial *Pneumocystis* pneumonia (PCP) among immunocompromised patients. A laboratory-developed real-time polyermase chain reaction (PCR) assay was validated for PJ detection to improve diagnosis of PCP.

METHODS: Forty stored bronchoalveolar lavage (BAL) samples (20 known PJ positive [PJ+] and 20 known PJ negative [PJ–]) were initially tested using the molecular assay. Ninety-two sequentially collected BAL samples were then analyzed using an immunofluorescence assay (IFA) and secondarily tested using the PJ real-time PCR assay. Discrepant results were resolved by retesting BAL samples using another real-time PCR assay with a different target. PJ real-time PCR assay performance was compared with the existing gold standard (ie, IFA) and a modified gold standard, in which a true positive was defined as a sample that tested positive in two of three methods in a patient suspected to have PCP.

RESULTS: Ninety of 132 (68%) BAL fluid samples were collected from immunocompromised patients. Thirteen of 92 (14%) BALs collected were PJ+ when tested using IFA. A total of 40 BAL samples were PJ+ in the present study including: all IFA positive samples (n=13); all referred PJ+ BAL samples (n=20); and seven additional BAL samples that were IFA negative, but positive using the modified gold standard. Compared with IFA, the PJ real-time PCR had sensitivity, specificity, and positive and negative predictive values of 100%, 91%, 65% and 100%, respectively. Compared with the modified gold standard, PJ real-time PCR had a sensitivity, specificity, and positive and negative predictive values of 100%.

CONCLUSION: PJ real-time PCR improved detection of PJ in immunocompromised patients.

Key Words: *Diagnosis; Immunocompromised; P jirovecii; Pneumocystis pneumonia; Real-time PCR*

Mise au point et validation d'un test de réaction en chaîne par polymérase en temps réel du *Pneumocystis jirovecii* pour diagnostiquer une pneumonie à *Pneumocystis*

HISTORIQUE : Le *Pneumocystis jirovecii* (PJ), un champignon pathogène, provoque une grave pneumonie à *Pneumocystis* interstitielle (PPC) chez les patients immunodéprimés. Les chercheurs ont validé un test de réaction en chaîne par polymérase (PCR) en temps réel pour détecter le PJ et ainsi améliorer le diagnostic de PPC.

MÉTHODOLOGIE : Les chercheurs ont d'abord vérifié 40 prélèvements de liquide bronchoalvéolaire (LBA) entreposés (20 cas positifs connus au PJ [PJ+] et 20 cas négatifs connus au PJ [PJ–]) au moyen du test moléculaire. Ils ont ensuite analysé 92 prélèvements séquentiels de LBA au moyen d'un test par immunofluorescence (IFA), puis d'un test de PCR en temps réel du PJ. Ils ont résolu les résultats divergents au moyen d'un nouveau test par PCR en temps réel des prélèvements de LBA axée sur une autre cible. Ils ont comparé le résultat du test de PCR en temps réel du PJ à la référence absolue (l'IFA) et à une référence modifiée, dans laquelle un véritable cas positif désignait un prélèvement positif par deux méthodes sur trois chez un patient atteint d'une PPC présumée.

RÉSULTATS : Quatre-vingt-dix prélèvements de LBA (68 %) sur 132 provenaient de patients immunodéprimés. Treize prélèvements de LBA (14 %) sur 92 étaient PJ+ d'après l'IFA. Dans la présente étude, 40 prélèvements de LBA étaient PJ+, y compris tous les prélèvements positifs à l'IFA (n=13), tous les prélèvements de LBA PJ+ aiguillés (n=20) et sept autres prélèvements de LBA négatifs à l'IFA, mais positifs selon la référence modifiée. Par rapport à l'IFA, la PCR en temps réel du PJ avait une sensibilité, une spécificité et des valeurs prédictives positive et négative de 100 %, 91 %, 65 % et 100 %, respectivement. Par rapport à la référence modifiée, la PCR en temps réel du PJ avait une sensibilité, une spécificité et des valeurs prédictives positive et négative de 100 %.

CONCLUSION : La PCR en temps réel du PJ en améliore la détection chez les patients immunodéprimés.

*P*neumocystis jirovecii (PJ) is an opportunistic fungal pathogen that causes *Pneumocystis* pneumonia (PCP) in humans (1). PCP is an important cause of mortality and morbidity in patients with immunosuppression, particularly among those with HIV infection (2-4). Severe PCP pneumonia has an in-hospital mortality between 7% to 11%; however, in critically-ill patients, it can be as high as 29% to 62%, especially where an etiological diagnosis is delayed (5). Although the incidence of PCP in HIV-infected patients has decreased with the advent of anti-retroviral therapy and chemoprophylaxis (6), its incidence among the non-HIV immunocompromised population has increased (7). Early diagnosis and treatment is critical for survival of all patients diagnosed with PCP, regardless of HIV status (8). Laboratory detection of PJ in lower respiratory samples must be highly sensitive and specific, so as not to miss any potential cases of PCP, while still being able to avoid unnecessary antimicrobial treatment in patients with asymptomatic colonization.

Many clinical microbiology laboratories continue to rely on direct microscopic detection of the cyst form of *Pneumocystis* in stained lower

[1]*Division of Microbiology, Calgary Laboratory Services, Departments of Pathology & Laboratory Medicine,* [2]*Division of Medical Microbiology and* [3]*Medicine, Alberta Health Services and the University of Calgary, Calgary, Alberta, and Department of Pathology & Laboratory Medicine,* [4]*Division of Medical Microbiology,* [5]*St Paul's Hospital and the University of British Columbia, Vancouver, British Columbia*
Correspondence: Dr Deirdre L Church, Division of Microbiology, Calgary Laboratory Services, 9-3535 Research Road Northwest, Calgary, Alberta T2L 2K8 e-mail deirdre.church@cls.ab.ca

respiratory tract samples (9,10). Laboratory-developed molecular methods have recently been reported, and have a higher sensitivity for the detection of PJ in lower respiratory tract samples compared with microscopy (11-14). Due to a lower cyst burden, diagnosis of PCP may be difficult using microscopic methods for immunocompromised patients without HIV infection, and in HIV-infected patients receiving antiretroviral therapy. Conventional staining and microscopic examination of bronchoalveolar lavage (BAL) fluid ranged between 70% and 92% in non-HIV infected immunocompromised patients, while the sensitivity for sputa was even lower, between 38% and 53% (14,15). Although several laboratory-developed qualitative PJ real-time polymerase chain reaction (PCR) assays had been reported for the diagnosis of PCP (16-20), at the time of the present study, no commercial molecular assays were available (21). The present study describes the clinical and laboratory development, and validation of a unique qualitative PJ real-time PCR assay for the rapid detection of PCP.

METHODS

Clinical setting

Calgary Laboratory Services (CLS) is a large regional centralized laboratory that provides diagnostic testing for infectious diseases for a population of approximately 1.5 million in Calgary and southern Alberta. Approximately 1200 BAL fluid samples are submitted each year from immunocompromised patients for PJ detection. Immunocompromised patients in the present study included those with solid organ or hematopoietic stem cell transplants, HIV or malignancy (solid/haematological). Demographical data and brief clinical history were initially obtained for each enrolled patient through completed laboratory requisitions, which included the patient's age, sex, date of birth and reason for immune compromise including the presence of neutropenia. The CLS study microbiologist (DLC) also subsequently reviewed positive PJ real-time PCR results with the attending physician to determine whether that positive result correlated with the presence of PCP versus asymptomatic colonization.

Sample collection

A total of 132 BAL fluid samples were collected from patients in whom PCP was considered in the differential diagnosis and tested during the study. Forty BAL fluid samples collected between 2006 and 2012 were obtained (20 known PJ positive [PJ+] and 20 known PJ negative [PJ–]) from St Paul's Hospital, Vancouver, British Columbia, designated as the referral laboratory (RL). All BAL samples from the RL were initially analyzed using microscopic examination after staining, and secondarily tested using their laboratory developed PJ real-time PCR assay (see Methods). Aliquots of the BAL fluid samples were then stored frozen at −80°C until referral. Another 92 BAL fluid samples were sequentially collected retrospectively at CLS between May 2011 and September 2012. Aliquots of the BAL fluid samples were frozen at −80°C after initially being tested using an immunofluorescence assay (IFA). Storage of multiple sample aliquots allowed later use in discrepant analysis without an additional freeze-thaw. If multiple BAL fluid samples were stored from the same patient, each was tested individually and not pooled.

Microscopic examination

All BAL fluid samples from the RL were initially analyzed using Toluidine Blue O stain (22) and/or a modified Gomori's methenamine silver borate stain and microscopic examination. All of the BAL fluid samples collected at CLS were initially tested using a commercial direct IFA. The Genetic Systems Monofluor *Pneumocystis* (Meridian Bioscience Inc, USA) immunofluorescence assay was performed according to the manufacturer's instructions.

CLS PJ real-time PCR assay

The BAL fluid samples were centrifuged before DNA extraction. DNA was extracted from stored BAL samples (180 µL aliquot) using the QuickGene 810 on the DNA Tissue Mode program according to

the manufacturer's protocol (FujiFilm Life Sciences, Japan). The QuickGene 810 extraction procedure typically yields 100 µL of eluent. A DNA purity check of the extract was performed by measuring the 260/280 nm ratio using a spectrophotometer (ND-100, NanoDrop Technologies Inc, USA), which consistently yielded 260 nm to 280 nm ratios of approximately 1.8. Aliquots (10 µL) of the DNA extract were stored frozen at −80°C.

Five microlitres of this DNA extract was used for each real-time PCR assay. The PJ real-time PCR assay was based on a previously described method with a positive cut-off cycle threshold (Ct) ≤37 (23). Integrated DNA Technologies (www.idtdna.com) supplied the hybridization probe and primers specific for the mitochondrial large subunit (mtLSU) ribosomal RNA gene of PJ. The forward primer (mtLSU FWD: 5'-TGG TAA GTA GTG AAA TAC AAA TCG G–3' [start = 178, stop = 203]) and the reverse primer (mtLSU REV: 5'–ACT CCC TCG AGA TAT TCA GTG C–3' [start = 277, stop = 299]) were identical to those previously published (18). However, the sequence of the hybridization probe (mtLSU PRB: 5'–/56-FAM/ ACT AGG ATA / ZEN/TAG CTG GTT TTC TGC GA/3IABkFQ/–3') and the fluorescent dyes used to tag the 5' and 3' probe ends differed from those previously published (23). PJ real-time PCR reactions contained 20 µL SmartMix HM Mastermix (5 Smart Mix beads, one QC bead, 185 µL of Sigma H_2O and 5 µL of each of the primers and the probe) and 5 µL purified DNA. During each run, a PJ DNA positive control and a template negative control were included. The SmartCycler (Cepheid, USA) program followed 50 cycles of 10 s at 95°C, 10 s at 60°C and 10 s at 72°C.

A positive patient sample that was IFA and PJ real-time PCR positive (ie, with an estimated 1×10^5 copies/mL) was used to estimate the assay's limit of detection. The BAL sample was serially diluted approximately 10,000-fold that of the original material before the PJ real-time PCR became negative (ie, no amplification signal above baseline). The dilution series of samples were also repeatedly tested (ie, up to six times) using the real-time PCR assay to establish the reproducibility of the Ct values for PJ+ samples over the range of dilutions in which PJ was detected (ie, 1:2, up to 1: approximately 10,000). Clinical BAL fluid samples were also tested in duplicate on three separate days to establish the precision of the assay, including two negative and three positive samples within the low, mid and high Ct range of the assay.

RL PJ real-time PCR assay

The St Paul's Hospital laboratory-developed PJ real-time-PCR assay was adapted from one previously published (19). Briefly, 400 µL of BAL fluid in phosphate-buffered saline was extracted with 10 µL of internal amplification control according to the total nucleic acid isolation blood protocol using a Roche Magna Pure Compact instrument (Roche Molecular Diagnostics, USA) and eluted in 100 µL. Respiratory samples containing thick mucus were pretreated with proteinase K (25 µL 1 g/mL) and sodium dodecyl sulfate then lysed using zirconium beads (150 µL 2.4 mm) and silica beads (50 µL 0.1 mm) (Biospec Products, USA) before DNA extraction. Primers and fluorescence resonance evergy transfer probes were previously described, and were designed to detect a 166-base pair region of the *cdc2* gene of PJ (19). PCR was performed on 5 µL of DNA extract using the LightCycler-FastStart DNA Master Hybridization Probes kit (Roche Diagnostics, Canada) in the presence of 4 mmol/L $MgCl_2$ using the Light Cycler 2.0 (Roche Diagnostics, Canada). Melting curve analysis was performed at the end of the *cdc2* PCR amplification to confirm positives. All primers and probes were synthesized by Metabion (Germany).

Data analysis

All patient information and PJ test results were entered into an Excel spreadsheet (Microsoft Corporation, USA) in an anonymous nonnominal fashion using the patient study number. Descriptive statistics were performed using standard methods. Performance of the CLS PJ real-time PCR assay was compared with the IFA as the existing gold standard during the study period. Discrepancies between IFA and the CLS PJ real-time PCR assay were resolved by secondarily testing the discrepant BAL samples with the PJ real-time PCR used by the RL (see Methods). The modified gold standard (ie, a true positive result) was defined as a BAL sample that tested positive according to both molecular assays and/or IFA in a patient suspected of having PCP. The presence of PCP was not only defined by the PJ test, but also after clinical review of each patient by DLC with the attending physician. Performance of each test was calculated using standard statistical methods with the modified gold standard. All statistical analyses were performed using standard methods with Analyze-It software version 2.6.1 (Microsoft Corporation, USA).

Ethics

Once obtained, all clinical information was handled in an anonymous fashion in the working dataset at each site. BAL samples from the RL were provided in an anonymous fashion to ensure patient confidentiality. The study was granted ethics approval by the Conjoint Health Research Ethics Board at the University of Calgary/Alberta Health Services (Calgary, Alberta) and St Paul's Hospital/University of British Columbia (Vancouver, British Columbia) Ethics Review Boards.

RESULTS

Patient population

A total of 132 BAL samples from 127 patients were analyzed in the present study. Almost all of the 20 PJ+ samples sent from the RL were collected from HIV infected individuals (19 of 20 [95%]); the remaining patient was receiving corticosteroids due to a central nervous system lymphoma. Most of the 20 PJ– BAL samples from the RL were also collected from immunocompromised patients (19 of 20 [95%]), including eight patients with HIV infection, nine transplant patients, one patient with myelodysplasia and one patient with systemic vasculitis being treated with immunosuppressive agents.

A total of 92 BAL samples from 87 patients were collected by CLS; both a right and left BAL fluid sample were tested for five patients. According to the clinical history provided on the laboratory requisition, 50 of 87 (57.5%) of the study samples were collected from immunocompromised patients including: nine who had HIV (18%), 23 who were solid-organ transplant recipients (46%), two who had received previous hematopoietic stem cell transplantation (4%) and 14 with malignancies (28%). The remaining 4% of the sample order requisitions did not provide descriptions of the cause of their immunosuppression.

CLS PJ real-time PCR assay validation

The PJ real-time PCR was initially used to test the 40 clinical samples (20 known PJ+ and 20 known PJ–) from the RL, with consistent results. The developed molecular assay could detect the approximately 1:10,000 diluted sample estimated to contain 10 cysts of organism per 2 μL, yielding an estimated limit of detection of at least 10 copies per PCR. Amplification of the serially diluted BAL fluid sample (ie, estimated to contain 1×10^5 cysts) generated Ct values of 20 for a 1:2 dilution, up to 37 for the 1:10,000 dilution. The CLS real-time PCR assay also provided excellent reproducibility. Both PJ– BAL fluid samples repeatedly tested negative including a Ct value of 0 on separate runs repeated on different days, and in two carryover runs performed back to back on the same day. The three PJ+ BAL fluid samples also repeatedly tested positive with a mean (± SD) Ct value of 20.85±0.13, 20.78±0.08, 21.2±0.12, 21.8±0.12 and 21.9±0.19, respectively, for the individual samples on two separate runs repeated on different days, and in two carryover runs performed back to back on the same day. When CLS PJ real-time PCR was performed on the 40 clinical samples (20 known PJ+ and 20 known PJ– samples) sent from the RL, similar results were found for all samples.

Figure 1 compares range and CIs for the PJ real-time assay Ct compared with the detection of PJ cysts using IFA. The 95% upper CI for PJ+ BAL fluid samples that were detected by both the IFA and

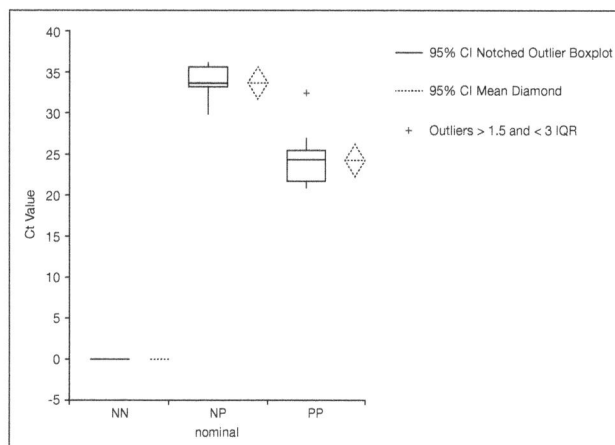

Figure 1) *Comparison of the* Pneumocystis jirovecii *(PJ) real-time polymerase chain reaction (PCR) assay to that of immunofluorescence assay (IFA) to confirm the diagnostic cut-off of the assay. Ct Cycle threshold; IQR Interquartile range; NN Negative according to both IFA and PJ real-time PCR; NP Negative according to IFA and positive according to PJ real-time PCR; PP Positive according to both IFA and PJ real-time PCR*

molecular assays was 26 cycles. The lower and upper 95% CIs for BAL fluid samples that were PJ– according to IFA, but PJ+ according to molecular assay, was 30 and 37 cycles, respectively. Therefore, the reportable range for the PJ real-time assay was established as follows: Ct ≤30 cycles = true positive PJ result; Ct ≥30 but <37 = low positive result that may be indicative of early infection or colonization in which clinical correlation is required to establish the presence of disease; and >37 = negative result.

The clinical performance of the PJ real-time PCR assay was compared with both the IFA and the modified gold standard. PJ cysts were detected in a total of 13 of 92 (15%) BAL fluid samples. Twelve of 13 (92.3%) of these PJ+ samples were derived from immunocompromised patients, while the clinical history for the last sample only mentioned pneumonia. Eight patients had HIV infection, three had a malignancy, and one had immunosuppression for an unspecified reason. All of the BAL fluid samples that were PJ+ according to IFA were also positive according to the molecular assay with Ct values ≤30 cycles. Another seven samples from six patients that were PJ– according to IFA, were PJ+ according to the PJ real-time PCR assay. The Ct values for these discrepant samples were all >30 but <37 (ie, 30.9, 33.9, 35.9, 33.6, 36.1, 33.2 and 34.9). Clinical review regarding these results with the attending physician enabled these results to be correlated with the presence of PCP in all cases. Two of these samples were taken from a patient (ie, right lower lobe and left lower lobe samples) with interstitial lung disease receiving high-dose steroids who was considered to have early infection. The remaining five patients had clinical PCP, and included one patient with HIV infection, one with a brain tumour receiving high-dose steroids, one hematopoietic stell cell transplantation patient with severe hypoxemia, one patient with interstitial lung disease and one patient with new-onset fever and pneumonia in whom HIV infection was suspected but not yet confirmed. One other BAL fluid sample from a patient receiving renal dialysis was PJ– according to IFA, but provided a very late Ct value (42.8) according to molecular testing. Because there was no evidence of PCP on clinical review, this result was called a true negative according to the PJ real-time PCR assay.

All of the seven BAL fluid samples that provided discrepant results between IFA (negative) and the CLS PJ real-time PCR assay (positive) were also PJ+ according to the RL real-time PCR assay. Table 1 summarizes the performance of the IFA and PJ real-time PCR assays for diagnosis of PCP. Although the IFA assay was highly specific, it was less sensitive than the molecular assay at diagnosing PCP. The IFA

Table 1
Performance of the immunofluorescence and *Pneumocystis jirovecii* (PJ) real-time polymerase chain reaction (PCR) assays for diagnosis of pneumonia*

Detection method	Positive	Negative	Total
IFA[†]			
Positive	13	0	13
Negative	7	72	79
Total	20	72	92
PJ real-time PCR[‡]			
Positive	20[§]	0	20
Negative	0	72	72
Total	20	72	92

Data presented as n. *True positive = bronchoalveolar lavage (BAL) positive according to immunofluorescence assay (IFA) and the PJ real-time PCR assay or IFA negative but both PJ real-time PCR assays positive in a patient with Pneumocystis pneumonia. †Sensitivity=13/20 (65%), specificity=72/72 (100%), positive predictive value (PPV)=13/13 (100%), negative predictive value (NPV)=72/79 (91.1%). ‡Sensitivity=20/20 (100%), specificity=72/72 (100%), PPV=20/20 (100%), NPV=72/72 (100%). §Two BAL fluid samples were tested from the same patient who was considered to have early PJ infection

also produced a lower negative predictive value because it was false negative in six patients with PCP and one who was suspected of having early PJ infection.

Performance of the PJ real-time PCR assay was similar in immunocompromised patients with HIV and those who were immune suppressed for other reasons. For the IFA, the sensitivity among non-HIV infected patients was slightly higher at 70.59% with the specificity preserved at 100%. Of the nine HIV positive patients, eight had a positive IFA test, and the ninth sample was positive based on the modified gold standard and a clinical diagnosis of PCP. The IFA test resulted in higher sensitivity (88.89%) for HIV patients, with 100% specificity.

DISCUSSION

We described a laboratory-developed real-time assay for the highly reliable detection of PJ from BAL fluid. Overall, the method can be performed the same day the sample is received and has a turnaround time of 2.5 h including DNA extraction, and has an overall increase in sensitivity of 35% over our existing IFA method. The present study confirms that PCR is more sensitive than staining and microscopic examination of BAL samples to diagnose PCP (17,24-28). The PJ real-time PCR developed and validated during the present study was highly sensitive and specific at diagnosing PCP in immunocompromised patients, particularly those without HIV infection. Real-time PCR detection of PJ is more rapid than conventional PCR, and reduces the potential for carry-over contamination run-to-run because the reaction is performed in a closed system. Real-time PCR also offers a high degree of objectivity that cannot be obtained by staining and microscopic examination of a BAL sample. In our laboratory, even highly experienced technologists would have difficulty calling the IFA positive when few cysts were present. This was also reflected in the performance of the IFA compared with the PJ real-time assay in our study. The sensitivity of IFA in our study was highest among HIV infected individuals (88.89%), which was similar to the molecular assay, although IFA was falsely negative in one patient with PCP. The sensitivity of IFA was lower when analyzing BAL samples from non-HIV immunocompromised patients (70.6%), and considerably less than the molecular assay when all patient samples were considered (65%).

The higher sensitivity of molecular detection of PJ in BAL fluid samples is consistent with the results of other studies (17,24-28). A systematic review that evaluated PJ PCR assays testing BAL fluid samples revealed an overall sensitivity of 98.3% and specificity of 91% for all of the studies included in their analysis (27), and highlighted that

one can expect false-positive PCR tests to occur in patients with no clinical evidence of PCP. All positive PCR results should, therefore, by correlated with the patient's clinical symptoms and radiological evidence of PCP; however, a negative PCR result essentially allows the diagnosis to be ruled out if controls perform to specification and PCR inhibition has not occurred (27,29). A more recent meta-analysis of reported molecular assays that included real-time PCR for PJ detection from BAL fluid samples produced a similar overall sensitivity of 98% but a higher specificity of 93% (29). Our study also confirmed the high inter-laboratory agreement among real-time PCR assays previously used for the detection of PJ (30).

Although there were no false-positive PJ real-time PCR tests in our study, previously reported validations of other laboratory developed qualitative molecular assays for PJ detection have found false-positive tests due to the higher sensitivity of molecular methods (23,31,32). Therefore, a diagnostic cut-off should be established, such as what occurred in our study, for the reportable range of the real-time PCR assay, that includes true positive, a 'grey-zone' for low-level positives, which may represent early infection or asymptomatic colonization and negative results. Clinical correlation of the results of our PJ real-time PCR assay with the presence of PCP validated that the established cut-offs for a true positive (ie, Ct ≤30) and low positive (ie, Ct >30 but <37) accurately diagnosed the presence of PCP. All of the patients with low positive PJ real-time PCR results who were negative according to IFA were confirmed to have definite PCP or suspected early infection (one patient) on clinical review. Confirmation that these seven discrepant BAL results were true positives was also documented by testing them using a second *Pneumocystis* gene target, the *cdc2* gene, by the RL. The second positive real-time PCR result, using another independent molecular method, further supported the presence of this fungal organism in the patient's sample.

Although the use of qualitative real-time PCR for PJ detection would improve our ability to rapidly and accurately diagnose PCP in our jurisdiction and our molecular assay demonstrated complete agreement with the RL's assay, standardized diagnostic performance across laboratories awaits the development of a quantitative PJ real-time PCR assay (33). A commercial quantitative PJ real-time PCR assay used in combination with serum (1,3)-β-D-glucan may enable improved differentiation of patients with PJ colonization and those with early or suppressed PCP infection (34,35), and also enhance therapeutic monitoring of PCP resolution while receiving treatment.

ACKNOWLEDGEMENTS: This study was supported by a Calgary Laboratory Services Research Grant that was awarded through a competitive peer-review process. The work was completed as part of an Internal Medicine residency project (A Ambasta). The work was presented as a poster presentation at the IDWeek Meeting, October 8 to 12, 2014, Philadelphia, Pennsylvania.

DISCLOSURES: The authors have no conflicts of interest to declare.

REFERENCES

1. Redhead SA, Cushion MT, Frenkel JK, Stringer JR. *Pneumocystis* and *Trypanosoma cruzi*: Nomenclature and typifications. J Eukaryot Microbiol 2006;53:2-11.
2. Kaplan JE, Benson C, Holmes KK, Brooks JT, Pau A, Masur H. Guidelines for prevention and treatment of opportunistic infections in HIV-infected adults and adolescents: Recommendations from CDC, the National Institutes of Health, and the HIV Medicine Association of the Infectious Diseases Society of America. MMWR 2009;58:1-207.
3. Calderon EJ, Gutierrez-Rivero S, Durand-Joly I, Dei-Cas E. *Pneumocystis* infection in humans: Diagnosis and treatment. Exp Rev Anti-Infect Ther 2010;8:683-701.
4. Kovacs JA, Masur H. Evolving health effects of *Pneumocystis*: One hundred years of progress in diagnosis and treatment. JAMA 2009;301:2578-85.

5. Morris A, Norris KA. Colonization by *Pneumocystis jiroveciii* and its role in disease. Clin Microbiol Rev 2012;25:297-317.

6. Kelley CF, Checkley W, Mannino DM, Franco-Paredes C, Del Rio C, Holguin F. Trends in hospitalizations for AIDS-associated *Pneumocystis jiroveciii* pneumonia in the United States (1986 to 2005). Chest 2009;136:190-7.

7. Mansharamani NG, Garland R, Delaney D, Koziel H. Management and outcome patterns for adult *Pneumocystis carinii* pneumonia, 1985 to 1995: Comparison of HIV-associated cases to other immunocompromised states. Chest 2000;118:704-711.

8. Asai N, Motojima S, Ohkuni Y, et al. Early diagnosis and treatment are crucial for the survival of *Pneumocystis pneumonia* patients without human immunodeficiency virus infection. J Infect Chemother 2012;18:898-905.

9. Procop GW, Haddad S, Quinn J, et al. Detection of *Pneumocystis jirovecii* in respiratory specimens by four staining methods. J Clin Microbiol 2004; 42:3333-5.

10. Silva RM, Bazzo ML, Borges AA. Induced sputum versus bronchoalveolar lavage in the diagnosis of *Pneumocystis jirovecii* pneumonia in human immunodeficiency virus-positive patients. Braz J Infect Dis 2007;11:549-53.

11. Wakefield AE, Stewart TJ, Moxon ER, Marsh K, Hopkin JM. Infection with *Pneumocystis carinii* is prevalent in healthy Gambian children. Trans R Soc Trop Med Hyg 1990;84:800-2.

12. Wakefield AE, Guiver L, Miller RF, Hopkin JM. DNA amplification on induced sputum samples for diagnosis of *Pneumocystis carinii* pneumonia. Lancet 1991;337:1378-1379.

13. Cartwright CP, Nelson NA, Gill VJ. Development and evaluation of a rapid and simple procedure for detection of *Pneumocystis carinii* by PCR. J Clin Microbiol 1994;32:1634-8.

14. Caliendo AM, Hewitt PL, Allega JM, Keen A, Ruoff KL, Ferraro MJ. Performance of a PCR assay for detection of *Pneumocystis carinii* from respiratory specimens. J Clin Microbiol 1998;36:979-82.

15. Lipschik GY, Gill VJ, Lundgren JD, et al. Improved diagnosis of *Pneumocystis carinii* infection by polymerase chain reaction on induced sputum and blood. Lancet 1992;340:203-6.

16. Flori P, Bellete B, Durand F, et al. Comparison between real-time PCR, conventional PCR and different staining techniques for diagnosing *Pneumocystis jirovecii* pneumonia from bronchoalveolar lavage specimens. J Med Microbiol 2004;53:603-7.

17. Arcenas RC, Uhl JR, Buckwalter SP, et al. A real-time polymerase chain reaction assay for detection of *Pneumocystis* from bronchoalveolar lavage fluid. Diagn Microbiol Infect Dis 2006;54:169-75.

18. Huggett JF, Taylor MS, Kocjan G, et al. Development and evaluation of a real-time PCR assay for detection of *Pneumocystis jiroveciii* DNA in bronchoalveolar lavage fluid of HIV-infected patients. Thorax 2008;63:154-9.

19. Wilson JW, Limper AH, Grys TE, Karre T, Wengenack NL, Binnicker MJ. *Pneumocystis jirovecii* testing by real-time polymerase chain reaction and direct examination among immunocompetent and immunosuppressed patient groups and correlation to disease specificity. Diagn Microbiol Infect Dis 2011;69:145-52.

20. Hauser PM, Bille J, Lass-Florl C, et al. Multicenter, prospective clinical evaluation of respiratory samples from subjects at risk for *Pneumocystis jiroveciii* infection by use of a commercial real-time PCR assay. J Clin Microbiol 2011;49:1872-78.

21. McTaggart LR, Wengenack NL, Richardson SE. Validation of the MycAssay Pneumocystis kit for detection of *Pneumocystis jiroveciii* in bronchoalveolar lavage specimens by comparison to a laboratory standard of direct immunofluorescence microscopy, real-time PCR, or conventional PCR. J Clin Microbiol 2012;50:1856-9.

22. Gosey LL, RM Howard, FG Witebsky, et al. Advantages of a modified Toluidine Blue I stain and bronchoalveolar lavage for the diagnosis of *Pneumocystis carinii* pneumonia. J Clin Microbiol 1985;22:803-7.

23. Botterel F, Cabaret O, Foulet F, Cordonnier C, Costa JM, Bretagne S. Clinical significance of quantifying *Pneumocystis jiroveciii* DNA by using real-time PCR in bronchoalveolar lavage fluid from immunocompromised patients. J Clin Microbiol 2012;50:227-31.

24. Galan F, Oliver JL, Roux P, Poirot JL, Bereziat G. Detection of *Pneumocystis carinii* DNA by polymerase chain reaction compared to direct microscopy and immunofluorescence. J Protozool 1991;38:199S-200S.

25. Chawla K, Martena S, Gurung B, Mukhopadhyay C, Varghese GK, Bairy I. Role of PCR for diagnosing *Pneumocystis jiroveciii* pneumonia in HIV-infected individuals in a tertiary care hospital in India. Ind J Pathol Microbiol 2011;54:326-9.

26. Takahashi T, Goto M, Endo T, et al. *Pneumocystis carinii* carriage in immunocompromised patients with and without human immunodeficiency virus infection. J Med Microbiol 2002;51:611-4.

27. Fan LC, Lu HW, Cheng KB, Li HP, Xu JF. Evaluation of PCR in bronchoalveolar lavage fluid for diagnosis of *Pneumocystis jiroveciii* pneumonia: A bivariate meta-analysis and systematic review. PloS one 2013;8:e73099.

28. Summah H, Zhu YG, Falagas ME, Vouloumanou EK, Qu JM. Use of real-time polymerase chain reaction for the diagnosis of *Pneumocystis* pneumonia in immunocompromised patients: A meta-analysis. Chin Med J 2013;126:1965-73.

29. Hauser PM, Blanc DS, Bille J, Nahimana A, Francioli P. Carriage of *Pneumocystis carinii* by immunosuppressed patients and molecular typing of the organisms. AIDS 2000;14:461-3.

30. Linssen CF, Jacobs JA, Beckers P, et al. Inter-laboratory comparison of three different real-time PCR assays for the detection of *Pneumocystis jirovecii* in bronchoalveolar lavage fluid samples. J Med Microbiol 2006;55:1229-35.

31. Lu Y, Ling G, Qiang C, et al. PCR diagnosis of *Pneumocystis* pneumonia: A bivariate meta-analysis. J Clin Microbiol 2011;49:4361-3.

32. Olsson M, Elvin K, Lofdahl S, Linder E. Detection of *Pneumocystis carinii* DNA in sputum and bronchoalveolar lavage samples by polymerase chain reaction. J Clin Microbiol 1996;34:2052.

33. Maillet M, Maubon D, Brion JP, et al. *Pneumocystis jiroveciii* (Pj) quantitative PCR to differentiate Pj pneumonia from Pj colonization in immunocompromised patients. Eur J Clin Microbiol Infect Dis 2014;33:331-6.

34. Matsumura Y, Ito Y, Iinuma Y, et al. Quantitative real-time PCR and the (1→3)-beta-D-glucan assay for differentiation between *Pneumocystis jiroveciii* pneumonia and colonization. Clin Microbiol Infect 2012;18:591-7.

35. Damiani C, Le Gal S, Da Costa C, Virmaux M, Nevez G, Totet A. Combined quantification of pulmonary *Pneumocystis jiroveciii* DNA and serum (1→3)-beta-D-glucan for differential diagnosis of *Pneumocystis* pneumonia and *Pneumocystis* colonization. J Clin Microbiol 2013;51:3380-8.

17

Usefulness of previous methicillin-resistant *Staphylococcus aureus* screening results in guiding empirical therapy for *S aureus* bacteremia

Anthony D Bai BHSc[1], Lisa Burry PharmD[2,3], Adrienne Showler MD[4,5], Marilyn Steinberg RN[2],
Daniel Ricciuto MD[4,5,6,7], Tania Fernandes PharmD[8], Anna Chiu BScPhm[8], Sumit Raybardhan BScPhm MPH[9],
George A Tomlinson PhD[4,10], Chaim M Bell MD PhD[2,4,10,11], Andrew M Morris MD SM[2,4,5,10]

AD Bai, L Burry, A Showler, et al. Usefulness of previous methicillin-resistant *Staphylococcus aureus* screening results in guiding empirical therapy for *S aureus* bacteremia. Can J Infect Dis Med Microbiol 2015;26(4):201-206.

BACKGROUND: *Staphylococcus aureus* bacteremia (SAB) is an important infection. Methicillin-resistant *S aureus* (MRSA) screening is performed on hospitalized patients for infection control purposes.
OBJECTIVE: To assess the usefulness of past MRSA screening for guiding empirical antibiotic therapy for SAB.
METHODS: A retrospective cohort study examined consecutive patients with confirmed SAB and previous MRSA screening swab from six academic and community hospitals between 2007 and 2010. Diagnostic test properties were calculated for MRSA screening swab for predicting methicillin resistance of SAB.
RESULTS: A total of 799 patients underwent MRSA screening swabs before SAB. Of the 799 patients, 95 (12%) had a positive and 704 (88%) had a negative previous MRSA screening swab. There were 150 (19%) patients with MRSA bacteremia. Overall, previous MRSA screening swabs had a positive likelihood ratio of 33 (95% CI 18 to 60) and a negative likelihood ratio of 0.45 (95% CI 0.37 to 0.54). Diagnostic accuracy differed depending on mode of acquisition (ie, community-acquired, nosocomial or health care-associated infection) (P<0.0001) and hospital (P=0.0002). At best, for health care-associated infection, prior MRSA screening swab had a positive likelihood ratio of 16 (95% CI 9 to 28) and a negative likelihood ratio of 0.27 (95% CI 0.17 to 0.41).
CONCLUSIONS: A negative prior MRSA screening swab cannot reliably rule out MRSA bacteremia and should not be used to guide empirical antibiotic therapy for SAB. A positive prior MRSA screening swab greatly increases likelihood of MRSA, necessitating MRSA coverage in empirical antibiotic therapy for SAB.

Key Words: *Antimicrobial stewardship; Empirical antimicrobial therapy; MRSA screening; Sensitivity; Specificity; Staphylococcus aureus bacteremia*

L'utilité d'un dépistage antérieur du *Staphylococcus aureus* résistant à la méthicilline pour orienter le traitement empirique de la bactériémie à *S. aureus*

HISTORIQUE : La bactériémie à *Staphylococcus aureus* (BSA) est une infection grave. Les patients hospitalisés subissent un dépistage du *S. aureus* résistant à la méthicilline (SARM) afin de prévenir les infections.
OBJECTIF : Évaluer l'utilité d'un dépistage antérieur du SARM pour orienter l'antibiothérapie empirique de la BSA.
MÉTHODOLOGIE : Les chercheurs ont effectué une étude de cohorte rétrospective dans six hôpitaux universitaires et hôpitaux généraux entre 2007 et 2010 auprès de patients consécutifs atteints d'une BSA confirmée ayant déjà subi un prélèvement de dépistage du SARM. Ils ont calculé les propriétés des tests diagnostiques par prélèvement pour diagnostiquer le SARM et prédire la résistance de la BSA à la méthicilline.
RÉSULTATS : Au total, 799 patients avaient déjà subi des prélèvements pour dépister le SARM avant une BSA. De ce nombre, 95 (12 %) ont présenté un résultat positif et 704 (88 %) avaient déjà subi un prélèvement pour dépister le SARM. Cent cinquante patients (19 %) avaient une bactériémie à SARM. Dans l'ensemble, les prélèvements antérieurs pour dépister le SARM avaient un ratio de probabilité positif de 33 (95 % IC 18 à 60) et négatif de 0,45 (95 % IC 0,37 à 0,54). La précision diagnostique différait en fonction du mode d'acquisition (origine non nosocomiale, origine nosocomiale ou association aux soins de santé) (P<0,0001) et de l'hôpital (P=0,0002). Dans le meilleur des cas, en présence d'une infection associée aux soins de santé, un prélèvement antérieur pour dépister un SARM s'associait à un ratio de probabilité positif de 16 (95 % IC 9 à 28) et négatif de 0,27 (95 % IC 0,17 à 0,41).
CONCLUSIONS : Un prélèvement antérieur négatif au SARM ne permet pas d'écarter une bactériémie par le SARM avec fiabilité et ne devrait pas orienter l'antibiothérapie empirique de la BSA. Un prélèvement antérieur positif au SARM accroît considérablement la probabilité de SARM, ce qui oblige à en tenir compte pour l'antibiothérapie empirique de la BSA.

*S*taphylococcus aureus is a leading cause of bloodstream infections and is associated with a high mortality of 10% to 30% (1-4). Methicillin-resistant *S aureus* (MRSA) is highly prevalent. In Canada, it is estimated that 27% of all S aureus bacteremia (SAB) are MRSA; however, prevalence varies greatly depending on the region (5). MRSA bacteremia results in higher mortality, longer hospital stay and increased cost compared with methicillin-susceptible *S aureus* (MSSA) (6,7).

The decision to initiate an antibiotic with activity against MRSA in empirical therapy of suspected bacteremia is complex. For MRSA bacteremia, vancomycin is the standard antimicrobial agent, because

[1]*Faculty of Medicine, University of Ottawa, Ottawa;* [2]*Mount Sinai Hospital;* [3]*Leslie Dan Faculty of Pharmacy;* [4]*Department of Medicine;* [5]*Division of Infectious Diseases, University of Toronto, Toronto;* [6]*Lakeridge Health, Oshawa;* [7]*Department of Medicine, Queen's University, Kingston;* [8]*Trillium Health Partners, Mississauga;* [9]*North York General Hospital;* [10]*University Health Network;* [11]*Institute for Clinical Evaluative Sciences, Toronto, Ontario*
Correspondence: Dr Andrew M Morris, Mount Sinai Hospital, 600 University Avenue, Suite 415, Toronto, Ontario M5G 1X5.
e-mail amorris@mtsinai.on.ca

β-lactam antibiotics are ineffective (8). Early empirical antibiotic therapy with MRSA coverage in MRSA bacteremia resulted in better clinical outcomes including lower mortality (9). However, vancomycin is inferior to β-lactam antibiotics in treating MRSA bacteremia (10,11). Furthermore, use of vancomycin increases antimicrobial resistance, such as vancomycin-resistant enterococci (12). Finally, use of vancomycin in the treatment of MRSA bacteremia is associated with risk for nephrotoxicity (8). In clinical practice, empirical vancomycin for suspected bacteremia is not universally used and not added unless there is an increased risk for MRSA (13-15). Ideally, empirical vancomycin is warranted only when the probability of MRSA is sufficiently high.

MRSA screening is usually performed in hospitals for infection control purposes. However, MRSA colonization may predict infection and, therefore, MRSA status may help guide empirical therapy in SAB (16,17). We conducted a retrospective cohort study to identify the clinical utility of past MRSA screening swab in predicting methicillin resistance for patients with SAB.

METHODS

Study design

The present study used data from a larger retrospective cohort study of SAB at six acute-care academic and community hospitals in the Greater Toronto Area (Ontario) from April 1, 2007 to April 1, 2010 (18). Research ethics board approval was obtained from each institution.

Consecutive patients were included in the study if they had ≥1 positive blood culture for S aureus and an MRSA screening swab was performed before blood culture susceptibility results. The MRSA screening swab may have been at a current or previous admission. Only the most recent MRSA screening swab was considered. Patients <18 years of age were excluded. Patients were only included in the study once, using the first positive blood culture as the index.

Data sources

Data were obtained from patients' medical records at each site and entered into a standardized case report form. Variables collected from patient medical records included patient age, sex, hospital site, admitting service, date of MRSA screening swab collection, date and time of positive blood culture, date of admission and mode of acquisition.

MRSA screening procedure

MRSA screening criteria were similar for all sites according to Ontario provincial guidelines (19). Patients were screened if they satisfied any of the following criteria: any known history of colonization with antibiotic-resistant organism; any known history of contact with a patient known to be colonized with an antibiotic-resistant organism; admission to a health care facility in the past 12 to 24 months; or unable to provide information regarding any of the aforementioned risk factors.

For all sites, swab samples were obtained from the nares and rectum, as well as any insertion site or open wounds. Laboratory confirmation of MRSA was similar for all sites. MRSA swabs were incubated in MRSA selective media at 35°C or 37°C for approximately 24 h. Isolates were identified as S aureus if the rapid S aureus agglutination test and/or the tube coagulase test were positive. Methicillin resistance was confirmed using positive PBP2a agglutination testing and/or susceptibility testing (oxacillin screen plate or Vitek2 XL system AST-GP67 cards [Biomérieux, USA]) according to Clinical and Laboratory Standards Institute guidelines (20).

Blood culture procedure

Blood collection and culture were similar for all sites. Blood culture bottles were incubated at 35°C for a maximum of five days. Direct Gram staining was performed on all positive blood cultures, which were then subcultured onto blood agar plates. Blood agar plates were incubated at 35°C for two days. S aureus was identified when Gram staining showed Gram-positive cocci in clusters and tube coagulase test was positive. Methicillin resistance was determined by the same method used for MRSA screening.

Covariates

Potential covariates being considered included patient age (18 to 30, 31 to 45, 46 to 60, 61 to 75, 76 to 90 or >90 years of age), sex, hospital site, admitting service (medical, surgical or intensive care unit), time from MRSA screening swab collection to blood culture collection, time from admission to blood culture collection, MRSA screen with blood culture collection on same admission and mode of acquisition (community-acquired, nosocomial or health care-associated infection). The time from MRSA screening to blood culture collection was categorized into three groups: <2 days, two to 14 days and >14 days (21). Modes of acquisition, including community acquired, health care associated and nosocomial, were based on standard definitions (22).

Empirical antibiotic therapy

Empirical antibiotic therapy was defined as antibiotics started within three days of blood culture collection before full susceptibility results of the blood culture were known. Empirical MRSA coverage was considered to include intravenous vancomycin, quinupristin-dalfopristin or daptomycin.

Statistical analysis

Diagnostic properties of the MRSA screening swab were determined. MRSA screening was considered to be the test, and methicillin susceptibility of the first S aureus blood culture was considered the criterion standard. For sensitivity, specificity and predictive values, the 95% CIs were calculated using the Wilson method (23). In other analyses, when 2×2 diagnostic test tables had a cell with zero in it, 0.5 was added for calculation of diagnostic properties. For likelihood ratios, the 95% CI was also calculated (24).

Potential covariates were examined using a multivariable logistic regression model to identify variables related to differences in sensitivity and specificity, as described by Coughlin et al (25). In the logistic model, the dependent variable was the MRSA screen result and the methicillin susceptibility of the blood culture was entered as an independent variable along with other covariates. Potential covariates were as listed. Both sensitivity and specificity could be derived from the coefficients of the independent variables in the model (25). Several methods were used to confirm the significant covariates including univariate selection based on P value, full model with all covariates, as well as forward and backward stepwise regression based on the Akaike information criterion and likelihood ratio test.

To adjust for the significant covariates identified in the previous step (mode of acquisition and hospitals) from the multivariable logistic regression, the study population was stratified according to mode of acquisition. Within each subgroup, a random effects bivariate model (26) was used to calculate a summary estimate of sensitivity and specificity from the six different hospitals. The CIs for the likelihood ratios from the bivariate model were derived from a Monte Carlo simulation of 2000 samples.

Probability of post-test MRSA at different MRSA prevalence was calculated and plotted based on the pooled nonadjusted positive and negative likelihood ratios using the following formulas:

$$\text{Pre-test odds of MRSA} = \frac{\% \text{ MRSA prevalence}}{100\% - \% \text{ MRSA prevalence}}$$

$$\text{Post-test odds of MRSA} = \begin{array}{l} \text{pre-test odds of MRSA} \\ \times \text{ likelihood ratio} \\ \text{(positive or negative)} \end{array}$$

$$\text{Post-test probability of MRSA} = \frac{\text{post-test odds of MRSA}}{\text{(post-test odds of MRSA} + 1)}$$

All reported CIs were two-sided 95% intervals and all tests were two-sided with a 5% significance level. All analyses were performed using R version 3.0.1 (R Foundation for Statistical Computing, Austria). Bivariate summary estimates of diagnostic properties were performed using R package mada.

TABLE 1
Patient characteristics

Characteristic	All sites (n=799)
Age, years, median (interquartile range)	66.0 (52.0–79.0)
Male sex	501 (63)
Hospital site	
A	121 (15)
B	102 (13)
C	223 (28)
D	167 (21)
E	68 (9)
F	118 (15)
Hospital admission service	
Medical	498 (62)
Surgical	166 (21)
Intensive care unit	134 (17)
Other	1 (0.1)
Mode of acquisition	
Community acquired	190 (24)
Health care associated	296 (37)
Nosocomial	297 (37)
Unable to determine	16 (2)
Susceptibility of initial *Staphylococcus aureus* positive blood culture	
MRSA	150 (19)
Results of MRSA screening swab	
Positive	95 (12)
Negative	704 (88)
Time course of MRSA screening to blood culture, days	
MRSA screens performed before susceptibility report	799 (100)
MRSA screening to susceptibility report, median (IQR)	6.0 (3.0–18.0)
MRSA screening to culture collection, median (IQR)*	1.0 (0.0–12.0)
Culture collection to susceptibility report, median (IQR)	3.4 (2.9–5.2)

*Data presented as n (%) unless otherwise indicated. *Data available for 797 patients. MRSA Methicillin-resistant S aureus*

TABLE 2
Diagnostic properties of methicillin-resistant *Staphlycoccus aureus* (MRSA) screening in predicting methicillin susceptibility in *S aureus* blood culture

	Overall (n=799)	Community acquired (n=190)	Health care associated (n=296)	Nosocomial (n=297)
True positive*, n	84	8	44	32
True negative†, n	638	169	232	223
False positive‡, n	11	1	8	1
False negative§, n	66	12	12	41
Sensitivity	56 (48–64)	40 (22–61)	79 (66–87)	44 (33–55)
Specificity	98 (97–99)	99 (97–100)	97 (94–98)	100 (98–100)
PPV	88 (80–93)	89 (57–99)	85 (73–92)	97 (85–100)
NPV	91 (88–93)	93 (89–96)	95 (92–97)	85 (80–88)
PLR (95% CI)	33 (18–60)	68 (9–516)	24 (12–47)	98 (14–706)
NLR (95% CI)	0.45 (0.37–0.54)	0.60 (0.42–0.86)	0.22 (0.13–0.37)	0.56 (0.46–0.69)
Bivariate sensitivity¶		43 (25–64)	74 (61–84)	49 (26–72)
Bivariate specificity¶		98 (94–99)	95 (92–97)	98 (94–99)
Bivariate PLR (95% CI)¶		18 (6–51)	16 (9–28)	21 (7–57)
Bivariate NLR (95% CI)¶		0.58 (0.38–0.77)	0.27 (0.17–0.41)	0.53 (0.29–0.77)

*Data presented as % (95% CI) unless otherwise indicated. *Positive MRSA screening swab and MRSA blood culture; †Negative MRSA screening swab and MRSA blood culture ‡Positive MRSA screening swab and MRSA blood culture §Negative MRSA screening swab and MRSA blood culture ¶Bivariate summary estimate for each mode of acquisition. NLR Negative likelihood ratio; NPV Negative predictive value; PLR Positive likelihood ratio; PPV Positive predictive value*

RESULTS

There were 799 patients who underwent a MRSA screening swab before the susceptibility results of the initial positive blood culture were known (Table 1). Of all MRSA screening swabs, 448 (56%) were performed within two days of blood culture collection; 167 (21%) within two to 14 days; 182 (23%) within >14 days; and two had missing data. The minimum time from MRSA screening swab to the susceptibility results of the initial positive blood culture was one day. Given the minimum time of one day, and the fact that processing of MRSA screening swab took 24 h, all patients in the study were assumed to have MRSA screening swab results available before or at the same time as when the methicillin susceptibility results of the initial positive blood culture were known.

Diagnostic test characteristics

These results allowed for the determination of diagnostic test characteristics for the MRSA screen in predicting methicillin resistance of the initial positive blood culture (Table 2). Diagnostic test properties are shown for each hospital site in Appendix 1.

Hospital sites and mode of acquisition (community-acquired, nosocomial or health care-associated infection) were statistically significant covariates in the final multivariable logistic regression model (Table 3). Age, sex, admitting service, time from MRSA screen to blood culture collection, time from admission to blood culture collection, and MRSA screen with blood culture collection on same admission were not significant covariates. Univariate selection based on P value and stepwise regressions all derived the same model.

For each mode of acquisition, a bivariate summary estimate of sensitivity, specificity and likelihood ratios were calculated from the six sites (Table 2).

The utility of MRSA screening results was modelled for different prevalences of MRSA by plotting post-test probability of MRSA, based on observed pooled and unadjusted positive and negative likelihood ratios (Figure 1).

Empirical MRSA coverage

Of 150 patients with MRSA bacteremia, 59 (39%) had empirical MRSA coverage and 91 (61%) did not. Of 91 patients with MRSA bacteremia with inappropriate empirical antibiotic therapy, 42 (46%) had a positive prior MRSA screening swab.

DISCUSSION

Our multicentre retrospective cohort study at six acute-care academic and community hospitals examined consecutive patients with SAB. From the 799 patients studied, we found that the MRSA screening swabs preceded the susceptibility results of the initial positive blood culture by a median of six days, which may have helped guide empirical antibiotic therapy.

Mode of acquisition was an important covariate for the diagnostic accuracy of the MRSA screen. The positive likelihood ratio for mode of acquisition was high, ranging from 16 to 21, regardless of how the infection was acquired. A positive likelihood ratio >10 is considered to be clinically helpful (27). Therefore, a positive MRSA screening swab may help guide treatment because the risk of methicillin resistance for SAB is increased markedly. The negative likelihood ratio ranged from 0.27 to 0.58 for different modes of acquisition. A negative likelihood ratio from 0.2 to 0.5 makes a small change to the probability of disease (27). Therefore, a negative MRSA screening swab result is not useful in ruling out MRSA bacteremia.

TABLE 3
Final logistic regression model* for probability of a positive methicillin-resistant *Staphylococcus aureus* (MRSA) screening test

Covariate	OR (95% CI)	P	P†
MRSA status on blood culture	197.47 (84.71–527.55)	<0.0001	<0.0001
Hospital site			0.0002
D	Reference		
A	0.99 (0.34–2.76)	0.9796	
B	0.57 (0.17–1.82)	0.3510	
C	0.25 (0.09–0.65)	0.0049	
E	0.06 (0.01–0.29)	0.0008	
F	0.20 (0.05–0.72)	0.0172	
Mode of acquisition			<0.0001
Community	Reference		
Health care associated	6.94 (2.38–22.55)	0.0007	
Nosocomial	1.13 (0.39–3.43)	0.8228	

*The logistic model used MRSA swab result as the dependent variable. The independent variables included methicillin susceptibility of blood culture along with the covariates listed above. CIs are likelihood ratio-based CIs. Both sensitivity and specificity can be derived from the coefficients of the model, as described by Coughlin et (26). The model used listwise deletion and included 780 patients with no missing data; †Values of the likelihood ratio test

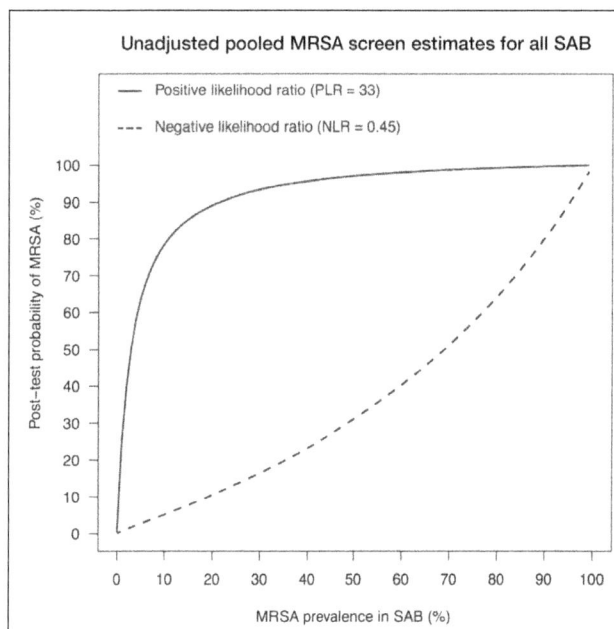

Figure 1) *Post-test probability of methicillin-resistant* Staphylococcus *aureus (MRSA) at different MRSA prevalence in* S aureus *bacteremia. NLR Negative likelihood ratio; PLR Positive likelihood ratio; SAB* S aureus *bacteremia*

There are few studies investigating the diagnostic accuracy of MRSA screening. The majority examined diagnostic accuracy of MRSA screening in the context of all clinical infections including non-*S aureus* infections (28,29). In contrast, we examined the diagnostic accuracy of MRSA swabs in SAB. One study by MacFadden et al (21) examined diagnostic accuracy of MRSA swabs in all *S aureus* infections including nonbacteremic infections. The overall specificity in our study was similar to their study, although our overall sensitivity was lower. The differences may be attributed partially to the types of clinical isolates included. Their study included isolates from both sterile and nonsterile sites that were treated with antistaphylococcal antibiotics, which could include colonization samples that were not clinical infections. In comparison, our study only included *S aureus*-positive blood cultures as clinical infections. As well, MacFadden et al (21) reported results from a single academic centre whereas the present study involved a diverse group of six academic and community hospitals. One of our study sites was also where MacFadden et al conducted their study, but there was no overlap of data between the two studies.

The present study had several strengths, including its size as the largest study, in examining the diagnostic accuracy of MRSA screening swabs in SAB. The study was conducted across many sites, both academic and community hospitals, enhancing its generalizability. In addition, methicillin susceptibility of *S aureus* determined from blood culture was an appropriate and independent standard that was uniformly performed in all patients regardless of MRSA screening swab results. Finally, the inclusion of only blood cultures growing *S aureus*, reflecting sterile site growth, ensured that all infections were true clinical infections and not colonization.

The present study had several limitations that merit discussion. First, as a retrospective chart review in which assessors of MRSA screening swab results were not blinded to the MRSA blood culture results, there could be potential information bias. However, the laboratory tests were determined and reported independent of other test results, making this unlikely. Second, there appeared to be heterogeneity in terms of diagnostic properties among MRSA hospital sites. The heterogeneity among different hospital sites might have been a result of minor differences in MRSA screening criteria, patient population at hospital sites and different rates of intrahospital MRSA transmission. However, the bivariate summary estimate accounts for this difference among hospital sites and

provides a more conservative estimate of diagnostic properties. Moreover, the heterogeneity exists mainly in sites with fewer patients where corrections of adding 0.5 to all cells needed to be made. Sites with a greater number of patients had more consistent results. Finally, previous data have shown that different MRSA genotypes have a different probabilities of causing SAB. Unfortunately, we did not collect any information on MRSA genotypes. However, MRSA genotype may not be clinically important, in that treatment of MRSA is the same regardless of MRSA genotypes in clinical practice and MRSA genotype is not considered in hospital infection control practices currently.

Our study identified the mode of acquisition as a possible significant covariate for diagnostic accuracy of MRSA screening. It may be that health care-associated infections were mostly associated with intravenous and hemodialysis therapy, and that these infections were strongly associated with pre-existent MRSA colonization. In contrast, for community-acquired and nosocomial infections, patients were more likely to be newly colonized with MRSA and, thus, were less likely to be detected by prior MRSA screening. Unlike the previous study (21), time from MRSA screening to blood culture collection was not a significant predictor. This is likely due to the fact that events such as mode of acquisition of infection and hospitalization play a more significant role in MRSA colonization and infection than the length of time. Mode of acquisition was not considered in the previous study (21).

Our study results have important clinical implications. A negative MRSA screen result does not significantly decrease the probability of MRSA bacteremia. The poor sensitivity and low negative likelihood ratio results in many false negatives. In these false-negative cases with MRSA bacteremia, withholding antibiotics with activity against MRSA based on negative MRSA screening swab may greatly increase the risk for mortality (9). Therefore, a negative MRSA screening swab is not useful and should not be considered in the decision of MRSA coverage for empirical antibiotic therapy. On the other hand, a positive prior MRSA screen rules in MRSA and empirical intravenous antibiotics with activity against MRSA should be started. In our cohort, 91 of 150 (61%) patients with MRSA bacteremia did not receive empirical MRSA coverage based on clinical judgment. In these 91 patients, the rule of a positive MRSA screen necessitating anti-MRSA empirical coverage would result in empirical MRSA coverage being added to 42 (46%) of the 91 MRSA bacteremia cases in which empirical MRSA coverage was originally missed. Following the same rule, MRSA empirical coverage would only be added to 11 (2%) of the 649 patients with MSSA bacteremia. Thus, this rule would significantly increase the rate of correct empirical MRSA coverage in MRSA bacteremia cases while adding minimal unnecessary anti-MRSA empirical coverage in MSSA bacteremia cases.

Our findings demonstrate that screening tests for infection control purposes can provide valuable, clinically relevant information for making treatment decisions.

DISCLOSURES: The present study was largely unfunded. The Mount Sinai Hospital Antimicrobial Stewardship Program is supported by an unrestricted educational grant from Pfizer Canada, which partially supports the employment of a research coordinator (M Steinberg). A Mount Sinai Hospital Department of Medicine Summer Studentship Award funded A Bai. A Morris receives partial salary support for his antimicrobial stewardship activities from Mount Sinai Hospital and University Health Network. A Canadian Institutes of Health Research/Canadian Patient Safety Institute Chair in Patient Safety and Continuity of Care supports C Bell.

APPENDIX 1
Patient and diagnostic characteristics for each hospital site

Characteristic	Hospital site					
	A (n=121)	B (n=102)	C (n=223)	D (n=167)	E (n=68)	F (n=118)
Age, years, median (Interquartile range)	65 (46–80)	76 (63–84)	67 (55–78)	59 (49–70)	70 (56–79)	63 (53–78)
Male sex	71 (59)	52 (51)	144 (65)	119 (71)	44 (65)	71 (60)
Hospital admission service						
Medical	80 (66)	74 (73)	116 (52)	110 (66)	44 (65)	74 (63)
Surgical	22 (18)	11 (11)	52 (23)	37 (22)	12 (18)	32 (27)
Intensive care unit	19 (16)	17 (17)	54 (24)	20 (12)	12 (18)	12 (10)
Other	0 (0)	0 (0)	1 (0.5)	0 (0)	0 (0)	0 (0)
Mode of acquisition						
Community	32 (26)	30 (29)	42 (19)	30 (18)	20 (29)	36 (31)
Health care associated	43 (36)	42 (41)	80 (36)	80 (48)	23 (34)	28 (24)
Nosocomial	45 (37)	29 (28)	93 (42)	55 (33)	22 (32)	53 (45)
Unable to determine	1 (1)	1 (1)	8 (4)	2 (1)	3 (4)	1 (1)
MRSA on blood culture	28 (23)	19 (19)	51 (23)	24 (14)	13 (19)	15 (13)
Positive MRSA screening	22 (18)	16 (16)	25 (11)	23 (14)	3 (4)	6 (5)
Diagnostic test						
True positive, n	20	13	21	21	3	6
True negative, n	91	80	168	141	55	103
False positive, n	2	3	4	2	0	0
False negative, n	8	6	30	3	10	9
Sensitivity, % (95% CI)	71 (53–85)	68 (46–85)	41 (29–55)	88 (69–96)	25 (10–51)	41 (21–64)
Specificity, % (95% CI)	98 (93–99)	96 (90–99)	98 (94–99)	99 (95–100)	99 (92–100)	100 (96–100)
PLR (95% CI)	33 (8–134)	19 (6–60)	18 (6–49)	63 (16–250)	28 (2–511)	85 (5–1429)
NLR (95% CI)	0.29 (0.16–0.53)	0.33 (0.17–0.64)	0.60 (0.48–0.76)	0.13 (0.04–0.37)	0.76 (0.56–1.03)	0.60 (0.40–0.90)

Data presented as n (%) unless otherwise indicated. MRSA Methicillin-resistant Staphylococcus aureus; *NLR Negative likelihood ratio; PLR Positive likelihood ratio*

REFERENCES

1. Landrum ML, Neumann C, Cook C, et al. Epidemiology of *Staphylococcus aureus* blood and skin and soft tissue infections in the US military health system, 2005-2010. JAMA 2012;308:50-9.
2. Jenkins TC, Price CS, Sabel AL, Mehler PS, Burman WJ. Impact of routine infectious diseases service consultation on the evaluation, management, and outcomes of *Staphylococcus aureus* bacteremia. Clin Infect Dis 2008;46:1000-8.
3. Wyllie DH, Crook DW, Peto TE. Mortality after *Staphylococcus aureus* bacteraemia in two hospitals in Oxfordshire, 1997-2003: Cohort study. BMJ 2006;333:281.
4. Chang FY, MacDonald BB, Peacock JE, et al. A prospective multicenter study of *Staphylococcus aureus* bacteremia: incidence of endocarditis, risk factors for mortality, and clinical impact of methicillin resistance. Medicine (Baltimore) 2003;82:322-32.
5. Zhanel GG, DeCorby M, Adam H, et al. Prevalence of antimicrobial-resistant pathogens in Canadian hospitals: Results of the Canadian Ward Surveillance Study (CANWARD 2008). Antimicrob Agents Chemother 2010;54:4684-93.
6. Cosgrove SE, Sakoulas G, Perencevich EN, Schwaber MJ, Karchmer AW, Carmeli Y. Comparison of mortality associated with methicillin-resistant and methicillin-susceptible *Staphylococcus aureus* bacteremia: A meta-analysis. Clin Infect Dis 2003;36:53-9.
7. Cosgrove SE, Qi Y, Kaye KS, Harbarth S, Karchmer AW, Carmeli Y. The impact of methicillin resistance in *Staphylococcus aureus* bacteremia on patient outcomes: mortality, length of stay, and hospital charges. Infect Control Hosp Epidemiol 2005;26:166-74.
8. Hidayat LK, Hsu DI, Quist R, Shriner KA, Wong-Beringer A. High-dose vancomycin therapy for methicillin-resistant *Staphylococcus aureus* infections: efficacy and toxicity. Arch Intern Med 2006;166:2138-44.
9. Paul M, Kariv G, Goldberg E, et al. Importance of appropriate empirical antibiotic therapy for methicillin-resistant *Staphylococcus aureus* bacteraemia. J Antimicrob Chemother 2010;65:2658-65.
10. Kim SH, Kim KH, Kim HB, et al. Outcome of vancomycin treatment in patients with methicillin-susceptible *Staphylococcus aureus* bacteremia. Antimicrob Agents Chemother 2008;52:192-7.
11. Schweizer ML, Furuno JP, Harris AD, et al. Comparative effectiveness of nafcillin or cefazolin versus vancomycin in methicillin-susceptible *Staphylococcus aureus* bacteremia. BMC Infect Dis 2011;11:279.
12. Fridkin SK, Edwards JR, Courval JM, et al. The effect of vancomycin and third-generation cephalosporins on prevalence of vancomycin-resistant enterococci in 126 U.S. adult intensive care units. Ann Intern Med 2001;135:175-83.
13. Mermel LA, Farr BM, Sherertz RJ, et al. Guidelines for the management of intravascular catheter-related infections. Clin Infect Dis 2001;32:1249-72.
14. Mermel LA, Allon M, Bouza E, et al. Clinical practice guidelines for the diagnosis and management of intravascular catheter-related infection: 2009 Update by the Infectious Diseases Society of America. Clin Infect Dis 2009;49:1-45.

15. Mackenzie I, Lever A. Management of sepsis. BMJ 2007;335:929-32.
16. Huang SS, Platt R. Risk of methicillin-resistant *Staphylococcus aureus* infection after previous infection or colonization. Clin Infect Dis 2003;36:281-85.
17. Davis KA, Stewart JJ, Crouch HK, Florez CE, Hospenthal DR. Methicillin-resistant *Staphylococcus aureus* (MRSA) nares colonization at hospital admission and its effect on subsequent MRSA infection. Clin Infect Dis 2004;39:776-82.
18. Bai AD, Showler A, Burry L, et al. Impact of infectious disease consultation on quality of care, mortality and length of stay in *Staphylococcus aureus* bacteremia: Results from a large multicenter cohort study. Clin Infect Dis 2015;60:1451-61.
19. Ontario Agency for Health Protection and Promotion, Provincial Infectious Diseases Advisory Committee (PIDAC). Annex A– Screening, testing and surveillance for antibiotic-resistant organisms (AROs) in all health care settings. Routine practices and additional precautions in all health care settings. Toronto: Queen's Printer for Ontario, Toronto, 2013.
20. Clinical and Laboratory Standards Institute. Performance standards for antimicrobial susceptibility testing, 17th edn. Wayne: Clinical and Laboratory Standards Institute, 2007.
21. Macfadden DR, Elligsen M, Robicsek A, Ricciuto DR, Daneman N. Utility of prior screening for methicillin-resistant *Staphylococcus aureus* in predicting resistance of S. aureus infections. CMAJ 2013;185:E725-E730.
22. Friedman ND, Kaye KS, Stout JE, et al. Health care-associated bloodstream infections in adults: a reason to change the accepted definition of community-acquired infections. Ann Intern Med 2002;137:791-7.
23. Wilson EB. Probable inference, the law of succession, and statistical inference. J Amer Stat Assoc 1927;22:209-12.
24. Simel DL, Samsa GP, Matchar DB. Likelihood ratios with confidence: Sample size estimation for diagnostic test studies. J Clin Epidemiol 1991;44:763-70.
25. Coughlin SS, Trock B, Criqui MH, Pickle LW, Browner D, Tefft MC. The logistic modeling of sensitivity, specificity, and predictive value of a diagnostic test. J Clin Epidemiol 1992;45:1-7.
26. Reitsma JB, Glas AS, Rutjes AW, Scholten RJ, Bossuyt PM, Zwinderman AH. Bivariate analysis of sensitivity and specificity produces informative summary measures in diagnostic reviews. J Clin Epidemiol 2005;58:982-90.
27. Jaeschke R, Guyatt GH, Sackett DL. Users' guides to the medical literature. III. How to use an article about a diagnostic test. B. What are the results and will they help me in caring for my patients? The Evidence-Based Medicine Working Group. JAMA 1994;271:703-7.
28. Harris AD, Furuno JP, Roghmann MC, et al. Targeted surveillance of methicillin-resistant *Staphylococcus aureus* and its potential use to guide empiric antibiotic therapy. Antimicrob Agents Chemother 2010;54:3143-8.
29. Sarikonda KV, Micek ST, Doherty JA, Reichley RM, Warren D, Kollef MH. Methicillin-resistant *Staphylococcus aureus* nasal colonization is a poor predictor of intensive care unit-acquired methicillin-resistant Staphylococcus aureus infections requiring antibiotic treatment. Crit Care Med 2010;38:1991-5.

18

Improving public health policy through infection transmission modelling: Guidelines for creating a Community of Practice

Seyed M Moghadas PhD[1], Margaret Haworth-Brockman MSc[2], Harpa Isfeld-Kiely MA[2], Joel Kettner MD[2]

SM Moghadas, M Haworth-Brockman, H Isfeld-Kiely, J Kettner. Improving public health policy through infection transmission modelling: Guidelines for creating a Community of Practice. Can J Infect Dis Med Microbiol 2015;26(4):191-195.

BACKGROUND: Despite significant research efforts in Canada, real application of modelling in public health decision making and practice has not yet met its full potential. There is still room to better address the diversity of the Canadian population and ensure that research outcomes are translated for use within their relevant contexts.

OBJECTIVES: To strengthen connections to public health practice and to broaden its scope, the Pandemic Influenza Outbreak Research Modelling team partnered with the National Collaborating Centre for Infectious Diseases to hold a national workshop. Its objectives were to: understand areas where modelling terms, methods and results are unclear; share information on how modelling can best be used in informing policy and improving practice, particularly regarding the ways to integrate a focus on health equity considerations; and sustain and advance collaborative work in the development and application of modelling in public health.

METHOD: The Use of Mathematical Modelling in Public Health Decision Making for Infectious Diseases workshop brought together research modellers, public health professionals, policymakers and other experts from across the country. Invited presentations set the context for topical discussions in three sessions. A final session generated reflections and recommendations for new opportunities and tasks.

CONCLUSIONS: Gaps in content and research include the lack of standard frameworks and a glossary for infectious disease modelling. Consistency in terminology, clear articulation of model parameters and assumptions, and sustained collaboration will help to bridge the divide between research and practice.

Key Words: *Communities of Practice; Infectious disease terminology; Knowledge translation; Mathematical modelling; Policy decision-making; Public health*

L'amélioration des politiques de santé publique par la modélisation de la transmission des infections : des directives pour créer une communauté de pratique

HISTORIQUE : Malgré l'ampleur des recherches au Canada, la mise en œuvre de la modélisation n'a pas encore atteint son plein potentiel en santé publique dans la prise de décision et la pratique. Il y a matière à mieux intégrer la diversité de la population canadienne et d'utiliser les résultats de la recherche dans les contextes pertinents.

OBJECTIFS : Pour renforcer les liens avec l'exercice de la santé publique et en élargir la portée, l'équipe de *Pandemic Influenza Outbreak Research Modelling* s'est associée au Centre de collaboration nationale des maladies infectieuses pour organiser un atelier national. Cet atelier visait à déterminer les secteurs où la terminologie, les méthodo-logies et les résultats de la modélisation manquent de clarté, à transmettre de l'information sur l'utilisation optimale de la modélisation pour étayer les politiques et améliorer la pratique, notamment en accordant plus d'importance aux questions d'équité en santé, et à maintenir et faire progresser la collaboration pour élaborer et mettre en œuvre la modélisation en santé publique.

MÉTHODOLOGIE : L'atelier sur l'utilisation de la modélisation mathématique dans la prise de décision relative aux maladies infectieuses en santé publique a réuni des chercheurs modélisateurs, des professionnels de la santé publique, des décideurs et d'autres experts du pays. Les conférenciers ont mis en contexte les discussions dans le cadre de trois séances. Une dernière séance a suscité des réflexions et des recommandations sur les futures tâches et possibilités.

CONCLUSIONS : Les lacunes en matière de contenu et de recherche incluent l'absence de cadres standardisés et de glossaire de la modélisation des maladies infectieuses. Une terminologie uniforme, la formulation claire des paramètres et des hypothèses de modélisation ainsi qu'une collaboration soutenue contribueront à corriger l'écart entre la recherche et la pratique.

The International Society for Pharmacoeconomics and Outcomes Research defines a mathematical model as a framework "representing some aspects of reality at a sufficient level of detail to inform a clinical or policy question" (1). Mathematical, computational and statistical models and techniques have been applied in the Canadian public health system, especially after the 2003 severe acute respiratory syndrome (SARS) epidemic, but it is unclear to what degree their outcomes have been used to shape policy and improve practice. Furthermore, the diversity of the Canadian population has not been adequately addressed in public health models, and research outcomes are often not translated for use within their relevant contexts. To improve the applicability and impact of models in public health, it is necessary to understand areas where modelling results are unclear, the value of a common language between modelling and public health, and how to sustain and enhance the application of modelling in public health.

Established during the early stages of the 2009 H1N1 pandemic in Canada, the Pandemic Influenza Outbreak Research Modelling (Pan-InfORM) team has a mandate to develop innovative modelling frameworks and knowledge translation methods that inform public health by linking theory, policy and practice. Aligned with its mandate, on October 6 and 7, 2014, Pan-InfORM held its fourth biannual workshop (2-4) cohosted by the National Collaborating Centre for Infectious Diseases. This workshop brought together public health

[1]*Agent-Based Modelling Laboratory, York University, Toronto, Ontario;* [2]*National Collaborating Centre for Infectious Diseases, Winnipeg, Manitoba*
Correspondence: Dr Seyed M Moghadas, Agent-Based Modelling Laboratory, York University, Toronto, Ontario M2J 1P3.
e-mail moghadas@yorku.ca

practitioners and leading research modellers (a list of attendees is available at <http://pan-inform.yorku.ca/events/pan-inform-workshop-2014/participants.html>) to enhance cross-discipline communications by providing a forum for knowledge to flow freely in a 'jargon-free' setting. The expected outcome was to identify the infrastructure, expertise and resources necessary to establish a 'Communities of Practice' (CoP) network. The CoP concept, initially developed by Jean Lave and Etienne Wenger, refers to groups of people who share a concern, a set of problems or a passion about something they do, and learn how to do it better by interacting regularly (5-8). The proposed CoP, as a new initiative to be catalyzed from this workshop, would offer new approaches to addressing problems at different levels of health care and population health and enable the development of strategic plans to move evidence to action. An important role for this CoP is to develop a common language that can be used in understanding the outcomes of health research and disease modelling.

The workshop objectives were to: understand areas where modelling terms, methods and results are unclear; share information on how modelling can best be used in informing policy and improving practice, particularly regarding the ways to integrate a focus on health equity considerations; and sustain and advance collaborative work in the development and application of modelling in public health.

The two-day event unfolded in four sessions. The first two, "Modelling in public health: Opportunities and challenges" and "Mathematical modelling in public health practice", helped to set the context regarding scientific methods and research applications, particularly for the evaluation of research uptake and provided public health perspectives on the utility of modelling in decision making. The third session, "Muddling through modelling: Communication, common language and health equity", spurred discussion regarding the need for common language between researchers and knowledge users, to improve the use of modelling study results. This included foundational issues regarding access to data and the involvement of indigenous and other community representation. In the final session, "Developing our network and communities of practice", participants reflected on earlier presentations and discussions to clarify what is needed to continue collaboration and knowledge exchange that can increase the value of research modelling in public health.

The presentations and discussions that ensued created compelling arguments that the most prominent and observable outcomes can be achieved when communication barriers between disciplines are eliminated. The present report discusses key presentations and discussions that took place, and summarizes the outcomes and action plans that emerged from the workshop.

Setting the context: opportunities and challenges for modelling in public health

Sessions 1 and 2 of the workshop began with a presentation regarding the development of infectious diseases modelling in Canada. Before the 2003 SARS epidemic, modelling activities were largely driven by research interests of individuals or small groups, with a significant emphasis on the theoretical aspects of exploring complex mathematical phenomena. For the most part, these activities were carried out in isolation, with minimal communication and engagement with public health professionals and policymakers (2). During and following the SARS epidemic, various groups of disease modellers were formed to engage with, and develop models for application to public and population health in more specific contexts. Despite the importance and relevance of these initiatives, knowledge translation remained a challenge that the Pan-InfORM was established in part to address (9).

The Canadian Institutes of Health Research supported the establishment of Pan-InfORM to address the limited knowledge exchange between modelling researchers and those who could potentially make use of models to inform health policy and improve practice. Since its inception, Pan-InfORM has undertaken several national initiatives for knowledge brokering, including the evaluation of Canada's response to the spring and winter waves of the novel H1N1 pandemic,

identification of strategies for protecting vulnerable populations from emerging infectious diseases, and development of approaches that can enrich existing links with Aboriginal health organizations and foster multijurisdictional collaborative efforts in Canada (2-4).

In Canada, public health decision making occurs within orders of government at all levels. Situations are often very complex for a number of reasons including the availability and adequacy of health resources; inconsistent or absent evidence regarding the effectiveness and cost effectiveness of intervention strategies; pressure from the public, media and government under which public health must operate; other competing public health services; and ethical considerations to balance the protection of community health against individuals' rights and freedoms. Other pertinent challenges include the lack of data to estimate potential outcomes of a public health program, paralysis resulting from having too much information on occasion, differing opinions and short timelines. In this context, as one presenter put it, there are three questions decision makers face: what is the benefit of the public health program or intervention; who will benefit from the program and; is the program cost-effective? Often, the evidence to answer these questions is not available in a timely manner.

Ideally, one would address these questions by investigating the effects experimentally. However, controlled trials may not be feasible or ethical, and can also be time consuming, laborious, expensive or inconclusive. Models provide a useful tool to overcome these challenges and systematically evaluate possible effects by using existing data and knowledge, generating quantitative outcomes and mapping out interdependencies that may be key factors for determining policy needs. Given these capabilities, models can be used to identify key uncertainties in the parameters and generate qualitative predictions, such as the effect of behavioural changes on the trends and distribution of an infection in the population. Indeed, the overarching goal of modelling is to support evidence-based public health policy.

To enhance the utility of models, communication and collaboration between modellers and public health leaders must take place early in a decision making process. Models are more valuable when end users are engaged in formulating the questions because models are built so that they truly reflect a public health question. End users who understand a model are likely to be better able to assess the results. During the construction and validation of a model, the relevance and importance of input parameters must be understood, and the sources for their values and ranges, uncertainty about the parameters, and sensitivity of the model outcomes with respect to parameter variation and original model assumptions, must be determined. New knowledge generated by a model should address the target question and be translated and disseminated for uptake and action appropriate to the context. Furthermore, when data are limited, it is essential to quantify any uncertainty in parameterization, because different sets of parameters may fit equally well. Ideally, the process to improve the model structure and its outcomes is iterative.

The value of direct conversations between modellers and public health leaders, in particular with regard to the availability and access to data and other critical information that are essential for model inputs of real-time scenarios (10), was exemplified in the use of modelling and the implementation of model recommendations for antiviral use and vaccination in Canada's response to the 2009 H1N1 pandemic (11,12). Table 1 summarizes key issues presented and discussed for modelling in public health during the workshop.

Muddling through modelling: finding a common language

The International Society for Pharmacoeconomics and Outcome Research guidelines highlight the importance of a common language for drafting a health decision question and addressing it through a modelling framework. The guidelines for transparency and validation state:

> Every model should have non-technical documentation that is freely accessible to any interested reader. At a minimum, it should describe in nontechnical terms, the type of model and

TABLE 1
Summary of issues arising from presentations and discussions on the use of modelling in public health

Areas of concern or interest	Consensus discussion	Recommendations
Applying models in public health	Modelling has an important place in public health policy and practice. The utilization of modelling has been far less that its potential in the Canadian context	Create a national infrastructure or network in Canada to develop useful and applicable models based on realistic assumptions and quality data
Closer working relationships	Collaboration, engagement and exchange between modellers, and policymakers are needed to facilitate iterative processes that optimize the value and understanding of models and their results	Identify partners at the provincial level within acute care, emergency services and public health divisions. Formalize exchange processes for regular communication and education
Applying health equity and other lenses	Limited attention has been paid to using health equity or sex and gender analyses. The availability of Aboriginal-specific information has been inconsistent at best	Modellers and users can be called on to create model frameworks and ask questions that will provide better information about where there are inequities and inequalities. Involve the people who understand equity issues
Data quality and access	Access to good-quality, population level data is essential to validate a model and its outcomes. Such data may not necessarily be available or accessible in a timely fashion during an emerging infectious disease	Evaluate data quality and the type of information provided by surveillance for its potential to be used for research modelling. Engage with provinces to determine the nature and availability of data required for modelling
Coherent and consistent descriptions of diseases as well as modelling terminology	Across 13 jurisdictions, public health in Canada does not have universal definitions or natural histories of diseases, such as tuberculosis, to input in models	Undertake the work needed to standardize descriptions, which can inform a standard lexicon of terminology and protocols for infectious disease modelling
Cost effectiveness	Public health personnel and governments do not have enough information about the economics of interventions for comprehensive decision making	Strengthen the existing infrastructure (eg, Canadian Immunization Registry Network, National Advisory Committee on Immunization) to include economic modelling that will inform policy decisions
Standardization of approaches	To develop useful models, three aspects of the modelling will need to be standardized: what (ie, frameworks that are context specific and take into account the population demographic and geographic characteristics); who (ie, involvement of policymakers, knowledge users and modellers with relevant expertise), and how (ie, develop an iterative process from the formulation of health policy questions to the dissemination of model outcomes)	A Communities of Practice network can be tasked with the standardization of this process to ensure that synergies exist when models are formulated to inform clinical or health policy decisions
Roles and responsibilities	Clarification on the roles of health agencies and jurisdictions are needed to engage partners from academic institutes, government health organizations and health industries	National Collaborating Centre for Infectious Diseases will lead the initiative to forge the linkages and develop appropriate channels and effective methods of communication between the involved partners
Capacity	Some jurisdictions lack modelling capacity. There is also a lack of information about which modellers are available to work with public health and their expertise	A centralized list or network could contribute to greater capacity for public health jurisdictions. Develop opportunities for public health personnel to learn more about models and their value

intended applications; funding sources; structure of the model; inputs, outputs, other components that determine the model's function and their relationships; data sources, validation methods and results; and limitations (1).

Good communication flows to and from knowledge producers and users, and requires a common language to build effective partnerships and understanding of the groups' respective concerns. There are a number of challenges to developing a common language: determining a common lexicon; understanding priorities and contributions, which may shift depending on the political climate or population health status; asking the right questions that are appropriate to the given context; knowing the right audience; and being able to communicate findings to others outside the research community.

The lack of such common language may have been an impediment to addressing key parameters in 'determinants of health' and 'health equity'. In the Canadian context, one needs to take into account differential health status and population structure of First Nations, Inuit and Métis people, population-level patterns of abuse, poverty and historical trauma, challenges regarding access to health services in rural and remote areas, and limits in identifying "vulnerable" populations in available datasets with no real markers. Building partnerships and an iterative exchange allows for goals and facts to be clearly identified, and outcomes to be assessed for their value to inform decisions about the potential benefits and risks of policy development and program delivery.

Effective partnerships require willingness and commitment, alignment of values, mechanisms to engage early and continuously, and plans to regularly review goals, objectives, roles, and responsibilities and outcomes.

Developing commonalities in modelling research and application
A recent review of literature highlights the inconsistency in definitions and interpretations of epidemiological terms in several modelling studies and the need for common language to sustain and enhance the application of models in public health (13). The review found that disparate outcomes and interpretations for policy decisions may arise from inconsistent use of terms in model structures, even when the assumptions and input parameters are identical. Discrepancies in how terms are used for modelling are generally associated with two main reasons. First, it is often assumed that the particular terms are well defined or well understood. For example, 'infectiousness' and 'infectious' were found to be used interchangeably; the former describes a characteristic of the disease and/or how readily the disease is transmitted, while the latter describes a patient state (13). Second, definitions of some terms have drifted over time as understanding of the mechanisms of disease processes and control has evolved. For example, the way terms such as 'prevention', 'protection' and 'reduced susceptibility' are used related to communicable disease may lead to different results depending how they are used in modelling. Developing a common

TABLE 2
Summary of challenges and actions identified to improve consistency in terminology in public health modelling

Opportunities and strengths a Community of Practice can provide

Develop a unified infrastructure to inform complex decision making and improve health practice based on quality data, evidence and scientific knowledge

Avoid duplication, use resources wisely and harness power of complementary disciplines to work collaboratively to common goals

Develop and foster the use of a common language for modelling in public health, and help identify similarities and differences in modelling approaches and their outcomes

Identify research priorities and data gaps (it is important to note that the lack of evidence and/or data may provide opportunities to exploit factors that affect model outcomes and their policy consequences. These opportunities can enhance our learning and, more importantly, may suggest novel data collection, better models and improved collaborations through a Community of Practice)

Facilitate data sharing and critical information in a timely fashion

Help address diversity of Canadian contexts

Identify relevant partners and stakeholders and engage them in formulating research questions

Integrate resources for knowledge translation and bidirectional communication

Increase uptake of knowledge and promote best practices for modelling collaborations

Community of Practice members

Exchange key documents, resources, and expertise

Evaluate research outcomes, and synthesize theoretical and practical knowledge gained from national and international collaboration

Organize targeted efforts for integrating modelling, surveillance, planning and decision making

Partnerships

Community of Practice will support the development of partnerships with federal/provincial/territorial health agencies and departments in Canada and other relevant organizations by enabling exchanges of information on the type of evidence used in decision making; assess the policy relevance of research outcomes; and support dissemination and implementation of the health policy recommendations

Research and knowledge translation priorities for modelling

Intervention strategies for outbreaks of influenza and other respiratory pathogens (eg, tuberculosis, pertussis)

Potential benefits of immunization of target groups (eg, school-aged children, or health care workers)

School closures strategies during emerging diseases with consideration of population characteristics

Cost-effectiveness of immunization programs

Strategies for early identification and treatment of active tuberculosis

Priorities for modelling consistency

Develop a glossary of definitions of terms used in modelling consistent with dictionary of terms for infectious disease epidemiology

Develop conceptual frameworks for natural history model of important diseases using standard terminologies

Provide guidelines and develop criteria for assessing the quality and relevance of databases for modelling

Develop guidelines for review and assessment of modelling research quality and the relevance to public health policy and practice in Canadian contexts

Host organization

National Collaborating Centre for Infectious Diseases

language will help to reduce possible variation in study results produced by different research communities. This will in turn decrease misinterpretation of the outcomes by allowing for comparisons of scientific evidence from multiple disciplines involving health research, and helping knowledge users and policymakers to better understand research outcomes and their applicability to policy and practice.

TABLE 3
Summary of final discussion session with action plans for further interaction and integration through a Community of Practice

Challenges

Inadequate methods and/or analysis for applying results to public health policy

Lack of evidence and/or data

Variability and uncertainty of model outcomes (results)

Validation and applicability of the results

Inadequate collaborative research or expertise

Insufficient knowledge translation and communication

Consensus

Need for consistent use of infectious disease terms in modelling studies

Need for greater use of modelling approaches and results beyond scientific discoveries

Action plans

Develop a process to standardize terms to be used in modelling of infectious diseases

Develop plans to generate and translate new knowledge with engagement of relevant stakeholders

Formalize the structures and linkages initiated by the Pandemic Influenza Outbreak Research Modelling team to tackle a wider range of public health issues facing Canadians

There are other factors responsible for variation in model findings, including different strategies or approaches and assumptions, different population demographic variables, and the objectives for evaluating policy effectiveness that can vary from one situation to another. The latter can be exemplified in two recent studies on the effectiveness of school closure during pandemic influenza outbreaks. When assessing the effect of school closure strategies in reducing community attack rates, Halder et al (14) found that due to the difficulty in determining the true degree of epidemic spread and its severity in the early stages of an outbreak, a strategy of individual school closures would be more effective than simultaneous closures across a region. The outcomes are drawn from an agent-based simulation model of Albany, a small community in Western Australia with a population of approximately 30,000 individuals. In contrast, to evaluate the impact of local reactive school closures on critical care provision in the United Kingdom population setting, House et al (15) concluded that school closures should be coordinated in time (simultaneous) and location (all schools within a school district) to become an effective strategy to reduce infection transmission and, consequently, relieve capacity pressures of hospital intensive care unit admissions. The population demographics and the objectives for closing schools are distinctly different between the two studies, suggesting that different modelling approaches are required for measuring the effectiveness of school closures.

Understanding scenario-specific outcomes and their applications requires a critical evaluation to address the following questions:

- Is the methodology appropriate for the specific population setting?
- Do the assumptions and parameters address the reality of demographic and geographic characteristics?
- Can the outcomes be compared with other studies and validated with observed data?
- How generalizable are the outcomes to address different scenarios or population settings?

A consensus emerged during the workshop regarding the need to develop a common language for modelling to enhance its application in a public health context and promote bidirectional communication (Table 2). To address this need, the fourth session of the workshop provided an opportunity for participants to discuss the establishment and potential impact of a Community of Practice.

FINAL DISCUSSION

During the final discussion session, a number of important issues related to the development of a CoP network were discussed, including its structure and governance, leadership and research capacity, memberships and partnerships, strategic plans for sustainability and resources, and the impact and uptake of outcomes (Table 3).

CONCLUDING REMARKS

The October 2014 national workshop propelled new discussion on the value of mathematical models in public health planning and the need for greater cohesion and collaboration among stakeholders. The workshop concluded with a consensus among participants that there is work to be done and a willingness to continue to work together. The creation of a common lexicon is a tangible, initial task that should be undertaken as an immediate response to the workshop discussions.

We expect that through sustained cross-disciplinary dialogues, a CoP will initially produce a 'book of terminology' that describes current usage and proposes common terminology (community standards) in different areas, including medical and infectious diseases epidemiology, public health and disease modelling. This reference book can then be updated regularly when new terms need clarification for shared understanding and agreement in use. Furthermore, in times of uncertainty, the virtual CoP network will provide opportunities to access, analyze, synthesize and utilize reliable information and databases in a timely fashion, and drive a broad consensus around plausible alternatives and integrated courses of action. It is also true, however, that ongoing discussions between modellers and public health personnel will help to clarify language use and break down perceived barriers.

Postscript

Within a number of weeks after the workshop, a new virtual Community of Practice, created by National Collaborating Centre for Infectious Diseases through LinkedIn, called mod4PH (modelling for public health) (16) was launched generating questions and comments to further the workshop discussions. The online network is open to new public health and research members.

AUTHORS' CONTRIBUTIONS: S Moghadas wrote the first draft of the manuscript. M Haworth-Brockman, H Isfeld-Kiely and J Kettner contributed to, revised and prepared the final version. All authors have read and approved the article.

ACKNOWLEDGEMENTS: The workshop was supported by the Canadian Institutes of Health Research (Dissemination Event Grant FRN 137233), National Collaborating Centre for Infectious Diseases, and International Centre for Infectious Diseases. Funding is also made possible through a contribution from the Public Health Agency of Canada through the NCCID. The authors thank all the participants for their significant contributions to the workshop.

DISCLOSURES: SM declares no competing interests. MHB, HIK, and JK are members of the National Collaborating Centre for Infectious Diseases, which partially supported the workshop.

REFERENCES

1. Caro JJ, Briggs AH, Siebert U, Kuntz KM, ISPOR-SMDM Modeling Good Research Practices Task Force. Modeling good research practices-overview: A report of the ISPOR-SMDM Modeling Good Research Practices Task Force-1. Med Dec Making 2012;32:667-77.
2. Moghadas SM, Pizzi NJ, Wu J, Yan P. Managing public health crises: The role of models in pandemic preparedness. Influenza Other Respir Viruses 2009;3:75-9.
3. Moghadas SM, Pizzi NJ, Wu J, Tamblyn SE, Fisman DN. Canada in the face of the 2009 H1N1 pandemic. Influenza Other Respir Viruses 2011;5:83-8.
4. Richardson KL, Driedger MS, Pizzi NJ, Wu J, Moghadas SM. Indigenous populations health protection: A Canadian perspective. BMC Public Health 2012;12:1098.
5. Braithwaite J, Westbrook JI, Ranmuthugala G, et al. The development, design, testing, refinement, simulation and application of an evaluation framework for communities of practice and social-professional networks. BMC Health Serv Res 2009;9:162.
6. Lathlean J, le May A. Communities of practice: An opportunity for interagency working. J Clin Nurs 2002;11:394-8.
7. Wenger E. Communities of Practice: Learning, Meaning and Identity. New York: Cambridge University Press; 1998.
8. Wenger E, McDermott R, Snyder W. Cultivating Communities of Practice. Boston, MA: Harvard Business School Press; 2002.
9. Pandemic Influenza Outbreak Research Modelling Team (Pan-InfORM), Fisman D. Modelling an influenza pandemic: A guide for the perplexed. CMAJ 2009;181:171-3.
10. Arino J, Bauch C, Brauer F, et al. Pandemic influenza: Modelling and public health perspectives. Math Biosci Eng 2011;8:1-20.
11. CIHR Institute of Infection and Immunity, Internal Assessment for 2011 International Review. 2011, Available at <www.cihr-irsc.gc.ca/e/43717.html> (Accessed on November 1, 2014).
12. Public Health Agency of Canada. 2009. Annex E. The Use of Antiviral Drugs During a Pandemic. 2009, Available at <www.phac-aspc.gc.ca/cpip-pclcpi/ann-e-eng.php> (Accessed on November 1, 2014).
13. Moghadas S, Laskowski M. Review of terms used in modelling influenza infection. NCCID 2014;1-39.
14. Halder N, Kelso JK, Milne GJ. Developing guidelines for school closure interventions to be used during a future influenza pandemic. BMC Infect Dis 2010;10:221-2334-10-221.
15. House T, Baguelin M, Van Hoek AJ, et al. Modelling the impact of local reactive school closures on critical care provision during an influenza pandemic. Proc Biol Sci 2011;278:2753-60.
16. Modelling for Public Health (mod4PH) <www.linkedin.com/groups?gid=6787233&goback=.bzo_*1_*1_*1_*1_*1_*1_*1_*1_national*5collaborating*5centre*5for*5infectious*5diseases&trk=rr_grp_name> (Accessed on February 23, 2015).

19

Low awareness but positive attitudes toward fecal transplantation in Ontario physicians

Madison Dennis MD[1], Mary Jane Salpeter RN BHA[2], Susy Hota MSc MD[1,2,3]

M Dennis, MJ Salpeter, S Hota. Low awareness but positive attitudes toward fecal transplantation in Ontario physicians. Can J Infect Dis Med Microbiol 2015;26(1):30-32.

BACKGROUND: Despite mounting evidence supporting fecal transplantation (FT) as a treatment for recurrent *Clostridium difficile* infection (CDI), adoption into clinical practice has been slow.
OBJECTIVE: To determine the health literacy and attitudes of academic physicians in Toronto and infectious disease physicians in Ontario toward FT as a treatment for recurrent CDI, and to determine whether these are significant barriers to adoption.
METHODS: Surveys were distributed to 253 general internists, infectious diseases specialists, gastroenterologists and family physicians.
RESULTS: The response rate was 15%. More than 60% of physicians described themselves as being 'not at all' or 'somewhat' familiar with FT. Of the 76% of physicians who had never referred a patient for FT, the most common reason (50%) was lack of awareness of where to access the treatment. The 'ick factor' accounted for only 13% of reasons for not referring. No respondent believed that the procedure was too risky to consider.
CONCLUSION: Despite general poor health literacy on FT, most physicians sampled share similar positive attitudes toward the treatment.

Key Words: *Fecal transplantation; Physician attitudes; Physician health literacy; Recurrent* Clostridium difficile *infection*

La transplantation fécale peu connue, mais accueillie positivement par les médecins ontariens

HISTORIQUE : Malgré les données croissantes en appui à la transplantation fécale (TF) pour traiter l'infection à *Clostridium difficile* (ICD) récurrente, son adoption est lente en pratique clinique.
OBJECTIF : Déterminer les connaissances et les attitudes des médecins universitaires de Toronto et des infectiologues de l'Ontario envers la TF pour traiter l'ICD récurrente et déterminer si elles constituent d'importants obstacles à leur adoption.
MÉTHODOLOGIE : Des sondages ont été distribués à 253 internistes généraux, infectiologues, gastroentérologues et médecins de famille.
RÉSULTATS : Le taux de réponse s'élevait à 15 %. Plus de 60 % des médecins se décrivaient comme « pas du tout » ou « quelque peu » familiers avec la TF. Des 76 % de médecins qui n'avaient jamais orienté un patient vers une TF, 50 % affirmaient manquer de connaissance quant à l'accès au traitement. Le facteur« peu ragoûtant » ne constituait que 13 % des raisons de ne pas aiguiller les patients. Aucun répondant ne trouvait l'intervention trop risquée pour être envisagée.
CONCLUSION : Malgré le peu de connaissances générales sur la TF, la plupart des médecins interrogés avaient les mêmes attitudes positives envers le traitement.

Recurrent *Clostridium difficile* infection (RCDI) is associated with high morbidity and mortality (1). Current standard treatments leave 30% of patients with further recurrences (2). One alternative therapy is fecal transplantation (FT), in which stool from a healthy, screened donor is administered to the recipient by nasojejunal tube, enema or colonoscopy. Several case reports and series have demonstrated promising results for FT as a treatment for RCDI (3). A recent systematic review of 317 patients involved in 27 case series found a success rate of 92% for FT with no adverse events (4). A randomized controlled trial also demonstrated that FT initially cured 81% of patients; 94% of patients were cured after repeat infusion, and no significant adverse events were observed (5).

Despite this, FT is still not commonly used. Many articles list the inherently unappealing nature of FT – the 'ick factor' – as a reason why patients would be opposed to it, but they provide no evidence for this claim (6,7). One survey examining patient attitudes toward FT reported that while patients found the treatment unappealing, >81% were open to it; when recommended by their physicians, this number increased to 94% (8).

In Canada, several hospitals have not supported FT. It has been proposed that it is health care personnel, not patients, who object to FT (9,10). It has even been suggested that physicians' negative attitudes act as a main barrier to FT adoption (11). One brief questionnaire study investigating physician attitudes found that 86% of physicians would refer patients to a FT centre (12). The present study aims to better understand physician referral patterns, health literacy and attitudes toward FT in Ontario, clarifying barriers to adopting the procedure more widely.

METHODS

The present study was performed in Ontario between February and April 2011. An electronic survey was created using SurveyMonkey. An introduction and link to the survey was sent via e-mail, using current listservs from the University of Toronto (Toronto, Ontario) department heads and the Ontario Medical Association, to 120 general internists at the University of Toronto, 78 infectious disease specialists at the Ontario Medical Association, and 31 gastroenterologists and 24 family physicians at three academic hospitals in Toronto, Ontario. One reminder e-mail was sent.

[1]*Faculty of Medicine, University of Toronto;* [2]*Department of Infection Prevention and Control, University Health Network;* [3]*Division of Infectious Diseases, Department of Medicine, University of Toronto, Toronto, Ontario*
Correspondence: Dr Susy Hota, Infection Prevention and Control, Toronto General Hospital, 9th floor Munk Wing, Room 800, 200 Elizabeth Street, Toronto, Ontario M5G 2C4. e-mail susy.hota@uhn.on.ca

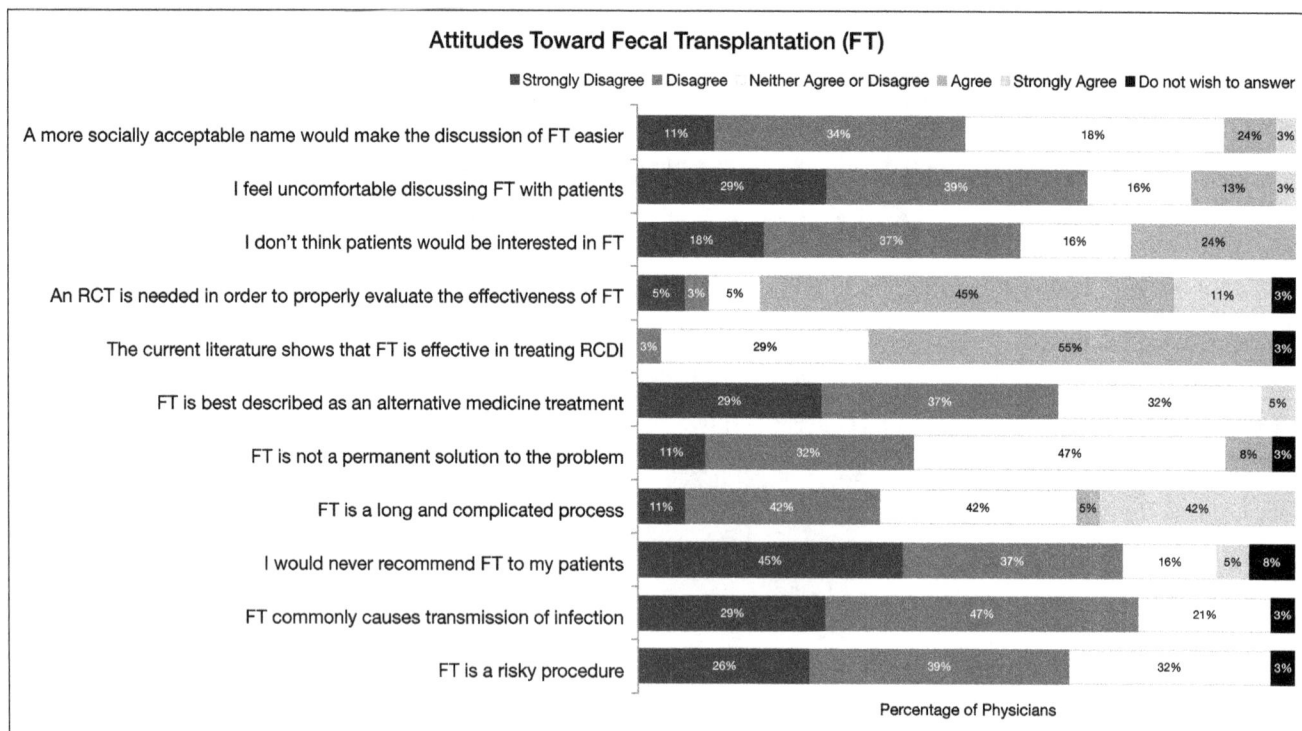

Attitudes Toward Fecal Transplantation (FT)

■ Strongly Disagree ■ Disagree ▒ Neither Agree or Disagree ▓ Agree ░ Strongly Agree ■ Do not wish to answer

A more socially acceptable name would make the discussion of FT easier — 11%, 34%, 18%, 24%, 3%

I feel uncomfortable discussing FT with patients — 29%, 39%, 16%, 13%, 3%

I don't think patients would be interested in FT — 18%, 37%, 16%, 24%

An RCT is needed in order to properly evaluate the effectiveness of FT — 5%, 3%, 5%, 45%, 11%, 3%

The current literature shows that FT is effective in treating RCDI — 3%, 29%, 55%, 3%

FT is best described as an alternative medicine treatment — 29%, 37%, 32%, 5%

FT is not a permanent solution to the problem — 11%, 32%, 47%, 8%, 3%

FT is a long and complicated process — 11%, 42%, 42%, 5%, 42%

I would never recommend FT to my patients — 45%, 37%, 16%, 5%, 8%

FT commonly causes transmission of infection — 29%, 47%, 21%, 3%

FT is a risky procedure — 26%, 39%, 32%, 3%

Percentage of Physicians

Figure 1) *Attitudes toward fecal transplantation. RCDI Recurrent* Clostridium difficile *infection; RCT Randomized controlled trial*

The survey contained five domains: demographic information; past experience with RCDI; knowledge regarding FT; attitudes toward FT; and exploring ways to improve understanding of FT. Multiple-choice responses were used to evaluate knowledge, and attitudes were assessed using a series of Likert-style questions and one open-ended question. The questionnaire was pilot tested and modified for readability, interpretability and face validity. Institutional research ethics board approval was obtained. Standard descriptive statistics were used to analyze the data from the survey. Open-ended questions were qualitatively analyzed for recurring themes.

RESULTS

Of the 253 surveys disseminated, 39 (15%) physicians completed the survey: four (17%) family physicians; 23 (19%) general internists; three (10%) gastroenterologists; and nine (12%) infectious disease specialists. The majority of survey participants were male (67%), general internists (59%) and practicing in Toronto (82%) at academic centres (87%).

In the past five years, 82% of respondents saw >20 cases of C *difficile* infection and 36% saw >10 cases of RCDI. Eighteen percent of surveyed physicians had referred patients for FT.

Physicians surveyed first heard about FT from their colleagues (34%) and from the medical literature (29%). When asked to report their own health literacy by selecting from 'not at all familiar', 'somewhat familiar', 'fairly familiar' and 'very familiar', >60% of physicians described themselves as being not at all or somewhat familiar with FT.

There was no clear consensus on when to use FT. Five percent of surveyed physicians believed that FT should be first-line therapy; 11% believed it should be used after the first recurrence; 47% after the second recurrence; 8% after the third recurrence; and 26% only as a last resort. Interestingly, no physician believed that FT should never be used.

Respondents were asked to select reasons for not referring for FT. Of the 76% of physicians who have never referred, the most common reason (50%) was they were unaware of where to access the treatment. Other frequently cited reasons were: that physicians believed they did not know enough about the treatment (20%); the 'ick factor' (13%); and the procedure was not supported by their hospital (13%). Only a

small number of physicians did not refer because they assumed the patient was not open to the treatment (7%) or because there was not enough scientific evidence (3%). No physician chose not to refer because the treatment was too risky.

Figure 1 presents the results of surveyed physician attitudes toward FT. Most physicians agreed with the statements: "The current literature shows that FT is effective in treating RCDI" and "A randomized controlled trial (RCT) is needed to properly evaluate the effectiveness of FT". Notably, the survey was conducted before publication of an RCT on FT. There was less agreement regarding the discomfort around FT.

The final question was open ended and asked how to improve physician knowledge and understanding of FT. The main themes were that the surveyed physicians were interested in receiving information and wanted key articles to be sent electronically.

DISCUSSION

The present survey was the first to study Ontario physician attitudes toward FT as a treatment for RCDI. Our findings suggest that the majority of Ontario physicians surveyed who see patients with RCDI have positive attitudes toward FT, and the main barrier to referral is a lack of health literacy.

Physician health literacy was self-reported to be quite low, with most surveyed physicians believing they were 'not at all' or 'somewhat' familiar with literature and media articles surrounding FT. Additionally, the top two reasons for not referring patients for FT were that physicians were unaware of where to access the treatment and they believed they lacked knowledge on the treatment.

An unanticipated finding of the study was that, despite general poor health literacy on FT, most surveyed physicians shared similar positive attitudes about the effectiveness and safety of the treatment. No respondent agreed with the statements that FT was a risky procedure or that it commonly caused transmission of infection. Interestingly, these are the two main reasons that hospitals in Canada are rejecting the use of FT (10).

While most surveyed physicians agree that FT is effective and safe, a significant minority of physicians felt uncomfortable discussing FT, did not believe their patients would be interested in it and believed a more socially acceptable name would make the discussion easier. For some physicians, these negative attitudes prevented them from referring patients for FT, with 13% not referring because of the 'ick factor' and 7% because they assume the patient would not be open to it.

Our findings on physician attitudes are similar to a recently published article investigating physician attitudes toward FT that surveyed physicians in New Hampshire and Texas, USA (13). Their study also found that only a small number of physicians did not refer for FT because of safety concerns (7%) or lack of efficacy (4%). However, they found that most physicians did not refer for FT because it was not 'the right clinical situation' (33%), and logistical and institutional barriers accounted for only 23% compared with 63% in our study (physicians not knowing where to access FT and FT not being supported in their hospital). They also found that physicians greatly overestimate the intensity of patient aversion. This may account for our study finding that 24% of physicians agree that patients would not be interested in FT, despite a patient survey finding that up to 94% of patients would consider FT.

Our study was limited by a low response rate (15%). Additional limitations include selection bias; 18% of surveyed physicians had prescribed FT, indicating that those less familiar with RCDI and FT may not have completed the study. There was also a sampling bias because most groups were accessed through academic networks. Finally, the majority of physicians who responded to the survey were from academic institutions in one large city. Although this population provides important insight into the attitudes and referring practices of physicians, it is important to survey more family physicians and physicians from the surrounding communities.

Finally, the present study was conducted before the publication of an RCT on FT for RCDI. It is unclear whether the results of this trial, which was stopped early, have affected physicians' attitudes and health literacy on the subject. The overall landscape of FT has been rapidly changing in terms of the overall published evidence, the regulatory landscape, the rise in at-home FT and increasing media coverage. For these reasons, it would be interesting to repeat our survey to evaluate the impact of all these factors on physician attitudes.

FUNDING: This study was supported by internal funds from the Department of Infection Prevention and Control, University Health Network, Toronto, Ontario.

DISCLOSURE: Susy Hota has served on an advisory board for Cubist Pharmaceuticals.

REFERENCES

1. Loo VG, Poirier L, Miller MA, et al. A predominantly clonal multi-institutional outbreak of *Clostridium difficile*-associated diarrhea with high morbidity and mortality. N Engl J Med 2005;353:2442-9.
2. McFarland LV, Elmer GW, Surawicz CM. Breaking the cycle: Treatment strategies for 163 cases of recurrent *Clostridium difficile* disease. Am J Gastroenterol 2002;97:1769-75.
3. Borody TJ, Warren EF, Leis SM, Surace R, Ashman O, Siarakas S. Bacteriotherapy using fecal flora: Toying with human motions. J Clin Gastroenterol 2004;38:475-84.
4. Gough E, Shaikh H, Manges AR. Systematic review of intestinal microbiota transplantation (fecal bacteriotherapy) for recurrent *Clostridium difficile* infection. Clin Infect Dis 2011;53:994-1002.
5. Van Nood E, Vrieze A, Nieuwdorp M, et al. Duodenal infusion of donor feces for recurrent *Clostridium difficile*. N Engl J Med 2013;368:407-15.
6. Kelly CP, LaMont JT. *Clostridium difficile* – more difficult than ever. N Engl J Med 2008;359:1932-40.
7. McFarland LV. Renewed interest in a difficult disease: *Clostridium difficile* infections – epidemiology and current treatment strategies. Curr Opin Gastroenterol 2009;25:24-35.
8. Zipursky JS, Sidorsky TI, Freedman CA, Sidorsky MN, Kirkland KB. Patient attitudes toward the use of fecal microbiota transplantation in the treatment of recurrent *Clostridium difficile* infection. Clin Infect Dis 2012;55:1652-8.
9. Floch MH. Fecal bacteriotherapy, fecal transplant, and the microbiome. J Clin Gastroenterol 2010;44:529-30.
10. Glauser W. Risk and rewards of fecal transplants. CMAJ 2011;183:541-2.
11. Brandt LJ. Fecal microbiota transplantation: Patient and physician attitudes. Clin Infect Dis 2012;55:1659-60.
12. Jiang ZD, Hoang LN, Lasco TM, Garey KW, Dupont HL. Physician attitudes toward the use of fecal transplantation for recurrent *Clostridium difficile* infection in a metropolitan area. Clin Infect Dis 2013;56:1059-60.
13. Zipursky JS, Sidorsky TI, Freedman CA, Sidorsky MN, Kirkland KB. Physician attitudes towards the use of fecal microbiota transplantation for the treatment of recurrent *Clostridium difficile* infection. Can J Gastroenterol Hepatol 2014;28:319-24.

20

Value of an aggregate index in describing the impact of trends in antimicrobial resistance for *Escherichia coli*

David M Patrick MD FRCPC MHSc[1,2], Catharine Chambers MSc[1], Dale Purych MD[3,4], Mei Chong MSc[1], Diana George MSc[1], Fawziah Marra BSc PharmD FCSHP[5]

DM Patrick, C Chambers, D Purych, M Chong, D George, F Marra. Value of an aggregate index in describing the impact of trends in antimicrobial resistance for *Escherichia coli*. Can J Infect Dis Med Microbiol 2015;26(1):33-38.

BACKGROUND: Drug resistance indexes (DRIs) quantify the cumulative impact of antimicrobial resistance on the likelihood that a given pathogen will be susceptible to antimicrobial therapy.
OBJECTIVE: To derive a DRI for community urinary tract infections caused by *Escherichia coli* in British Columbia for the years 2007 to 2010, and to examine trends over time and across patient characteristics.
METHODS: Indication-specific utilization data were obtained from BC PharmaNet for outpatient antimicrobial prescriptions linked to diagnostic information from physician payment files. Resistance data for *E coli* urinary isolates were obtained from BC Biomedical Laboratories (now part of LifeLabs Medical Laboratory Services). DRIs were derived by multiplying the rate of resistance to a specific antimicrobial by the proportional rate of utilization for that drug class and aggregating across drug classes. Higher index values indicate more resistance.
RESULTS: Adaptive-use DRIs remained stable over time at approximately 18% (95% CI 17% to 18%) among adults ≥15 years of age and approximately 28% (95% CI 26% to 31%) among children <15 years of age. Similar results were observed when proportional drug use was restricted to the baseline year (ie, a static-use model). Trends according to age group suggest a U-shaped distribution, with the highest DRIs occurring among children <10 years of age and adults ≥65 years of age. Males had consistently higher DRIs than females for all age groups.
CONCLUSIONS: The stable trend in adaptive-use DRIs over time suggests that clinicians are adapting their prescribing practices for urinary tract infections to local resistance patterns. Results according to age group reveal a higher probability of resistance to initial therapy among young children and elderly individuals.

Key Words: *Antimicrobial resistance; Drug resistance index;* Escherichia coli

La valeur d'un indice composite pour décrire les effets des tendances de résistance antimicrobienne à l'*Escherichia coli*

HISTORIQUE : Les indices de pharmacorésistance (IPR) quantifient l'effet cumulatif de la résistance antimicrobienne sur la probabilité qu'un pathogène donné soit susceptible à un traitement antimicrobien.
OBJECTIF : Dériver l'IPR des infections urinaires d'origine non nosocomiale causées par l'*Escherichia coli* en Colombie-Britannique entre 2007 et 2010 et examiner les tendances au fil du temps et selon les caractéristiques des patients.
MÉTHODOLOGIE : Les données sur les indications d'utilisation, tirées du système PharmaNet de la Colombie-Britannique relativement aux prescriptions d'antimicrobiens, étaient liées à l'information diagnostique prélevée dans les dossiers d'honoraires des médecins. Les données de résistance reliées aux isolats urinaires d'*E coli* provenaient des *BC Biomedical Laboratories* (qui font désormais partie des *LifeLabs Medical Laboratory Services*). Les IPR étaient dérivés en multipliant le taux de résistance à un antimicrobien précis au taux proportionnel d'utilisation de cette classe de médicament et en les regroupant entre les classes de médicaments. Des indices de valeur plus élevés indiquaient une plus forte résistance.
RÉSULTATS : Les IPR à utilisation adaptée demeuraient stables au fil du temps, à environ 18 % (95 % IC 17 % à 18 %) chez les adultes de 15 ans et plus, et à environ 28 % (95 % IC 26 % à 31 %) chez les enfants de moins de 15 ans. Les chercheurs ont observé des résultats similaires lorsque l'utilisation proportionnelle des médicaments était restreinte à l'année de référence (modèle à utilisation statique). Les tendances en fonction des groupes d'âge laissent supposer une répartition en U, les IPR les plus élevés se produisant chez les enfants de moins de dix ans et les adultes de 65 ans et plus. Dans tous les groupes d'âge, les hommes présentaient un IPR plus élevé que les femmes.
CONCLUSIONS : D'après la tendance stable des IPR à utilisation adaptée au fil du temps, les cliniciens adaptent leurs pratiques de prescription pour le traitement des infections urinaires aux profils de résistance locaux. Les résultats en fonction des groupes d'âge révèlent une plus forte probabilité de résistance à la thérapie initiale chez les jeunes enfants et les personnes âgées.

Urinary tract infections (UTIs) are common bacterial infections that affect both pediatric and adult patients in community and hospital settings. *Escherichia coli* is the most predominant uropathogen, causing approximately 80% of uncomplicated cystitis in adult females (1-3). Treatment of acute uncomplicated cystitis typically involves oral therapy with nitrofurantoin, with alternative therapies including cefixime, trimethoprim-sulfamethoxazole (TMP-SMX), trimethoprim or ciprofloxacin (4). However, the increasing proportion of uropathogens that are resistant to recommended antibiotic treatments challenges the appropriate care and management of UTIs and limits the potential benefits of these drugs (5,6).

Evidence from national surveillance programs in Canada suggests that antimicrobial resistance among uropathogens has increased in recent years (7-9). In British Columbia (BC), there has been a nine-fold increase in the proportion of *E coli* isolates nonsusceptible to ciprofloxacin from 1999 to 2011, with the highest resistance rates

[1]*British Columbia Centre for Disease Control;* [2]*School of Population and Public Health, University of British Columbia, Vancouver;* [3]*LifeLabs Medical Laboratory Services;* [4]*Fraser Health Authority, Surrey;* [5]*Faculty of Pharmaceutical Services, University of British Columbia, Vancouver, British Columbia*

Correspondence: Dr David M Patrick, BC Centre for Disease Control, 655 West 12th Avenue, Vancouver, British Columbia V5Z 4R4. e-mail david.patrick@bccdc.ca

observed among elderly age groups (10). In 2011, more than one-quarter (27%) of E coli isolates in BC were resistant to ciprofloxacin, more than one-quarter (26%) were resistant to TMP-SMX and almost one-half (46%) were resistant to ampicillin (10). Risk factors for developing a drug-resistant UTI include having had a previous UTI, previous antimicrobial exposure, recent hospitalization, long-term care residence, male sex, older age and comorbidities such as diabetes (11-15).

Ongoing surveillance of antimicrobial resistance trends is necessary to assess the overall burden of antimicrobial resistance over time and to derive empirical treatment guidelines for bacterial infections. However, conveying this information in an understandable and cohesive manner to policymakers and health care practitioners is challenging, particularly when resistance rates are examined separately for each drug and when trends are inconsistent across drug classes (16). Further challenges arise when these trends are interpreted in the absence of information on the proportional use of antimicrobials used to treat a given infection, or the availability and relative effectiveness of alternative treatments (16). A drug resistance index (DRI) can overcome these challenges by aggregating resistance to multiple drug classes into a single composite measure for a given bacterial species or type of infection. The purpose of the present analysis was to calculate a DRI for community UTIs caused by E coli in BC for the years 2007 to 2010, and to examine DRI trends over time and across patient demographics.

METHODS

Data sources

Antimicrobial utilization data were obtained from the BC PharmaNet database of outpatient prescriptions for oral antimicrobials for systematic use for the years 2007 to 2010. The PharmaNet database includes records of all outpatient prescriptions dispensed from community pharmacies to BC residents. It excludes over-the-counter medications, medications administered to inpatients in acute care hospitals, medication samples dispensed at a physician's office, and medications administered for veterinary or agricultural use. Antimicrobial utilization data were classified according to the WHO's Anatomical Therapeutic Chemical classification system (17).

To derive indication-specific antimicrobial utilization rates, antimicrobial prescription records were linked to diagnostic codes from the BC Medical Services Plan (MSP) files. The MSP files contain data for all medically necessary services provided by fee-for-service practitioners to BC residents covered under the provincial insurance program. Prescription records were linked to MSP records based on matching patient and physician identifiers when the prescription dispensing date occurred within five days of the practitioner service date. In instances in which more than one MSP record was extracted, the record with the most recent service date was used. Indications were defined according to the *International Classification of Diseases, Ninth Edition* (ICD-9) (18). PharmaNet-MSP linked data were restricted to ICD-9 diagnostic codes for cystitis (595) and its subcodes (595.0, 595.1, etc).

Antimicrobial resistance data for E coli urinary isolates were obtained from BC Biomedical Laboratories Ltd (part of LifeLabs Medical Service Laboratories as of 2013), a community-based laboratory practice serving the Vancouver Coastal and Fraser Health Authorities in BC, for the years 2007 to 2010. Testing of isolates conformed to Clinical and Laboratory Standards Institute guidelines (19).

Annual population estimates used in the calculation of antimicrobial utilization rates were obtained from the BC Health Data Warehouse (20).

Analysis

Analyses were performed separately for adults ≥15 years of age and children <15 years of age. In adults, antimicrobial utilization rates were calculated as the defined daily dose (DDD) per 1000 population per day, where DDD represents the average maintenance dose per day

for a drug used in its main indication in adults (17). In children, antimicrobial utilization rates were calculated as the total number of prescriptions per 1000 population per day because antimicrobial dosing in pediatric patients varies according to weight.

An adaptive-use DRI for E coli was calculated according to methods adapted from Laxminarayan and Klugman (16) using the formula:

$$R = \sum_k p_k^t q_k^t$$

where p_k^t is the rate of resistance to drug class k at time t and q_k^t is the proportional rate of use for drug class k used to treat cystitis at time t. Higher index values indicate more resistance.

For contrast, a 'static use' model was used to measure the hypothetical DRI trend had proportional antimicrobial use remained unchanged over time (16). Differences between static and observed adaptive DRIs help gauge the contributions of physician-adaptation to preserving the value of initial empirical therapy. The static DRI was calculated using the proportional rate of use for drug class k fixed to the baseline year of the analysis. To ensure comparability of results with those of previous studies, a sensitivity analysis was also performed using overall prescription data for any indication rather than prescription data specifically for the treatment of cystitis.

Anatomical Therapeutic Chemical drug classes were restricted to drug classes relevant to the treatment of UTIs caused by E coli, where data were available. These included: penicillins with extended spectrum (J01CA), first-generation cephalosporins (J01DB), third-generation cephalosporins (J01DD), fluoroquinolones (J01MA), nitrofuran derivatives (J01XE) and sulphonamide/trimethoprim combinations (J01EE). An isolate was considered to be resistant to a drug class if it was found to be nonsusceptible to at least one antimicrobial agent within that class (21). It should be noted that cefotaxime resistant cut-off ranges were modified in 2010, but that standards otherwise remained constant throughout the study period.

Stratified analyses were performed according to patient demographic characteristics (ie, age group and sex). Trends in DRIs were assessed using the nonparametric Spearman Rank test. Percentile CIs were calculated using nonparametric bootstrap methods with m=1000 simulations performed on an approximately 10% sample (PharmaNet = 47,782 observations; BC Biomedical = 13,166 observations) drawn at random from the full datasets. Ethics approval for the present analysis was obtained from the Clinical Research Ethics Board at the University of British Columbia (Vancouver, British Columbia). All analyses were performed using SAS version 9.2 (SAS Institute, USA).

RESULTS

Among both patient populations, the highest resistance rates were observed for ampicillin (43.8% for adults and 46.9% for children) in the baseline year, followed by cephalothin (25.8% and 20.1%), TMP-SMX (25.1% and 26.2%) and ciprofloxacin (22.7% and 7.1%). Resistance rates for cefotaxime (11.8% and 6.5%) and nitrofuratoin (3.3% and 1.3%) remained relatively low for both patient populations across all study years. For adults, resistance rates were generally stable over time despite a trend toward increasing resistance to fluoroquinolones (P>0.05) (Figure 1A). For children, resistance rates for ampicillin significantly decreased over time (rho=−1.00; P<0.01), while resistance rates for ciprofloxacin significantly increased (rho=1.00; P<0.01) (Figure 1B). Resistance rates for all other included drug classes were stable (P>0.05).

Among adults, fluoroquinolones comprised the largest proportional use at 37.9% in the baseline year, followed by nitrofuran derivatives (32.1%) and sulphonamide/trimethoprim combinations (21.4%) (Figure 2A). Proportional use of fluoroquinolones (rho=−1.00; P<0.01) and sulphonamide/trimethoprim combinations (rho=−1.00; P<0.01) significantly decreased during the study period, corresponding to a significant increase in the proportional use of nitrofuran derivatives (rho=1.00; P<0.01).

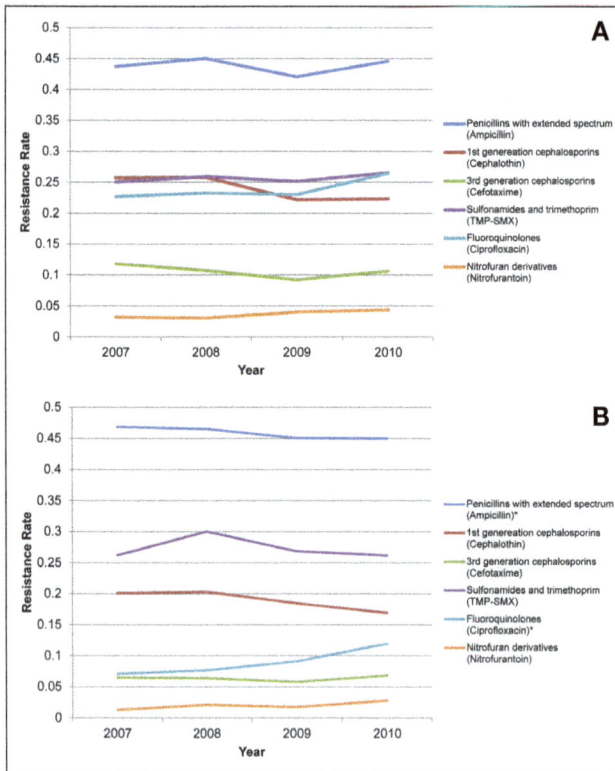

Figure 1) *Proportion of* Escherichia coli *urinary isolates nonsusceptible to relevant drug classes in British Columbia among adults ≥15 years of age (**A**) and children <15 years of age (**B**). *Trends over time are statistically significant according to nonparametric Spearman Rank test. TMP-SMX Trimethoprim-sulfamethoxazole*

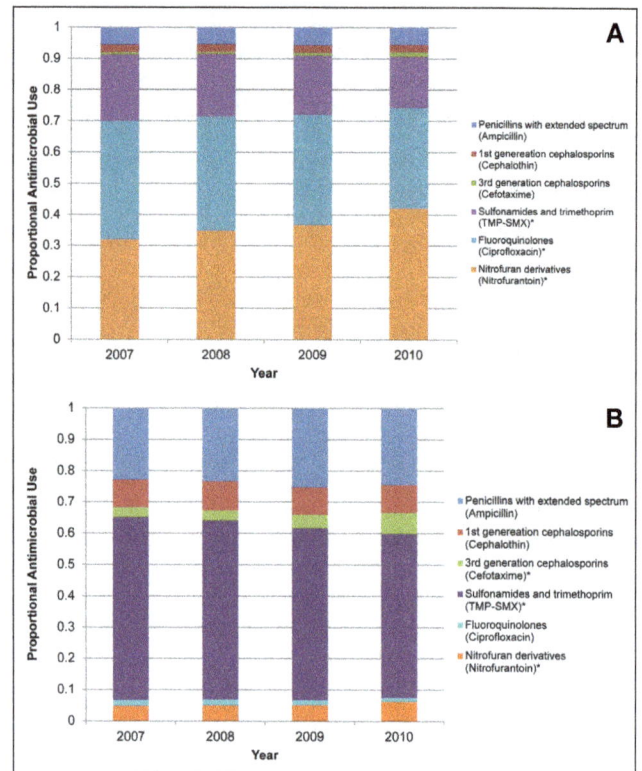

Figure 2) *Proportional rate of antimicrobial use for cystitis in British Columbia among adults ≥15 years of age (**A**) and children <15 years of age (**B**). *Trends over time are statistically significant according to nonparametric Spearman Rank test. TMP-SMX Trimethoprim-sulfamethoxazole*

Among children, sulphonamide/trimethoprim combinations comprised the largest proportional drug use at >50% across all study years (Figure 2B). A significant decreasing trend in proportional use was observed for sulphonamide/trimethoprim combinations over time (rho=−1.00; P<0.001), while significant increasing trends were observed for third-generation cephalosporins (rho=1.00; P<0.001) and nitrofuran derivatives (rho=1.00; P<0.001).

Among adults, the adaptive-use DRI, when averaged across all study years, was 0.18 (95% CI 0.17 to 0.18) and remained stable over time (rho=−0.80; P=0.20) (Figure 3A). The static-use DRI increased from 0.18 (95% CI 0.17 to 0.19) in 2007 to 0.20 (95% CI 0.19 to 0.21) in 2010; however, the overall trend was not significant (rho=0.80; P=0.20). DRI values for the static-use model did not significantly differ from the adaptive-use model over the four years of study, as indicated by the overlapping 95% CIs. DRI values did not dramatically differ when total number of prescriptions (versus DDDs) was used to calculate proportional antimicrobial use for adults (data not shown).

Among children, the adaptive-use DRI peaked at 0.30 (95% CI 0.25 to 0.35) in 2008 then declined to 0.27 (95% CI 0.22 to 0.32) in 2010; however, this trend was not significant (rho=−0.40; P=0.60) (Figure 3B). Nearly identical DRI values were observed for the static-use model.

Fluoroquinolones and sulphonamide/trimethoprim combinations made the largest contribution to the DRI among adults across all years, while among children the trend in DRI values was predominantly driven by sulphonamide/trimethoprim combinations and penicillins with extended spectrum (Table 1). Other drug classes had relatively less impact on DRI trends among both adults and children. Analyses according to age group and sex show that DRI values were consistently higher among males than females across all age groups (Figure 4). For adults, there was a significant increasing trend from 0.09 (95% CI 0.08 to 0.11) among those 15 to 19 years of age to 0.32 (95% CI

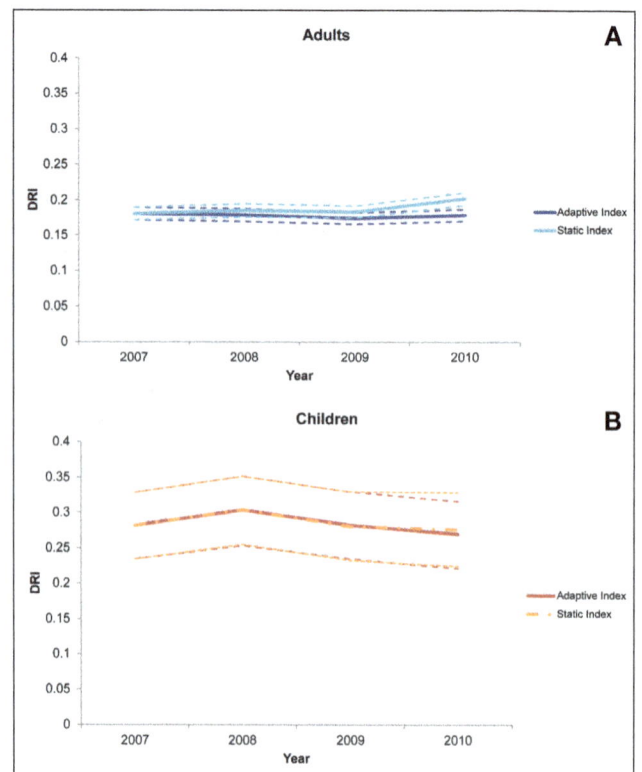

Figure 3) *Adaptive- and static-use drug resistance indexes (DRIs) for* Escherichia coli *with 95% CIs (shown as dashed lines) in British Columbia among adults ≥15 years of age (**A**) and children <15 years of age (**B**)*

TABLE 1
Resistance rates for *Escherichia coli* urinary isolates and proportional rates of antimicrobial use for cystitis among adults ≥15 years of age and children <15 years of age in British Columbia, 2007–2010

Drug class (antibiotic)	Resistance rate (A), %	Proportional antimicrobial use (B), %	Drug resistance index (A*B)	95% CI for drug resistance index
Adults				
Penicillins with extended spectrum (ampicillin)	44.3	5.5	0.02	
First-generation cephalosporins (cephalothin)	24.3	2.4	0.01	
Third-generation cephalosporins (cefotaxime)	10.6	0.9	0.00	
Sulfonamides and trimethoprim (TMP-SMX)	25.8	19.1	0.05	
Fluoroquinolones (ciprofloxacin)	24.7	35.3	0.09	
Nitrofuran derivatives (nitrofurantoin)	3.8	36.7	0.01	
Sum			0.18	0.17–0.18
Children				
Penicillins with extended spectrum (ampicillin)	45.8	23.9	0.11	
First-generation cephalosporins (cephalothin)	19.3	9.1	0.02	
Third-generation cephalosporins (cefotaxime)	6.2	4.4	0.00	
Sulfonamides and trimethoprim (TMP-SMX)	27.1	55.6	0.15	
Fluoroquinolones (ciprofloxacin)	9.2	1.6	0.00	
Nitrofuran derivatives (nitrofurantoin)	2.0	5.4	0.00	
Sum			0.28	0.26–0.31

TMP-SMX Trimethoprim-sulfamethoxazole

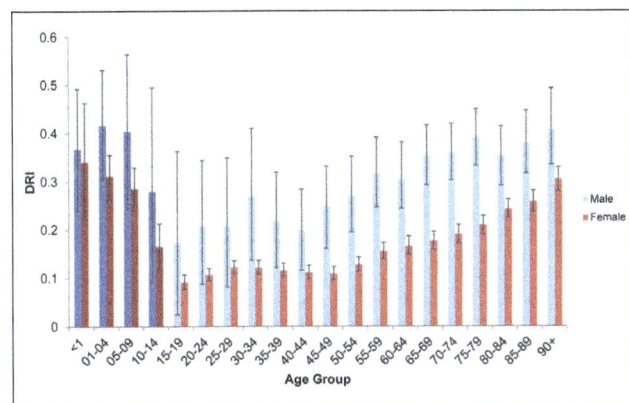

Figure 4) *Adaptive-use drug resistance index (DRI) with 95% CIs for Escherichia coli in British Columbia according to age group and sex*

0.29 to 0.34) among those >90 years of age (rho=0.95; P<0.01). For children, there was a significant declining trend from 0.35 (95% CI 0.27 to 0.43) among those <1 year of age to 0.17 (95% CI 0.13 to 0.22) among those 10 to 14 years of age (rho=−1.00; P<0.01).

Sensitivity analysis
A sensitivity analysis was performed using overall, rather than indication-specific, prescription data to calculate proportional drug use. Among both patient populations, penicillins with extended spectrum were the most frequently used antimicrobial class for any indication in the baseline year (43.4% for adults and 75.0% for children), followed by fluoroquinolones (22.1% and 0.4%, respectively), first-generation cephalosporins (14.8% and 12.4%, respectively), sulphonamide/trimethprim combinations (11.5% and 9.6%, respectively), nitrofuran derivatives (7.5% and 0.4%, respectively) and third-generation cephalosporins (0.7% and 2.2%, respectively). Among adults, the adaptive-use DRI was significantly higher at 0.31 (95% CI 0.31 to 0.32) when overall prescription data were used. The adaptive-use DRI remained stable over time (rho=0.40; P=0.60) and did not significantly differ from the static-use model. Among children, the adaptive-use DRI was significantly higher at approximately 0.40 (95% CI 0.37 to 0.43) when overall prescription data were used and remained stable over time (rho=−0.80; P=0.20).

DISCUSSION
The DRI reflects the proportion of prescriptions for *E coli* cystitis in a population that uses a drug to which the organism is not susceptible. Our findings show that the overall DRI value for community *E coli* urinary isolates, when averaged across study years, is 18% (95% CI 17% to 18%) among adults ≥15 years of age. This value is lower than the *E coli* DRI of 30% (95% CI 29% to 32%) reported by Laxminarayan and Klugman (16) for 2006, likely because our study used indication-specific antimicrobial utilization data, which will more accurately reflect the tailored selection of antimicrobials for the treatment of UTIs. Sensitivity analyses based on overall prescribing for any indication found DRI values more consistent with previously reported values at 31% (95% CI 31% to 32%), largely driven by the greater proportional use of extended-spectrum penicillins. Our analyses were stratified according to age group, which may also partially explain the discrepancy with previous findings. While resistance rates were similar between adults ≥15 years of age and children <15 years of age, the higher proportional use of extended-spectrum pencillins and sulphonamide/trimethoprim combinations among children increased the relative contribution of these drug classes to the age-specific DRI. For children, the overall DRI value across all study years was 28% (95% CI 26% to 31%). Geographical variability may also be a factor because resistance rates are known to be significantly higher in the United States in comparison with Canada (8,9).

Adaptive-use DRI trends remained stable over time, and DRI values based on a static-use model that fixes proportional antimicrobial use to the baseline year did not significantly differ from an adaptive-use model. However, even over this short study period, the static index appears to be trending upward. A contrast between the value of the observed adaptive and static DRI is consistent with physicians increasing the proportionate use of nitrofurantoin. Physicians appear to have been increasing their use of this drug at the expense of TMP-SMX and ciprofloxacin. This change could be in response to evolving guidelines, emphasis in continuing education sessions or individual physician attention to antibiograms. Whatever the driver, physicians may be adapting prescribing practices to local resistance patterns (16). However, the limited availability of data makes it difficult to assess long-term trends. Others have noted rising resistance rates over time associated with the clonal spread of virulent, multidrug-resistant strains (7,22), including extended-spectrum beta-lactamase-producing strains of community-acquired *E coli* (23,24). A longer duration of surveillance will be required to monitor the impact of extended-spectrum beta-lactamase-producing *E coli* strains on DRI trends in BC.

Consistent with recent guidelines (4,25), our data suggest that nitrofurantoin is an appropriate treatment for acute uncomplicated cystitis given its low observed resistance rates. While this may be good news for cystitis, nitrofurantoin is not indicated for the treatment of pyelonephritis due to inadequate concentrations achieved in renal tissues and should not be used if early pyelonephritis is suspected (4,25). Despite earlier research suggesting that nitrofurantoin has lower clinical cure rates and more side effects than traditional first-line agents, namely TMP-SMX and fluoroquinolones (26), more recent studies suggest that empirical treatment with nitrofurantoin is as effective as these drugs (25). Given the concerning resistance trends observed for ciprofloxacin and TMP-SMX, our findings support calls made by others for more judicious use of these drugs (8,25-27). Routine testing data were not available for our study period for other, alternative treatments for UTIs, such as fosfomycin, which has only recently become available again in Canada.

DRI trends according to age group suggest a U-shaped distribution with the lowest rates occurring among adults <50 years of age and the highest rates occurring among young children and the elderly. Elderly adults are at greater risk for developing a drug-resistant infection, likely as a result of cumulative lifetime exposure to antimicrobials, particularly to fluoroquinolones, higher frequency and longer duration of hospital stays, increased likelihood of developing complicated infections and increased prevalence of comorbidities (7,11,12,14). While acute, uncomplicated UTIs are generally self-limiting and not associated with long-term medical sequelae in adults in the absence of underlying conditions (1,28), among pediatric patients, UTIs can be associated with significant morbidity, including impaired renal function and end-stage renal disease (28,29).

Males had consistently higher DRI values than females across all age groups, a finding that is consistent with resistance trends observed nationally (7-9). These trends are largely driven by the greater proportional use of fluoroquinolones for cystitis and the higher rates of ciprofloxacin resistance among men (data not shown). The high prevalence of complicated UTIs among men, combined with the longer duration of therapies and older age at diagnosis, likely explains the higher observed resistance rates (7,30,31). In children, this sex difference is likely the result of congenital abnormalities, which are more prevalent among males than females (29,30).

The present study extends previous work in this area in a number of important ways. Access to prescription drug use through BC PharmaNet allows for examination of antimicrobial utilization in community settings for the entire population of BC. We have adopted standardized methods of measuring antimicrobial use in units of DDDs (17) and established linkage methodologies to connect antimicrobial prescriptions to ICD-9 diagnostic codes to derive indication-specific antimicrobial prescribing (32,33). However, despite these strengths, certain limitations should be acknowledged. Prescription data from PharmaNet are restricted to oral antimicrobials dispensed in outpatient settings. While these data comprehensively measure prescription use in the community – the main focus of our study – they do not capture antimicrobial use for agents that are administered parenterally

and/or primarily used in inpatient settings. As a result, utilization rates for certain drug classes may be underestimated in our study or, in the case of carbapenems and aminoglycosides, excluded completely. The accuracy of data on indication-specific prescribing will depend on the manner in which physicians code the diagnosis when billing. We focused on the majority of UTIs for which a cystitis code (ICD-9 595) was coded to assure specificity of that diagnosis in describing treatment patterns, UTIs identified by less specific codes (eg, ICD-9 599) were excluded. Nonetheless, our linked data analysis reflects patterns of prescription for an entire population. BC Biomedical Laboratories are located in only two of five of the regional health authorities in BC, and, although one of the largest laboratory service providers in BC, they are not the sole provider of outpatient laboratory services in these areas. However, we have observed only limited variation in prescribing by region in BC. Future analyses will begin with more complete sampling of laboratory data through collaboration with broader laboratory systems.

Routine susceptibility testing of penicillins with beta-lactamase inhibitors (eg, amoxicillin-clavulanate) was only performed from 2009 onwards; consequently, this antimicrobial class was excluded from our analysis to ensure comparability of DRI values over time. Culture samples are generally not indicated for young, otherwise healthy, premenopausal women. As such, isolates may be more representative of certain patient populations with higher resistance rates such as those with complicated UTIs (7-9). Finally, DRIs for adults and children in the present analysis may not be directly comparable due to differences in their calculations (refer to the Methods section).

CONCLUSIONS

DRIs improve our ability to quantify and communicate the cumulative impact of antimicrobial resistance on the likelihood that an organism will be susceptible to initial antimicrobial treatment. For clinicians, they provide information on the effectiveness of alternative treatment regimens and the relative adaptability of these treatments to local resistance patterns. For policymakers and other nonexpert groups, DRIs function as an important communication tool for translating knowledge about antimicrobial resistance into practice. Our findings show that the overall DRI value for community UTIs caused by *E coli* in BC is 18% for adults and 28% for children for the years 2007 to 2010. The likelihood that a UTI caused by *E coli* will be susceptible to initial antimicrobial therapy is highest among adult females, while concerning DRI values were observed among young children and the elderly. Further work is required to develop a DRI to summarize the impact of resistance on all relevant pathogens causing UTI in a population.

ACKNOWLEDGEMENTS: The authors thank collaborators who provided data required to conduct this study: the BC Ministry of Health and BC Biomedical Laboratories Ltd (part of LifeLabs Medical Service Laboratories Ltd as of 2013). The authors also acknowledge Ramanan Laxminarayan and Nikolay Braykov at the Center for Disease Dynamics, Economics and Policy in Washington, DC for their input on the methods.

INSTITUTION FROM WHICH WORK ORIGINATED: BC Centre for Disease Control.

REFERENCES

1. Foxman B. The epidemiology of urinary tract infection. Nat Rev Urol 2010;7:653-60.
2. Nicolle LE. Uncomplicated urinary tract infection in adults including uncomplicated pyelonephritis. Urol Clin North Am 2008;35:1-12.
3. Ronald A. The etiology of urinary tract infection: Traditional and emerging pathogens. Am J Med 2002;113(Suppl 1A):14S-9S.
4. Blondel-Hill E, Fryters S. Bugs and Drugs: An Antimicrobial/Infectious Disease Reference, 2012 edn. Edmonton: Alberta Health Services, 2012.
5. Cohen ML. Epidemiology of drug resistance: Implications for a post-antimicrobial era. Science 1992;257:1050-5.

6. Kunin CM. Resistance to antimicrobial drugs – a worldwide calamity. Ann Intern Med 1993;118:557-61.
7. Karlowsky JA, Lagace-Wiens PR, Simner PJ, et al. Antimicrobial resistance in urinary tract pathogens in Canada from 2007 to 2009: CANWARD surveillance study. Antimicrob Agents Chemother 2011;55:3169-75.
8. Zhanel GG, Hisanaga TL, Laing NM, et al. Antibiotic resistance in outpatient urinary isolates: Final results from the North American Urinary Tract Infection Collaborative Alliance (NAUTICA). Int J Antimicrob Agents 2005;26:380-8.
9. Zhanel GG, Hisanaga TL, Laing NM, et al. Antibiotic resistance in *Escherichia coli* outpatient urinary isolates: Final results from the

North American Urinary Tract Infection Collaborative Alliance (NAUTICA). Int J Antimicrob Agents 2006;27:468-75.

10. British Columbia Centre for Disease Control. Antimicrobial resistance trends in the province of British Columbia, 2011. Vancouver: Communicable Disease Prevention and Control Services, British Columbia Centre for Disease Control, 2012.

11. Ben Ami R, Rodriguez-Bano J, Arslan H, et al. A multinational survey of risk factors for infection with extended-spectrum beta-lactamase-producing enterobacteriaceae in nonhospitalized patients. Clin Infect Dis 2009;49:682-90.

12. Colodner R, Rock W, Chazan B, et al. Risk factors for the development of extended-spectrum beta-lactamase-producing bacteria in nonhospitalized patients. Eur J Clin Microbiol Infect Dis 2004;23:163-7.

13. Colodner R, Kometiani I, Chazan B, Raz R. Risk factors for community-acquired urinary tract infection due to quinolone-resistant E. coli. Infection 2008;36:41-5.

14. Sotto A, De Boever CM, Fabbro-Peray P, Gouby A, Sirot D, Jourdan J. Risk factors for antibiotic-resistant Escherichia coli isolated from hospitalized patients with urinary tract infections: A prospective study. J Clin Microbiol 2001;39:438-44.

15. Wright SW, Wrenn KD, Haynes ML. Trimethoprim-sulfamethoxazole resistance among urinary coliform isolates. J Gen Intern Med 1999;14:606-9.

16. Laxminarayan R, Klugman KP. Communicating trends in resistance using a drug resistance index. BMJ Open 2011;1:e000135.

17. WHO Collaborating Centre for Drug Statistics Methodology. Guidelines for ATC classification and DDD assignment, 2012. Oslo: World Health Organization, 2011.

18. American Medical Association. International Classification of Diseases, 9th Revision, Clinical Modification. 1997.

19. Clinical and Laboratory Standards Institute. Performance standards for antimicrobial susceptibility testing: 19th information supplement. CLSI document M100-S19. Wayne: Clinical and Laboratory Standards Institute, 2009.

20. BC Stats. Population projections. <www.bcstats.gov.bc.ca/StatisticsBySubject/Demography/PopulationProjections.aspx> (Accessed January 9, 2013).

21. Magiorakos AP, Srinivasan A, Carey RB, et al. Multidrug-resistant, extensively drug-resistant and pandrug-resistant bacteria: An international expert proposal for interim standard definitions for acquired resistance. Clin Microbiol Infect 2012;18:268-81.

22. Gupta K. Addressing antibiotic resistance. Am J Med 2002;113(Suppl 1A):29S-34S.

23. Nicolas-Chanoine MH, Blanco J, Leflon-Guibout V, et al. Intercontinental emergence of Escherichia coli clone O25:H4-ST131 producing CTX-M-15. J Antimicrob Chemother 2008;61:273-81.

24. Pitout JD, Nordmann P, Laupland KB, Poirel L. Emergence of Enterobacteriaceae producing extended-spectrum beta-lactamases (ESBLs) in the community. J Antimicrob Chemother 2005;56:52-9.

25. Gupta K, Hooton TM, Naber KG, et al. International clinical practice guidelines for the treatment of acute uncomplicated cystitis and pyelonephritis in women: A 2010 update by the Infectious Diseases Society of America and the European Society for Microbiology and Infectious Diseases. Clin Infect Dis 2011;52:e103-e120.

26. Hooton TM, Bradley SF, Cardenas DD, et al. Diagnosis, prevention, and treatment of catheter-associated urinary tract infection in adults: 2009 International Clinical Practice Guidelines from the Infectious Diseases Society of America. Clin Infect Dis 2010;50:625-63.

27. Naber KG, Schito G, Botto H, Palou J, Mazzei T. Surveillance study in Europe and Brazil on clinical aspects and Antimicrobial Resistance Epidemiology in Females with Cystitis (ARESC): Implications for empiric therapy. Eur Urol 2008;54:1164-75.

28. Stamm WE. Scientific and clinical challenges in the management of urinary tract infections. Am J Med 2002;113(Suppl 1A):1S-4S.

29. Ma JF, Shortliffe LM. Urinary tract infection in children: Etiology and epidemiology. Urol Clin North Am 2004;31:517-26.

30. Neal DE, Jr. Complicated urinary tract infections. Urol Clin North Am 2008;35:13-22.

31. Nicolle LE. Complicated urinary tract infection in adults. Can J Infect Dis Med Microbiol 2005;16:349-60.

32. Fuertes EI, Henry B, Marra F, Wong H, Patrick DM. Trends in antibiotic utilization in Vancouver associated with a community education program on antibiotic use. Can J Public Health 2010;101:304-8.

33. McKay RM, Vrbova L, Fuertes E, et al. Evaluation of the Do Bugs Need Drugs? program in British Columbia: Can we curb antibiotic prescribing? Can J Infect Dis Med Microbiol 2011;22:19-24.

21

Parents' and adolescents' willingness to be vaccinated against serogroup B meningococcal disease during a mass vaccination in Saguenay–Lac-St-Jean (Quebec)

Eve Dubé PhD[1,2,3], Dominique Gagnon MSc[1], Denis Hamel MSc[1], Sylvie Belley MD[4], Hélène Gagné Bsinf[4], Nicole Boulianne MSc Bsinf[1,2,3], Monique Landry MD[5], Julie A Bettinger PhD[6]

E Dubé, D Gagnon, D Hamel, et al. Parents' and adolescents' willingness to be vaccinated against serogroup B meningococcal disease during a mass vaccination in Saguenay–Lac-St-Jean (Quebec). Can J Infect Dis Med Microbiol 2015;26(3):163-167.

A mass vaccination campaign with the 4CMenB vaccine (Bexsero®; Novartis Pharmaceutical Canada Inc) was launched in a serogroup B endemic area in Quebec. A telephone survey was conducted to assess parental and adolescent opinions about the acceptability of the vaccine. Intent to receive the vaccine or vaccine receipt was reported by the majority of parents (93%) and adolescents (75%). Meningitis was perceived as being a dangerous disease by the majority of parents and adolescents. The majority of respondents also considered the 4CMenB vaccine to be safe and effective. The main reason for positive vaccination intention or behaviour was self-protection, while a negative attitude toward vaccination in general was the main reason mentioned by parents who did not intend to have their child vaccinated. Adolescents mainly reported lack of interest, time or information, and low perceived susceptibility and disease severity as the main reasons for not intending to be vaccinated or not being vaccinated.

Key Words: *4CMenB vaccine; Adolescents; Children; Meningococcal serogroup B vaccine; Vaccine acceptability*

La volonté des parents et des adolescents de se faire vacciner contre la méningococcie du sérogroupe B pendant une vaccination de masse au Saguenay–Lac-St-Jean (Québec)

Une campagne de vaccination de masse avec le vaccin 4CMenB (Bexsero®; Novartis Pharma Canada Inc.) a été lancée dans une région du Québec endémique au sérogroupe B. Un sondage téléphonique afin d'évaluer l'acceptabilité du vaccin par les parents et les adolescents a été réalisé. La majorité des parents (93 %) et des adolescents (75 %) ont déclaré avoir l'intention de se faire vacciner / de faire vacciner leur enfant ou l'avoir déjà fait. La majorité des parents et des adolescents percevaient la méningite comme dangereuse et considéraient le vaccin 4CMenB comme sécuritaire et efficace. La protection de l'enfant était la principale raison d'accepter le vaccin chez les parents, tandis qu'une attitude négative envers la vaccination en général était la principale raison que donnaient les parents qui n'avaient pas l'intention de faire vacciner leur enfant. Les adolescents déclaraient surtout un manque d'intérêt, de temps ou d'information, la perception d'être peu susceptibles à la maladie et la perception que la maladie n'était pas très grave comme principales raisons de ne pas s'être fait vacciner ou de ne pas avoir l'intention de le faire.

In Canada, invasive meningococcal disease (IMD) is endemic with outbreaks caused by virulent *Neisseria meningitidis* clones. The incidence of IMD varies considerably depending on the different serogroups, age groups, geographical areas and time periods. Before 2005, most cases of IMD were caused by serogroup C (1). In recent years, the incidence of serogroup C disease has declined significantly due to the introduction of meningococcal C conjugate vaccine into routine immunization programs for infants, children and adolescents (2-4).

Since the widespread use of the meningococcal C conjugate vaccine, serogroup B infection now makes up the greatest proportion of reported IMD cases in Quebec (5). Between 2003 and 2010, 72% of all cases of meningococcal disease were due to serogroup B meningococci (6) and the province reported the highest incidence of serogroup B IMD across Canada. Important disparities in incidence occur among different regions in Quebec. In the area of Saguenay–Lac-St-Jean, the incidence of serogroup B IMD is seven times higher than in other areas in the province (5). Therefore, with the licensure in December 2013 of a new vaccine against meningococcal serogroup B (4CMenB, Bexsero®,

Novartis Pharmaceutical Canada Inc.) (7), the Quebec Immunization Committee (CIQ) recommended vaccination of individuals from two months to 20 years of age residing in Saguenay–Lac-St-Jean to control the incidence of IMD caused by serogroup B (5). A targeted vaccination campaign was started on May 4, 2014.

In the context of the targeted mass vaccination campaign against meningococcal serogroup B disease in Saguenay–Lac-St-Jean, the objective of the present study was to assess the knowledge, attitudes and intention of parents of eligible children and of adolescents targeted to receive the 4CMenB vaccine over time. The present article describes the first phase of the study.

METHODS

Study design

The first phase of the present longitudinal study was conducted at the beginning of the mass vaccination campaign to assess the determinants of parents' intention to have their child vaccinated with the 4CMenB vaccine (or adolescents' intention to receive the 4CMenB

[1]*Institut national de santé publique du Québec;* [2]*Centre de recherche du CHU de Québec;* [3]*Université Laval, Québec;* [4]*Direction de santé publique du Saguenay–Lac-St-Jean, Chicoutimi;* [5]*Ministère de la santé et des Services sociaux, Montréal, Québec;* [6]*Vaccine Evaluation Center, BC Children's Hospital, University of British Columbia, Vancouver, British Columbia*
Correspondence: Dr Eve Dubé, 2400 D'Estimauville, Québec, Québec G1E 7G9. e-mail eve.dube@inspq.qc.ca

TABLE 1
Parents' and adolescents' self-reported vaccine status

	All recommended vaccines	Some vaccines only	No vaccine	Do not know
Parents of children:				
2 months to <5 years of age	88.3 (84.42–92.17)	9.5 (6.00–13.02)	1.7 (0.00–3.42)	0.5 (0.00–1.17)
5 years to <12 years of age	96.2 (93.45–98.90)	3.6 (0.91–6.29)	0.2 (0.00–0.67)	0.0
12 years to <16 years of age	91.2 (86.62–95.86)	7.9 (3.54–12.17)	0.0	0.9 (0.00–2.69)
Total (parents)	92.5 (90.40–94.53)	6.5 (4.58–8.46)	0.6 (0.06–1.21)	0.4 (0.00–0.87)
Adolescents	65.8 (57.98–73.64)	29.0 (21.56–36.52)	0.7 (0.00–2.19)	4.4 (0.93–7.89)

Data presented as % (95% CI)

vaccine). A professional research and polling firm (SOM Recherches et Sondages) handled recruitment and data collection. Computer-assisted telephone interviews were performed from May 9 to May 17, 2014. The sample was constituted using random-digit dialling methodology (8). The households and potential respondent in the household were both randomly selected. When the selected person was <16 years of age, the person in charge of health decisions for the selected child responded to the survey questionnaire, while participants ≥16 years of age answered for themselves. Eligibility criteria were: to be either the main caregiver of at least one child between two months and 15 years of age or between 16 and 20 years of age; and to live or study in Saguenay–Lac-St-Jean at the time of the survey. To participate, respondents had to be able to answer a French questionnaire. The target was to enroll 875 respondents to provide a precision of ±5% for the most conservative variable estimation.

The study was evaluated positively with regard to its methodology by the Ethics Review Board (ERB) of the CHU de Québec, but was exempted from complete evaluation by the ERB due to article 2.5 of the Tri-Council Policy Statement on Ethical Conduct for Research Involving Humans in Canada (9). Before beginning the interview, respondents were informed about the objectives and the sponsors of the survey, and verbal consent was obtained.

Survey instrument
The survey instrument was developed only in French and included questions to measure the respondents' knowledge and attitudes about IMD and the 4CMenB vaccine as well as the respondents' intention to have their child vaccinated (or, for adolescents, to be vaccinated themselves) and main reasons for intending or not intending to receive the 4CMenB vaccine. Most of the questions used a four-point Likert scale ranging from "totally agree" to "totally disagree". Open-ended questions were used to collect reasons for vaccinating or not vaccinating. The survey questionnaire was developed based on questions used in similar studies (10-12). Before initiation of the study, the survey was reviewed by public health practitioners, physicians and nurses involved in the mass campaign for content validity. Questions perceived to be ambiguous were modified or removed. The survey questionnaire was also pretested with 10 respondents and additional clarifications were made in the wording of some questions. Standard sociodemographic variables were collected (for parents: age, level of education as well as age and sex of the child; for adolescents: main occupation, level of education). The survey instrument is available on request.

Data analysis
Expansion weights were assigned to ensure that the results were representative of the target population by adjusting for disproportionate sampling and nonresponse bias. Weighting included a calibration that was applied to each respondent in the sample, based on sociodemographic characteristics drawn from the data contained in the Quebec immunization registry developed specifically for the campaign as well as from census data.

Descriptive statistics were generated for all variables. For each estimate, 95% CIs were calculated. Comparison between respondent groups according to demographic characteristics (age and sex of the child, level of parents' education, etc) were performed using χ^2 or Fisher's exact tests

as appropriate. Beliefs and attitudes about meningococcal B vaccination were analyzed to explore the associated factors with vaccination intention. Percent of agreement was dichotomized in agree (totally agree, somewhat agree) versus disagree (somewhat disagree and totally disagree). A multivariate logistic regression model was used to determine variables independently associated with the adolescent's intention not to be vaccinated with the 4CMenB. Dependent and explanatory variables were dichotomized. The verbatim wording of the open-ended questions was transcribed by the interviewers and submitted to content analysis. Qualitative data were organized into main coded themes and concepts belonging to a similar theme were regrouped. These themes were updated and revised until no new properties, dimensions or relationships emerged during analysis. This content analysis was first performed using Word processing software and then imported into SAS version 9.3 (SAS Institute, USA) when completed. All statistical analyses were performed using SAS version 9.3. All tests were considered to be statistically significant at the threshold of 5% (P<0.05).

RESULTS
The response rate was 72% and 887 interviews were completed (703 interviews with parents of children between two months and 16 years of age and 184 with adolescents ≥16 years of age). More than one-half of parents were between 30 and 39 years of age (54%). Almost two-thirds of parents had a university (32%) or collegial degree (31%). Almost all adolescents were in school. The majority of parents reported that their child had received all recommended vaccines (92%), whereas 66% of adolescents reported this. Less than 1% of parents and adolescents mentioned not receiving any vaccine (Table 1). A higher proportion of parents of children five to 12 years of age reported that their child was fully vaccinated compared with parents of children <5 years of age or >12 years of age.

Overall, most parents (99%) and adolescents (90%) knew that a vaccination campaign against meningitis was launched in their region. Among adolescents, more girls than boys were aware of the campaign (98% versus 83%; P=0.0001). The majority of parents (93%) intended to have their child vaccinated with the 4CMenB vaccine or had already done so (Table 2). A higher proportion of parents of children <5 years of age did not know whether they would have their child vaccinated with the 4CMenB vaccine. Approximately 75% of adolescents also intended to be vaccinated or had received the 4CMenB vaccine (Table 2). A positive association between self-reported complete vaccination status for other recommended vaccines and intention to receive the 4CMenB vaccine (or being already vaccinated) was observed, for both parents and adolescents.

The main reason cited by parents for intending to have or having had their child vaccinated with the 4CMenB vaccine was to protect him/her against meningitis. The desire to be protected against meningitis was also the main reason stated by adolescents who intended to receive or had received the vaccine. General trust in vaccines, the perception that the benefits of the 4CMenB outweighed the risks, and knowing someone who suffered from meningitis were others reasons for vaccination reported by parents and adolescents. In addition, some adolescents indicated ease of access to the 4CMenB vaccine and that it was free as reasons for intending to be or being vaccinated. The most

TABLE 2
Intention to receive the 4CMenB vaccine

	Intend to receive	Do not intend to receive	Vaccinated with 4CMenB vaccine	Do not know
Parents of children:				
2 months to <5 years of age	54.9 (48.98–60.78)	3.4 (1.11–5.72)	34.9 (29.29–40.46)	6.8 (3.63–10.03)
5 years to <12 years of age	90.3 (85.85–94.78)	4.3 (1.18–7.38)	4.5 (1.32–7.69)	0.9 (0.00–2.15)
12 years to <16 years of age	91.8 (87.56–96.13)	1.5 (0.00–3.09)	2.1 (0.00–4.26)	4.5 (1.07–7.99)
Total (parents)	79.5 (76.42–82.67)	3.3 (1.74–4.90)	13.5 (10.96–15.97)	3.7 (2.22–5.11)
Adolescents	50.7 (42.50–58.97)	22.1 (15.12–29.00)	22.4 (15.64–29.21)	4.8 (1.23–8.33)

Data presented as % (95% CI)

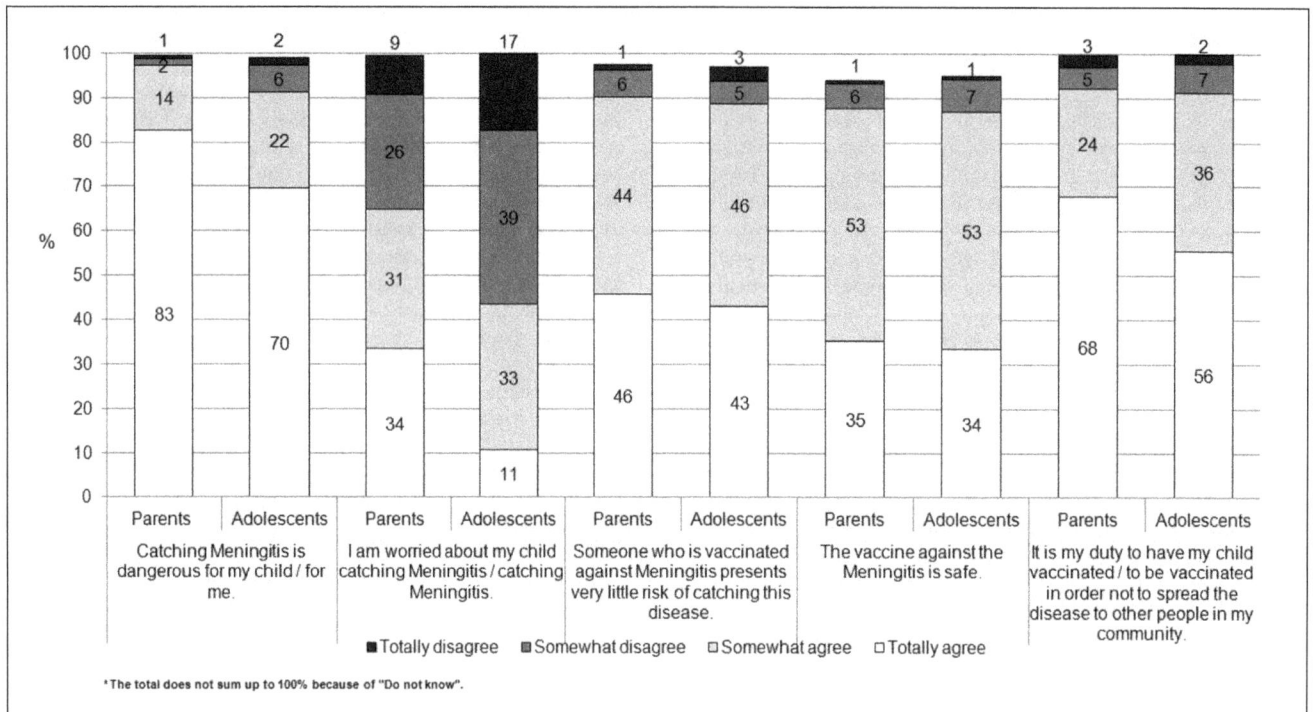

Figure 1) *Parents' and adolescents' knowledge, attitudes and beliefs regarding invasive meningococcal disease and the 4CMenB vaccine**

frequent reason mentioned by parents who did not intend to have their child vaccinated was opposition to vaccination in general. For adolescents, lack of interest, time or information about the vaccine and low perceived susceptibility to infection and perceived low disease severity were the main reasons cited by adolescents who did not intend to be vaccinated.

The results of questions assessing respondents' knowledge, beliefs and attitudes regarding IMD and the 4CMenB vaccine are illustrated in Figure 1. Generally, the majority of respondents considered IMD to be a severe disease and were worried about their own or their child's susceptibility to it. Most respondents also perceived 4CMenB vaccine to be safe and effective. Five percent of adolescents and 6% of parents answered "I don't know" to the question about the vaccine's safety. More than 90% of respondents also considered that it was their duty to receive the vaccine or to vaccinate their child to prevent the transmission of meningitis to others in their community.

Parents who were less educated (high school diploma or less) were more worried that their child could contract meningitis when compared with parents with a college or university degree (78%, 62% and 57%, respectively, P<0.0001). In addition, among adolescents, more girls than boys were worried about the risk of contracting meningitis (57% versus 29%, P=0.0002).

Because almost all parents intended to have or had their child vaccinated, it was not possible to perform multivariate analyses. However,

a multivariate regression analysis was performed to identify the factors associated with adolescents' intention not to be vaccinated. The results of this multivariate analysis are presented in Table 3. Not being aware of the vaccination campaign, believing that the 4CMenB was not safe and not believing that it was a duty to be vaccinated to prevent the spread of infection in the community were associated with the intention not to be vaccinated with the 4CMenB vaccine.

DISCUSSION

Results of the first phase of our study indicated that the majority of respondents were aware of the mass vaccination campaign against meningococcal serogroup B disease that was going on in Saguenay–Lac-St-Jean. This is not surprising given that the survey was conducted two weeks after the official announcement of the campaign, which was highly publicized in local media (13-16).

Our results illustrated a high willingness to receive the new 4CMenB in the context of a targeted mass campaign. More than nine of 10 parents indicated an intention to have their child vaccinated or had already done so. Almost three of four adolescents surveyed indicated an intention to receive the vaccine or had received it. As in other studies, our results indicate a strong association between having received all recommended vaccines and intending to receive the new vaccine (17,18).

Our results mirror findings from prelicensure trials that showed a high level of acceptability for the vaccine (17-26). Because it can

TABLE 3
Factors associated with adolescents' intention not to receive the 4CMenB vaccine

	Adjusted OR*	95% CI	P
Have you heard about a vaccination campaign against meningitis that is ongoing in your region? *(No)*	18.45	4.79–71.13	<0.0001
Catching meningitis is dangerous for me *(Disagree)*	1.72	0.35–8.45	0.5045
I am worried about catching meningitis *(Disagree)*	2.91	0.95–8.92	0.0617
Someone who is vaccinated against meningitis presents very little risk of catching this disease *(Disagree)*	1.20	0.16–8.90	0.8561
The vaccine against meningitis is safe *(Disagree)*	25.17	5.13–123.46	<0.0001
It is my duty to be vaccinated in order not to spread the disease to other people in my community *(Disagree)*	9.41	2.11–42.09	0.0033

Adjusted OR with all items in the model.

arise in an unpredictable manner, develop rapidly and lead to serious consequences, meningitis has characteristics that increase the population's perception of risk (27). Meningitis was perceived as being a dangerous disease by the majority of parents and adolescents surveyed. The death due to serogroup B meningitis of a 16-year-old adolescent living in Saguenay–Lac-St-Jean in spring 2014, before the launch of the campaign, was covered extensively by the media and has probably contributed to the perceived risk of the disease in the public (28-30). In fact, approximately two-thirds of parents reported that they were worried about the risk for their child contracting the disease. Although adolescents between 15 and 20 years of age have high rates of IMD (31), fewer adolescents were concerned about their own risk for contracting meningitis.

Different studies have shown that new vaccines are likely to engender doubts and concerns (17,32,33). For instance, in a recent pan-Canadian survey, one-half of the parents were concerned that new vaccines are not as safe as older vaccines, and one-third believed that children today receive too many vaccines (34). The fact that the 4CMenB vaccine is new did not have an important influence on its acceptability by parents and adolescents in our study. A minority of respondents have cited the novelty of the vaccine as a reason for not intending to be vaccinated. In the particular context of an endemic situation, the perceived threat of the disease may outweigh the perceived risks associated with new vaccines (35,36).

Clinical trials showed the 4CMenB vaccine to be more reactogenic than vaccines routinely used in Quebec, which we hypothesized could have a negative impact on its acceptability (37,38). We anticipated that (real or perceived) side effects after the first dose, such as pain and fever, could compromise the acceptability of the subsequent doses and even have a negative impact on the acceptability of other routine vaccines (39-42). For instance, the results of one study on vaccination against seasonal influenza highlighted the reduced acceptability of a second dose of the vaccine on the basis of the severity of side effects perceived by parents after the first dose (39). The second phase of our study will provide additional information on this issue.

The present study had both strengths and limitations. The response rate of 72% is well above rates typically obtained with telephone surveys (43,44). Other strengths of the present study were the use of random-digit dialling methodology for data collection and the use of case-weights to adjust for disproportionate sampling and non-response bias. However, similar to most surveys, we cannot exclude the potential of socially desirable responses, which is the tendency of respondents to reply in a manner that will be viewed favourably by others. The survey was conducted only in French; however, <1% of the contacted households did not participate due to a language barrier. We used a telephone survey, which resulted in a recruitment bias toward more educated individuals and against the young and new residents of a community with no household telephone number (43). However, it is known that in Quebec most families with young children are residents of the same community for several years and most of them have a household telephone number. In 2013, 89% of Quebecers households with children reported using a landline telephone (45). Finally, because of the gap between intention and behaviour (46,47), our findings are limited by the fact that our survey was conducted at the beginning of the campaign. To conclude, the first phase of the present study has indicated high acceptance of the new 4CMenB vaccine at the beginning of the mass campaign in Saguenay–Lac-St-Jean. Intention to receive the vaccine was high, as was perceived severity and susceptibility of the disease. The second phase of the study, which will be conducted in March and April 2015, after the end of the campaign, will provide additional information on the determinants of acceptance of the vaccine. It will then be possible to describe the determinants for having received one, all or none of the recommended doses of the 4CMenB vaccine. We will also be able to assess the potential impact of adverse events after the first dose (real or perceived) on the acceptability of the subsequent doses and of other scheduled vaccines.

ACKNOWLEDGEMENTS: This study was financially supported by Quebec Ministry of Health. The authors thank Zhou Zhou and Laurie Costa, CHU de Québec Research Center, for their assistance with data analysis.

REFERENCES
1. Sadarangani M, Scheifele DW, Halperin SA, et al. The impact of the meningococcal serogroup C conjugate vaccine in Canada between 2002 and 2012. Clin Infect Dis 2014;59:1208-15.
2. Bettinger JA, Scheifele DW, Halperin SA, et al. Evaluation of meningococcal serogroup C conjugate vaccine programs in Canadian children: Interim analysis. Vaccine 2012;30:4023-7.
3. Halperin SA, Bettinger JA, Greenwood B, et al. The changing and dynamic epidemiology of meningococcal disease. Vaccine 2012;30(Suppl 2):B26-36.
4. De Wals P. Analysis of mortality following a mass immunization campaign with serogroup C meningococcal conjugate vaccine. Vaccine 2009;27:5730.
5. De Wals P, Deceuninck G, Dubé E, et al. Avis sur la pertinence d'une intervention visant à contrôler une incidence élevée d'infections invasives à méningocoque de sérogroupe B dans l'Est du Québec. Québec: Institut national de santé publique du Québec, March 2014.
6. Zhou J, Lefebvre B, Deng S, et al. Invasive serogroup B *Neisseria meningitidis* in Quebec, Canada, 2003-2010: Persistence of the ST-269 clone since it first emerged in 2003. J Clin Microbiol 2012;50:1545-51.
7. Novartis Pharmaceutical Canada Inc. BEXSERO® Multicomponent Meningococcal B Vaccine (recombinant, absorbed). Québec: Novartis Pharmaceutical Canada Inc, December 6, 2013.
8. Brick JM. Random-digit dialing (RDD). In: Lavrakas P, ed. Encyclopedia of Survey Research Methods. Thousand Oaks: SAGE Publications Inc, 2008:676-9.
9. Canadian Institute of Health Research, Natural Sciences and Engineering Research Council of Canada and Social Sciences and Humanities Research Ethics Special Working Committee. Tri-Council Policy Statement: Ethical Conduct for Research Involving Humans. December 2014.
10. Krawczyk A, Knauper B, Gilca V, et al. Parents' decision-making about the human papillomavirus vaccine for their daughters: I. Quantitative results. Hum Vaccin Immunother 2015;11:330-6.
11. Dube E, Bettinger JA, Halperin B, et al. Determinants of parents' decision to vaccinate their children against rotavirus: Results of a longitudinal study. Health Educ Res 2012;27:1069-80.

12. Dube E, De Wals P, Gilca V, et al. New vaccines offering a larger spectrum of protection against acute otitis media: Will parents be willing to have their children immunized? Int J Pediatr Otorhinolaryngol 2009;73:987-91.

13. Thibeault J. Campagne de vaccination massive dans la région. InfoSaguenay. April 23, 2014.

14. La Haye J. La campagne de vaccination contre le méningocoque débutera le 5 mai. Journal L'Étoile du Lac. April 28, 2014.

15. Girard C. Campagne de vaccination contre le méningocoque de type B. Le Courrier du Saguenay. April 22, 2014.

16. Savoie-Soulières M. Vaste campagne de vaccination contre la méningite de type B. Radio Canada. April 22, 2014.

17. Bedford H, Lansley M. More vaccines for children? Parents' views. Vaccine 2007;25:7818-23.

18. Marshall H, Clarke M, Sullivan T. Parental and community acceptance of the benefits and risks associated with meningococcal B vaccines. Vaccine 2013;32:338-44.

19. CBG Health Research Limited. Evaluation of meningococcal B immunisation national roll-out. 2006. <www.health.govt.nz/system/files/documents/publications/menzb-implementation-evaluation-nov06.pdf> (Accessed April 7, 2014).

20. Watson PB, Yarwood J, Chenery K. Meningococcal B: Tell me everything you know and everything you don't know. New Zealanders' decision-making regarding an immunisation programme. N Z Med J 2007;120:U2751.

21. Bland M, Clear GM, Grogan A, Hoare K, Waldock J. Mum's the word: Factors that influenced young adults' participation in the New Zealand Meningococcal B immunisation programme. N Z Med J 2009;122:30-8.

22. Bakhache P, Rodrigo C, Davie S, et al. Health care providers' and parents' attitudes toward administration of new infant vaccines – a multinational survey. Eur J Pediatr 2013;172:485-92.

23. Dubé E, Defay F, Sauvageau C, Lavoie F, Gilca V. Priorités en vaccination chez les professionnels de la santé du Québec. Données non publiées 2010.

24. Cohen R, Levy C, Bechet S, Elbez A, Corrard F. How pediatricians and GP consider the implementation of meningococcal B vaccination in France? Arch Pediatr 2012;19:1379-85.

25. Fisher W, Bettinger J, Gilca V, et al. Understanding parental acceptance of a novel meningococcal serogroup B vaccine for infants. Milan: 31st Annual Meeting of the European Society for Paediatric Infectious Diseases, May 28 to June 1, 2013.

26. Rodrigo C, Bakhache P, Rose M, et al. Parental awareness and knowledge about invasive meningococcal disease: Results of a multinational survey. 30th Annual Meeting of the European Society For Paediatric Infectious Diseases; May 8 to 12; Thessaloniki, Greece, 2012.

27. Slovic P. Perception of risk. Science 1987;236:280-5.

28. Lavoie S. Un ado de 16 ans succombe à la méningite. TVA Nouvelles. February 24, 2014.

29. Bégin S. Terassé par la méningite. La Presse. February 24, 2014.

30. Radio Canada. Cas mortel de méningite. Radio Canada. February 23, 2014.

31. Gilca R, Deceuninck G, Lefebvre B, et al. The changing epidemiology of meningococcal disease in Quebec, Canada, 1991-2011: Potential implications of emergence of new strains. PLoS One 2012;7:e50659.

32. Gust DA, Darling N, Kennedy A, Schwartz B. Parents with doubts about vaccines: Which vaccines and reasons why. Pediatrics 2008;122:718-25.

33. Freed GL, Clark SJ, Butchart AT, Singer DC, Davis MM. Parental vaccine safety concerns in 2009. Pediatrics 2010;125:654-9.

34. Ekos Research Associates Inc. Survey of Parents on Key Issues Related to Immunization. Ottawa: Public Health Agency of Canada, September 2011.

35. Chen RT, DeStefano F, Pless R, et al. Challenges and controversies in immunzation safety. Infect Dis Clin North Am 2001;15:21-39.

36. Chen RT, Rastogi SC, Mullen JR, et al. The Vaccine Adverse Event Reporting System (VAERS). Vaccine 1994;12:542-50.

37. Robinson JL. La vaccination contre le méningocoque du sérogroupe B : ce que le praticien doit savoir. Paediatr Child Health 2014;19:95-8.

38. European Medicines Agency. European public assessment report for Bexsero. <ema.europa.eu/Find_medicine/Human Medicines/European public assessment reports> (Accessed April 12, 2013).

39. Broos N, van Puijenbroek EP, van Grootheest K. Fever following immunization with influenza A(H1N1) vaccine in children. Drug Saf 2010;33:1109-15.

40. Mak DB, Carcione D, Joyce S, Tomlin S, Effler PV. Paediatric influenza vaccination program suspension: Effect on childhood vaccine uptake. Aust N Z J Public Health 2012;36:494-5.

41. Parrella A, Gold M, Marshall H, et al. Parental views on vaccine safety and future vaccinations of children who experiences an adverse event following routine of seasonal influenza vaccination in 2010. Hum Vaccin Immunother 2012;8:662-7.

42. Flood EM, Ryan KJ, Rousculp MD, et al. Parent preferences for pediatric influenza vaccine attributes. Clin Pediatr (Phila) 2011;50:338-47.

43. Dillman DA, Smyth JD, Christian LM, eds. Internet, mail, and mixed-mode surveys – The tailored design method, 3rd edn. Hoboken: John Wiley & Sons, 2009.

44. Environics Research Group. Canadian Adult National Immunization Coverage (NICS) Survey – 2010 – Québec. Ottawa: ministère de la Santé et des Services sociaux du Québec, February 2011.

45. CEFRIO. NETendances 2013 – Les modes de communication au Québec à travers les génération. 2013.

46. Webb TL, Sheeran P. Does changing behavioral intentions engender behavior change? A meta-analysis of the experimental evidence. Psychol Bull 2006;132:249-68.

47. Sheeran P. Intention-behavior relations: A conceptual and empirical review. Eur Rev Soc Psychol 2002;12:1-36.

22

Preventing ophthalmia neonatorum

Dorothy L Moore, Noni E MacDonald; Canadian Paediatric Society, Infectious Diseases and Immunization Committee

DL Mooore, NE MacDonald; Canadian Paediatric Society, Infectious Diseases and Immunization Committee. Preventing ophthalmia neonatorum. Paediatr Child Health 2015;20(2):93-96.

The use of silver nitrate as prophylaxis for neonatal ophthalmia was instituted in the late 1800s to prevent the devastating effects of neonatal ocular infection with *Neisseria gonorrhoeae*. At that time – during the preantibiotic era – many countries made such prophylaxis mandatory by law. Today, neonatal gonococcal ophthalmia is rare in Canada, but ocular prophylaxis for this condition remains mandatory in some provinces/territories. Silver nitrate drops are no longer available and erythromycin, the only ophthalmic antibiotic eye ointment currently available for use in newborns, is of questionable efficacy. Ocular prophylaxis is not effective in preventing chlamydial conjunctivitis. Applying medication to the eyes of newborns may result in mild eye irritation and has been perceived by some parents as interfering with mother-infant bonding. Physicians caring for newborns should advocate for rescinding mandatory ocular prophylaxis laws. More effective means of preventing ophthalmia neonatorum include screening all pregnant women for gonorrhea and chlamydia infection, and treatment and follow-up of those found to be infected. Mothers who were not screened should be tested at delivery. Infants of mothers with untreated gonococcal infection at delivery should receive ceftriaxone. Infants exposed to chlamydia at delivery should be followed closely for signs of infection.

Key Words: *Chlamydia; Gonococcus; Neonatal ophthalmia; Prophylaxis; Screening in pregnancy; STIs*

La prévention de la conjonctivite néonatale

Le nitrate d'argent a commencé à être utilisé en prophylaxie à la fin des années 1800 pour prévenir les effets dévastateurs de l'infection oculaire à *Neisseria gonorrhoeae* du nouveau-né. À cette époque où les antibiotiques n'existaient pas, cette prophylaxie avait force de loi dans de nombreux pays. De nos jours, la conjonctivite gonococcique du nouveau-né est rare au Canada, mais la prophylaxie oculaire demeure obligatoire dans certaines provinces et certains territoires. Les gouttes de nitrate d'argent ne sont plus en marché, tandis que l'efficacité de l'érythromycine, le seul onguent antibiotique actuellement offert pour les nouveau-nés, est douteuse. La prophylaxie oculaire ne prévient pas la conjonctivite à *Chlamydia* avec efficacité. L'application de médicaments dans les yeux des nouveau-nés peut provoquer une irritation oculaire bénigne. Pour certains parents, cette pratique nuit à l'attachement entre la mère et son nourrisson. Les médecins qui s'occupent de nouveau-nés devraient plaider pour la suppression des lois qui obligent la prophylaxie oculaire. Parmi les moyens plus efficaces de prévenir la conjonctivite néonatale, soulignons le dépistage de la gonorrhée et de la *Chlamydia* chez toutes les femmes enceintes et le traitement et le suivi de celles qui sont infectées. Les femmes qui n'ont pas été soumises au dépistage devraient l'être à l'accouchement. Les nourrissons de mères chez qui on décèle, à l'accouchement, une gonococcie non traitée devraient recevoir de la ceftriaxone. Ceux exposés à la *Chlamydia* lors de l'accouchement devraient faire l'objet d'un suivi étroit pour déceler tout signe d'infection.

The present statement replaces a statement on neonatal ophthalmia published in 2002 by the Canadian Paediatric Society's Infectious Diseases and Immunization Committee.(1) This update is indicated because in Canada, the epidemiology and antibiotic susceptibility of *Neisseria gonorrhoeae*, as well as the availability of products for prophylaxis, have all changed, raising concerns about the utility of the previously recommended strategy.

Neonatal ophthalmia, a relatively common illness, is defined as conjunctivitis occurring within the first four weeks of life.(2) Originally, this term only referred to cases caused by *N gonorrhoeae*, but the term currently encompasses any conjunctivitis in this age group. *N gonorrhoeae* now accounts for <1% of reported cases of neonatal ophthalmia in the United States, while that due to *Chlamydia trachomatis* ranges from 2% to 40%. Other bacteria such as *Staphylococcus* species, *Streptococcus* species, *Haemophilus* species and other Gram-negative bacterial species account for 30% to 50% of cases.(2) Much less commonly, neonatal conjunctivitis is caused by viral infections (herpes simplex, adenovirus, enteroviruses). Infectious conjunctivitis must be distinguished from eye discharge secondary to blocked tear ducts and from conjunctivitis due to exposure to chemical or other irritants.

In most instances, neonatal ophthalmia is a mild illness. The exception is ophthalmia due to infection with *N gonorrhoeae*.(2) Without preventive measures, gonococcal ophthalmia occurs in 30% to 50% of infants exposed during delivery(3-5) and may progress quickly to corneal ulceration, perforation of the globe and permanent visual impairment.(6) Infants at increased risk for gonococcal ophthalmia are those whose mothers are at risk for sexually transmitted infections (STIs).(7)

Historically, the purpose of prophylaxis for neonatal ophthalmia was to prevent devastating neonatal eye infection due to *N gonorrhoeae*. Silver nitrate prophylaxis against *N gonorrhoeae* ophthalmia neonatorum, first used by Dr Carl Credé in 1880,(6) was a significant preventive medicine triumph at a time when there was no effective treatment available for gonorrhea. Nevertheless, silver nitrate was not a perfect agent because it caused transient chemical conjunctivitis in 50% to 90% of infants.(8) Also, some parents were concerned that the practice could interfere with mother-infant bonding.(9) Silver nitrate eye drops are no longer available in Canada. Tetracycline and erythromycin ointments have been considered to be acceptable alternatives for preventing gonococcal ophthalmia. (2,10) However, *N gonorrhoeae* strains isolated in Canada in 2012 showed considerable resistance to these agents, with tetracycline at 30% and erythromycin at 23%.(11) Whether this resistance can be overcome by the high local antibiotic levels achieved by topical

Correspondence: Canadian Paediatric Society, 2305 St Laurent Boulevard, Ottawa, Ontario K1G 4J8. E-mail info@cps.ca, website www.cps.ca

application is unknown, and there are no recent studies of the efficacy of ophthalmia prophylaxis with these agents.

In Canada, erythromycin has been the only antibiotic eye ointment available for use in neonates since tetracycline ophthalmic ointment became unavailable. Povidone-iodine has been considered for prophylaxis,(12) but this agent may not be effective(13,14) and has been associated with a 5% rate of chemical conjunctivitis.(15) Gentamicin ointment was used for newborn ocular prophylaxis during a shortage of erythromycin ointment in the United States in 2009, but resulted in reports of severe ocular reactions.(16,17) Other ophthalmic antibiotic preparations have not been evaluated in newborns. Therefore, it is questionable whether universal ocular prophylaxis for neonatal gonococcal ophthalmia remains an effective option in Canada. Of note, universal ocular prophylaxis was abandoned decades ago in several high-income countries including Denmark, Norway, Sweden and the United Kingdom. One study from the United Kingdom showed that this change did not increase the rate of blindness due to gonococcal ophthalmia.(18) However, the Canadian Medical Protective Association established that in 2013, neonatal ocular prophylaxis was required by law in Alberta, British Columbia, Ontario, Prince Edward Island and Quebec. In British Columbia, prophylaxis may be waived if a parent makes a written request. In New Brunswick, the law requiring prophylaxis was repealed in 2009. No current legislation was found for the remaining provinces and territories.(19,20)

Infants born to women with untreated chlamydia infection at delivery have a 50% risk of acquiring chlamydia, a 30% to 50% risk of developing neonatal conjunctivitis and a 10% to 20% risk of developing chlamydia pneumonia.(21) Topical ocular prophylaxis does not prevent transmission from mother to infant, does not reliably prevent neonatal conjunctivitis and does not prevent pneumonia.(10,22-26) Oral erythromycin prophylaxis of infants born to untreated mothers has been used in the past but has not been recommended since the association between erythromycin and pyloric stenosis was recognized.(27) Routine prenatal screening for C trachomatis and treatment of identified infections during pregnancy is the preferred option for preventing neonatal conjunctivitis and other infections in newborns caused by this organism. Close clinical follow-up of exposed infants is recommended.(2,28) The Public Health Agency of Canada recommends testing conjunctival and nasopharyngeal secretions of symptomatic infants and treating those who show positive results.(28)

A recent meta-analysis concluded that evidence from randomized and quasirandomized trials regarding the efficacy of prophylactic agents used to prevent gonococcal and chlamydia conjunctivitis was not of high quality. Moreover, all of the agents reviewed had clinically significant failure rates.(18)

Rates of neonatal ophthalmia caused by N gonorrhoeae and C trachomatis declined significantly in North America through the 1980s due to the decreased prevalence of these infections in the general population, and the institution of routine prenatal screening and treatment of these STIs in pregnancy.(18,19) In the United States in 2002, the rate of neonatal ophthalmia was 8.5 per 100,000 births.(18) National surveillance of neonatal ophthalmia was discontinued in Canada in 2000 because of low incidence.(29) Current rates of infection can be estimated from reported cases of chlamydia and gonorrhea in infants <1 year of age, for whom the average national rate between 2000 and 2011 was six per 100,000 for chlamydia infection and 0.5 per 100,000 for gonorrhea.(30) In Ontario, the combined rate of chlamydia and gonococcal ophthalmia in 2004 was 4.5 per 100,000.(18) There were no reported cases of neonatal gonococcal ophthalmia in Alberta between 2005 and 2013, but rates of chlamydial ophthalmia ranged from 0 to 12.2 per 100,000 per year, with a reported rate of 7.5 per 100,000 in 2013.(31) In areas of the world where prenatal screening and treatment are not available and prevalence of gonococcal infections is high, vision loss from neonatal gonococcal ophthalmia continues to occur and ocular prophylaxis with silver nitrate continues to be an important and cost-effective intervention.(4,32)

If ocular prophylaxis *must* be given to comply with provincial/territorial regulations, 0.5% erythromycin base can be used and may be effective in some cases, depending on the antibiotic sensitivity of circulating strains. Povidone-iodine or gentamicin ointment should not be used because of high rates of adverse topical effects.(2,7) To prevent potential cross-contamination, single-use tubes of erythromycin are used. Before administration, each eyelid is wiped gently with sterile cotton to remove foreign matter and to permit adequate eversion of the lower lid. A line of antibiotic ointment, sufficiently long to cover the entire lower conjunctival area, is placed in each lower conjunctival sac, taking care to prevent injury to the eye or the eyelid from the tip of the tube. The closed eyelids are massaged gently to help spread the ointment. After 1 min, excess ointment is gently wiped from the eyelids and surrounding skin with sterile cotton.

RECOMMENDATIONS

To prevent neonatal ophthalmia caused by N gonorrhoeae and C trachomatis, the Canadian Paediatric Society recommends the following:

Neonatal ocular prophylaxis:

- Neonatal ocular prophylaxis with erythromycin, the only agent currently available in Canada for this purpose, may no longer be useful and, therefore, should not be routinely recommended.
- Paediatricians and other physicians caring for newborns, along with midwives and other health care providers, should become familiar with local legal requirements concerning ocular prophylaxis.
- Paediatricians and other physicians caring for newborns should advocate to rescind ocular prophylaxis regulations in jurisdictions in which this is still legally mandated.
- Jurisdictions in which ocular prophylaxis is still mandated should assess their current rates of neonatal ophthalmia and consider other, more effective preventive strategies, as outlined below.

Screening and treatment of pregnant women:

- All pregnant women should be screened for N gonorrhoeae and C trachomatis infections at the first prenatal visit.
- Those who are infected should be treated during pregnancy, tested after treatment to ensure therapeutic success and tested again in the third trimester or, failing that, at time of delivery. Their partners should also be treated. Women who test negative but are at risk for acquiring infection later in pregnancy should be screened again in the third trimester.(2,7,28,33) Rescreening for N gonorrhoeae, C trachomatis and other STIs should be considered in the third trimester for women who are not in a stable monogamous relationship.
- Processes should be in place to ensure communication between physicians and others caring for a woman during pregnancy, and those who will care for her newborn. Information regarding maternal STI screening, treatment and risk factors is crucial to the well-being of the newborn, and must be available to all health care providers caring for the newborn at and following delivery.
- Pregnant women who were not screened during pregnancy should be screened for N gonorrhoeae and C trachomatis at delivery, using the most rapid tests available.(7,28)

Managing newborns exposed to N gonorrhoeae:

- A system should be established to ensure that all infants born to mothers found to have untreated N gonorrhoeae infection at delivery are treated.
- If the mother's test results are not available at discharge, a plan must be in place to ensure that she can be contacted promptly if the results are positive. The mother must also be advised to watch her infant for eye discharge in the first week of life and told whom to contact immediately if this symptom develops, or if the child is unwell in any way. When there is doubt about maternal compliance with this recommendation and the mother is considered to be at risk for gonococcal infection, administering one dose of ceftriaxone should be considered for the infant before discharge.

- Infants born to women with untreated *N gonorrhoeae* infection at the time of delivery, including those born by Caesarian section,(34) should be tested and treated immediately without waiting for test results.(28)
  - Infants exposed to *N gonorrhoeae* who appear to be *healthy* at birth, both term and preterm, should have a conjunctival culture for *N gonorrhoeae* and receive a single dose of ceftriaxone (50 mg/kg to a maximum of 125 mg) intravenously or intramuscularly. The preferred diluent for intramuscular ceftriaxone is 1% lidocaine without epinephrine (0.45 mL/125 mg). This intervention is both safe and effective. Biliary stasis from ceftriaxone is not considered to be a risk with a single dose. (Ceftriaxone is contraindicated in newborns receiving intravenous calcium. A single dose of cefotaxime [100 mg/kg given intravenously or intramuscularly] is an acceptable alternative.)
  - If the exposed infant is *unwell* in any way, blood and cerebrospinal fluid cultures should also be performed. Infants with established gonococcal disease require additional investigation and therapy in consultation with a specialist in paediatric infectious diseases.(2,7,28)

Managing newborns exposed to C *trachomatis*:

- Infants born either vaginally or by Caesarian section to mothers with an untreated chlamydia infection should be closely monitored for symptoms (eg, conjunctivitis, pneumonitis) and treated if infection occurs.(2,7,28) Routine cultures should not be performed on asymptomatic infants.
- Prophylaxis of exposed newborns is not recommended because of the association of macrolides with pyloric stenosis, but may be considered when infant follow-up cannot be guaranteed.(7,28)

ACKNOWLEDGEMENTS: This statement has been reviewed by the Community Paediatrics and Fetus and Newborn Committees of the Canadian Paediatric Society, as well as by the Public Health Agency of Canada's Canadian STI Guidelines Expert Working Group and representatives from the Society of Obstetricians and Gynaecologists of Canada.

REFERENCES

1. Canadian Paediatric Society, Infectious Diseases and Immunization Committee. Recommendations for the prevention of neonatal ophthalmia. Paediatr Child Health 2002;7(7):480-3.
2. American Academy of Pediatrics. Prevention of neonatal ophthalmia. In: Pickering LK, Baker CJ, Kimberlin DW, Long SS, eds. Red Book: 2012 Report of the Committee on Infectious Diseases, 29th ed. Elk Grove Village, IL. American Academy of Pediatrics, 2012:880-2.
3. Laga M, Plummer FA, Nzanze H, et al. Epidemiology of ophthalmia neonatorum in Kenya. Lancet 1986;2(8516):1145-9.
4. Galega FP, Heymann DL, Nasah BT. Gonococcal ophthalmia neonatorum: The case for prophylaxis in tropical Africa. Bull World Health Organ 1984;62(1):95-8
5. Davidson HH, Hill JH, Eastman NJ. Penicillin in the prophylaxis of ophthalmia neonatorum. J Am Med Assoc 1951;145(14):1052-5.
6. Forbes GB, Forbes GM. Silver nitrate and the eye of the newborn. Credé's contribution to preventive medicine. Am J Dis Child 1971;121(1):1-3.
7. U.S. Centers for Disease Control and Prevention. Sexually transmitted diseases treatment guidelines, 2010. MMWR 2010;59(No. RR-12): www.cdc.gov/std/treatment/2010/default.htm (Accessed November 27, 2014).
8. Nishida H, Risenberg HM. Silver nitrate ophthalmic solution and chemical conjunctivities. Pediatrics 1975;56(3):368-73.
9. Butterheld PM, Emdh RN, Svejda MJ. Does the early application of silver nitrate impair maternal attachment? Pediatrics 1981;67(5):737-8.
10. Laga M, Plummer FA, Piot P, et al. Prophylaxis of gonococcal and chlamydial ophthalmia neonatorum. A comparison of silver nitrate and tetracycline. N Engl J Med 1988;318(11):653-7.
11. Public Health Agency of Canada, National Microbiology Laboratory. National surveillance of antimicrobial susceptibilities of *Neisseria gonorrhoeae*. Annual Summary 2012: http://publications. gc.ca/collections/collection_2014/aspc-phac/HP57-3-2012-eng.pdf (Accessed November 27, 2014).
12. Isenberg SJ, Apt L, Wood M. A controlled trial of povidone-iodine as prophylaxis against ophthalmia neonatorum. N Engl J Med 1995;332(9):562-6.
13. Ali Z, Khadije D, Elahe A, Mohammad M, Fateme Z, Narges Z. Prophylaxis of ophthalmia neonatorum comparison of betadine, erythromycin and no prophylaxis. J Trop Pediatr 2007; 53(6):388-92.
14. Ramirez-Ortiz MA, Rodriguez-Almaraz M, Ochoa-Diazlopez H, Diaz-Prieto P, Rodriguez-Suárez RS. Randomised equivalency trial comparing 2.5% povidone-iodine drops and ophthalmic chloramphenicol for preventing neonatal conjunctivitis in a trachoma endemic area in southern Mexico. Br J Ophthalmol 2007;91(11):1430-4.
15. David M, Rumelt S, Weintraub Z. Efficacy comparison between povidone iodine 2.5% and tretracycline 1% in prevention of ophthalmia neonatorum. Ophthalmology 2011;118(7):1454-8.
16. Binenbaum G, Bruno CJ, Forbes BJ, et al. Periocular ulcerative dermatitis associated with gentamicin ointment prophylaxis in newborns. J Pediatr 2010;156(2):320-1.
17. Nathawad R, Mendez H, Ahmad A, et al. Severe ocular reactions after neonatal ocular prophylaxis with gentamicin ophthalmic ointment. Pediatr Infect Dis J 2011;30(2):175-6.
18. Darling EK, McDonald H. A meta-analysis of the efficacy of ocular prophylactic agents used for the prevention of gonococcal and chlamydial ophthalmia neonatorum. J Midwifery Womens Health 2010;55(4):319-27.
19. Gray J. Executive Director, Canadian Medical Protective Agency. June 2013. Personal communication.
20. Wong T. Director, Professional Guidelines and Public Health Practice Division, Centre for Communicable Diseases and Infection Control, Public Health Agency of Canada. June 2013, Personal communication.
21. Hammerschlag MR. Chlamydial and gonococcal infections in infants and children. Clin Infect Dis 2011;53(Suppl 3):S99-102.
22. Rettig PJ, Patamasucon P, Siegal JD. Postnatal prophylaxis of chlamydial conjunctivitis. JAMA 1981;246(20):2321-2.
23. Bell TA, Sandström KI, Gravett MG, et al. Comparison of ophthalmic silver nitrate solution and erythromycin ointment for prevention of natally acquired *Chlamydia trachomatis*. Sex Transm Dis 1987;14(4):195-200.
24. Chen JY. Prophylaxis of ophthalmia neonatorum: Comparison of silver nitrate, tetracycline, erythromycin and no prophylaxis. Pediatr Infect Dis J 1992;11(12):1026-30.
25. Hammerschlag MR, Cummings C, Roblin PM, Williams TH, Delke I. Efficacy of neonatal ocular prophylaxis for the prevention of chlamydial and gonococcal conjunctivitis. N Engl J Med 1989;320(12):769-72.
26. Black-Payne C, Bocchini JA Jr, Cedotal C. Failure of erythromycin ointment for postnatal ocular prophylaxis of chlamydial conjunctivitis. Pediatr Infect Dis J 1989;8(8):491-5.
27. Rosenman MB, Mahon BE, Downs SM, Kleiman MB. Oral erythromycin prophylaxis vs watchful waiting in caring for newborns exposed to *Chlamydia trachomatis*. Arch Pediatr Adolesc Med 2003;157(6):565-71.
28. Public Health Agency of Canada, Centre for Communicable Diseases and Infection Control. Canadian guidelines on sexually transmitted infections: The evergreen edition. Updated January 2010: www.phac-aspc.gc.ca/std-mts/sti-its/guide-lignesdir-eng.php (Accessed November 27, 2014).
29. Public Health Agency of Canada. Notifiable Diseases On-Line. Gonococcal ophthalmia neonatorum. Number of Reported Cases, Canada, 1990 to 1999: http://dsol-smed.phac-aspc.gc.ca/dsol-smed/ ndis/disease2/gon-eng.php (Accessed November 27, 2014).
30. Public Health Agency of Canada. Notifiable Diseases On-Line: http://dsol-smed.phac-aspc.gc.ca/dsol-smed/ndis/charts.php?c=gb (Accessed November 27, 2014).

31. Alberta Health Services, Centralized STI Services, February 2014, personal communication.

32. Laga M, Meheus A, Piot P. Epidemiology and control of gonococcal ophthalmia neonatorum. Bull World Health Organ 1989;67(5):471-8.

33. Public Health Agency of Canada. Canadian guidelines on sexually transmitted infections. Supplementary statement for recommendations related to the diagnosis, management, and follow-up of pregnant women. March 2014: www.phac-aspc.gc.ca/std-mts/sti-its/cgsti-ldcits/preg-ence-eng.php (Accessed November 27, 2014).

34. Diener B. Cesarean section complicated by gonococcal ophthalmia neonatorum. J Fam Pract 1981;13(5):739-44.

CPS INFECTIOUS DISEASES AND IMMUNIZATION COMMITTEE

Members: *Natalie A Bridger* MD; *Jane C Finlay* MD *(past member)*; *Susanna Martin* MD *(Board Representative)*; *Jane C McDonald* MD; *Heather Onyett* MD; *Joan L Robinson* MD *(Chair)*; *Marina I Salvadori* MD *(past member)*; *Otto G Vanderkooi* MD

Liaisons: *Upton D Allen* MBBS, *Canadian Pediatric AIDS Research Group*; *Michael Brady* MD, *Committee on Infectious Diseases, American Academy of Pediatrics*; *Charles PS Hui* MD, *Committee to Advise on Tropical Medicine and Travel (CATMAT), Public Health Agency of Canada*; *Nicole Le Saux* MD, *Immunization Monitoring Program, ACTive (IMPACT)*; *Dorothy L Moore* MD, *National Advisory Committee on Immunization (NACI)*; *Nancy Scott-Thomas* MD, *College of Family Physicians of Canada*; *John S Spika* MD, *Public Health Agency of Canada*

Consultant: *Noni E MacDonald* MD

Principal authors: *Dorothy L Moore* MD, *Noni E MacDonald* MD

23

Subacute bacterial endocarditis caused by *Cardiobacterium hominis*: A case report

Davie Wong MD[1], Julie Carson MD[2,3], Andrew Johnson MD[4]

D Wong, J Carson, A Johnson. Subacute bacterial endocarditis caused by *Cardiobacterium hominis*: A case report. Can J Infect Dis Med Microbiol 2014;25(1):41-43.

Cardiobacterium hominis, a member of the HACEK group of organisms, is an uncommon but important cause of subacute bacterial endocarditis. First-line therapy is a third-generation cephalosporin due to rare beta-lactamase production. The authors report a case involving endovascular infection due to *C hominis* that initially tested resistant to third-generation cephalosporins using an antibiotic gradient strip susceptibility method (nitrocephin negative), but later proved to be susceptible using broth microdilution reference methods (a 'major' error). There are limited studies to guide susceptibility testing and interpretive breakpoints for *C hominis* in the medical literature, and the present case illustrates some of the issues that may arise when performing susceptibility testing for fastidious organisms in the clinical microbiology laboratory.

Key Words: Cardiobacterium hominis; *Etest*; *Infective endocarditis*

Une endocardite bactérienne subaiguë causée par le *Cardiobacterium hominis* : un rapport de cas

Le *Cardiobacterium hominis*, qui appartient aux organismes du groupe HACEK, est une cause d'endocardite bactérienne subaiguë peu fréquente, mais importante. La céphalosporine de troisième génération en est le traitement de première ligne, en raison d'une rare production de bêta-lactamase. Les auteurs rendent compte d'un cas d'infection endovasculaire à *C hominis* qui a d'abord été considéré comme résistant aux céphalosporines de troisième génération d'après la méthode de susceptibilité par bandelette contenant un gradient d'antibiotique (négative à la nitrocéphine), mais qui s'y est révélé susceptible selon les méthodes de microdilution de référence (une erreur « majeure »). Peu de publications traitent des études pour orienter les tests de susceptibilité et les seuils d'interprétation du *C hominis*, et le présent cas démontre quelques problèmes qui peuvent surgir lors de tests de susceptibilité d'organismes difficiles à isoler au laboratoire de microbiologie clinique.

CASE PRESENTATION

A 47-year-old man was admitted to hospital with worsening malaise, fatigue, drenching night sweats, anorexia and a 15 kg weight loss. Four months previously, he developed dyspnea, orthopnea, exertional chest heaviness and a single episode of hemoptysis, for which he had been empirically treated with two 10-day courses of oral antibiotics (cefuroxime, then clarithromycin). Transient swelling, erythema and tenderness over his shins ensued, followed by numbness of his fingers and the left side of his body. These neurological symptoms had improved, but not resolved, at presentation. A dental procedure (unknown) had been performed 12 months before symptom onset.

On examination, he appeared unwell. His temperature was 36.8°C, heart rate 80 beats/min, blood pressure 95/50 mmHg, respiratory rate 18 breaths/min and oxygen saturation 99% on 3 L nasal prongs. Cardiovascular examination revealed a soft S2, an S3, a grade II/VI aortic systolic ejection murmur and a grade III/VI diastolic decrescendo murmur at the left lower sternal border, without signs of congestive heart failure. Fundoscopic examination revealed changes consistent with hypertension, but did not demonstrate retinal hemorrhages or Roth's spots. Oral hygiene was unremarkable. There was a tender area of induration on the palm of his left hand and the dorsum of his left foot (Figure 1A), but no erythema nodosum. The spleen was palpable.

Abnormal laboratory investigations included a white blood cell count of 14.1×10^9/L (normal values 4×10^9/L to 11×10^9/L), neutrophils 11×10^9/L (normal values 2×10^9/L to 8×10^9/L), a normocytic, normochromic anemia with a hemoglobin level of 117 g/L (normal level 137 g/L to 180 g/L) and elevated inflammatory markers (C-reactive protein level 64 mg/L [normal level 0 mg/L to 8 mg/L] and erythrocyte sedimentation rate 28 mm (normal value 0 mm to 10 mm). Three temporally distinct sets of blood cultures were obtained,

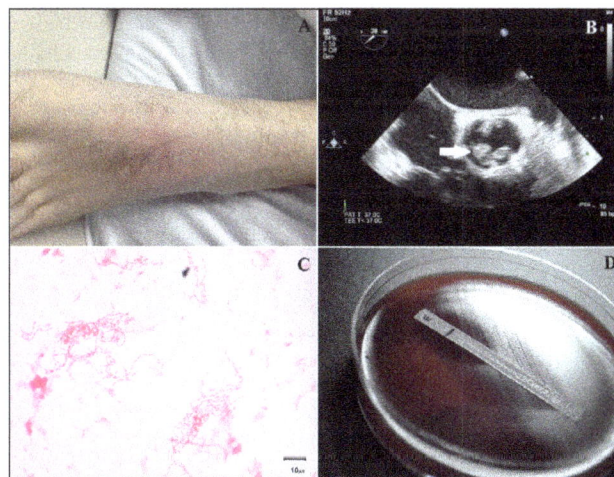

Figure 1) A *Focal area of induration on dorsum of left foot.* **B** *Transesophageal echocardiogram (parasternal short axis view) demonstrating a bicuspid aortic valve with a large vegetation.* **C** *Gram stain of blood culture demonstrating Gram-negative bacilli consistent with Cardiobacterium hominis.* **D** *Etest (bioMérieux Canada, Inc) results for ceftriaxone with a double zone of inhibition at a minimum inhibitory concentration of 0.023 µg/mL and 16 µg/mL. Bacteria within the intermediate zone of inhibition could not be cultured*

and empirical therapy with intravenous vancomycin and ceftriaxone was initiated. Magnetic resonance angiography of the brain and a transesophageal echocardiogram were obtained.

[1]*Internal Medicine, University of Manitoba, Winnipeg, Manitoba;* [2]*Section of Microbiology, Department of Pathology and Laboratory Medicine, University of Calgary;* [3]*Calgary Laboratory Services;* [4]*Section of Infectious Diseases, Department of Medicine, University of Calgary, Calgary, Alberta*

Correspondence: Dr Julie Carson, Calgary Laboratory Services, 9 – 3535 Research Road Northwest, Calgary, Alberta T2L 2K8. e-mail julie.carson@cls.ab.ca

TABLE 1
Summary of minimum inhibitory concentrations for *Cardiobacterium hominis* isolates

Antibiotic	Minimum inhibitory concentration (µg/mL) by method and media			CLSI interpretive criteria (µg/mL)	
	Etest-MHB	Etest-BBA	BMD-CAMHB-LHB*	Sensitive	Resistant
Penicillin	0.5	≤0.016	≤0.06	≤1	≥4
Ampicillin	0.094	0.023	≤0.06	≤1	≥4
Amoxicillin-clavulanate	0.5[†]	0.023[†]	≤0.5/0.25	≤4/2	≥8/4
Imipenem	0.032	0.006	No data	≤0.5	≥2
Meropenem	0.006	≤0.002	≤0.06	≤0.5	≥2
Ceftriaxone	16	0.016	≤0.25	≤2	–
Cefotaxime	32	0.094	≤0.25	≤2	–
Levofloxacin	0.012	0.008	≤0.25	≤2	≥8
Trimethoprim-sulfamethoxazole	0.094[‡]	0.016[†]	≤0.25/4.75	≤0.5/9.5	≥4/76

Clinical Laboratory Standards Institute methodology (CLSI); †Amoxicillin concentration; ‡Trimethoprim concentration. BMD Broth microdilution; BBA Brucella blood agar; CAMHB-LHB Cation-adjusted Mueller-Hinton broth with 5% lysed horse blood; MHB Mueller-Hinton agar with 5% sheep blood

DIAGNOSIS

Transesophageal echocardiogram demonstrated a 1.7 cm vegetation on a previously unrecognized bicuspid aortic valve, with severe aortic insufficiency (Figure 1B). Magnetic resonance angiography of the brain revealed a focus of restricted diffusion in the corpus callosum, concerning for an infarct. By 48 h, all blood cultures yielded a Gram-negative bacillus (oxidase positive, catalase negative and urease negative) identified as *Cardiobacterium hominis* (Figure 1C). The identification was confirmed by matrix-assisted laser desorption ionization time-of-flight (Vitek MS) and the Vitek NH identification card (bioMérieux Canada Inc, Canada). At the time of aortic valve replacement, both native aortic leaflets were markedly thickened and a perivalvular abscess was observed at the aortic valve root, which subsequently grew *C hominis*.

Initial Etest (bioMérieux Canada Inc) results, using Mueller-Hinton agar supplemented with 5% defibrinated sheep blood (MHB), demonstrated resistance to ceftriaxone and cefotaxime (Figure 1D). The nitrocefin-based test (Nitrocefin SR112, Oxoid Microbiology Products, USA) for beta-lactamase production was negative. Subsequently, broth microdilution (BMD) in cation-adjusted Mueller-Hinton broth supplemented with 5% lysed horse blood (CAMHB-LHB) as well as Etest susceptibilities using *Brucella* blood agar (1) demonstrated susceptibility to all agents tested (Table 1).

DISCUSSION

Endovascular infection with *C hominis*, a member of the HACEK group of microorganisms (*Haemophilus* species, *Actinobacillus actinomycetemcomitans*, *Cardiobacterium hominis*, *Eikenella corrodens* and *Kingella* species), is usually insidious in onset, with a prolonged subacute course characterized by leukocytosis, anemia, splenomegaly, embolic phenomena, congestive heart failure and weight loss (2). Dental work (as well as routine oral hygiene/quality of dentition) and bicuspid aortic valve are both well-documented risk factors for developing infective endocarditis due to HACEK microorganisms (2). Our patient typified these characteristics.

Although *C hominis* is of relatively low virulence, endovascular infection complicates 95% of all cases of bacteremia, with the aortic valve being most commonly affected (3,4). Almost one-half of patients require valve replacement. Peripheral and central nervous system emboli occur frequently in *C hominis* endocarditis, noted in 51% and 21% of cases, respectively, especially when the aortic valve is involved (3,5,6). Extravascular infection is unusual (7). Prognosis is generally favourable, with a 93% cure rate for both native and prosthetic valve infection (3). A third-generation cephalosporin is the drug of choice for infection with HACEK organisms (8).

In our patient, initial minimum inhibitory concentration determinations using Etest methodology on MHB agar demonstrated resistance to third-generation cephalosporins (nitrocephin negative). This complicated early management of the patient because it appeared to preclude the use of first-line therapy for *C hominis* endocarditis.

Repeat testing with Clinical and Laboratory Standards Institute (CLSI)-approved reference methods (1) demonstrated susceptibility to third-generation cephalosporins. We were unable to reproduce this 'major' error with other recent *C hominis* isolates (n=5) in our laboratory (data not shown).

Penicillin resistance due to beta-lactamase production has been documented in *C hominis* (9,10), but cephalosporin resistance has only been described in a single case report (9) based on disc diffusion testing. Guidelines for susceptibility testing of fastidious organisms, including the HACEK group, are relatively new (1). For *Cardiobacterium* species, the recommended testing method is BMD in CAMBH-LHB (as for pneumococcus and other fastidious organisms). Although not endorsed by CLSI, many laboratories use Etest or other gradient strip methodologies for ease of use and accessibility. In the present case, use of a non-CLSI-approved antibiotic gradient strip susceptibility testing methodology resulted in a 'major' error. The risk of a 'very major' error cannot be ascertained.

The likely cause of the 'major' error was the use of an antibiotic gradient susceptibility testing method with media (MHB) not adequately validated in microbiological studies. MHB agar has previously been used in agar dilution and Etest methodologies for other HACEK-group organisms (11-13). The Etest application guide recommends using either *Brucella* blood agar or Mueller-Hinton agar with 1% hemoglobin and 1% IsoVitalex (BD, USA) for HACEK organisms (14); however, the cited literature provides no data on the use of Mueller-Hinton agar for susceptibility testing of *C hominis*. Penicillinase or cephalosporinase production appeared to be unlikely based on a negative nitrocefin test. A subpopulation of *C hominis* with isolated resistance to cephalosporins due to specific penicillin-binding protein mutations (as has been described in *Streptococcus pneumoniae* [15]) was also considered to be unlikely given that the intermediate zones did not grow when subcultured to another agar plate and the repeated susceptibility testing using BMD did not show any evidence of resistance.

Returning to the case, the patient received six weeks of intravenous ceftriaxone following his aortic valve replacement, rather than a standard four-week course (8), because of his septic cerebral embolus. Repeat echocardiography demonstrated complete resolution of his perivalvular abscess and a properly functioning prosthetic aortic valve. His neurological symptoms continued to improve, although he still had residual left-sided numbness at three-month follow-up. This case highlights both the typical clinical presentation of endovascular infection with *C hominis* and the potential issues that may arise when performing susceptibility testing for fastidious organisms in the clinical microbiology laboratory.

ACKNOWLEDGEMENTS: The authors thank Dr Johann Pitout for his assistance in this case.

REFERENCES

1. Clinical Laboratory Standards Institute. Methods for Antimicrobial dilution and disk susceptibility testing of infrequently isolated or fastidious bacteria; Approved Guideline – Second Edition. CLSI document M45-A2. Wayne: Clinical and Laboratory Standards Institute, 2010.
2. Steinberg JP, Burd EM. Other Gram-negative and Gram-variable bacilli. In: Mandell GL, Bennett JE, Dolin R, eds. Principles and Practice of Infectious Diseases, 7th edn. Philadelphia: Elsevier, 2010:3019.
3. Malani AN, Aronoff DM, Kauffman CA. *Cardiobacterium hominis* endocarditis: Two cases and a review of the literature. Eur J Clin Microbiol Infect Dis 2006;25:587-95.
4. Chambers ST, Murdoch D, Morris A, et al. HACEK infective endocarditis: Characteristics and outcomes from a large, multi-national cohort. PLoS One 2013;8:e63181.
5. Chentanez T, Khawcharoenporn T, Chokrungvaranon N, et al. *Cardiobacterium hominis* endocarditis presenting as acute embolic stroke: A case report and review of the literature. Heart Lung 2011;40:262-9.
6. Lena TS, De Meulemeester C. A case of infective endocarditis caused by *C. hominis* in a patient with HLAB27 aortitis. Can J Neurol Sci 2009;36:385-7.
7. Wormser GP, Bottone EJ. *Cardiobacterium hominis*: Review of microbiologic and clinical features. Rev Infect Dis 1983;5:680-91.
8. Baddour LM, Wilson WR, Bayer AS, et al. Infective endocarditis: Diagnosis, antimicrobial therapy, and management of complications: A statement for healthcare professionals from the Committee on Rheumatic Fever, Endocarditis, and Kawasaki Disease, Council on Cardiovascular Disease in the Young, and the Councils on Clinical Cardiology, Stroke, and Cardiovascular Surgery and Anesthesia, American Heart Association. Circulation 2005;111:394-434.
9. Le Quellec, Bessis D, Perez C, et al. Endocarditis due to β-lactamase-producing *Cardiobacterium hominis*. Clin Infect Dis 1994;19:994-5.
10. Lu PL, Hsueh PR, Hung CC, et al. Infective endocarditis complicated with progressive heart failure due to β-lactamase-producing *Cardiobacterium hominis*. J Clin Microbiol 2000;38:2015-7.
11. Maurissen W, Eyskens B, Gewillig M, et al. Beta-lactamase-positive *Cardiobacterium hominis* strain causing endocarditis in a pediatric patient with tetralogy of Fallot. Clin Microbiol News 2008;30:132-3.
12. Yagupsky P, Katz O, Peled N. Antibiotic susceptibility of *Kingella kingae* isolates from respiratory carriers and patients with invasive infections. J Antimicrob Chemother 2001;47:191-3.
13. Goldstein EJ, Cherubin CE, M Shulman. Comparison of microtiter broth dilution and agar dilution methods for susceptibility testing of *Eikenella corrodens*. Antimicrob Agents Chemother 1983;23:42-5.
14. Kugler KC, Biedenbach DJ, Jones RN. Determination of the antimicrobial activity of 29 clinically important compounds tested against fastidious HACEK group organisms. Diagn Microbiol Infect Dis 1999;34:73-6.
15. Smith AM, Botha RF, Koornhof HJ, Klugman KP. Emergence of a pneumococcal clone with cephalosporin resistance and penicillin susceptibility. Antimicrob Agents Chemother 2001;45:2648-50.

24

A confirmed case of toxic shock syndrome associated with the use of a menstrual cup

Michael A Mitchell MD[1], Steve Bisch MD[2], Shannon Arntfield MD FRCSC[2],
Seyed M Hosseini-Moghaddam MD MPH FRCPC[1]

MA Mitchell, S Bisch, S Arntfield, SM Hosseini-Moghaddam.
A confirmed case of toxic shock syndrome associated with the
use of a menstrual cup. Can J Infect Dis Med Microbiol
2015;26(4):218-220.

Menstrual cups have been reported to be an acceptable substitute for
tampons. These flexible cups have also been reported to provide a
sustainable solution to menstrual management, with modest cost savings and no significant health risk.

The present article documents the first case of toxic shock syndrome
associated with the use of a menstrual cup in a woman 37 years of age,
using a menstrual cup for the first time. Toxic shock syndrome and the
literature on menstrual cups is reviewed and a possible mechanism for
the development of toxic shock syndrome in the patient is described.

Key Words: *Feminine hygiene products*; *Menstrual cups*; Staphylococcus
aureus; *Toxic shock syndrome*; *Vaginal cups*

Un cas confirmé de syndrome du choc toxique causé par l'utilisation de la coupe menstruelle

Les coupes menstruelles sont considérées comme un substitut acceptable
des tampons. Ces coupes flexibles sont également considérées comme
une solution durable pour gérer les menstruations, entraînant de
modestes économies, sans risque important pour la santé.

Le présent article rend compte du premier cas de syndrome du
choc toxique chez une femme de 37 ans, qui utilisait une coupe men-
struelle pour la première fois. Les chercheurs analysent le syndrome
du choc toxique et les publications sur les coupes menstruelles et
décrivent un mécanisme possible d'apparition du syndrome du choc
toxique chez la patiente.

CASE PRESENTATION

A 37-year-old Caucasian woman presented to the emergency department with a two-day history of fevers, conjunctival hyperemia, abdominal cramps, myalgias, vaginal discharge and diffuse erythroderma
prominent on her upper thorax, inner thighs and perineum. She had
a history of Hashimoto's thyroiditis and chronic menorrhagia.

Ten days before her presentation, she began using The DivaCup
(Diva International Inc, USA), a brand of menstrual cup for menstrual
blood collection (Figure 1). She used appropriate hygiene when hand-
ling and changing the cup, but retrospectively reported causing a small
abrasion during one of her initial insertions. Her subsequent menses
became heavier and longer than normal. By day 7, she noticed an
episode of black vaginal discharge followed two days later by yellow
purulent discharge along with subjective fevers, at which point she
stopped using the menstrual cup. She presented to the emergency
department the following day, after continuing to feel unwell.

On initial examination, she looked unwell and had an oral temperature of 37.2°C, blood pressure of 98/65 mmHg and a heart rate of
132 beats/min. No other obvious source of sepsis was found during
physical examination. Despite receiving aggressive intravenous fluid
resuscitation and antibiotic therapy, including linezolid and piperacillin-
tazobactam, she remained hypotensive for the next 24 h. Vaginal
examination revealed yellow discharge and mild menstrual bleeding,
but no cervical motion tenderness. The menstrual cup was not present
because it had been removed before presenting to hospital. Her blood
and urine cultures, methicillin-resistant *Staphylococcus aureus* screening, *Clostridium difficile* toxin assay and nasopharyngeal swab for respiratory viruses were negative (Table 1).

During the next 24 h, the patient clinically deteriorated; she had a
temperature of 39.1°C, a blood pressure of 76/45 mmHg and a heart
rate of 137 beats/min. She continued to receive aggressive intravenous
fluids and was transferred to a high-acuity observational unit.
Postadmission day 2, the patient developed a generalized morbilliform
rash. The Infectious Diseases services were consulted. Subsequently,
intravenous clindamycin was added to her antibiotic regimen with
probable diagnosis of menstrual toxic shock syndrome (TSS).

Within 24 h of receiving clindamycin, her blood pressure had significantly improved. Desquamation of her skin rash began on postadmission
day 4. The patient remained stable on her antibiotic regimen, ultimately
being discharged in good health eight days postadmission. She remained
stable for the next two weeks, at which point she was seen at the
Infectious Diseases Outpatient Clinic at University Hospital, London
Health Sciences Centre (London, Ontario). Control cultures including
nasal swab for *S aureus* remained negative.

DISCUSSION

Menstrual TSS

The term 'toxic shock syndrome' was first coined in 1978 in a *Lancet*
publication describing the symptom complex in children eight to
17 years of age with an acute febrile illness (1). It did not come to
public attention until 1980, when an association between TSS and
young menstruating women using tampons was discovered (2). Risk
factors included the use of high-absorbency tampons and prolonged,
continual usage (3). Cases occurring in men and nonmenstruating
women were thereafter identified and it was recognized that TSS
can occur in any population. There has been a recently published

[1]Department of Medicine; [2]Department of Obstetrics and Gynecology, Western University, London, Ontario, Canada
Correspondence: Dr Seyed M Hosseini-Moghaddam, Transplant Infectious Diseases, Assistant Professor, Department of Medicine, Western
University, London Health Sciences Centre, B3-420, St. Joseph's Hospital, 268 Grosvenor Street, London, Ontario N6A 4V2.
e-mail seyed.hosseini@lhsc.on.ca

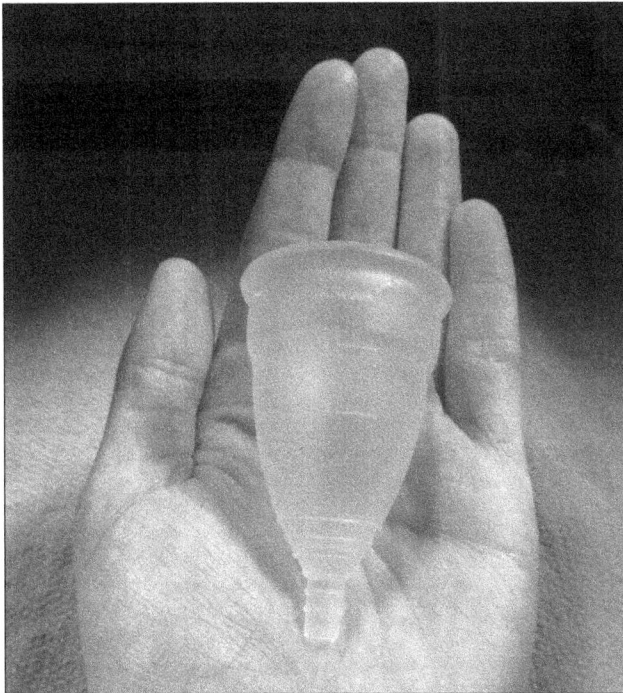

Figure 1) *The DivaCup (Diva International Inc, USA) (a brand of menstrual cup)*

TABLE 1
Laboratory results from initial assessment

Parameter (normal range)	Result
White blood cell count (4.0–10.0×10⁹/L)	23.6×10⁹/L
Hemoglobin (115–160 g/L)	72 g/L
Platelets 1(50–400×10⁹/L)	107×10⁹/L
International normalized ratio (0.9–1.1)	1.8
Fibrinogen (2.0–4.0 g/L)	4.79 g/L
Creatinine (<100 μmol/L)	106 μmol/L
Creatine kinase (<167 U/L)	346 U/L
Blood urea nitrogen (<8.3 mmol/L)	2.8 mmol/L
Alanine aminotransferase (<33 U/L)	52 U/L
Aspartate aminotransferase (<32 U/L)	72 U/L
Total bilirubin (3.4–17.1 μmol/L)	61.3 μmol/L
Potassium (3.5–5.0 mmol/L)	3.0 mmol/L
Magnesium (0.65–1.05 mmol/L)	0.34 mmol/L
Ionized calcium (1.09–1.30 mmol/L)	1.05 mmol/L
Urinalysis	20–30 leukocytes/high power field
Total beta human chorionic gonadotropin	Negative (<1 IU/L)
Blood cultures	Negative ×2
Urine culture	Negative

TABLE 2
Centers for Disease Control and Prevention (Georgia, USA) 2011 case definition for toxic shock syndrome (other than *Streptococcus*) (5)

Clinical criteria

An illness with the following clinical manifestations:

- Fever: temperature ≥102.0°F (≥38.9°C)
- Rash: diffuse macular erythroderma
- Desquamation: one to two weeks after onset of rash
- Hypotension: systolic blood pressure ≤90 mmHg for adults or less than fifth percentile for children <16 years of age

Multisystem involvement (≥3 of the following organ systems):

- Gastrointestinal: vomiting or diarrhea at onset of illness
- Muscular: severe myalgia or creatine phosphokinase level at least twice the upper limit of normal
- Mucous membrane: vaginal, oropharyngeal or conjunctival hyperemia
- Renal: blood urea nitrogen or creatinine at least twice the upper limit of normal for laboratory or urinary sediment with pyuria (≥5 leukocytes per high-power field) in the absence of urinary tract infection
- Hepatic: total bilirubin, alanine aminotransferase enzyme or asparate aminotransferase enzyme levels at least twice the upper limit of normal for laboratory
- Hematological: platelets <100,000/mm³
- Central nervous system: disorientation or alterations in consciousness without focal neurological signs when fever and hypotension are absent

Laboratory criteria for diagnosis

Negative results on the following tests, if obtained:

- Blood or cerebrospinal fluid cultures blood culture may be positive for *Staphylococcus aureus*
- Negative serologies for Rocky Mountain spotted fever, leptospirosis or measles

Case classification

Probable

- A case that meets the laboratory criteria and in which four of the five clinical criteria described above are present

Confirmed

- A case that meets the laboratory criteria and in which all five of the clinical criteria described above are present, including desquamation, unless the patient dies before desquamation occurs

---

report of recurrent TSS in a 15-year-old girl even after she ceased to use tampons (4).

Increased public awareness and change in the composition of tampons to less-absorbent materials led to a substantial decrease in the incidence of menstrual TSS over the next decade (3).

Menstrual TSS is a severe, multisystem, toxin-mediated disease associated with multiorgan failure (Table 2) (5). Considering these criteria, the clinical findings of our patient and her laboratory data fulfill the criteria of a 'confirmed' case.

S aureus TSS toxin 1 (TSST-1) is responsible for multiorgan failure in nearly all (95%) patients with menstrual TSS. (6). This toxin acts as a superantigen, stimulating excessive and nonconventional T cell

activation and, subsequently, cytokine expression (7). Superantigens bypass normal major histocompatibility complex-restricted antigen recognition and activate 30% of host T cells, while conventional antigen presentation activates only approximately 0.01% of the host T cell population (8). Eventually, significant cytokine release causes multiorgan failure. Detection of TSST-1 is not required for the diagnosis of TSS and this test is only available in some research laboratories.

Treatment includes active fluid resuscitation, early use of vasopressors and appropriate antimicrobial therapy. Clindamycin has been demonstrated to reduce the expression of superantigens (9). Theoretically, clindamycin suppresses the protein synthesis and, as a result, more effectively inhibits toxin production compared with vancomycin, which inhibits cell wall synthesis. Linezolid has also been successfully used to treat nonmenstrual TSS and has been shown to decrease TSST-1 production (10). To our knowledge, we report the first case of menstrual TSS that was successfully treated with combination of linezolid and clindamycin. Although rapid clinical improvement has been previously described with the use of linezolid in TSST-1-producing *S aureus*, our patient remained hypotensive while receiving linezolid (10). Her blood pressure significantly improved only after the addition of clindamycin. She did not require intravenous immunoglobulin. Although both clindamycin and linezolid inhibit bacterial protein synthesis and, therefore, toxin production, our patient remained hypotensive until clindamycin was included in her antibiotic regimen. Further experimental and comparative studies are required to determine the inhibitory effects of these two medications against TSST-1.

Menstrual cups

Menstrual cups are a reusable alternative to conventional tampons. Designed to collect rather than absorb menstrual flow, they are made of silicone and worn internally (Figure 1). In a recent multicentre randomized controlled trial by Howard et al (11), the use of tampons was compared with The DivaCup in a total of 110 women. The results demonstrated that overall satisfaction was higher among users of The DivaCup, with 91% of users stating they would continue using it. The present case report identified increased vaginal irritation with The DivaCup compared with tampons, but was not powered to detect a difference in infectious complications (11).

Tierno (12) explained the probable reasons for the association between hyperabsorbable tampons and TSS as follows:

1. Accumulation of blood in the polyester foam cubes and chips of carboxymethylcellulose.
2. Increase of vaginal pH in menstruation from 4.2 to around 7.4.
3. Existence of both oxygen and carbon dioxide in the vagina during menstruation.

These three main factors provide a condition for S aureus growth. In a narrative review, Vostral (13), concluded that the gelled carboxymethylcellulose, in essence, acted like agar in a petri dish, providing a medium on which the bacteria may grow. Menstrual cups are made of silicone or rubber, and carboxymethylcellulose is not used in their structure. Silicone itself does not support microbiological growth. However, because of accumulation of blood, menstrual cups appear to provide a medium for bacterial growth with the same three conditions mentioned above. Menstrual blood in the uterine environment is sufficient to promote the growth of S aureus in the lower genital tract. As such, the menstrual cup appears to provide a necessary milieu for S aureus growth during menstruation. Our patient began using the menstrual cup approximately 10 days before presentation. This duration appears to be sufficient for S aureus growth. High placement of a previously handled cup, an abundant volume of menstrual blood and mucosal irritation within the vagina may be considered as other probable contributing factors.

To our knowledge, the present report is the first to detail the association between a menstrual cup and menstrual TSS. We present here a rare case in a 37-year-old woman who met all six Centers for Disease Control and Prevention (Georgia, USA) criteria (5) for confirmed TSS after wearing a menstrual cup for the first time.

DISCLOSURES: The authors have no financial disclosures or conflicts of interest to declare.

REFERENCES

1. Todd J, Fishaut M, Kapral F, et al. Toxic-shock syndrome associated with phage-group-I Staphylococci. Lancet 1978;2:1116-8.
2. Reingold AL, Hargrett NT, Shands KN, et al. Toxic shock syndrome surveillance in the United States, 1980 to 1981. Ann Intern Med 1982;96:875-80.
3. Reingold AL, Broome CV, Gaventa S, et al. Risk factors for menstrual toxic shock syndrome: Results of a multistate case-control study. Rev Infect Dis 1989;11 Suppl 1:S35-42.
4. Tremlett W, Michie C, Kenol B, et al. Recurrent menstrual toxic shock syndrome with and without tampons in an adolescent. Pediatr Infect Dis J 2014;33:783-5.
5. Centers for Disease Control and Prevention. Toxic shock syndrome (other than Streptococcal) (TSS) 2011 Case Definition. <www.cdc.gov/nndss/script/casedef.aspx?CondYrID=869&DateP ub=1/1/2011%2012:00:00%20AM > (Accessed December 1, 2014).
6. Parsonnet J, Hansmann MA, Delaney ML, et al. Prevalence of toxic shock syndrome toxin 1-producing Staphylococcus aureus and the presence of antibodies to this superantigen in menstruating women. J Clin Microbiol 2005;43:4628-34.

7. Lappin E, Ferguson AJ. Gram-positive toxic shock syndromes. Lancet Infect Dis 2009;9:281-90.
8. Llewelyn M, Cohen J. Superantigens: Microbial agents that corrupt immunity. Lancet Infect Dis 2002;2:156-62.
9. Sriskandan S, McKee A, Hall L, et al. Comparative effects of clindamycin and ampicillin on superantigenic activity of Streptococcus pyogenes. J Antimicrob Chemother 1997;40:275-7.
10. Stevens DL, Wallace RJ, Hamilton SM, et al. Successful treatment of staphylococcal toxic shock syndrome with linezolid: A case report and in vitro evaluation of the production of toxic shock syndrome toxin type 1 in the presence of antibiotics. Clin Infect Dis 2006;42:729-30.
11. Howard C, Rose CL, Trouton K, et al. FLOW (finding lasting options for women): Multicentre randomized controlled trial comparing tampons with menstrual cups. Can Fam Physician 2011;57:208-15.
12. Tierno P. The secret life of germs: Observations and lessons from a microbe hunter. New York: Pocket Books, 2004:79-80.
13. Vostral SL. Rely and Toxic Shock Syndrome: A technological health crisis. Yale J Biol Med 2011;84:447-59.

25

Bacterial communities in neonatal feces are similar to mothers' placentae

Xu-Dong Dong PhD[1,2,3]*, Xiao-Ran Li PhD[2]*, Jian-Jun Luan MM[2], Xiao-Feng Liu MS[2], Juan Peng MS[3], Yi-Yong Luo PhD[2], Chen-Jian Liu PhD[2]

X-D Dong, X-R Li, J-J Luan, et al. Bacterial communities in neonatal feces are similar to mothers' placentae. Can J Infect Dis Med Microbiol 2015;26(2):90-94.

BACKGROUND: The gut microbiota plays an important role in human health. It is essential to understand how the composition of the gut microbiota in neonates is established.
OBJECTIVES: To investigate the nature of the microbial community in the first feces of newborn infants compared with the mothers' placentae and vaginas.
METHODS: One infant who was delivered via Cesarean section was compared with an infant who was delivered vaginally. Bar-coded pyrosequencing of 16S ribosomal RNA genes was used to investigate the bacterial community composition and structure of each site.
RESULTS: Neonatal feces of both infants had similar bacterial communities, and they were similar to the mother's placenta regardless of the method of delivery. The vaginal bacterial community differed between the two mothers, but not different sites within the vagina. The bacteria in the neonatal feces and the mothers' placentae demonstrated considerably higher diversity compared with the vaginas. The family *Lactobacillaceae* dominated in the vaginal samples, while the most abundant family in the fecal and placental samples was *Micrococcineae*.
CONCLUSIONS: These results may provide new directions for the study of infant gut microbial formation.

Key Words: *Bacterial community; Neonates' feces; Placenta; Vagina*

Les communautés bactériennes des fèces néonatales similaires à celles du placenta de la mère

HISTORIQUE : Le microbiote intestinal joue un rôle important dans la santé humaine. Il est essentiel de comprendre comment il s'établit chez les nouveau-nés.
OBJECTIFS : Examiner la structure et la composition de la communauté microbienne des premières fèces des nouveau-nés par rapport à celles du placenta et du vagin de la mère.
MÉTHODOLOGIE : Les chercheurs ont comparé un nourrisson né par césarienne à un nourrisson né par voie vaginale. Ils ont utilisé le pyroséquençage à code-barres des gènes d'ARN ribosomique 16S pour examiner la composition et la structure de la communauté bactérienne de chaque foyer.
RÉSULTATS : Les fèces des nouveau-nés contenaient des communautés bactériennes similaires, qui étaient également similaires à celles du placenta de la mère, quel que soit le mode d'accouchement. La communauté bactérienne vaginale n'était pas la même chez les deux mères, mais étaient similaires dans les différents foyers du vagin. Les bactéries contenues dans les fèces néonatales et le placenta de la mère ont démontré une beaucoup plus grande diversité que celles des vagins. La famille de *Lactobacillaceae* dominait dans les échantillons vaginaux, tandis que la famille des *Micrococcineae* était plus abondante dans les échantillons fécaux et placentaires.
CONCLUSIONS : Ces résultats fournissent de nouvelles voies pour étudier la formation de la flore microbienne intestinale du nourrisson.

The gut microbiota harbours a vast array of microbes and provides important metabolic capabilities (1-4). Thus, it is important to understand how the composition of the gut microbiota in neonates is established. Bifidobacteria and lactobacilli are considered to be the most important health-beneficial bacteria for the human host, whereas bacteria such as staphylococci and clostridia are potential pathogens (5,6).

For a long time, the healthy human fetus was believed to develop in a bacteria-free environment, and the presence of bacteria was considered to be a serious threat to the growing fetus; however, this is no longer considered to be correct. The presence of bacteria may lead to inflammation, but there are some bacteria whose presence does not appear to harm the developing fetus (7). Bacterial infection is a frequent cause of preterm labour, and neonatal sepsis was believed to be caused by infections that that originate during pregnancy or perinatally (8,9). However, it has now become apparent that bacteria are quite often present in the placenta in normal pregnancies. In one study that examined 195 placentas, intracellular bacteria were detected in the placental basal plate in 27%; bacteria were present in placentas from preterm as well as from full-term gestations (10). Neonates are exposed to a wide variety of microbes, which are mostly provided by the mother during

and after the passage through the birth canal (11). Today, many human infants are not exposed to vaginal microbes at birth because they are delivered by Cesarean section. In previous studies, researchers focused on the effects of these delivery methods. Gronlund et al (12) demonstrated that the establishment of primary gut flora in infants born by Cesarean section was delayed. Furthermore, as supported by other studies, the infant gut microbiota largely reflects the delivery modes (5,11,13). In another study, Dominguez-Bello et al (11) found that neonates harboured bacterial communities that were undifferentiated across multiple body habitats, regardless of the method of delivery; these results also showed that the mother's vaginal and skin surface microbiota affected neonatal gut bacterial communities. At the same time, Trosvik et al (4) described the infant gut ecological dynamic using a combination of nonlinear data modelling and simulations of the early infant gut colonization processes, and confirmed that different delivery modes did not affect the phylum composition in the infant gut. These studies focused on the bacterial communities of the mother's vagina or skin.

The aim of the present study was to investigate whether the microbial communities of the first feces of neonates were similar to the mothers' vaginal or placental communities. Samples were taken from two sites in

*Xu-Dong Dong and Xiao-Ran Li contributed equally to this work
[1]Faculty of Environmental Science and Engineering; [2]Faculty of Life Science and Technology, Kunming University of Science and Technology, Chenggong; [3]Department of Obstetrics, First People Hospital of Yunnan Province, Kunming, Yunnan, China
Correspondence: Chen-Jian Liu, Faculty of Life Science and Technology, Kunming University of Science and Technology, Chenggong, Kunming 650500, Yunnan, China.e-mail newstaar8@hotmail.com

TABLE 1
Analysis of operational taxonomic units (OTUs) in eight samples

Sample	Sequences, n	Average sequence length, bp	OTUs, n, 97% (99%)	Singletons	Coverage, %	ACE, n, 97% (99%)	Chao1, n, 97% (99%)
Mother 1*							
Vagina side	405	558	12 (55)	6	99	20 (1673)	16 (619)
Vagina posterior	557	551	10 (75)	6	99	37 (700)	18 (336)
Placenta	1001	533	87 (269)	57	94	395 (2287)	187 (1040)
Infant's first feces	296	532	34 (91)	25	92	103(554)	77 (383)
Mother 2[†]							
Vagina side	668	558	39 (130)	24	96	141 (1038)	74 (511)
Vagina posterior	1035	565	49 (185)	32	97	263 (1578)	120 (773)
Placenta	498	532	71 (179)	42	92	211 (1227)	133 (584)
Infant's first feces	507	531	41 (124)	29	94	274 (1101)	99 (464)

*ACE Abundance-based coverage estimator; *Vaginal delivery; [†]Cesarean section delivery*

the mothers' vaginas, as well as from the placentae and the first feces of neonates. The composition and structure of the bacterial communities were analyzed using bar-coded pyrosequencing by amplifying the V3-V6 regions of the bacterial 16S ribosomal RNA (rRNA) gene.

METHODS

Sampling

Specimens were collected one day before childbirth by wiping the posterior and side wall of the vagina with sterile cotton swabs. The placentas were collected after childbirth in delivery room or operating room to ensure sterility. The placenta samples were collected using sterile centrifuge tubes immediately after delivery of the placenta. To avoid the placenta being contaminated by the vagina, samples were collected from the inner surface of the placenta. The first feces of the neonates were also collected in the delivery room using sterile cotton swabs. All samples were immediately stored at −20°C. Sterile cotton swabs in the same environment were also analyzed as negative controls. Both mothers were 29 years of age and neither had experienced bacterial vaginosis during pregnancy. Both mothers and neonates did not receive any antibiotic treatment. Mother 1 delivered vaginally and mother 2 via Cesarean section. Ethics approval was granted by the First People Hospital of Yunnan Province, Yunnan, China.

DNA extraction and purification

Samples were stored at −20°C before DNA extraction. The cotton swabs were used for DNA extraction. Total DNA was extracted from 1 g samples of placenta or feces, or one cotton swab as previously described (14), with minor modifications. Briefly, samples were simultaneously treated with lysozyme (1 mg/mL) and lyticase (0.16 mg/mL). Subsequently, samples were treated with sodium dodecyl sulfate (1%) and cetrimonium bromide (1%). Three liquid nitrogen freeze/thaw cycles were also performed to ensure the homogeneity of lysed cell samples. The concentration of extracted DNA was determined using a spectrophotometer (NanoDrop ND 1000, Thermo Fisher, USA).

Polymerase chain reaction amplification and pyrosequencing

In all polymerase chain reaction (PCR) amplifications, reactions were performed with rTaq MasterMix (TaKaRa, China) with a total volume of 50 μL and approximately 50 ng DNA template. A modified primer set (338F and 907R) was generated according to a metagenomic database (15). All PCR programs consisted of an initial 5 min denaturation at 95°C, followed by 30 cycles of denaturation at 94°C for 1 min, annealing at 53°C for 1 min, extension at 72°C for 1.5 min and a final elongation step of 10 min at 72°C. To obtain similar numbers of sequences from each sample, an equivalent amount of each purified PCR product was mixed for sequencing using the Genome Sequencer FLX System (Roche, Switzerland). Sequences were preprocessed to assess the overall quality, and classified using bar codes and primer sequences. All pyrosequencing samples were extracted using the specified bar code for each sample. Sequences containing 'N' or those <350 bp were excluded.

Classification and phylogenetic analysis

Classification information of all 16S rRNA gene sequences was determined with the Silva v108 database using the mothur program v.1.25.1 (www.mothur.org/wiki/Main_Page). The operational taxonomic units (OTUs) of the 16S rRNA gene sequences were determined using a 3% cut-off. To determine the phylogenetic position of the 16S rRNA genes, sequences were compared with available database sequences via a BLAST search; related sequences were obtained from the National Center for Biotechnology Information nonredundant database. The taxonomic information was further confirmed by the online analysis tool EzTaxon (16). Phylogenetic trees were constructed via MEGA version 4.0 (17) using the neighbour-joining method (18).

Diversity index analysis

Richness and diversity statistics were calculated using the mothur program v.1.25.1, including the abundance-based coverage estimator (ACE) (19,20) and the bias-corrected Chao1 (21). The estimated coverage of the 16S rRNA gene sequences was calculated as:

$$C = (1 - [n_1/N]) \times 100$$

in which n_1 is the number of singleton sequences, and N is the total number of sequences (22).

Community analysis

Microbial community similarity analyses were conducted using the weighted pair group method with arithmetic averages (WPGMA) clustering and principal component analysis (PCA) using the online UNIFRAC program (23), which measures the molecular evolutionary distances of the sequences and is able to compare the relationships among microbial communities.

Nucleotide sequences accession numbers

The sequences were available in the short read archive of the National Center for Biotechnology Information, using the accession number SRA060045.

RESULTS

Analysis of OTU richness

In the eight samples obtained from the two mothers/neonates, a total of 4967 (mean [± SD] sequence numbers 621±268) pyrosequencing samples were used for analysis. The estimated OTU numbers according to ACE and Chao1 were generated to allow for 3% sequence dissimilarities of 16S rRNA gene (Table 1). Based on a 97% cutoff, the numbers of the estimated OTUs ranged from 10 to 87, with an average of 43. The higher OTU numbers appeared in both placental samples. The OTU numbers in four samples from mother 2 were higher than those in mother 1. In all samples, the estimated coverage was >90%. The ACE and Chao1 estimates were calculated to compare the diversities and richness of the bacterial communities. Those indexes showed higher bacterial genotype diversities in fecal and placental samples compared with those recovered in vaginal samples in the present study.

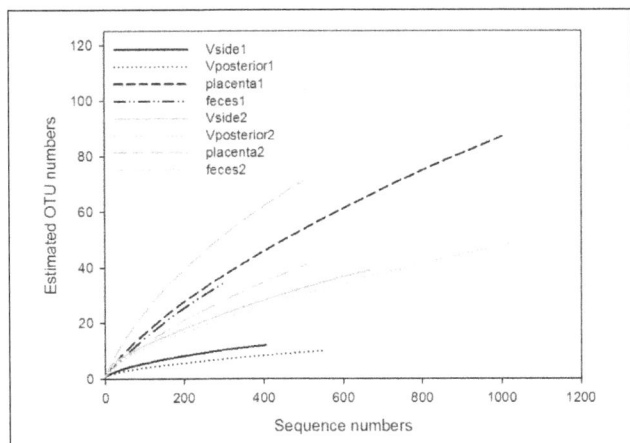

Figure 1) *Rarefaction curves of the pyrosequencing sequences in samples from the mothers and neonates. The phylotypes were determined using a 97% similarity cutoff. OTU Operational taxonomic unit; V Vagina*

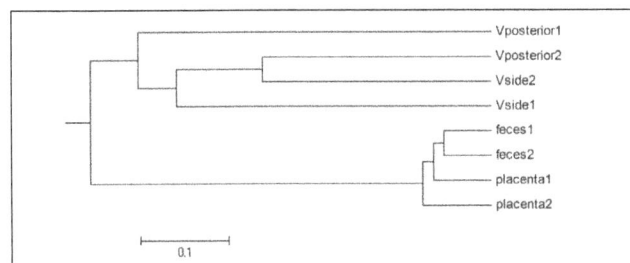

Figure 2) *Weighted pair group method with arithmetic averages (WPGMA) cluster of the samples from the mothers and neonates. V Vagina*

Rarefaction analysis was then performed for each sample (Figure 1). This analysis clearly showed that in both mothers/neonates, placental samples showed the highest diversity, followed by fecal samples.

Comparison of bacterial communities between neonatal first feces and mothers' vaginas and placentae

To investigate the establishment of neonatal gut bacterial communities, the bacterial communities of each mother's vagina and placenta were compared with the first feces of their neonates. The WPGMA tree showed that the bacteria in fecal and placental samples were distinct from those in the vaginal samples (Figure 2). Furthermore, fecal bacteria were more similar between the two infants than with each respective mother's placenta, while bacteria in the vaginal samples showed individual characteristics.

Figure 3 presents the PCA plots of the comparison of bacterial communities. These results clearly confirmed the WPGMA cluster. In the PCA analysis, the bacterial communities in fecal and placental samples were very similar.

Taxonomic identification and phylogenetic analysis

Given the robust evidence that the bacterial community structures of the neonatal gut were similar to the mother's placenta (Figures 1 and 2), the authors sought to identify the bacterial taxa that were contributing to this environment. According to the Silva taxonomic information, a total of eight phyla were detected in the present study, of which only four were detected in vaginal samples. More than 90% of the sequences could be assigned to the family level, and 37 families were observed (Figure 4). The major families in the vaginal samples were completely different from those in the feces and placental samples. In vaginal samples, the majority of 16S rRNA gene sequences belonged to the family *Lactobacillaceae*, followed by *Micrococcineae*. Approximately 1% of the sequences from the vagina of mother 2 were assigned to the family *Bifidobacteriaceae*, which was not detected in mother 1. As in the placental and fecal samples, the

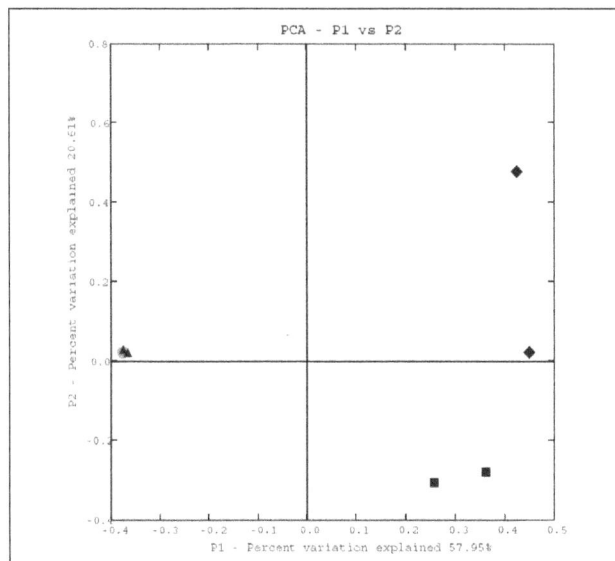

Figure 3) *Principal coordinate analysis (PCA) plots based on UniFrac analysis of bacterial communities. The scatterplots were for the first two principal components. Diamond: vaginal samples from mother 1; square: vaginal samples from mother 2; triangle: fecal and placenta samples from mother/neonate 1; circle: fecal and placenta samples from mother/neonate 2*

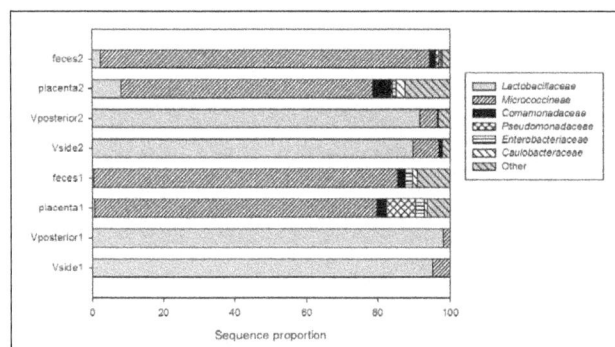

Figure 4) *The sequence proportion of the major families (>1%) in samples from the mothers and neonates. V Vagina*

proportions of the families *Lactobacillaceae* and *Micrococcineae* were opposite to those in vaginal samples. In addition to the families mentioned above, the families *Comamonadaceae*, *Pseudomonadaceae* and *Enterobacteriaceae* were also found in placental and fecal samples.

A total of 343 OTUs from eight samples were identified based on a 3% cut-off. OTUs containing >1% of sequences in each sample were used to construct the phylogenetic tree (Figure 5). In vaginal samples, the most abundant OTUs in the samples from the two mothers were all similar to *Lactobacillus crispatus* (NR_041800), among which >90% of 16S rRNA gene sequences could be assigned to this group (OTUs Vside1_1, 96% and Vbehind1_1, 93%) in the vaginal samples from mother 1. In vaginal samples from mother 2, these proportions were 65% and 70%, respectively. In vaginal samples from mother 2, OTUs (Vside2_3, 8% and Vbehind2_2, 16%) were similar to *Lactobacillus* species detected in human vaginal samples. Twelve percent of sequences could be assigned to the OTU Vside2_2 with a 98% similarity to *Lactobacillus hominis* (FR681902). Placental and fecal samples showed similar bacterial community compositions. The OTUs of placenta1_1 (77%), placenta2_1 (68%), feces1_1 (84%) and feces2_1 (86%) showed more than 97% similarity to one another; these were assigned to *Cellulosimicrobium* species via phylogenetic analysis. Only one OTU, placenta2_3 (6%), was similar to the most abundant OTUs in the vaginal samples. The OTU feces2_3 (2%) was similar to *Lactobacillus*

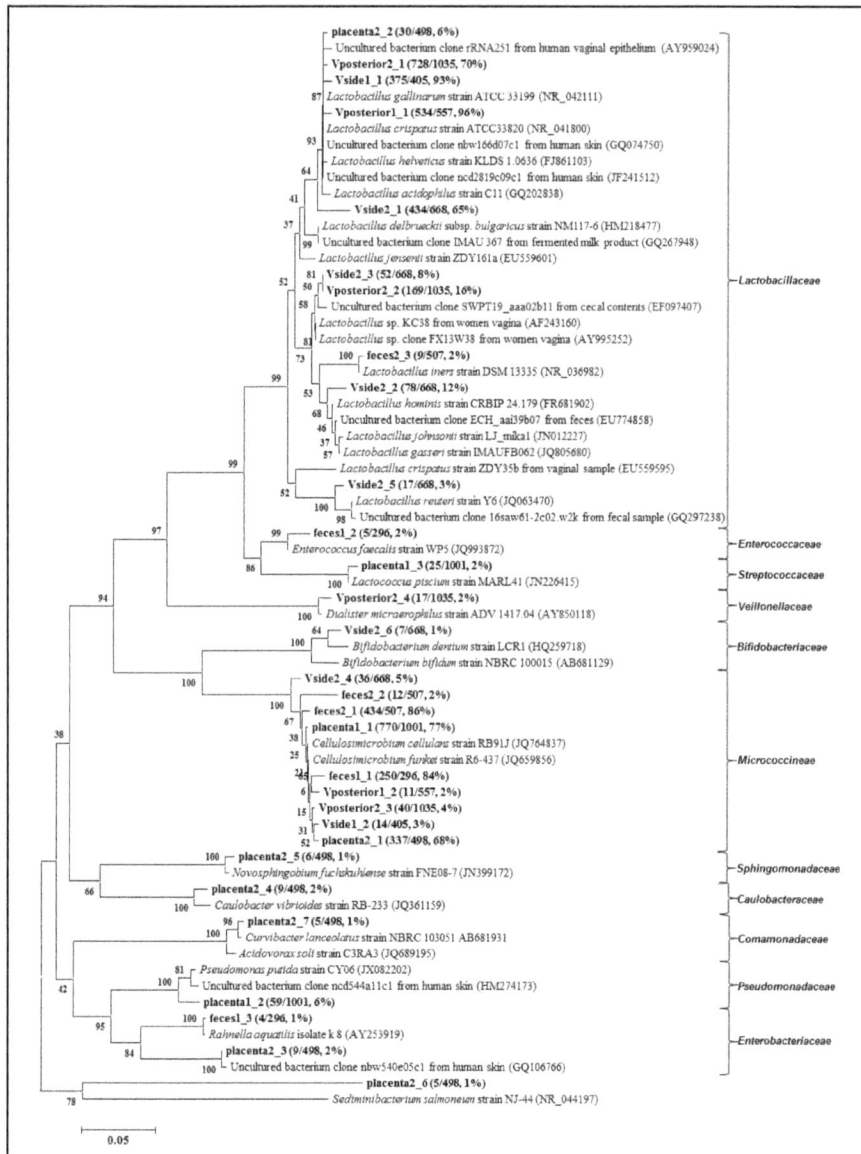

Figure 5) *Phylogenetic tree of the 16S ribosomal RNA gene sequences (>1%) and their phylogenetic relatives. The tree was constructed using the neighbour-joining method. Numbers on nodes indicate bootstrap values (1000 resamplings). The scale bar indicates 0.05 nucleotide substitutions per nucleotide position. The operational taxonomic units obtained in the present study are shown in bold. V Vagina*

iners (NR_036982). All sequences were then classified using the online analysis tool EzTaxon (16). Approximately 3% of the 16S rRNA gene sequences were <97% similar to those of cultured bacteria.

DISCUSSION

The importance of human gastrointestinal microbiota and the establishment of gut microbiota in early infancy has received considerable attention in recent years (3,4,6,12,24,25). It is now known that fetal development does not occur in a sterile environment. Thus, the first bacterial colonization of the fetus may be from the placenta during gestation. A recent study characterized a low-abundance but metabolically rich microbiome composed of nonpathogenic commensal microbiota, which were most similar to the human oral microbiome (26). In this study, 16S rRNA gene-based OTU analyses revealed associations of the placental microbiome with a remote history of antenatal infection, such as urinary tract infection in the first trimester, as well as with preterm birth (26). Many studies have focused on the effects of the delivery modes on the gut microbiota of infants (11,12); the delivery mode was found to have no effect on the formation of infant gut microbiota in many studies (11,13). These studies provided rich information on the formation of the infant gut microbiota, and also confirmed that the developmental environment of the fetus was not sterile. In the present study, an analysis using bar-coded pyrosequencing was conducted to compare the bacterial communities among the first feces of neonates and the placentas and vaginas of the mothers who had given birth through either vaginal delivery or Cesarean section. Similar to previous studies, we found that the environment in which a human fetus develops is not sterile, and the bacterial specimens in the first feces of neonates were similar to the mothers' placentae regardless of the method of delivery. The results provided useful information for further studies investigating the relationship between the neonatal gut microbiota and the mothers' vaginal or placental communities.

Our results also revealed that placental bacterial communities had a higher diversity than vaginal bacterial communities (Figure 1), and the read numbers that were obtained may be sufficient to elucidate all of the bacterial communities in the placentae in the present study, according to the rarefaction curves and coverage. The bacterial communities in the first feces of the neonates also showed higher diversity than those of the vaginas.

The bacterial community composition indicated that the bacteria in the feces may have come from the mothers' placentae. However, the bacterial composition in fecal and placental samples were unlike either of the vaginas (27-29) or infant fecal samples from previous studies (4,12,13,30). The neonatal first feces and mothers' placentae had their own unique bacterial community composition. In vaginal bacterial communities, lactobacilli are recognized as bioindicators in healthy women, and bacterial vaginosis is characterized by a loss of most *Lactobacillus* species (31,32). In the fecal samples in the present study, only 2% of sequences of neonate 2 were classified as *L iners* strain DSM 13335 (NR_036982) (33), which was first isolated from human urine. In addition, 6% of placental sequences from neonate 2 could be assigned to *L crispatus* strain ATCC33820 (NR_041800). Both of these strains were recognized as normal flora in a healthy vagina (27,34). In previous studies investigating the infant fecal bacterial community, the phyla *Firmicutes* and *Bacteroides* were recognized as dominant in the human gut (4,24). However, the majority of fecal and placental bacteria were identified as *Cellulosimicrobium cellulans* or *Cellulosimicrobium funkei* belonging to the phylum *Actinobacteria*, which was considered to have cellulose decomposition capabilities (35) as well as alkaline protease production (36). Human placentae provide nutrition and food to fetuses in utero, and bacterial communities may be one sources of these nutrients. Similar to other vaginal studies (27-29,31,32,34,37), the vaginal bacterial community composition observed in the present study was dominated by *Lactobacillus* species.

Because the results of the present study have further confirmed that the fetal developmental environment is not sterile, we compared the bacterial communities among the first feces of neonates and the mothers' vaginas and placentae to understand the origin of the microbial communities in the first feces of neonates. There were some limitations to the present study. The lower number of samples compared with other studies investigating human vaginal or fecal bacterial communities limited the results of the present study. In future studies, a sufficient number of samples should be analyzed to compare the influencing factors of placental and neonatal fecal bacteria composition and structures. In addition, many studies have shown that even full-length 16S rRNA gene sequences were not suitable to identify sequences at the species level, especially in the family *Lactobacillaceae* (5,38). In the present study, similar results were observed; 16S rRNA gene sequences could be only identified accurately at the genus level. Thus, in future studies, a combination of other molecular markers is necessary to clarify the exact bacterial composition and community succession. However, our results have demonstrated that the family *Lactobacillaceae* is not the dominant bacteria in the first feces of neonates; thus, the role of the family *Micrococcineae* in the neonatal gut should receive more attention in future studies. It would be interesting to confirm whether *Micrococcineae* lead to preterm labour and neonatal sepsis, or are helpful for the reconstruction of neonatal intestinal flora.

REFERENCES

1. Stappenbeck TS, Hooper LV, Gordon JI. Developmental regulation of intestinal angiogenesis by indigenous microbes via Paneth cells. Proc Natl Acad Sci U S A 2002;99:15451-5.
2. Frank DN, Amand ALS, Feldman RA, Boedeker EC, Harpaz N, Pace NR. Molecular-phylogenetic characterization of microbial community imbalances in human inflammatory bowel diseases. Proc Natl Acad Sci U S A 2007;104:13780-5.
3. Li M, Wang B, Zhang M, et al. Symbiotic gut microbes modulate human metabolic phenotypes. Proc Natl Acad Sci U S A 2008;105:2117-22.
4. Trosvik P, Stenseth NC, Rudi K. Convergent temporal dynamics of the human infant gut microbiota. ISME J 2010;4:151-8.
5. Penders J, Thijs C, Vink C, et al. Factors influencing the composition of the intestinal microbiota in early infancy. Pediatrics 2006;118:511-21.
6. Rastall RA. Bacteria in the gut: Friends and foes and how to alter the balance. J Nutr 2004;134:2022S-2026S.
7. Wassenaar TM, Panigrahi P. Is a foetus developing in a sterile environment? Lett Appl Microbiol 2014;59:572-9.
8. Goldenberg RL, Hauth JC, Andrews WW. Intrauterine infection and preterm delivery. N Engl J Med 2000;342:1500-7.
9. Heron M. Deaths: Leading causes for 2010. Natl Vital Stat Rep 2013;62:1-96.
10. Stout MJ, Conlon B, Landeau M, et al. Identification of intracellular bacteria in the basal plate of the human placenta in term and preterm gestations. Am J Obstet Gynecol 2013;208:226.e1-7.
11. Dominguez-Bello MG, Costello EK, Contreras M, et al. Delivery mode shapes the acquisition and structure of the initial microbiota across multiple body habitats in newborns. Proc Natl Acad Sci U S A 2010;107:11971-5.
12. Gronlund MM, Lehtonen OP, Eerola E, Kero P. Fecal microflora in healthy infants born by different methods of delivery: Permanent changes in intestinal flora after cesarean delivery. J Pediatr Gastroenterol Nutr 1999;28:19-25.
13. Favier CF, de Vos WM, Akkermans AD. Development of bacterial and bifidobacterial communities in feces of newborn babies. Anaerobe 2003;9:219-29.
14. Schmidt TM, DeLong EF, Pace NR. Analysis of a marine picoplankton community by 16S rRNA gene cloning and sequencing. J Bacteriol 1991;173:4371-8.
15. Mao D-P, Zhou Q, Chen C-Y, Quan Z-X. Coverage evaluation of universal bacterial primers using the metagenomic datasets. BMC Microbiol 2012;12:66.
16. Chun J, Lee J-H, Jung Y, et al. EzTaxon: A web-based tool for the identification of prokaryotes based on 16S ribosomal RNA gene sequences. Int J Syst Evol Microbiol 2007;57:2259-61.
17. Tamura K, Dudley J, Nei M, Kumar S. MEGA4: Molecular evolutionary genetics analysis (MEGA) software version 4.0. Mol Biol Evol 2007;24:1596-9.
18. Saitou N, Nei M. The neighbor-joining method: A new method for reconstructing phylogenetic trees. Mol Biol Evol 1987;4:406-25.
19. Chao A, Lee SM. Estimating the number of classes via sample coverage. J Am Statist Ass 1992;87:210-7.
20. Chao A, Hwang W-H, Chen Y-C, Kuo C-Y. Estimating the number of shared species in two communities. Stat Sin 2000;10:227-46.
21. Lee SM, Chao A. Estimating population size via sample coverage for closed capture-recapture models. Biometrics 1994;50:88-97.
22. Good IJ. The population frequencies of species and the estimation of population parameters. Biometrika 1953;40:237-64.
23. Lozupone C, Knight R. UniFrac: A new phylogenetic method for comparing microbial communities. Appl Environ Microbiol 2005;71:8228-35.
24. Turnbaugh PJ, Hamady M, Yatsunenko T, et al. A core gut microbiome in obese and lean twins. Nature 2009;457:480-7.
25. Gosalbes MJ, Durbán A, Pignatelli M, et al. Metatranscriptomic approach to analyze the functional human gut microbiota. PLoS ONE 2011;6:e17447.
26. Aagaard K, Ma J, Antony KM, Ganu R, Petrosino J, Versalovic J. The placenta harbors a unique microbiome. Sci Transl Med 2014;6:237ra65
27. Jakobsson T, Forsum U. *Lactobacillus iners*: A marker of changes in the vaginal flora? J Clin Microbiol 2007;45:3145-5.
28. Oakley BB, Fiedler TL, Marrazzo JM, Fredricks DN. Diversity of human vaginal bacterial communities and associations with clinically defined bacterial vaginosis. Appl Environ Microbiol 2008;74:4898-909.
29. Aagaard K, Riehle K, Ma J, et al. A metagenomic approach to characterization of the vaginal microbiome signature in pregnancy. PLoS ONE 2012;7:e36466.
30. Albesharat R, Ehrmann MA, Korakli M, Yazaji S, Vogel RF. Phenotypic and genotypic analyses of lactic acid bacteria in local fermented food, breast milk and faeces of mothers and their babies. Syst Appl Microbiol 2011;34:148-55.
31. Yoshimura K, Morotomi N, Fukuda K, et al. Intravaginal microbial flora by the 16S rRNA gene sequencing. Am J Obstet Gynecol 2011;205:235.e1-9.
32. Srinivasan S, Hoffman NG, Morgan MT, et al. Bacterial communities in women with bacterial vaginosis: High resolution phylogenetic analyses reveal relationships of microbiota to clinical criteria. PLoS One 2012;7:e37818.
33. Falsen E, Pascual C, Sjoden B, Ohlen M, Collins MD. Phenotypic and phylogenetic characterization of a novel *Lactobacillus* species from human sources: Description of *Lactobacillus iners* sp. nov. Int J Food Microbiol 1999;49:217-21.
34. Vasquez A, Jakobsson T, Ahrne S, Forsum U, Molin G. Vaginal *Lactobacillus* flora of healthy Swedish women. J Clin Microbiol 2002;40:2746-9.
35. Huang S, Sheng P, Zhang H. Isolation and identification of cellulolytic bacteria from the gut of *Holotrichia parallela* larvae (Coleoptera: Scarabaeidae). Int J Mol Sci 2012;13:2563-77.
36. Ferracini-Santos L, Sato HH. Production of alkaline protease from *Cellulosimicrobium cellulans*. Braz J Microbiol 2009;40:54-60.
37. Marrazzo, JM. Interpreting the epidemiology and natural history of bacterial vaginosis: Are we still confused? Anaerobe 2011;17:186-90.
38. Li X-R, Ma E-B, Yan L-Z, et al. Bacterial and fungal diversity in the traditional Chinese liquor fermentation process. Int J Food Microbiol 2011;146:31-7.

A case series of third-trimester raltegravir initiation: Impact on maternal HIV-1 viral load and obstetrical outcomes

I Boucoiran MD MSc[1,2], K Tulloch PharmD[1], N Pick MD[3], F Kakkar MD MPH[4,5], J van Schalkwyk MD[1,2], D Money MD[1,2], M Boucher MD[5,6]

I Boucoiran, K Tulloch, N Pick, F Kakkar, J van Schalkwyk, D Money, M Boucher. A case series of third-trimester raltegravir initiation: Impact on maternal HIV-1 viral load and obstetrical outcomes. Can J Infect Dis Med Microbiol 2015;26(3):145-150.

OBJECTIVE: To describe the impact of initiating raltegravir (RAL)-containing combination antiretroviral therapy (cART) regimens on HIV viral load (VL) in pregnant women who have high or suboptimal VL suppression late in pregnancy.

METHODS: HIV-infected pregnant women who started RAL-containing cART after 28 weeks' gestation from 2007 to 2013 were identified in two university hospital centres.

RESULTS AND DISCUSSION: Eleven HIV-infected women started RAL at a median gestational age of 35.7 weeks (range 31.1 to 38.0 weeks). Indications for RAL initiation were late presentation in pregnancy (n=4) and suboptimal VL suppression secondary to poor adherence or viral resistance (n=7). Mean VL at the time of RAL initiation was 73,959 copies/mL (range <40 to 523,975 copies/mL). Patients received RAL for a median of 20 days (range one to 71 days). The mean decline in VL from the time of RAL initiation to delivery was 1.93 log, excluding one patient who received only one RAL dose and one patient with undetectable VL at the time of RAL initiation. After eight days on RAL, 50% of the women achieved a VL <1000 copies/mL (the threshold for recommended Caesarean section to reduce the risk for perinatal transmission). There were no cases of perinatal HIV transmission.

CONCLUSION: The present study provides preliminary data to support the use of RAL-containing cART to expedite HIV-1 VL reduction in women who have a high VL or suboptimal VL suppression late in pregnancy, and to decrease the risk of HIV perinatal transmission while avoiding Caesarean section. Further assessment of RAL safety during pregnancy is warranted.

Key Words: *HIV-1; Integrase inhibitor; Pregnancy; Raltegravir; Viral load*

Une série de cas sur l'initiation du raltégravir au troisième trimestre : les répercussions de la charge virale du VIH-1 et les résultats obstétricaux

OBJECTIF : Décrire les répercussions de l'amorce d'une antirétrovirothérapie prophylactique associative (ARPA) contenant du raltégravir (RAL) sur la charge virale (CV) du VIH chez les femmes enceintes dont la suppression de la CV est élevée ou sous-optimale en fin de grossesse.

MÉTHODOLOGIE : Les chercheurs ont extrait le dossier des femmes enceintes infectées par le VIH qui avaient amorcé une ARAP contenant du RAL après 28 semaines de grossesse dans deux centres hospitaliers universitaires entre 2007 et 2013.

RÉSULTATS ET EXPOSÉ : Onze femmes infectées ont entrepris un traitement de RAL à une médiane de 35,7 semaines de grossesse (plage de 31,1 à 38,0 semaines). Les indications pour entreprendre le RAL étaient une présentation tardive au suivi de grossesse (n=4) et une suppression sous-optimale de la CV en raison d'un mauvais respect du traitement ou d'une résistance virale (n=7). La CV moyenne au début du traitement au RAL était de 73 959 copies/mL (plage de moins de 40 copies/mL à 523 975 copies/mL). Les patientes ont pris du RAL pendant une médiane de 20 jours (plage de un à 71 jours). La diminution moyenne de la CV entre le début du RAL et l'accouchement était de 1,93 log, à l'exception d'une patiente qui n'a reçu qu'une dose de RAL et d'une patiente dont la CV n'était pas décelable au moment d'entreprendre le RAL. Au bout de huit jours de RAL, 50 % des femmes présentaient une CV inférieure à 1 000 copies/mL (le seuil pour recommander une césarienne afin de réduire le risque de transmission périnatale). Il n'y a d'ailleurs eu aucun cas de transmission périnatale du VIH.

CONCLUSION : La présente étude fournit des données provisoires pour soutenir l'utilisation d'ARPA contenant du RAL afin d'accélérer la réduction de la CV du VIH-1 chez les femmes qui présentaient une CV élevée ou une suppression sous-optimale de leur CV pendant la grossesse, ainsi que pour réduire le risque de transmission périnatale du VIH tout en évitant une césarienne. Une évaluation plus approfondie de l'innocuité du RAL est justifiée pendant la grossesse.

The availability of combination antiretroviral therapy (cART) has drastically reduced the risk of HIV-1 perinatal transmission. With cART, undetectable viral loads (VL) are achievable, allowing for vaginal delivery and perinatal transmission rates of <1% to 2% in non-breastfeeding women (1,2). Before the use of antiretrovirals, the rate of HIV-1 perinatal transmission was 25% to 35% in North America, with more than one-half of the cases occurring during the late antenatal period and delivery (3). The risk of perinatal transmission is proportional to maternal plasma VL at delivery (4). Therefore, reaching maximal viral suppression before delivery is the main goal of antiretroviral treatment in pregnancy. To further reduce the risk of transmission, North American guidelines recommend elective Caesarean

[1]*Department of Obstetrics and Gynecology, University of British Columbia, BC Women's Hospital;* [2]*Women's Health Research Institute, BC Women's Hospital;* [3]*Division of Infectious Diseases, University of British Columbia, BC Women's Hospital, Vancouver, British Columbia;* [4]*Division of Infectious Diseases, Centre hospitalier universitaire Sainte-Justine and Department of Pediatrics, Faculty of Medicine, Université de Montréal;* [5]*Centre Maternel et Infantile sur le SIDA, Centre hospitalier universitaire Sainte-Justine;* [6]*Department of Obstetrics and Gynecology, Université de Montréal, Centre hospitalier universitaire Sainte-Justine, Montreal, Quebec*

Correspondence: Dr I Boucoiran, BC Women's Hospital and Health Centre, B327-4500 Oak Street, Box 42, Vancouver, British Columbia V6H 3N1 .e-mail isabelle@boucoiran.fr

delivery at 38 weeks' gestation for women when the last measured VL is >1000 copies/mL (4,5).

Late presentation of pregnant women with HIV, either due to limited or absent prenatal care or acquisition of HIV in late pregnancy, continues to occur and hinders the timely initiation of HIV perinatal transmission preventive measures (6). An Italian cohort study reported that 16% of new HIV-infection diagnoses during pregnancy occurred in the third trimester (7), and 20% of HIV-infected pregnant women presented beyond 28 weeks of pregnancy at the major HIV reference centre in Bahia, Brazil (8). Canadian data reported by the Perinatal HIV Surveillance Program found that between 1997 and 2011, 13% of the HIV-infected pregnant women received no antiretroviral therapy and 17% received <4 weeks of antiretrovirals (9). In 2011 in Canada, 10% of HIV-infected pregnant women had received none or <4 weeks of antiretrovirals. Because women continue to present in late pregnancy with suboptimal VL suppression despite the availability of cART, new therapeutic modalities are required to achieve a prompt decline of HIV VL to decrease the risk of perinatal transmission, potentially also obviating the need for an HIV-indicated Caesarean section.

Raltegravir (RAL) is an HIV-1 integrase strand transfer inhibitor that leads to potent viral suppression while maintaining a favourable adverse effect profile and minimal drug interactions (10). Its effectiveness to rapidly control HIV VL has been demonstrated in patients with drug resistance as well as in the antiretroviral-naive population (11-14). Although there are limited data regarding the use of RAL in pregnancy, there is increasing anecdotal evidence of its efficacy to rapidly reduce maternal VL when used as a part of cART regimens late in pregnancy, with few maternal side effects and no detrimental effects on the fetus (8,15-26).

The objective of our case series was to describe the impact of initiating RAL-containing cART regimens on HIV VL in pregnant women who have high or suboptimal VL suppression late in pregnancy.

METHODS
A retrospective review of two Canadian HIV perinatal databases (those of the Oak Tree Clinic at BC Woman's Hospital, Vancouver, British Columbia, and of the *Grossesse Avec Maladie Infectieuse* clinic at Sainte-Justine Hospital, Montreal, Quebec) was conducted to identify HIV-infected pregnant women who initiated treatment with RAL (400 mg twice per day orally) after 28 weeks' gestation. Data collected between 2007, the year when RAL became available, and December 2013 were reviewed. Each patient's chart was then retrospectively abstracted for data including RAL indication, tolerance and timing of exposure.

The standard of care in both clinics included treatment of HIV-infected pregnant women with cART regardless of baseline CD4 cell-count and HIV-1 VL, as well as assessment of the women's clinical, virological and immunological status every four weeks. Toxicity due to the antiretrovirals was monitored at these times. Infants were evaluated at least at birth, two weeks of age, one month of age and then every three to four months until 18 months of age. HIV-negative status in infants was defined presumptively by at least two negative HIV RNA polymerase chain reaction test results before four months of age, and confirmed by the absence of HIV-1 antibody at 18 months of age.

Maternal and neonatal adverse reactions were systematically addressed according to WHO criteria (27), with specific attention devoted to hematological and hepatic complications.

HIV-1 VL was measured either using the Ultrasensitive Amplicor HIV-1 Monitor Test or COBAS TaqMan HIV-1 Test, v1.0 (Roche Molecular Systems Inc, USA) for cases in Vancouver, and the Abott RealTime HIV-1 assay (Abbott Molecular Inc, USA) for cases in Montreal.

The study was approved by the institutional review board of each centre.

Statistics
A descriptive analysis of population characteristics was performed. Because of the non-normal distribution, median and range are reported.

A nonparametric survival analysis was then conducted to compute the time to achieve a VL <50 copies/mL and <1000 copies/mL, respectively. The statistical analysis was performed using R version 2.11.1 (R Core Team, 2013).

RESULTS
A total of 11 women who initiated RAL during the third trimester of their pregnancies were identified. Their clinical and laboratory characteristics are summarized in Table 1. The median age was 31 years (range 21 to 39 years). Five were antiretroviral-naive before pregnancy. Three women (cases 3, 5 and 7) had a new diagnosis of HIV during the current pregnancy. The median gestational age at their first clinic visit was 24 weeks (range seven to 35 weeks). The median duration of consistent cART received was 42 days (range seven to 202 days). No women had any previous exposure to RAL. Indications for RAL were late presentation in pregnancy (n=4) and suboptimal VL reduction secondary to poor adherence or viral resistance (n=7). All patients received RAL in combination with at least two other active antiretroviral agents, started at a median gestational age of 35.7 weeks (range 31.1 to 38.0 weeks). Exposure duration was a median of 20 days (range one to 71 days). Five women received <2 weeks of RAL.

The median gestational age at delivery was 38.7 weeks; one patient (case 9) delivered at 35 weeks in a context of spontaneous preterm labor. At the time of delivery, nine women had a HIV VL <1000 copies/mL, of which seven were <50 copies/mL. Figure 1 summarizes the typical VL evolution after RAL initiation.

Among the 11 women, three had a vaginal delivery, three had a Caesarean section for obstetrical indications and five had a Caesarean section to further decrease the risk of HIV perinatal transmission. Three of these Caesarean sections could have been avoided (ie, the VL was below threshold of 1000 copies/mL) if the HIV VL had been known at the time of the delivery.

Maternal RAL was discontinued after delivery in all 11 cases. There were no cases of HIV perinatal transmission observed in the in utero-exposed infants. One infant was believed to be breastfed (case 2). One infant (case 11) presented a transient symptomatic cardiac arrhythmia at birth, as well as unilateral hydronephrosis and skin abnormalities (nevus, four nipples), which were not prenatally diagnosed.

The following two cases were excluded from subsequent analysis:
- One woman (case 3) had an undetectable VL at RAL initiation. She was initially started with a combination regimen with zidovudine, lamivudine and ritonavir-boosted lopinavir at 28 weeks and four days. However, she had adherence issues in a context of a newly diagnosed HIV infection in pregnancy with hepatitis C coinfection and substance use. The woman was admitted for directly observed therapy and RAL was started at 33 weeks to rapidly suppress her VL. At the time of RAL initiation, the last available VL result (measured two weeks previously) was 1762 copies/mL, and the woman reported poor adherence to her cART regimen during this time period. Retrospectively, it was determined that at the time of RAL initiation, her VL was undetectable; however, because of concerns surrounding adherence and risk of resistance rise, RAL was pursued. The woman discharged herself from hospital for three days at approximately 35 weeks' gestation but returned with a positive urine cocaine screen. She had a vaginal delivery at 38 weeks and five days' gestation with a confirmed undetectable VL.
- One woman (case 10) received only one dose of RAL. Her pregnancy had been complicated by poor adherence and intolerance to cART. At 37 weeks' gestation, she was admitted for supervised cART, and her VL was found to be 232,245 copies/mL. As soon as this result was known, RAL was added to her regimen to attempt a rapid and maximal suppression of the HIV VL before delivery. However, 3 h after receiving the first dose of RAL the woman experienced spontaneous rupture of membranes and went into active labour.

In the remaining nine women, median VL at RAL initiation was 88,707 copies/mL (range 246 to 523,975 copies/mL; mean 73,959 copies/mL). The mean decline of VL from time of RAL

TABLE 1

Summary of the 11 patients who initiated raltegravir during the third trimester for HIV perinatal transmission prophylaxis

Case	Age, years	ART status	Coinfec-tion	ART used during pregnancy (in addition to RAL)	Indications for RAL initiation	GA at RAL initiation (weeks)	CD4 at RAL initiation (cells/mL)	VL at RAL initiation (copies/mL)	VL at delivery (copies/mL)	Exposure to RAL (days)	VL decrease ($\log_{10}$ copies/mL)	Mode of delivery	Peripartum prophy-laxis	Infant prophy-laxis	Infant HIV status
1	31	Exp	–	ABC+3TC +ATZ/r	VL rebound despite dose adjustment	34.1	437	1562	40	43	1.59	Urgent C-section for labour dystocia	AZT IV	AZT +3TC	Neg
2	24	Exp	–	AZT+3TC +LPV/r	VL rebound due to resistance	36.4	440	1003	41	8	1.39	Elective C-section for perinatal transmission prophylaxis	AZT IV	AZT +3TC	Neg
3	39	Naive	HCV	AZT+3TC +LPV/r	Late initiation of ART, fear of resistance due to compliance issues	33.4	308	<40	<40	34	0.00	Vaginal delivery	AZT IV	AZT +3TC	Neg
4	33	Exp	–	AZT+3TC +LPV/r	Late presentation	35.0	54	208,993	154	20	3.13	Elective C-section for perinatal transmission prophylaxis	AZT IV	AZT +3TC +LPV/r	Neg*
5	36	Naive	–	AZT+3TC +LPV/r	VL rebound despite adequate drug levels	35.7	357	246	<40	25	0.79	Emergent C-section for nonreassuring fetal heart rate and choriamnionitis	AZT IV	AZT +3TC	Neg*
6	34	Naive	–	AZT+3TC +LPV/r	Late presentation	36.3	132	523,975	1163	11	2.65	Elective C-section for perinatal transmission prophylaxis	AZT IV	AZT +3TC +NFV	Neg
7	35	Naive	–	AZT+3TC +LPV/r	VL rebound	37.6	484	695	<40	13	1.24	Vaginal delivery	AZT IV	AZT +3TC	Neg
8	21	Exp	–	AZT+3TC +LPV/r	Late presenta-tion, multi-class genotypic resistance	31.1	168	26,770	<40	71	2.83	Emergent C-section for nonreassuring fetal status and placental abruption	AZT IV	AZT +3TC	Neg
9	29	Exp	HCV	ABC+3TC +DRV/r, ABC+3TC +LPV/r	VL rebound after interruption of ART	34.0	210	32,830	338	7	1.99	Elective C-section for perinatal transmission prophylaxis	AZT IV + NVP po	AZT +3TC +NFV	Neg
10	29	Naive	HCV	TDF+FTC + ATZ/r	VL rebound after interruption of ART	38.0	50	15,153	15,153	1	NA	Elective C-section for perinatal transmission prophylaxis	AZT IV + NVP po	AZT +3TC +LPN/r	Neg
11	22	Naive	–	TDF+FTC + ATZ/r then ABC+3TC +ATZ/r	VL rebound after interruption of ART	36.0	600	2287	<40	35	1.76	Vaginal delivery	AZT IV	AZT	Neg

*Confirmatory HIV serology at 18 months is pending. 3TC Lamivudine; ABC Abacavir; ATZ/r Atazanavir/ritonavir; ART Antiretroviral therapy; AZT Zidovudine; C-section Caesarean section; DRV/r Darunavir/ritonavir; Exp Experienced; FTC Emtricitabine; GA Gestational age; HCV Hepatitis C virus; IV Intravenous; LPV/r Lopinavir/ritonavir; NA Not applicable; Neg Negative; NFV Nelfinavir; NVP Nevirapine; RAL Raltegravir; TDF Tenofovir; VL HIV RNA viral load

initiation to delivery was 1.93 $\log_{10}$ copies/mL (95% CI 1.32 to 2.53 $\log_{10}$ copies/mL) (Figure 1). In the four women who received <2 weeks of RAL, the mean VL decrease was 1.82 $\log_{10}$ copies/mL. In the four women who had an initial VL >4 $\log_{10}$ copies/mL, the mean decrease was 2.65 $\log_{10}$ copies/mL. After eight days on RAL, 50% of the women achieved a VL <1000 copies/mL (Figure 2). Similarly, 50% of the women achieved a VL <50 copies/mL after 26 days on RAL.

Only one maternal adverse event was observed (case 6). An asymptomatic elevation of liver enzyme levels (11- and fivefold the

upper limit of normal of alanine aminotransferase and aspartate aminotransferase, respectively) was noted in a woman for whom RAL was added to a combination of zidovudine, lamivudine and ritonavir-boosted lopinavir because of late presentation. The elevation of liver enzyme levels was first observed after five days on RAL, without signs of preeclampsia or cholestasis. The status regarding hepatitis A, B and C infections was confirmed to be negative. After RAL discontinua-tion, liver enzyme levels immediately began to decrease significantly. This case has previously been described by the authors' team (23).

TABLE 2

Summary of previous published case reports of raltegravir initiation during the third trimester of pregnancy

First author (reference), year	Number of cases	GA at RAL initiation, weeks, range	Exposure to RAL, days, range	HIV RNA at RAL initiation, copies/mL, range	HIV RNA at delivery, copies/mL,*	HIV RNA decrease, log$_{10}$ copies/mL, range	Undetectable viral load at delivery, n	Mode of delivery	Perinatal transmission, n
Pinnetti (15), 2010	1	38	9	75,584	260	2.46	0	C-section	0
McKeown (16), 2010	3	28–39	11–17	183–67,100	40–185	0.66–2.56	2	C-section	0
Taylor (18), 2010	5	33–34	17–46	51–48,884	<40–380	0.11–3.16	3	C-section	0
Lopez-Valera (19), 2012	1	35	28	1902	<50	1.58	1	Vaginal delivery	0
Westling (21), 2012	4	34–37	8–22	65,600–637,000	<20–2700	1.39–3.56	1	C-section	0
Nobrega (8), 2013	14	34–38	7–32 (median 17)	636–391,535 (median 35,364)	<50–457	0.84–3.90 (median 2.6)	7	13 C-sections, 1 vaginal delivery	1
Hegazi (24), 2013	1	29	71	1,740,000,000	208	6.92	0	C-section	0
Cha (25), 2013	1	33	35	106,110	200	2.72	0	C-section	0
De Hoffer (26), 2013	1	35	19	8903	<20	2.65	1	C-section	0

*Viral load the day of delivery or, if it was not reported, viral load the closest to the day of delivery. C-section Caesarean section; GA Gestational age; RAL Raltegravir

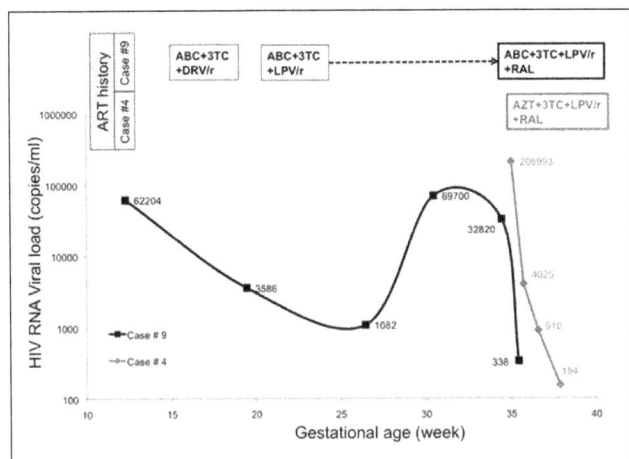

Figure 1) *Examples of HIV RNA viral load evolution after raltegravir (RAL) initiation late in pregnancy. Case 4: a 33-year-old woman from Haiti who had recently immigrated to Canada was first seen at the authors' clinic at 35 weeks' gestation. A combination of zidovudine (AZT), lamivudine (3TC), boosted lopinavir (LPV/r) and RAL was immediately started. An elective Caesarean section was performed at 38 weeks, after intravenous zidovudine. At delivery, the HIV viral load was retrospectively found to be 154 copies/mL. Case 9: a 29-year-old First Nations nulliparous woman coinfected with hepatitis C with a history of substance abuse was first seen at 10 weeks' gestation. Because of tolerance and adherence issues, her viral load was 32,820 copies/mL at 34 weeks' gestation. She was admitted to hospital for supervised combination antiretroviral drug therapy (ART) containing RAL and received a total of seven days of this regimen. An emergent Caesarean section was performed at 35 weeks' gestation in the context of preterm labour, after an intravenous loading dose of AZT and a single-dose of oral nevirapine 200 mg. At delivery, her HIV viral load was retrospectively found to be 338 copies/mL. Both newborns were uninfected. ABC Abacavir*

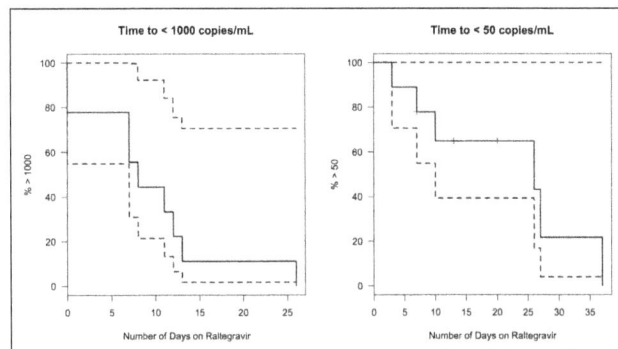

Figure 2) *Time to achieve a HIV viral load <1000 copies/mL and <50 copies/mL after raltegravir initiation during the third trimester (n=10). Dotted lines represent CIs*

DISCUSSION

In our experience, adding RAL to a cART regimen was useful in rapidly reducing HIV-1 VL to prevent perinatal transmission in women who have high VL or suboptimal suppression late in pregnancy.

Our findings are consistent with previously published cases of RAL use late in pregnancy, which are summarized in Table 2 (8,15-18,20-22,24-26,28). Among these, only one case of perinatal transmission has been reported (8); the clinical presentation in that case suggested in utero HIV transmission. No neonatal safety issues have been observed among the published cases.

We were able to confirm the drastic and rapid decrease of HIV VL after RAL initiation, and computed a median time to achieve VL <1000 copies/mL (eight days), information that will be useful in the clinical setting. However, the low number of subjects limits the generalizability of our findings. Moreover, important limitations of the present case series include the absence of data regarding resistance to integrase inhibitors among the women treated, and regarding maternal and neonatal RAL plasma concentrations. Published data indicate that, despite a reduction of RAL median area under the curve by approximately 50% during pregnancy (29), RAL readily crosses the placenta and achieves adequate concentrations in the neonate, with mean cord blood-maternal blood drug ratios of 1.5 (range 0.32 to 9.5) (15,16,22,28). Else et al (30) found that RAL achieves the highest placental/neonatal concentration among available antiretroviral medications. Explanations for effective placental transfer of RAL include its relatively low protein binding and small molecular weight, as well as its favourable pH-dependent lipophilicity, which results in increased amount of ionized drug in the fetal circulation (11,22,30,31). A high cord:maternal serum ratio reflects a high placental transfer but also a neonatal accumulation. The ability of fetuses to metabolize and eliminate RAL on their own is likely limited by the immaturity of UGT-glucuronidation pathways (22,32).

We observed a 1.82 log$_{10}$ copies/mL decrease in HIV VL within two weeks of receipt of a RAL-containing cART regimen, which is faster than the mean time of approximately five weeks to suppression that is typically observed with traditional cART (33). This finding is consistent with the VL reductions (2 log$_{10}$ copies/mL within 10 to 14 days of receipt of a RAL-based regimen) observed in randomized controlled trials using RAL-based regimens (12-14) and in observational studies investigating RAL administration late in pregnancy (8,15,16,18,21).

The reported case of liver toxicity (23) is, to our knowledge, the second that has been described with RAL use in pregnancy (29). Although hepatotoxicity is one of the well-recognized side effects of antiretroviral drugs, it has not been commonly associated with RAL therapy, with increase of aspartate aminotransferase and alanine aminotransferase levels >5 times the upper limit of normal seen in only 5% of exposed individuals (31,34). Sufficient data are not yet available to conclude whether the risk of hepatotoxicity is higher in pregnancy. Close follow-up of liver enzyme levels in pregnant women treated with RAL would be prudent until more safety data are available.

RAL has not been associated with any congenital anomalies (31). The infant who was diagnosed with cardiac arrhythmia, unilateral hydronephrosis and skin anomalies had been exposed to RAL in utero for 35 days, starting at 36 weeks' gestation. Because of this timing, the congenital anomalies are not likely related to RAL exposure. However, safety data regarding RAL exposure in pregnancy are weak, and it remains a category C drug (31).

Considering the potential advantages of RAL noted above, it remains to be determined whether its ability to rapidly reduce VL in late pregnancy will reduce the need for Caesarean delivery and the rate of perinatal transmission for women who present near term with high VL. This would benefit HIV-infected women, particularly those with low CD4 cell counts, considering the increased risk of postpartum complications related to Caesarean delivery (35,36). An important factor to consider, however, is the availability of rapid HIV quantitative test to follow the VL and allow for a safe vaginal delivery. Indeed, in previously published cases of pregnant women treated with RAL (8,15,16,18,20-22,24-26) as well as in the three cases presented here, VL were retrospectively found to be <1000 copies/mL after Caesarean section was performed to decrease the risk of perinatal transmission. Availability of rapid HIV quantitative polymerase chain reaction would assist the clinician to better decide whether Caesarean delivery is indicated, according to their national guidelines (4,5).

CONCLUSIONS

Our findings support the consideration of the use of RAL to reduce the risk of perinatal transmission in late-presenting HIV-infected pregnant women and in women with VL rebound near term. However, long-term data are needed to assess the impact of RAL use for short-term therapy in the obstetrical setting on the resistance profile. Indeed, there is a legitimate concern about the effectiveness of future RAL-based regimens. Moreover, current Canadian (5) and United States perinatal guidelines (4) are permissive but do not advocate for RAL use in this setting due to the lack of established data. The results of two ongoing clinical trials (NCT01854762 and NCT01618305) will help to assess advantages of RAL compared with other antiretrovirals in pregnancy. Further research needs to be performed to understand the role of RAL in women with HIV acquisition in pregnancy, who are at even higher risk for perinatal transmission.

ACKNOWLEDGEMENTS: The authors thank Silvie Valois, research nurse at the *Centre Maternel Infantile sur le SIDA*, for her help in collecting the data. IB was funded by a scholarship of the Sainte-Justine foundation.

REFERENCES

1. Kourtis AP, Lee FK, Abrams EJ, Jamieson DJ, Bulterys M. Mother-to-child transmission of HIV-1: Timing and implications for prevention. Lancet Infect Dis 2006;6:726-32.
2. Forbes JC, Alimenti AM, Singer J, et al. A national review of vertical HIV transmission. AIDS 2012;26:757-63.
3. Connor EM, Sperling RS, Gelber R, et al. Reduction of maternal-infant transmission of human immunodeficiency virus type 1 with zidovudine treatment. Pediatric AIDS Clinical Trials Group Protocol 076 Study Group. N Engl J Med 1994;331:1173-80.
4. Panel on Treatment of HIV-Infected Pregnant Women and Prevention of Perinatal Transmission. Recommendations for use of antiretroviral drugs in pregnant HIV-1-infected women for maternal health and interventions to reduce perinatal HIV transmission in the United States. March 2014. <http://aidsinfo.nih.gov/contentfiles/lvguidelines/perinatalgl.pdf> (Accessed February 15, 2015).
5. Money D, Tulloch K, Boucoiran I, et al. Guidelines for the care of pregnant women living with HIV and interventions to reduce perinatal transmission: Executive summary. J Obstet Gynaecol Can 2014;36:721-51.
6. Read JS, Cohen RA, Hance LF, et al. Missed opportunities for prevention of mother-to-child transmission of HIV-1 in the NISDI Perinatal and LILAC cohorts. Int J Gynaecol Obstet 2012;119:70-5.
7. Floridia M, Ravizza M, Tamburrini E, et al. Diagnosis of HIV infection in pregnancy: Data from a national cohort of pregnant women with HIV in Italy. Epidemiol Infect 2006;134:1120-7.
8. Nobrega I, Travassos AG, Haguihara T, Amorim F, Brites C. Use of raltegravir in late-presenting, HIV-infected pregnant women. AIDS Res Hum Retroviruses 2013;29:1451-4.
9. Bitnun A, Lee T, Singer J, et al. Missed opportunities for the prevention of vertical HIV transmission (VT): Evidence from the Canadian Perinatal HIV Surveillance Program (CPHSP). Can J Infect Dis Med Microbiol 2013;24(Suppl A):P084
10. ACOG Committee Opinion No. 418: Prenatal and perinatal human immunodeficiency virus testing: Expanded recommendations. Obstet Gynecol 2008;112:739-42.
11. Rokas KE, Bookstaver PB, Shamroe CL, et al. Role of raltegravir in HIV-1 management. Ann Pharmacother 2012;46:578-89.
12. Grinsztejn B, Nguyen BY, Katlama C, et al. Safety and efficacy of the HIV-1 integrase inhibitor raltegravir (MK-0518) in treatment-experienced patients with multidrug-resistant virus: A phase II randomised controlled trial. Lancet 2007;369:1261-9.
13. Lennox JL, DeJesus E, Lazzarin A, et al. Safety and efficacy of raltegravir-based versus efavirenz-based combination therapy in treatment-naive patients with HIV-1 infection: A multicentre, double-blind randomised controlled trial. Lancet 2009;374:796-806.
14. Markowitz M, Morales-Ramirez JO, Nguyen BY, et al. Antiretroviral activity, pharmacokinetics, and tolerability of MK-0518, a novel inhibitor of HIV-1 integrase, dosed as monotherapy for 10 days in treatment-naive HIV-1-infected individuals. J Acquir Immune Defic Syndr 2006;43:509-15.
15. Pinnetti C, Baroncelli S, Villani P, et al. Rapid HIV-RNA decline following addition of raltegravir and tenofovir to ongoing highly active antiretroviral therapy in a woman presenting with high-level HIV viraemia at week 38 of pregnancy. J Antimicrob Chemother 2010;65:2050-2.
16. McKeown DA, Rosenvinge M, Donaghy S, et al. High neonatal concentrations of raltegravir following transplacental transfer in HIV-1 positive pregnant women. AIDS 2010;24:2416-8.
17. Jaworsky D, Thompson C, Yudin MH, et al. Use of newer antiretroviral agents, darunavir and etravirine with or without raltegravir, in pregnancy: A report of two cases. Antivir Ther 2010;15:677-80.
18. Taylor N, Touzeau V, Geit M, et al. Raltegravir in pregnancy: A case series presentation. Int J STD AIDS 2011;22:358-60.
19. Lopez-Varela E, Rojo-Conejo P, Blazquez-Gamero D, Gonzalez-Granado L. [Undetectable viral load after the addition of raltegravir in a 36 week pregnant adolescent with high-level HIV viraemia]. An Pediatr (Barc) 2012;76:296-7.
20. Hegazi A, McKeown D, Doerholt K, Donaghy S, Sadiq ST, Hay P. Raltegravir in the prevention of mother-to-child transmission of HIV-1: Effective transplacental transfer and delayed plasma clearance observed in preterm neonates. AIDS 2012;26:2421-3.
21. Westling K, Pettersson K, Kaldma A, Naver L. Rapid decline in HIV viral load when introducing raltegravir-containing antiretroviral treatment late in pregnancy. AIDS Patient Care STDS 2012;26:714-7.
22. Croci L, Trezzi M, Allegri MP, et al. Pharmacokinetic and safety of raltegravir in pregnancy. Eur J Clin Pharmacol 2012;68:1231-2.
23. Renet S, Closon A, Brochet MS, Bussieres JF, Boucher M. Increase in transaminase levels following the use of raltegravir in a woman with a high HIV viral load at 35 weeks of pregnancy. J Obstet Gynaecol Can 2013;35:68-72.

24. Hegazi A, Hay P. HIV seroconversion in the third trimester of pregnancy: Using raltegravir to prevent mother-to-child transmission. Int J STD AIDS 2013.

25. Cha A, Shaikh R, Williams S, Berkowitz LL. Rapid reduction in HIV viral load in late pregnancy with raltegravir: A case report. J Int Assoc Provid AIDS Care 2013:12:312-4.

26. De Hoffer L, Di Biagio A, Bruzzone B, et al. Use of raltegravir in a late presenter HIV-1 woman in advanced gestational age: Case report and literature review. J Chemother 2013;25:181-3.

27. World Health Organization. ARV drugs adverse events, case definition, toxicity grading and laboratory diagnosis. Geneva (Switzerland) 2008. <http://hivforumannals.org/index.php/annals/article/download/12/9> (Accessed May 28, 2015).

28. Clarke DF, Acosta EP, Rizk M, et al. Raltegravir Pharmacokinetics and Safety in Neonates (IMPAACT P1097). Atlanta: Conference on Retroviruses and Opportunistic Infections, March 2013.

29. Watts DH, Stek A, Best BM, et al. Raltegravir pharmacokinetics during pregnancy. J Acquir Immune Defic Syndr 2014;67:375-81.

30. Else LJ, Taylor S, Back DJ, Khoo SH. Pharmacokinetics of antiretroviral drugs in anatomical sanctuary sites: The fetal compartment (placenta and amniotic fluid). Antivir Ther 2011;16:1139-47.

31. Merck Canada Inc. Product monograph. ISENTRESS®. Kirkland, Quebec, 2013. <www.merck.ca/assets/en/pdf/products/ISENTRESS-PM_E.pdf> (Accessed May 28, 2015).

32. Brainard DM, Wenning LA, Stone JA, Wagner JA, Iwamoto M. Clinical pharmacology profile of raltegravir, an HIV-1 integrase strand transfer inhibitor. J Clin Pharmacol 2011;51:1376-402.

33. Patel D, Cortina-Borja M, Thorne C, Newell ML. Time to undetectable viral load after highly active antiretroviral therapy initiation among HIV-infected pregnant women. Clin Infect Dis 2007;44:1647-56.

34. Administration. UFaD. Highlights of Prescribing Information. Isentress (relategravir) Tablets 2009. <www.accessdata.fda.gov/drugsatfda_docs/label/2009/022145s004lbl.pdf> (Accessed May 28, 2015).

35. Read JS, Tuomala R, Kpamegan E, et al. Mode of delivery and postpartum morbidity among HIV-infected women: The women and infants transmission study. J Acquir Immune Defic Syndr 2001;26:236-45.

36. Louis J, Buhari MA, Allen D, Gonik B, Jones TB. Postpartum morbidity associated with advanced HIV disease. Infect Dis Obstet Gynecol 2006;2006:79512.

Empyema caused by *Clostridium bifermentans*: A case report

Safa Edagiz MD[1], Phil Lagace-Wiens MD[1,2], John Embil MD[3], James Karlowsky PhD[1,2], Andrew Walkty MD[1,2,3]

S Edagiz, P Lagace-Wiens, J Embil, J Karlowsky, A Walkty. Empyema caused by *Clostridium bifermentans*: A case report. Can J Infect Dis Med Microbiol 2015;26(2):105-107.

A case of pneumonia with associated empyema caused by *Clostridium bifermentans* is described. *C bifermentans* is an anaerobic, spore-forming, Gram-positive bacillus. This organism is infrequently reported as a cause of infection in humans, and older publications tended to regard it as nonpathogenic. However, in more recent reports, *C bifermentans* has been documented as a cause of septic arthritis, osteomyelitis, soft tissue infection, abdominal infections, brain abscess, bacteremia and endocarditis. The present case is the third reported case of empyema caused by *C bifermentans*, and it serves to further define the spectrum of illness due to this uncommon organism.

Key Words: Clostridium bifermentans; *Empyema*; *Pneumonia*

Un empyème causé par le *Clostridium bifermentans* : un rapport de cas

Les auteurs décrivent un cas de pneumonie associé à de l'empyème attribuable à un *Clostridium bifermentans*. Le *C bifermentans* est un bacille anaérobique sporulé Gram positif. Il est rarement signalé comme cause d'infection chez les humains, et les publications plus anciennes ont tendance à le considérer comme non pathogène. Cependant, dans des rapports plus récents, le *C bifermentans* est attesté comme cause d'arthrite septique, d'ostéomyélite, d'infection des tissus mous, d'infection abdominale, d'abcès du cerveau, de bactériémie et d'endocardite. Le présent cas, qui est le troisième cas déclaré d'empyème attribuable au *C bifermentans*, contribue à mieux définir le spectre de maladie causé par cet organisme peu courant.

CASE PRESENTATION

A 60-year-old man with a medical history significant only for an anxiety disorder presented to a community hospital in Winnipeg, Manitoba with a four-day history of increasing fatigue, weakness, cough and shortness of breath. The patient also complained of sharp right-sided pleuritic chest pain, as well as right upper quadrant abdominal pain associated with deep breathing. He denied nausea and vomiting. A review of systems was otherwise negative. The patient was a heavy smoker and reported occasional alcohol consumption. He denied the use of intravenous recreational drugs.

On physical examination at the time of presentation, the patient was noted to be febrile, with an oral temperature of 39.2°C. He was otherwise hemodynamically stable. The patient was edentulous. On respiratory examination, decreased air entry was noted in the right lower and middle lobes. Bronchial breath sounds were noted at the right lung base, and crepitations were heard with auscultation over the rest of the right lung. The abdomen was tender to palpation in the right upper quadrant. The remainder of the physical examination was unremarkable. Laboratory investigations performed on presentation demonstrated an elevated total leukocyte count (17.8×10^9 cells/L) with a neutrophil predominance (neutrophil count 16.12×10^9 cells/L). Blood cultures (aerobic and anaerobic) were negative. On chest radiography, a right-sided pneumothorax with right lower lobe consolidation and associated pleural fluid was apparent (Figure 1). The patient underwent a noncontrast computed tomography (CT) scan of the abdomen to rule out a subdiaphragmatic abscess in view of the right upper quadrant abdominal pain. No intra-abdominal abnormality was noted; however, the assessment did confirm a right-sided hydropneumothorax, with areas of pulmonary consolidation and loculated pleural fluid.

The patient was admitted to hospital. A chest tube was placed, and empirical antimicrobial therapy with a combination of levofloxacin and metronidazole was initiated. A sample of pleural fluid was submitted to the microbiology laboratory for further analysis. No polymorphonuclear cells or bacteria were observed on Gram stain. The aerobic culture did not demonstrate any bacterial growth following 72 h of incubation. However, after 48 h of incubation, a large Gram-positive spore-forming bacillus was recovered on anaerobic culture. The organism was subsequently identified as *Clostridium bifermentans* using a Vitek™ 2 ANC card (bioMérieux, Canada). Antimicrobial susceptibility testing was performed by E-test (bioMérieux, Canada), with minimum inhibitory concentrations interpreted according to 2012 Clinical and Laboratory Standards Institute breakpoints for anaerobic bacteria (1). The isolate was susceptible to amoxicillin-clavulanate, cefoxitin, clindamycin, meropenem, metronidazole and penicillin.

On the third day postadmission, the patient continued to complain of significant dyspnea and chest pain. A CT scan of the chest was performed with contrast and this demonstrated a right main pulmonary artery embolus. The patient clinically deteriorated and ultimately required admission to the intensive care unit. His antimicrobial therapy was changed to a combination of piperacillin-tazobactam and levofloxacin, and heparin was initiated as treatment for the pulmonary embolus. Fifteen days postadmission, the patient underwent a thoracotomy and decortication of the right lung. Empyema fluid obtained at the time of surgery was submitted to the microbiology laboratory. *C bifermentans* was once again recovered on anaerobic culture. Postoperatively, antimicrobial therapy with piperacillin-tazobactam alone was continued.

Following surgery, the patient experienced intermittent low-grade fevers (approximately 38°C) and ongoing hypoxia requiring 2 L of

[1]*Department of Medical Microbiology, University of Manitoba;* [2]*Diagnostic Services Manitoba;* [3]*Department of Internal Medicine, Section of Infectious Diseases, University of Manitoba, Winnipeg, Manitoba*
Correspondence: Dr Andrew Walkty, MS673B Microbiology, Health Sciences Centre, 820 Sherbrook Street, Winnipeg, Manitoba R3A 1R9. e-mail awalkty@dsmanitoba.ca

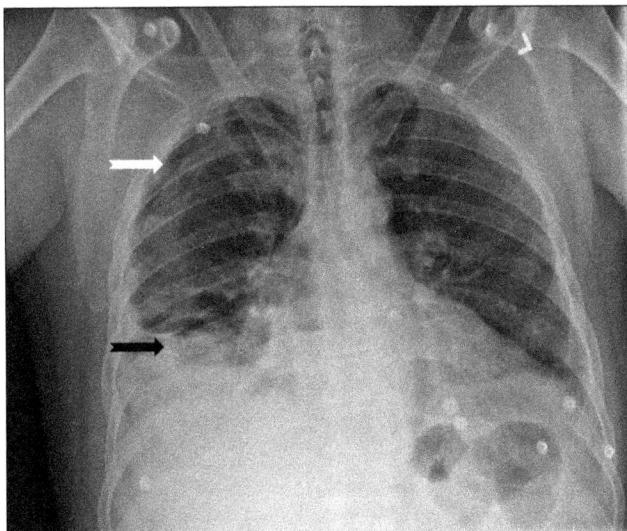

Figure 1) *Chest radiograph demonstrating a right-sided pneumothorax (white arrow) and right lower lobe consolidation (black arrow)*

oxygen via nasal prongs. Repeat chest radiography revealed a loculated right-sided pneumothorax with a small amount of fluid remaining in the empyema cavity. Twenty-nine days after the initial surgical procedure (44 days postadmission), the patient was taken back to the operating room for a second thoracotomy, right rib resection and empyema drainage. Lung tissue obtained at the time of this surgery for aerobic and anaerobic bacterial culture was found to be sterile. After the second surgery, the antimicrobial therapy was changed to a combination of ceftriaxone and metronidazole. An echocardiogram was performed, which did not demonstrate any evidence of endocarditis or other valvular pathology. The patient gradually improved over a period of several weeks. He was ultimately discharged home 76 days postadmission with a prescription for oral metronidazole to complete an additional 10 days of therapy as an outpatient (arbitrary treatment duration of six weeks following the final surgical drainage procedure).

DISCUSSION

Bacteria belonging to the genus *Clostridium* are anaerobic Grampositive rods with the ability to form endospores (2,3). More than 200 species and subspecies have been recognized to date. *Clostridium* species are ubiquitous in the environment. They may be found in soil, sewage, marine sediment and feces (2,3). *Clostridium* species are part of the normal flora of the intestinal tract of humans and other animals, and may also be isolated from the female genital tract and the oral mucosa (2).

C bifermentans was first described in 1902 under the name *Bacillus bifermentans sporogenes* (4). The name 'bifermentans' relates to the ability of this organism to ferment both carbohydrates and amino acids (5). It may be differentiated from other members of the genus *Clostridium*, in part, by a negative urease test, and positive indole and lecithinase tests (2). Older publications in the literature tended to regard *C bifermentans* as nonpathogenic (4,6). In somewhat dated animal studies involving mice and guinea pigs, *C bifermentans* did not demonstrate any lethal or dermatonecrotic properties (4,6). Furthermore, before 1970, only two cases of human infection due to this organism had been reported (7,8). These included a contaminated war wound with very poor documentation describing the infection, and a case of food poisoning (7,8). However, over the past three decades, several case reports have been published in the English language documenting a variety of clinical infectious due to this bacteria. *C bifermentans* has been described as a cause of septic arthritis, liver abscess following blunt abdominal trauma, abdominal abscess (in association with *Cardiobacterium hominis*), delayed brain abscess due to a

retained foreign body, metastatic osteomyelitis, soft tissue infection and endocarditis (7,9-15). Furthermore, in various published series of *Clostridium* species bacteremia, *C bifermentans* typically accounts for a small percentage of cases (16-18). It is likely that the increased reporting of this organism reflects, at least in part, improved laboratory methods for detection and identification.

Pleuropulmonary disease, including pneumonia and/or empyema, is an uncommon manifestation of infection due to *Clostridium* species in the absence of preceding trauma (19). Several clostridial species have been documented as a cause of pleuropulmonary infection, including *Clostridium perfringens*, *Clostridium sordellii*, *Clostridium sporogenes*, *Clostridium paraputrificum*, *Clostridium difficile*, *Clostridium septicum*, *Clostridium cadaveris* and *Clostridium tetani* (19-23). *C bifermentans* has only been reported as a cause of pulmonary infection/empyema in two other publications (24,25). Jonsson et al (24) described a 60-year-old man who presented with fever, cough and pleuritic chest pain. A large pleural effusion was demonstrated on chest radiography. Cultures of the pleural fluid grew *C bifermentans* and *Bacillus cereus*. The patient improved following thoracotomy with decortication and appropriate antimicrobial therapy. Misra and Hurst (25) reported a 41-year-old woman who presented with cough, hemoptysis and pleuritic chest pain. A lung scan performed on admission was consistent with pulmonary emboli and the patient was treated with heparin. She subsequently deteriorated in hospital, with repeat chest radiography demonstrating pulmonary infiltrates and a pneumothorax that appeared to communicate with a cavitary lesion in the chest. *C bifermentans* was recovered from blood and pleural fluid cultures. The patient succumbed to complications of the illness (25).

In both of the previously published cases of *C bifermentans* empyema as well as the current case, it is unclear whether infection occurred secondary to hematogenous spread, inhalation or aspiration of the organism, although inhalation was favoured in the report by Jonsson et al (24). The case presented here is similar to the case described by Misra and Hurst (25) in that the infection occurred in the setting of a pulmonary embolus. Given the reported low virulence of *C bifermentans*, it is tempting to speculate that tissue injury/infarction secondary to a pulmonary embolus may have predisposed our patient to develop this infection. A septic embolus would also be possible as a mechanism of infection, although blood cultures were negative. Unfortunately, the lack of an infused chest CT scan on presentation prevents determination of whether the pulmonary embolus was present at the start of the illness or whether it occurred in hospital once the infection was already established. Alternatively, the infection may have occurred secondary to aspiration, although the patient did not have any risk factors for aspiration specifically identified. It should be noted that the possibility of polymicrobial infection could not be completely excluded because all pleural fluid and tissue specimens were obtained after the start of antimicrobial therapy. Thus, the patient remained on broad-spectrum antimicrobials during his stay in hospital. The etiology of the pneumothorax in the present case also remains uncertain, as is its association (if any) with the development of infection. With the history of smoking, it is possible that our patient did, in fact, have underlying pulmonary disease, and this may have been a predisposing factor for the pneumothorax and/or the empyema.

CONCLUSION

The present report describes a case of pneumonia/empyema caused by *C bifermentans*. Infections due to *C bifermentans* are infrequently reported, potentially due to the relatively low virulence of this organism. Older publications tended to regard *C bifermentans* as nonpathogenic (4,6). However, in more recent reports, this organism has been documented as a cause of septic arthritis, osteomyelitis, soft tissue infection, abdominal infections, brain abscess, bacteremia and endocarditis (7,9-18). The present article describes the third reported case of empyema caused by *C bifermentans*, and serves to further define the spectrum of illness due to this uncommon organism.

REFERENCES

1. Clinical and Laboratory Standards Institute. Performance Standards for Antimicrobial Susceptibility Testing; Twenty-Second Informational Supplement. M100-S22. Wayne: Clinical and Laboratory Standards Institute, 2012.

2. Stevens DL, Bryant AM, Berger A, Von Eichel-Streiber C. Clostridium. In: Versalovic J, Carroll KC, Funke G, Jorgensen JH, Landry ML, Warnock DW, eds. Manual of Clinical Microbiology, 10th edn. Washington, DC: ASM Press, 2011:834-57.

3. Onderdonk AB, Garrett WS. Gas gangrene and other Clostridium-associated diseases. In: Mandell GL, Bennett JE, Dolin R, eds. Principles and Practice of Infectious Diseases, 7th edn. Philadelphia: Churchill Livingstone Elsevier, 2010:3103-9.

4. Brooks ME, Epps HBG. Taxonomic studies of the genus Clostridium: Clostridium bifermentans and C. sordellii. J Gen Microbiol 1958;21:144-55.

5. Vos PD, Garrity GM, Jones D, et al. (eds). Bergey's Manual of Systematic Bacteriology, 2nd edn. Volume 3: The Firmicutes. New York: Springer Science+Business Media, 2009:758.

6. Nishida S, Tamai K, Yamagishi T. Taxonomy of Clostridium bifermentans and Clostridium sordellii I. Their toxigenicity, urease activity, and sporulating potency. J Bacteriol 1964;88:1641-6.

7. Nolan B, Leers WD, Schatzker J. Septic arthritis of the knee due to Clostridium bifermentans. J Bone Joint Surg 1972;54-A:1275-8.

8. MacLennan JD. Anaerobic infections of war wounds in the Middle East. Lancet 1943;242:123-6.

9. Nachman S, Kaul A, Li KI, Slim MS, San Filippo JA, Van Horn K. Liver abscess caused by Clostridium bifermentans following blunt abdominal trauma. J Clin Microbiol 1989;27:1137-8.

10. Rechtman DJ, Nadler JP. Abdominal abscess due to Cardiobacterium hominis and Clostridium bifermentans. Rev Infect Dis 1991;13:418-9.

11. Pencek TL, Burchiel KJ. Delayed brain abscess related to a retained foreign body with culture of Clostridium bifermentans. J Neurosurg 1986;64:813-5.

12. Scanlan DR, Smith MA, Isenberg HD, Engrassia S, Hilton E. Clostridium bifermentans bacteremia with metastatic osteomyelitis. J Clin Microbiol 1994;32:2867-8.

13. Gorbach SL, Thadepalli H. Isolation of Clostridium in human infections: Evaluation of 114 cases. J Infect Dis 1975;131:S81-5.

14. Moyano R, Gomez-Mateos JM, Lozano de Leon F, Florez C, Jimenez-Ocana C, Gamboa F. Clostridium bifermentans: An exceptional agent of endocarditis. Clin Infect Dis 1994;18:837.

15. Kolander SA, Cosgrove EM, Molavi A. Clostridial endocarditis. Report of a case caused by Clostridium bifermentans and review of the literature. Arch Intern Med 1989;149:455-6.

16. Rechner PM, Agger WA, Mruz K, Cogbill TH. Clinical features of clostridial bacteremia: A review from a rural area. Clin Infect Dis 2001;33:349-53.

17. Leal J, Gregson DB, Ross T, Church DL, Laupland KB. Epidemiology of Clostridium species bacteremia in Calgary, Canada, 2000-2006. J Infect 2008;57:198-203.

18. Haddy RI, Nadkarni DD, Mann BL, et al. Clostridial bacteremia in the community hospital. Scand J Infect Dis 2000;32:27-30.

19. Patel SB, Mahler R. Clostridial pleuropulmonary infections: Case report and review of the literature. J Infect 1990;21:81-5.

20. Hudson DA, Gibb AP, Gill MJ. Empyema caused by Clostridium difficile. Can J Infect Dis 1999;10:170-1.

21. Stolk-Engelaar V, Verwiel J, Bongaerts G, Linsen V, Lacquet L, Cox A. Pleural empyema due to Clostridium difficile and Clostridium cadaveris. Clin Infect Dis 1997;25:160.

22. Granok AB, Mahon PA, Biesek GW. Clostridium septicum empyema in an immunocompetent woman. Case Rep Med 2010;231738.

23. Mayall BC, Snashall EA, Peel MM. Isolation of Clostridium tetani from anaerobic empyema. Pathology 1998;30:402-4.

24. Jonsson S, Clarridge J, Young EJ. Necrotizing pneumonia and empyema caused by Bacillus cereus and Clostridium bifermentans. Am Rev Respir Dis 1983;127:357-9.

25. Misra DP, Hurst DJ. Necrotising pneumonia and empyema caused by Clostridium bifermentans. Thorax 1980;35:310-11.

28

Pasteurella multocida non-native joint infection after a dog lick: A case report describing a complicated two-stage revision and a comprehensive review of the literature

Philip W Lam BScPhm MD[1], Andrea V Page BScH MSc MD FRCPC[1,2]

PW Lam, AV Page. *Pasteurella multocida* non-native joint infection after a dog lick: A case report describing a complicated two-stage revision and a comprehensive review of the literature. Can J Infect Dis Med Microbiol 2015;26(4):212-217.

Prosthetic joint infections (PJIs) are commonly caused by pathogens such as *Staphylococcus aureus* and coagulase-negative staphylococci; however, other microbial etiologies and specific risk factors are increasingly recognized. *Pasteurella multocida* is a Gram-negative coccobacillus that is part of the normal oral flora in many animals, and is particularly common in dogs and cats. PJIs caused by *P multocida* have been reported only rarely in the literature and typically occur in the context of an animal bite or scratch. The present article describes a *P multocida* joint infection that occurred after a dog lick and complicated a two-stage revision arthroplasty. A comprehensive review of the literature regarding *P multocida* PJIs follows.

Key Words: *Dog bite; Dog lick;* Pasteurella multocida, *Prosthetic joint infection*

L'infection à *Pasteurella multocida* non indigène d'une articulation léchée par un chien : rapport de cas d'une révision compliquée en deux étapes et analyse bibliographique approfondie

Les infections sur prothèse articulaire (IPA) sont souvent causées par des pathogènes comme le *Staphylococcus aureus* et les staphylocoques à coagulase négative. Cependant, on constate de plus en plus d'autres étiologies microbiennes et de facteurs de risque particuliers. Le *Pasteurella multocida*, un coccobacille à Gram négatif qui fait partie de la flore orale normale de nombreux animaux, est particulièrement courant chez les chiens et les chats. Peu d'IPA causées par le *P multocida* sont signalées dans les publications scientifiques, mais elles se produisent surtout après une morsure ou une griffure d'animal. Le présent article décrit une infection à *P multocida* qui s'est manifestée après que l'articulation a été léchée par un chien et une arthroplastie de révision compliquée en deux étapes. Une analyse bibliographique approfondie de l'IPA à *P multocida* suit.

Prosthetic joint infections (PJIs) are common, occurring in approximately 1% to 2% of all joint replacements (1). Bacterial seeding of the prosthetic joint can occur during surgery or afterward via hematogenous spread. Pathogens such as *Staphylococcus aureus* and coagulase-negative staphylococci account for the majority of PJIs; however, other factors, such as the joint involved, timing of infection postoperatively, and comorbidities, can influence the microbiology (1). Risk factors for PJIs include older age, diabetes, rheumatoid arthritis, immunosuppressive medications, malignancy and history of arthroplasty revision (1). Perioperative factors, such as hematoma formation, superficial surgical site infection, wound drainage and wound dehiscence, have also been identified as risk factors (1).

In the present report, we describe a two-stage revision arthroplasty that was complicated by a *Pasteurella multocida* joint infection following a dog lick, and present a comprehensive review of the literature surrounding *P multocida* PJIs.

CASE PRESENTATION

A 55-year-old woman presented to the emergency department with a five-day history of chills, progressive right hip pain and difficulty ambulating. Her medical history was significant for a right total hip arthroplasty eight years previously due to osteoarthritis and severe obesity. She experienced an acute postoperative wound infection requiring irrigation and debridement and a second infection two years later requiring a staged revision. One year before presentation, she began to experience a series of monomicrobial PJIs that were treated with a combination of surgery and antimicrobial therapy as follows: *Staphylococcus lugdunensis* (two-stage revision, ceftriaxone), *Klebsiella*

pneumoniae (irrigation and debridement with liner exchange, ciprofloxacin), coagulase-negative *Staphylococcus* (first stage of a planned two-stage revision with cement spacer, vancomycin) and *Candida albicans* (cement spacer exchange, fluconazole). Two months before presentation, she underwent excision of all hardware in the hip as part of a planned two-stage joint revision given recurrent infections with the cement spacer in situ. At that time, she received a six-week course of ertapenem for a joint infection with class A extended-spectrum beta-lactamase (ESBL)-producing *Escherichia coli*, with a vacuum-assisted wound dressing of the surgical site.

At presentation, she was afebrile, but examination of the right hip revealed a nonhealing, erythematous wound with purulent discharge. She had leukocytosis (13,320 cells/µL) and elevated inflammatory markers (erythrocyte sedimentation rate 68 mm/s, C-reactive protein 132 mg/L), and was immediately taken to the operating room for irrigation and debridement.

Diagnosis

Three of three operative cultures of synovial tissue and fluid were positive for *P multocida* (susceptible to ceftriaxone, imipenem, levofloxacin, meropenem, penicillin and trimethoprim/sulfamethoxazole) (Table 1) and *Corynebacterium striatum* (susceptible to vancomycin and gentamicin, resistant to erythromycin and penicillin) (Table 2). Bacterial identification was confirmed using fatty acid methyl ester analysis with gas chromatography, and susceptibilities were determined using Sensititre Susceptibility MIC Plates (TREK Diagnostic Systems, USA). Of note, she was also confirmed to be colonized with ESBL-producing organisms based on rectal swabs obtained as part of routine infection control screening practices then in place. On further

[1]Department of Medicine, University of Toronto; [2]Division of Infectious Diseases, Mount Sinai Hospital, Toronto, Ontario
Correspondence: Dr Andrea V Page, Mount Sinai Hospital, Suite 427, 600 University Avenue, Toronto, Ontario M5G 1X5.
e-mail apage@mtsinai.on.ca

TABLE 1
In vitro susceptibility profile of *Pasteurella multocida* isolate

Antimicrobial agent	Susceptibility	MIC, µg/mL
Ceftriaxone	Susceptible	≤0.03
Imipenem	Susceptible	≤0.5
Levofloxacin	Susceptible	≤0.03
Meropenem	Susceptible	≤0.06
Penicillin	Susceptible	0.12
Trimethroprim/sulfamethoxazole	Susceptible	≤0.06

MIC Minimum inhibitory concentration

TABLE 2
In vitro susceptibility profile of *Corynebacterium striatum* isolate

Antimicrobial agent	Susceptibility	MIC, µg/mL
Erythromycin	Resistant	≥4
Gentamicin	Susceptible	≤2
Penicillin	Resistant	8
Vancomycin	Susceptible	0.5

MIC Minimum inhibitory concentration

questioning, she was found to live with five dogs and two cats, and reported allowing her dogs to lick a superficial laceration on her right lower leg that she had sustained in a fall just before symptom onset; she denied allowing her pets to lick her surgical wound site. On the basis of her most recent culture results and known ESBL colonization, she was treated with intravenous vancomycin and ertapenem for six weeks. One month following admission, she was discharged to a rehabilitation facility with instructions to avoid close pet contact with any unhealed or open wounds. She responded well to antimicrobial therapy and a vacuum-assisted dressing. Two months later, the patient underwent the second stage of her planned two-stage revision, with hip prosthesis re-implantation without complications. She remains free of infection after 10 months of follow-up.

DISCUSSION

P multocida is a Gram-negative coccobacillus that is part of the normal oral flora in many animals, including domestic dogs and cats (2,3). Infections caused by *P multocida* may follow an animal bite or scratch, and range from cellulitis to septic arthritis and osteomyelitis (4). Respiratory infections can also occur, especially in patients with a history of pulmonary disease or immune suppression (4). Other less common infections include bacteremia, endocarditis, meningitis and intra-abdominal infections (4).

Although our case is unique in that infection occurred after excision arthroplasty in the midst of a two-stage revision, PJIs caused by *P multocida* have been reported in the literature and typically occur in the context of an animal bite or scratch. A comprehensive literature review revealed 32 documented cases of *P multocida* PJIs, all of which involved either the hip or knee joint (Table 3) (5-35).

Of the 32 documented cases, almost all patients had a history of animal contact, with 26 cases of soft tissue injury as a result. Twenty-two of the cases involved cats, while 10 cases involved dogs. Women have been shown to experience cat bites more frequently compared with men (36), and this may explain why 26 of the 32 reported cases of *P multocida* PJIs involved women. Known risk factors for PJIs that were also present in patients with *P multocida* PJIs included older age (mean 66.7 years), rheumatoid arthritis (11 of 32 patients [34.4%]), corticosteroid use (10 of 32 patients [31.3%]), other immunosuppressive therapy (two of 32 patients [6.3%]) and malignancy (one of 32 patients [3.1%]).

The presumed pathogenesis of *P multocida* PJIs following animal contact involves the inoculation of bacteria into soft tissues causing bacteremia and subsequent hematogenous seeding of prosthetic material. This is supported by the fact that most documented cases of *P multocida* PJI occur remote from prosthesis implantation (months to years) and shortly after animal contact (days to weeks) (Table 3). Only two cases documented animal contact >1 month before onset of clinical signs or symptoms (16,31).

Despite the importance of biofilm formation in the pathogenesis of typical PJIs, the characteristics of *P multocida* biofilm formation have not been well studied. Animal strains of *P multocida* have been shown to produce biofilms in vitro (37); however, in vivo evidence is lacking. Romanò et al (31) performed an in vitro spectrophotometric screening with positive control testing in their reported case of *P multocida* PJI but found no biofilm production in their isolate.

The case we presented represents only the sixth documented report of *P multocida* non-native joint infection following a dog lick, and the first to occur after excision arthroplasty. Our patient's extensive history of PJIs requiring multiple surgical revisions likely contributed to the increased risk for subsequent infections. Although the patient's hardware was surgically removed two months before presentation, underlying joint damage likely facilitated bacterial adhesion and infection. We suspect the patient's superficial laceration on the lower leg served as a portal of entry for bacteria from the dog's saliva, facilitating hematogenous spread and seeding of the damaged hip joint. Although direct inoculation of the surgical wound by a dog lick was possible, both the history and the presence of a vacuum dressing made this less likely.

P multocida infections following close pet contact have also occurred with other foreign materials including breast prostheses (38,39), vascular stent graft (40), peritoneal dialysis catheters (41) and hemodialysis lines (42). However, foreign material is not a prerequisite for infection, as illustrated by the present case (postexcision arthroplasty), as well as in three cases of respiratory pasteurellosis, which developed in patients providing palliative care to their pets (43). These cases demonstrate the importance of counselling patients about the risk for zoonotic infection and the steps that can be taken to potentially reduce this risk, including good hand hygiene after pet contact and before dressing changes, covering the wound at all times, avoiding direct pet contact with the surgical site or other wounds, and reporting any animal-induced wounds to a physician. Moreover, facilities that use animal-assisted interventions (also known as pet therapy) should ensure that institution-specific infection control policies are consistent with published guidelines (44) to minimize the risk for zoonotic infection.

Isolates of *P multocida* from human infections continue to be susceptible to most antibiotics including penicillin, amoxicillin-clavulanate, doxycycline, third-generation cephalosporins, fluoroquinolones and carbapenems (45-47). Infections caused by beta-lactamase producing *P multocida* have been reported in respiratory infections but remain uncommon (48,49). It is important to note that while most human isolates remain susceptible to beta-lactams, strains isolated from animals have demonstrated marked resistance to a variety of antibiotics (50). Furthermore, empirical treatment of a PJI in the context of a recent animal bite should be directed against a polymicrobial microbiota including Gram-positive and Gram-negative aerobes, and anaerobes, consistent with the expected oral flora of the animal.

Early cases of *P multocida* PJIs were treated with penicillin alone (6-9,11). Although there were more cases of treatment failure in this group, these patients were also less likely to be treated surgically (Table 3). More recent reports have successfully used a third-generation cephalosporin, beta-lactam/beta-lactamase inhibitor combination or fluoroquinolone in addition to surgical intervention. Interestingly, linezolid, an oxazolidinone with Gram-positive activity has been shown to demonstrate in vitro activity against *P multocida* (51). Ferguson et al (33) successfully treated a penicillin-allergic patient with *P multocida* PJI using a combination of linezolid and ciprofloxacin in conjunction with surgical debridement, joint lavage and replacement of the joint liner. It is unclear whether combination therapy is more effective than monotherapy for the treatment of *P multocida* PJIs, despite several case reports describing the successful use of dual antibiotics (13,20,22,25,26,30,31,33,35). Current guidelines recommend treating

TABLE 3
Literature review of documented *Pasteurella multocida* prosthetic joint infections

Author (reference), year	Age, years/ sex	Risk factors	Site	Time from prosthesis	Animal contact	Time to symptoms	Surgical intervention	Antibiotic treatment*	Outcome
Griffin et al (5), 1975	64/F	RA, CS	TKA	6 months	Cat scratch	2 days	None	Ampicillin	Cure
Maurer et al (6), 1975	55/F	RA, CS	TKA	Years	Dog lick	–	None	Penicillin ×2 weeks	Cure
Sugarman et al (7), 1975	33/F	RA, CS	TKA	5 weeks	Dog lick	–	None	Penicillin ×60 weeks	Failure, revision
Arvan and Goldberg (8), 1978	72/F	NR	TKA	4 months	Cat bite	1 week	Debridement, joint lavage and irrigation/suction drainage (2 weeks)	Penicillin ×55 weeks	Cure
Spagnuolo (9), 1978	72/F	NR	TKA	4 months	Cat bite	5 days	None	Penicillin ×6 weeks	Cure
Gomez-Reino et al (10), 1980	64/F	NR	TKA	3 years	Cat bite	1 day	None	Cephalothin ×6 weeks, cephalexin ×2 weeks	Failure, revision
Mellors and Schoen (11), 1984	68/F	RA, CS	B/L TKA	NR	Cat scratch	4 days	Joint lavage	Penicillin ×6 weeks	Cure
Orton and Fulcher (12), 1984	74/F	NR	B/L TKA	3 years	Cat bite	12 h	None	Ampicillin ×17 days, penicillin + tetracycline ×12 weeks	Failure, revision
Braithwaite and Giddins (13), 1992	48/F	Diabetes	THA	14 years	Cat bite	NR	Single stage revision	Penicillin + flucloxacillin ×6 weeks	Cure
Gabuzda and Barnett (14), 1992	88/F	NR	TKA	10 months	Cat bite	Days	Debridement, removal of prosthesis, placement of cement spacer	Ampicillin/sulbactam ×3 weeks, penicillin ×3 weeks	Cure
Guion and Sculco (15), 1992	45/F	RA, CS	TKA	2 years	Dog scratch	Days	Two-stage revision	Cefotaxime ×6 weeks	Cure
Antuna et al (16), 1997	73/F	RA	TKA	1 year	Dog bite	2 months	Single-stage revision	Ciprofloxacin ×10 weeks	Cure
Maradona et al (17), 1997	73/F	Diabetes	TKA	6 months	Dog bite	45 days	Debridement, joint lavage	Penicillin ×3 weeks, ciprofloxacin ×3 weeks	Cure
Takwale et al (18), 1997	57/F	RA, MTX, CS	THA	12 years	Cat scratch	1 day	Two-stage revision	Benzyl penicillin ×4 weeks, ciprofloxacin ×8 weeks	Cure
Chikwe et al (19), 2000	69/M	NR	THA	4 years	Dog contact	–	Two-stage revision	Unknown	Cure
Ciampolini et al (20), 2004	73/F	NR	TKA	14 months	Cat scratch	2 weeks	Two-stage revision	Benzyl penicillin + ciprofloxacin, amoxicillin + ciprofloxacin ×6 weeks	Cure
Mehta and Mackie (21), 2004	84/F	RA, CS	THA	15 years	Cat scratch	1 month	Single-stage revision	Benzyl penicillin ×1 week, ciprofloxacin ×7 weeks	Cure
Mehta and Mackie (21), 2004	57/F	RA, MTX, CS	THA	10 years	Cat scratch	NR	Two-stage revision	Benzyl penicillin ×4 weeks, ciprofloxacin ×8 weeks	Cure
Polzhofer et al (22), 2004	73/F	NR	TKA	6 months	Cat bite	Days	Arthroscopic debridement, synovectomy, irrigation/suction drainage (6 days)	Ampicillin/sulbactam + clindamycin ×3 weeks	Cure
Stiehl et al (23), 2004	63/M	NR	TKA	12 days	Dog contact, horse injury	–	Two-stage revision	Ciprofloxacin and piperacillin/tazobactam	Cure
Zebeede et al (24) 2004	41/F	SLE, APS, CS	TKA	2 years	Cat scratch	2 weeks	None	Ciprofloxacin ×12 weeks	Cure
Heym et al (25), 2006	72/F	NR	TKA	1 year	Dog lick	3 weeks	Synovectomy, removal with reimplantation	Doxycycline + amoxicillin ×8 weeks	Failure, revision
Serrano et al (26), 2007	79/M	NR	TKA	6 years	Cat scratch	NR	Joint lavage	Amoxicillin/clavulanate ×3 weeks, ciprofloxacin ×4 weeks + TMP/SMX ×12 weeks	Cure
Kadakia and Langkamer (27), 2008	80/F	Breast carcinoma	TKA	9 months	Cat bite	8–10 days	Arthroscopic joint lavage	Cefuroxime ×2 weeks, ciprofloxacin ×8 weeks	Cure

Continued on next page

TABLE 3 – CONTINUED
Literature review of documented *Pasteurella multocida* prosthetic joint infections

Author (reference), year	Age, years/ sex	Risk factors	Site	Time from prosthesis	Animal contact	Time to symptoms	Surgical intervention	Antibiotic treatment*	Outcome
Miranda et al (30), 2013	64/M	NR	TKA	1 year	Cat scratch/ bite	9 days	Joint lavage, debridement, replacement of spacer	Amoxicillin/clavulanate + levofloxacin ×6 weeks	Cure
Romanò et al (31), 2013	82/F	RA	TKA	10 years	Cat scratch	5 months	Debridement and replacement of tibial tray	Amoxicillin/clavulanate ×34 days + ciprofloxacin ×6 weeks	Cure
Subramanian et al (32), 2013	47/M	NR	TKA	23 days	Probable dog lick	–	Debridement, joint lavage and replacement of liner	Cefuroxime ×2 weeks, doxycycline ×6 weeks	Cure
Ferguson et al (33), 2014	67/F	NR	TKA	13 weeks	Dog lick	–	Debridement, joint lavage and replacement of insert	Linezolid ×4 weeks + ciprofloxacin ×8 weeks	Cure
Vélez et al (34), 2014	75/M	NR	TKA	16 months	Cat bite	2 days	Debridement, and replacement of spacer	Ampicillin/sulbactam ×4 weeks, amoxicillin/clavulanate ×24 weeks	Cure
Alsaffar and Gaur (35), 2014	74/F	NR	THA	26 years	Cat bite	4 days	Joint lavage	Amoxicillin + ciprofloxacin ×8 weeks	Cure

Antibiotics separated by commas denote subsequent change in antibiotics, antibiotics separated by plus sign denote concurrent use. APS Antiphospholipid antibody syndrome; B/L Bilateral; CS Corticosteroids; F Female; M Male; MTX Methotrexate; NR Not reported; RA Rheumatoid arthritis; SLE Systemic lupus erythematosus; THA Total hip arthroplasty; TKA Total knee arthroplasty

nonstaphylococcal PJIs with four to six weeks of antimicrobial therapy (52). Of the 29 case reports with documented duration of therapy, 27 were treated with at least four weeks of antibiotics and 16 were treated with >6 weeks of antibiotics (Table 3).

The present report represents the first case of *P multocida* joint infection successfully treated with ertapenem. The decision to treat with ertapenem was based on its documented efficacy in vitro against *P multocida* (45), the patient's positive ESBL screening swabs and history of PJI caused by ESBL-producing organisms and the ease of outpatient dosing. The presence of *C striatum* in all operative cultures also prompted treatment with vancomycin. In one study of the microbiology of infections after animal-induced injuries, *Corynebacterium* species accounted for 12% of aerobic bacteria isolated from infected dog bite wounds (53). However, *Corynebacterium* species are part of normal human skin flora and, therefore, may have entered the wound from the patient's skin postoperatively during prolonged wound healing.

The optimal surgical management of PJIs should be individualized. Our literature review demonstrated a wide spectrum of surgical interventions, including no intervention (seven of 32 patients [21.9%]), lavage only (four of 32 patients [12.5%]), debridement and lavage (four of 32 patients [12.5%]), debridement with replacement of exchangeable components (six of 32 patients [18.8%]), single-stage revision (four of 32 patients [12.5%]) and two-stage revision (six of 32 patients [18.8%]). Earlier case reports of *P multocida* PJIs were more likely to be treated nonoperatively. Of the seven patients treated nonoperatively, three (42.9%) failed antimicrobial therapy alone (7,10,12). The benefits of less-invasive interventions must be balanced with the risk of treatment failure. Algorithms have been developed by expert panels to identify patients with PJIs suitable for less-invasive interventions (52,54). Factors in the algorithm include duration of illness, extent of soft tissue infection, presence of coexisting illness, surgical risk, stability of implant and bacterial susceptibility to antibiotics (52,54). However, these algorithms do not specifically address PJIs associated with zoonotic pathogens. Our patient underwent irrigation and debridement because there was no prosthetic material present at the time of infection.

Several authors of previous case reports have advocated for the use of prophylactic antibiotics in all individuals with a prosthetic joint

who have sustained an animal bite, especially if other risk factors are present (such as rheumatoid arthritis or corticosteroid use). Proposed antibiotics include penicillin (9), oxacillin (12), amoxicillin (18), cefuroxime (18) and amoxicillin/clavulanate (20). Recent guidelines have recommended antibiotic prophylaxis in all individuals with bite wounds at high risk for developing infection, such as those with significant immunocompromise (diabetes, steroid use, HIV, peripheral vascular disease), advanced liver disease, edema of the affected area and wounds involving deeper structures (55). To our knowledge, the use of prophylactic antibiotics following an animal bite or scratch in individuals with a prosthetic joint has not been directly addressed.

CONCLUSION

The present report represents the sixth documented case of *P multocida* non-native joint infection following a dog lick, and the first to occur in the midst of a two-stage revision. The accompanying literature review of PJIs caused by *P multocida* is the most comprehensive performed to date and includes all 32 cases reported in the literature. While PJIs due to *P multocida* classically occur following an animal bite or scratch, our review highlights the fact that penetrating trauma is not a prerequisite for infection. It is important for clinicians to ask about animal exposure when evaluating a patient with a PJI, particularly if the infection has occurred remote from the surgery, so that the appropriate empirical therapy can be chosen. Our literature review also documented other risk factors that may increase the risk for *P multocida* PJI following an animal-induced wound, including rheumatoid arthritis, corticosteroids, other immunosuppressive therapy and malignancy. In light of the case presented here, it is reasonable to counsel patients about the risk for zoonotic infections of surgical wounds and the steps that can be taken to potentially reduce this risk, such as maintaining good hand hygiene after pet contact, keeping wounds covered, avoiding direct pet contact with any unhealed, uncovered or open wounds, and reporting all significant animal-induced wounds to a physician.

DISCLOSURES: The authors have no financial disclosures or conflicts of interest to declare.

REFERENCES

1. Tande AJ, Patel R. Prosthetic joint infection. Clin Microbiol Rev 2014;27:302-345.
2. Elliott DR, Wilson M, Buckley CMF, Spratt DA. Cultivable oral microbiota of domestic dogs. J Clin Microbiol 2005;43:5470-76.
3. Freshwater A. Why your housecat's trite little bite could cause you quite a fright: A study of domestic felines on the occurrence and antibiotic susceptibility of Pasteurella multocida. Zoonoses Public Health 2008;55:507-13.
4. Weber DJ, Wolfson JS, Swartz MN, Hooper DC. Pasteurella multocida infections. Report of 34 cases and review of the literature. Medicine (Baltimore) 1984;63:133-154.
5. Griffin AJ, Barber HM. Letter: Joint infection by Pasteurella multocida. Lancet 1975;1:1347-48.
6. Maurer KH, Hasselbacher P, Schumacher HR. Letter: Joint infection by Pasteurella multocida. Lancet 1975;2:409.
7. Sugarman M, Quismorio FP, Patzakis MJ. Letter: Joint infection by Pasteurella multocida. Lancet 1975;2:1267.
8. Arvan GD, Goldberg V. A case report of total knee arthroplasty infected by Pasteurella multocida. Clin Orthop Relat Res 1978;132:167-9.
9. Spagnuolo PJ. Pasteurella multocida infectious arthritis. Am J Med Sci 1978;275:359-63.
10. Gomez-Reino JJ, Shah M, Gorevic P, Lusskin R. Pasteurella multocida arthritis. Case report. J Bone Joint Surg Am 1980;62:1212-13.
11. Mellors JW, Schoen RT. Pasteurella multocida prosthetic joint infection. Ann Emerg Med 1985;14:617.
12. Orton DW, Fulcher WH. Pasteurella multocida: Bilateral septic knee joint prostheses from a distant cat bite. Ann Emerg Med 1984;13:1065-67.
13. Braithwaite BD, Giddins G. Pasteurella multocida infection of a total hip arthroplasty. A case report. J Arthroplasty 1992;7:309-10.
14. Gabuzda GM, Barnett PR. Pasteurella infection in a total knee arthroplasty. Orthop Rev 1992;21:601, 604-5.
15. Guion TL, Sculco TP. Pasteurella multocida infection in total knee arthroplasty. Case report and literature review. J Arthroplasty 1992;7:157-60.
16. Antuna SA, Mendez JG, Castellanos JL, Jimenez JP. Late infection after total knee arthroplasty caused by Pasteurella multocida. Acta Orthop Belg 1997;63:310-12.
17. Maradona JA, Asensi V, Carton JA, Rodriguez Guardado A, Lizon Castellano J. Prosthetic joint infection by Pasteurella multocida. Eur J Clin Microbiol Infect Dis 1997;16:623-25.
18. Takwale VJ, Wright ED, Bates J, Edge AJ. Pasteurella multocida infection of a total hip arthroplasty following cat scratch. J Infect 1997;34:263-64.
19. Chikwe J, Bowditch M, Villar RN, Bedford AF. Sleeping with the enemy: Pasteurella multocida infection of a hip replacement. J R Soc Med 2000;93:478-9.
20. Ciampolini J, Timperley J, Morgan M. Prosthetic joint infection by cat scratch. J R Soc Med 2004;97:441-2.
21. Mehta H, Mackie I. Prosthetic joint infection with Pasturella multocida following cat scratch: A report of 2 cases. J Arthroplasty 2004;19:525-527.
22. Polzhofer GK, Hassenpflug J, Petersen W. Arthroscopic treatment of septic arthritis in a patient with posterior stabilized total knee arthroplasty. Arthroscopy 2004;20:311-13.
23. Stiehl JB, Sterkin LA, Brummitt CF. Acute Pasteurella multocida in total knee arthroplasty. J Arthroplasty 2004;19:244-47.
24. Zebeede E, Levinger U, Weinberger A. Pasteurella multocida infectious arthritis. Isr Med Assoc J 2004;6:778-9.
25. Heym B, Jouve F, Lemoal M, Veil-Picard A, Lortat-Jacob A, Nicolas-Chanoine MH. Pasteurella multocida infection of a total knee arthroplasty after a "dog lick". Knee Surg Sports Traumatol Arthrosc 2006;14:993-7.
26. Serrano MT, Menéndez JN, García Bde L, Fernández ML. Infección de prótesis articular de rodilla por Pasteurella multocida. Enferm Infecc Microbiol Clin 2007;25:492.
27. Kadakia AP, Langkamer VG. Sepsis of total knee arthroplasty after domestic cat bite: Should we warn patients? Am J Orthop 2008;37:370-371.
28. Blanco JF, Pescador D, Martin JM, Cano C, Sanchez MD. Acute infection of total knee arthroplasty due to a cat scratch in a patient with rheumatoid arthritis. J Clin Rheumatol 2012;18:314-15.
29. Heydemann J, Heydemann JS, Antony S. Acute infection of a total knee arthroplasty caused by Pasteurella multocida: A case report and a comprehensive review of the literature in the last 10 years. Int J Infect Dis 2010;14(Suppl 3):e242-5.
30. Miranda I, Angulo M, Amaya JV. Acute total knee replacement infection after a cat bite and scratch: A clinical case and review of the literature. Rev Esp Cir Ortop Traumatol 2013;57:300-5.
31. Romanò CL, De Vecchi E, Vassena C, Manzi G, Drago L. A case of a late and atypical knee prosthetic infection by no-biofilm producer Pasteurella multocida strain identified by pyrosequencing. Pol J Microbiol 2013;62:435-8.
32. Subramanian B, Holloway E, Townsend R, Sutton P. Infected total knee arthroplasty due to postoperative wound contamination with Pasteurella multocida. BMJ Case Rep 2013;2013:10.1136/bcr-2013-009973.
33. Ferguson KB, Bharadwaj R, MacDonald A, Syme B, Bal AM. Pasteurella multocida infected total knee arthroplasty: A case report and review of the literature. Ann R Coll Surg Engl 2014;96:e1-4.
34. Velez FA, Laboy Ortiz IE, Lopez R, Sanchez A, Colon M, Hernan Martinez J. Pasteurella multocida: A nightmare for a replaced joint and the challenge to save it. Bol Asoc Med PR 2014;106:43-5.
35. Alsaffar L, Gaur S. Acute infection of a total hip arthroplasty by Pasteurella multocida successfully treated with antibiotics and joint washout. J Med Cases 2014;5:411-12.
36. MacBean CE, Taylor DM, Ashby K. Animal and human bite injuries in Victoria, 1998-2004. Med J Aust 2007;186:38-40.
37. Olson ME, Ceri H, Morck DW, Buret AG, Read RR. Biofilm bacteria: Formation and comparative susceptibility to antibiotics. Can J Vet Res 2002;66:86-92.
38. Johnson LB, Busuito MJ, Khatib R. Breast implant infection in a cat owner due to Pasteurella multocida. J Infect 2000;41:110-11.
39. Mathieu D, Rodriguez H, Jacobs F. Breast prosthesis infected by Pasteurella multocida. Acta Clin Belg 2008;63:351.
40. Silberfein EJ, Lin PH, Bush RL, Zhou W, Lumsden AB. Aortic endograft infection due to Pasteurella multocida following a rabbit bite. J Vasc Surg 2006;43:393-5.
41. Sol PM, van de Kar NC, Schreuder MF. Cat induced Pasteurella multocida peritonitis in peritoneal dialysis: A case report and review of the literature. Int J Hyg Environ Health 2013;216:211-13.
42. Boinett C, Gonzalez A. Pasteurella multocida septicaemia in a patient on haemodialysis. BMJ Case Rep 2009;2009:10.1136/bcr.01.2009.1492.
43. Myers EM, Ward SL, Myers JP. Life-threatening respiratory pasteurellosis associated with palliative pet care. Clin Infect Dis 2012;54:e55-7.
44. Writing Panel of Working Group, Lefebvre SL, Golab GC, et al. Guidelines for animal-assisted interventions in health care facilities. Am J Infect Control 2008;36:78-85.
45. Goldstein EJ, Citron DM, Merriam CV, Warren YA, Tyrrell K, Fernandez H. Comparative in vitro activity of ertapenem and 11 other antimicrobial agents against aerobic and anaerobic pathogens isolated from skin and soft tissue animal and human bite wound infections. J Antimicrob Chemother 2001;48:641-51.
46. Goldstein EJ, Citron DM, Merriam CV, Warren YA, Tyrrell KL, Fernandez HT. Comparative in vitro activity of faropenem and 11 other antimicrobial agents against 405 aerobic and anaerobic pathogens isolated from skin and soft tissue infections from animal and human bites. J Antimicrob Chemother 2002;50:411-20.
47. Lion C, Conroy MC, Carpentier AM, Lozniewski A. Antimicrobial susceptibilities of Pasteurella strains isolated from humans. Int J Antimicrob Agents 2006;27:290-93.
48. Lion C, Lozniewski A, Rosner V, Weber M. Lung abscess due to beta-lactamase-producing Pasteurella multocida. Clin Infect Dis 1999;29:1345-46.
49. Rosenau A, Labigne A, Escande F, Courcoux P, Philippon A. Plasmid-mediated ROB-1 beta-lactamase in Pasteurella multocida from a human specimen. Antimicrob Agents Chemother 1991;35:2419-22.
50. Kehrenberg C, Schulze-Tanzil G, Martel JL, Chaslus-Dancla E, Schwarz S. Antimicrobial resistance in pasteurella and mannheimia: epidemiology and genetic basis. Vet Res 2001;32:323-39.

51. Goldstein EJ, Citron DM, Merriam CV. Linezolid activity compared to those of selected macrolides and other agents against aerobic and anaerobic pathogens isolated from soft tissue bite infections in humans. Antimicrob Agents Chemother 1999;43:1469-74.

52. Osmon DR, Berbari EF, Berendt AR, et al. Executive summary: Diagnosis and management of prosthetic joint infection: Clinical practice guidelines by the Infectious Diseases Society of America. Clin Infect Dis 2013;56:1-10.

53. Abrahamian FM, Goldstein EJ. Microbiology of animal bite wound infections. Clin Microbiol Rev 2011;24:231-46.

54. Leone S, Borre S, Monforte A, et al. Consensus document on controversial issues in the diagnosis and treatment of prosthetic joint infections. Int J Infect Dis 2010;14 Suppl 4:S67-77.

55. Stevens DL, Bisno AL, Chambers HF, et al. Practice guidelines for the diagnosis and management of skin and soft tissue infections: 2014 update by the Infectious Diseases Society of America. Clin Infect Dis 2014;59:147-59.

29

Bacteremia due to *Pasteurella dagmatis* acquired from a dog bite, with a review of systemic infections and challenges in laboratory identification

Jianhui Xiong PhD[1], Sigmund Krajden MD[2,3,5], Julianne V Kus PhD[4,5], Prasad Rawte MSc[4], John Blondal MD[3], Mark Downing MD[2,3], Urszula Zurawska MD[3], William Chapman MD[1,5]

J Xiong, S Krajden, JV Kus, et al. Bacteremia due to *Pasteurella dagmatis* acquired from a dog bite, with a review of systemic infections and challenges in laboratory identification. Can J Infect Dis Med Microbiol 2015;26(5):273-276.

A case of bacteremia in a 74-year-old man, which was caused by *Pasteurella dagmatis* and complicated by thrombocytopenia, is presented. Microorganism identification was performed by the provincial reference laboratory using traditional biochemical profiling, complemented with both the sequencing of the 16S ribosomal RNA gene and matrix-assisted laser desorption/ionization time-of-flight mass spectrometry; antibiotic-susceptibility testing was also performed. After treatment with the appropriate antibiotics, the patient fully recovered. Systemic infections attributed to this organism are rarely reported in the literature. Other reported cases of bacteremia due to *P dagmatis* are reviewed and compared with the present case. The challenges of relying on standard automatic identification are discussed, with alternative methodologies provided.

Key Words: *16S rRNA gene sequencing; Bacteremia; Dog bite; Identification; MALDI-ToF MS; Pasteurella dagmatis; VITEK 2*

Une bactériémie à *Pasteurella dagmatis* contractée par une morsure de chien, une analyse des infections systémiques et les difficultés pour le dépistage en laboratoire

Les auteurs présentent un cas de bactériémie chez un homme de 74 ans, causé par un *Pasteurella dagmatis* et compliqué par une thrombocytopénie. Le laboratoire de référence provincial a identifié le microorganisme au moyen du profilage biochimique classique et l'a complété par le séquençage du gène de l'ARN ribosomique 16S et par la spectrométrie de masse à temps de vol par désorption-ionisation laser assistée par matrice. Le laboratoire a également effectué un test de susceptibilité aux antibiotiques. Après un traitement antibiotique pertinent, le patient s'est complètement rétabli. Les publications scientifiques contiennent peu de déclarations d'infections systémiques attribuées à cet organisme. D'autres cas de bactériémie à *P dagmatis* sont analysés et comparés à la présente situation. Les problèmes liés à l'identification automatique standard sont exposés et d'autres méthodologies sont proposées.

CASE PRESENTATION

A 74-year-old man startled his dog and sustained a penetrating bite to his hand. The dog then licked the blood off the injured extremity. A few days later, the patient developed fever, chills and weakness, resulting in a fall. He presented to the emergency room for assessment. Medical history and significant comorbidities included chronic obstructive pulmonary disease, hypertension, dyslipidemia and idiopathic dilated cardiomyopathy, Grade 3 left ventricle. No immunocompromising illnesses were present. Physical examination revealed a temperature of 40°C, with bronchial breath sounds and crackles heard in the left chest; the bite wound appeared improved. A chest x-ray revealed a left perihilar infiltrate. Peripheral white blood cell count was 15.5×10^9/L, neutrophils 13.4×10^9/L, hemoglobin 126 g/L and platelet nadir $14,000\times10^9$/L. The patient was admitted for further investigation and treatment. Blood cultures grew coagulase-negative *Staphylococcus*, which was considered to be a contaminant, and Gram-negative coccobacilli were later determined to be *Pasteurella dagmatis*. Treatment was initiated with oral azithromycin 500 mg per day and intravenous ceftriaxone 1 g every 24 h for five days. The patient defervesced within four days and his condition improved dramatically. Oral levofloxacin 500 mg was administered as step-down therapy for 10 days. The hematological abnormalities resolved. On follow-up three months later, he remained well.

Laboratory findings

Two sets of blood cultures were drawn 5 h apart from the patient on the day of admission using BD BACTEC PLUS aerobic/F and anaerobic/F bottles (Becton, Dickinson and Company, Canada). Three bottles produced Gram-negative coccobacilli with beaded ends in 14 h to 34 h, and one anaerobic/F bottle also produced Gram-positive cocci in clusters, which were subsequently identified as coagulase-negative staphylococci; this organism was considered to be a contaminant. The subcultures on blood agar plates produced tiny grey-brown creamy colonies, which did not grow on MacConkey agar. The Gram-negative coccobacilli were initially identified as *Pasturella pneumotropica* by the VITEK 2 system, software version 06.01 (BioMerieux, France) using the GN card, with bionumber 0001010210040001 and an excellent identification (probability 99%). Unusual bacteria such as this are routinely sent to the local reference laboratory (Public Health Ontario, Toronto, Ontario) for confirmation of identification and susceptibility testing. The susceptibility profile of the bacterium was interpreted by CLSI M45-A2 (1) (Table 1).The biochemical characteristics (Table 2), 16S ribosomal RNA (rRNA) gene polymerase chain reaction (PCR) and sequencing (below), as well as matrix-assisted laser desorption/ionization time-of-flight mass spectrometry (MALDI-ToF MS) were used for identification of the bacterium.

[1]*Department of Laboratory Medicine;* [2]*Division of Infectious Diseases;* [3]*Internal Medicine of St Joseph's Health Centre;* [4]*Public Health Ontario;* [5]*Department of Laboratory Medicine and Pathobiology, University of Toronto, Toronto, Ontario*

Correspondence: Dr Sigmund Krajden, Department of Internal Medicine, St Joseph's Health Centre, 30 The Queensway, Toronto, Ontario M6R 1B5 .e-mail krajds@stjoe.on.ca

TABLE 1
Antibiotic susceptibility of *Pasteurella dagmatis*

Antibiotic	Mininmum inhibitory concentration, mg/L	Interpretation
Penicillin	0.12	Sensitive
Ampicillin	≤2	Sensitive
Pipercillin/tazobactum	≤4	Sensitive
Cefazolin	≤4	Sensitive
Ceftazidime/ceftriaxone	≤1	Sensitive
Meropenem	≤0.25	Sensitive
Gentamicin/tobramycin	≤1	Sensitive
Ciprofloxacin	≤0.25	Sensitive
Levofloxacin	≤0.03	Sensitive
Trimetoprim/sulfamethoxazole	≤20	Sensitive

Analysis performed using VITEK 2 (BioMerieux, France) and agar dilution as per the Clinical and Laboratory Standards Institute (1)

TABLE 2
Key biochemical characteristics of *Pasteurella dagmatis*, *P stomatis* and *P pneumotropica*

	P dagmatis	P stomatis	P pneumotropica
Dextrose	+	+	n/a
Lactose	–	–	–
Sucrose	+	+	+
Xylose	–	–	+
Mannitol	–	–	–
Maltose	+	–	+
Arabinose	–	–	V
Sorbitol	–	–	–
Trelose	+	+	+
Dulcitol	–	–	–
Catalase	+	+	+
Oxidase	+	+	+
TSI slant/butt	+/+	+/+	+/+
Indole	+	+	+
Urea activity	+	–	+
Nitrate to nitrite	+	+	+
Motility	–	–	–
Ornithine	–	–	+
Arginine	–	–	n/a
Lysine	–	–	V
Ortho-nitrophenyl-β-galactoside	–	–	+

Data presented as positive (+) or negative (–). Reactions refer to reference 2. n/a Not available; V Variable;

Biochemical profile

Traditional biochemical testing was performed on the isolate and based on its profile was determined to be *P dagmatis* (2) (Table 2). Because this organism is not often encountered, alternate identification methods were also used to ensure a correct identification.

16S rRNA gene PCR/sequencing

16S rRNA gene PCR was performed at Public Health Ontario. A 736-base pair amplicon was generated (primers, forward: 5'-AGTTTGATCCTGGCTCAG–3'; Reverse: 5'-GGACTACCAGGGTATCTAAT–3') and sequenced using routine methods (3). The sequence was analyzed using National Center for Biotechnology Information basic local alignment search tool (4) and results were interpreted using CLSI MM18-A guidelines (5). The PCR product was 99% similar to six deposits within the nr/nt database with 99% to 100% coverage. Sequences with high

TABLE 3
Summary of reports involving bacteremia in humans with *Pasteuralla dagmatis* in the English literature

Patient age, years/sex	Animal bites	Diagnosis	Antibiotic Treatment	Outcome	Reference
78/male	None	Prosthetic valve endocarditis	Ceftriaxone	Survived	10
66/male	None	Septicemia	Penicillin	Recovered	11
51/male	Dog	Septicemia, diabetic foot	Penicillin	Resolved	12
55/female	Cat	Infectious endocarditis thrombocytopenia	Ceftriaxone	Survived	14
77/male	Cat	Prosthetic valve endocarditis	Ceftriaxone, penicillin	Recovered	15
56/female	Dog	Peritonitis, septicemia, cirrhosis	Benzypenicillin, ciprofloxacin, metronidazole	Passed away within 24 h	16

levels of homology to the query sequence included the type strain of *P dagmatis*, ATCC 43325/CCUG 12397 (99%; NR_042883.1 and M75051.1) and the type strain of *Pasteurella stomatis*, CCUG 17979 (99%; NR_042888.1). Based on CLSI MM18-A interpretation guidelines (5), due to the low level of demarcation of the sequence of the 16S rRNA gene between these species, the unknown bacteria may only be identified as *P dagmatis* or *P stomatis*. However, based on the biochemical profile (Table 2), this organism could not be *P stomatis* (which is urease and maltose negative, because the organism in question is urease and maltose positive); therefore, in the present case, the identification of the organism was *P dagmatis*.

MALDI-ToF MS

Single colonies of fresh organisms grown overnight were prepared using a modified formic acid extraction procedure and analyzed using the Bruker MALDI BioTyper (Bruker Daltonics, Germany) in duplicate using standard settings. The query spectra had a high level of similarity >2.0 (≥2.0 is an acceptable score for species-level identification) to *P dagmatis* spectra within the routine commercial database. The top five matches were to spectra from different strains of *P dagmatis* within the commercial database.

DISCUSSION AND LITERATURE REVIEW

P dagmatis is a relatively new species for many clinicians. It is a Gram-negative coccobacillus belonging to the *Pasteurellaceae* family, which is fermentative, aerobic, nonmotile, oxidase positive and penicillin-sensitive. This organism has been isolated from both dogs and cats as normal flora, and also reported as a pathogen in human infections. It was previously labeled as *Pasteurella* "gas", *Pasteurella* new species 1 or *P pneumotropica* type Henriksen, and was eventually reclassified as *P dagmatis* (6).

Bacteria from the *Pasteurellaceae* family cause zoonotic infections in humans, with *P multocida* and *P canis* being the most common *Pasturella* species reported in human infections (7,8). Infections caused by *Pasteurella* species are typically introduced by animals, particularly cat or dog bites, but also occasionally by other animals, and often manifest as skin or soft tissue infections (7-9). Sometimes, animal contact is not prominent in the initial patient history (10,11) (Table 3). The most probable route of transmission of *P dagmatis* infection in the present case was most likely the bite and licking of the patient's traumatized skin by his dog, as has been previously described (11,12). Continuous shedding of *P dagmatis* from asymptomatic animals (eg, in dog urine [13]) and whether it can be an indirect route of infection to human remains to be investigated.

While *Pasteurella* species are well recognized for causing skin or soft tissue infections, *P dagmatis* can also cause more serious disease, including infective and prosthetic valve endocarditis (10,14,15), septicemia (11,12,16), peritonitis (17), vertebral osteomyelitis (18,19), chronic bronchiectasis (20) and pneumonia (21), mainly in immunocompromised patients. A small number of case reports describing systemic human *P dagmatis* infections are listed in Table 3. Interestingly, while *Pasturella* species infrequently cause systemic infectious disease, in our review of the literature, when *P dagmatis* infections are reported, they appear to be frequently associated with severe disseminated infection including bacteremia. Coinfections of *P dagmatis* with another *Pasturella* species have also been observed (9,12,22); therefore, it is important for the laboratory to test multiple morphotypes from the plate to ensure that >1 *Pasturella* species is not present.

Similar to other *Pasturella* species, *P dagmatis* is typically highly susceptible to many antibiotics, particularly, the beta-lactams (Table 1). Early suspicion and timely laboratory diagnosis of *Pasturella* infection are crucial for a favourable clinical outcome.

Several reports have demonstrated that the VITEK 2 GN card misidentifies *P dagmatis* as *P pneumotropica* or *P canis*, despite an excellent identification probability (9,15,23,24). This is most likely because *P dagmatis* has not been included in the system database; as well, there has been a nomenclature change because *P dagmatis* was formerly grouped with *P pneumotropica*, type Henriksen. In a study that included 66 clinical *Pasturella* isolates and used *sodA* gene sequencing as a reference method, Zangenah et al (24) revealed that VITEK 2 only identified approximately 50% of *Pasturella* isolates correctly, while conventional biochemical tests and MALDI-ToF MS were able to correctly identify 94% and 89%, respectively. Interestingly, in the Zangenah et al (24) study, two *P dagmatis* isolates were not identified by VITEK MS MALDI-ToF (BioMerieux, France) and this limitation was also observed in our study (data not shown). The biological and genetic profiles among *P dagmatis*, *P pneumotropica* and *P stomatis* are very similar (Table 2); both a commercial biochemical identification system and the sequence analysis of a portion of the 16S rRNA gene were unable to differentiate between these species.

Correct identification was made using MALDI-ToF MS (MALDI Biotyper, Bruker, Germany) and was also supported by comparing the key biochemical characteristics among *P dagmatis*, *P pneumotropica* and *P stomatis* (Table 2). It is probable that many clinical isolates of *P dagmatis* have been misidentified due to the limitation of commercial biochemical identification systems, such as VITEK 2. Misidentification may have contributed to an underestimation of the frequency of this organism in clinical samples; however, the growing use of MALDI-ToF MS systems for microorganism identification in routine clinical microbiology laboratories may allow for a more accurate picture of how frequently *P dagmatis* causes infections. Correct identification is important for diagnosis and therapeutic management, and epidemiological monitoring of the transmission of *Pasturella* species, particularly for the systemic infections such as in the present case. Unfortunately, most routine methods available at hospital laboratories cannot identify the organism correctly.

CONCLUSION

P dagmatis can cause severe animal-associated infections in humans, mainly in immunocompromised individuals. To our knowledge, this is the first systemic *P dagmatis* infection reported in Canada. Clinical outcomes rely on early accurate laboratory confirmation and timely administration of effective antibiotic treatment. Conventional identification of *P dagmatis* using VITEK 2 can be misleading, probably due to the absence of this organism from the database; 16S rRNA gene sequence analysis and MALDI-ToF MS systems represent excellent options for identifying rarely encountered or difficult to identify organisms, such as members of the *Pasturellaceae* family. The present study re-emphasizes the need for continuously improving the database of automatic microbial identification systems.

ACKNOWLEDGEMENTS: The authors thank the microbiology laboratory staff from SJHC and PHOL for their help and support of this study.

DISCLOSURES: The authors have no financial relationships or conflicts of interest to declare.

REFERENCES

1. Clinical and Laboratory Standards Institute. Methods for antimicrobial dilution and disk susceptibility testing of infrequently isolated or fastidious bacteria; approved guideline – second edition. CLSI document M45-A2. Wayne: 19087-1898. Clinical and Laboratory Standards Institute; 2010.

2. Weyant R, Moss CW, Weaver RE, et al. Identification of unusual pathogenic Gram-negative aerobic and facultatively anaerobic bacteria. In: Hensyl WR, 2nd edn. Philadelphia: Lippincott Williams and Wilkins, 1996:445-67.

3. Knox M, Cevellos V, and Dean D. 16S ribosomal DNA typing for identification of pathogens in patients with bacterial keratitis. J Clin Microbiol 1998;36:3492-6.

4. Altschul SF, Gish W, Miller W, Myers EW, Lipman DJ. Basic local alignment search tool. J Mol Biol 1990;215:403-10.

5. Clinical and Laboratory Standards Institute. Interpretive criteria for identification of bacteria and fungi by DNA target sequencing; approved guideline – first edition. CLSI document MM18-A. Wayne: 19087-1898. Clinical and Laboratory Standards Institute; 2008.

6. Mutters R, Ihm P, Pohl S, Frederiksen W, Mannheim W. Reclassification of the genus *Pasteurella* trevisan 1887 on the basis of deoxyribonucleic acid homology, with proposals for the new species *Pasteurella dagmatis*, *Pasteurella canis*, *Pasteurella stomatis*, *Pasteurella anatis*, and *Pasteurella langaa*. Int J Sys Bacteriol 1985; 35:309-22.

7. Abrahamian FM, Goldstein EJC. Microbiology of animal bite wound infections. Clin Microbiol Rev 2011;24:231-46.

8. Talan DA, Citron DM, Abrahamian FM, Moran GJ, Goldstein EJC. Bacteriological analysis of infected dog and cat bites. N Engl J Med 1999;340:85-92.

9. Akahane T, Nagata M, Matsumoto T, et al. A case of wound dual infection with *Pasteurella dagmatis* and *Pasteurella canis* resulting from a dog bite – limitations of Vitek-2 system in exact identification of Pasteurella species. Eur J Med Res 2011; 16:531-6.

10. Rosenbach KA, Poblete J, Larkin I. Prosthetic valve endocarditis caused by *Pasteurella dagmatis*. South Med J 2001;94:1033-5.

11. Deschilder I, Gordts B, Van Landuyt H, Renders F, Selleslag D. *Pasteurella dagmatis* septicemia in an immunocompromised patient without a history of dog or cat bites. Acta Clin Belg J 2000;55:225-6.

12. Fajfar-Whetstone CJ, Coleman L, Biggs DR, Fox BC. *Pasteurella multocida* septicemia and subsequent *Pasteurella dagmatis* septicemia in a diabetic patient. J Clin Microbiol 1995;33:202-4.

13. Mosallanejad B, Avizeh R, Ghadiri AR, Moarrabi A, Naddaf H, Jamshidian M. First report of *Pasteurella dagmatis* isolation from a bitch urine in Iran. Iranian J Vet Res 2008;9:384-6.

14. Sorbello AF, O'Donnell J, Kaiser-Smith J, Fitzharris J, Shinkarow J, Doneson S. Infective endocarditis due to *Pasteurella dagmatis*: Case report and review. Clin Infect Dis 1994;18:336-8.

15. Strahm C, Goldenberger D, Gutmann M, Kuhnert P, Graber P. Prosthetic valve endocarditis caused by a *Pasteurella dagmatis*-like isolate originating from a patient's cat. J Clin Microbiol 2012;50:2818-9.

16. Ashley BD, Noone M, Dwarakanath AD, Malnick H. Fatal *Pasteurella dagmatis* peritonitis and septicaemia in a patient with cirrhosis: A case report and review of the literature. J Clin Pathol 2004;57:210-2.

17. Wallet F, Toure F, Devalckenaere A, Pagniez D, Courcol RJ. Molecular identification of *Pasteurella dagmatis* peritonitis in a patient undergoing peritoneal dialysis. J Clin Microbiol 2000;38:4681-2.

18. Garcia-Hejl C, Bigaillon C, Garcia C, et al. *Pasteurella dagmatis*: An unusal cause of vetebral osteomyelitis. J Pathobiol 2007;55:340-2.

19. Dupuy O, Garrabe E, Bordier L, et al. *Pasteurella dagmatis* spondylodiscitis in a diabetic patient. Revue de Medecine Interne 2006;27:803-4.

20. Allison K, Clarridge JE. Long-term respiratory tract infection with canine-associated *Pasteurella dagmatis* and *Neisseria canis* in a patient with chronic bronchiectasis. J Clin Microbiol 2005;43:4272-4.

21. Laurens C, Marouze N, Jean-Pierre H. *Staphylococcus pseudintermedius* and *Pasteurella dagmatis* associated in a case of community-acquired pneumonia. Medecine et Maladies Infectieuses 2012;42:129-31.

22. Zbinden R, Sommerhalder P, von Wartburg U. Co-isolation of *Pasteurella dagmatis* and *Pasteurella multocida* from cat-bite wounds. Eur J Clin Microbiol & Infect Dis 1988;7:203-4.

23. Guillard T, Duval V, Jobart R, et al. Dog bite wound infection by *Pasteurella dagmatis* misidentified as *Pasteurella pneumotropica* by automated system Vitek 2. Diag Microbiol and Infect Dis 2009;65:347-8.

24. Zangenah S, Güleryüz G, Boräng S, Ullberg M, Bergman P, Ozenci V. Identification of clinical *Pasteurella* isolates by MALDI-TOF – a comparison with VITEK 2 and conventional microbiological methods. Diag Microbiol and Infect Dis 2013;77:96-8.

30

Fidaxomicin: A novel agent for the treatment of *Clostridium difficile* infection

George G Zhanel PhD[1], Andrew J Walkty MD[1], James A Karlowsky PhD[1]

GG Zhanel, AJ Walkty, JA Karlowsky. Fidaxomicin: A novel agent for the treatment of *Clostridium difficile* infection. Can J Infect Dis Med Microbiol 2015;26(6):305-312.

BACKGROUND: Due to the limitations of existing treatment options for *Clostridium difficile* infection (CDI), new therapies are needed.
OBJECTIVE: To review the available data on fidaxomicin regarding chemistry, mechanisms of action and resistance, in vitro activity, pharmacokinetic and pharmacodynamic properties, efficacy and safety in clinical trials, and place in therapy.
METHODS: A search of PubMed using the terms "fidaxomicin", "OPT-80", "PAR-101", "OP-1118", "difimicin", "tiacumicin" and "lipiarmycin" was performed. All English-language articles from January 1983 to November 2014 were reviewed, as well as bibliographies of all articles.
RESULTS: Fidaxomicin is the first macrocyclic lactone antibiotic with activity versus *C difficile*. It inhibits RNA polymerase, therefore, preventing transcription. Fidaxomicin (and its active metabolite OP-1118) is bactericidal against *C difficile* and exhibits a prolonged postantibiotic effect (approximately 10 h). Other than for *C difficile*, fidaxomicin demonstrated only moderate inhibitory activity against Gram-positive bacteria and was a poor inhibitor of normal colonic flora, including anaerobes and enteric Gram-negative bacilli. After oral administration (200 mg two times per day for 10 days), fidaxomicin achieved low serum concentration levels but high fecal concentration levels (mean approximately 1400 µg/g stool). Phase 3 clinical trials involving adults with CDI demonstrated that 200 mg fidaxomicin twice daily for 10 days was noninferior to 125 mg oral vancomycin four times daily for 10 days in regard to clinical response at the end of therapy. Fidaxomicin was, however, reported to be superior to oral vancomycin in reducing recurrent CDI and achieving a sustained clinical response (assessed at day 28) for patients infected with non-BI/NAP1/027 strains.
CONCLUSION: Fidaxomicin was noninferior to oral vancomycin with regard to clinical response at the end of CDI therapy. Fidaxomicin has been demonstated to be as safe as oral vancomycin, but superior to vancomycin in achieving a sustained clinical response for CDI in patients infected with non-BI/NAP1/027 strains. Caution should be exercised in using fidaxomicin monotherapy for treatment of severe complicated CDI because limited data are available. Whether fidaxomicin is cost effective (due to its significantly higher acquisition cost versus oral vancomycin) depends on the acceptable willingness to pay threshold per quality-adjusted life year as a measure of assessing cost effectiveness.

Key Words: Clostridium difficile; *Fidaxomicin; Infection; Recurrence; Treatment*

La fidaxomicine : un nouvel agent pour traiter l'infection à *Clostridium difficile*

HISTORIQUE : Étant donné le peu de traitements de l'infection à *Clostridium difficile* (ICD), il faut en trouver de nouveaux.
OBJECTIF : Examiner les données sur les caractéristiques chimiques, les mécanismes d'action, la résistance, l'activité *in vitro*, les propriétés pharmacocinétiques et pharmacodynamiques, l'efficacité et l'innocuité de la fidaxomicine dans les essais cliniques, ainsi que la place qu'elle occupe dans les traitements.
MÉTHODOLOGIE : Les chercheurs ont fouillé dans PubMed à l'aide des termes *fidaxomicin*, *OPT-80*, *PAR-101*, *OP-1118*, *difimicin*, *tiacumicin* et *lipiarmycin*. Ils en ont extrait tous les articles en anglais entre janvier 1983 et novembre 2014, de même que les bibliographies de tous les articles.
RÉSULTATS : La fidaxomicine est la première lactone macrocyclique à résister au *C difficile*. Elle inhibe la polymérase de l'ARN et, par conséquent, en empêche la transcription. La fidaxomicine (et son métabolite actif, l'OP-1118) est bactéricide contre le *C difficile* et possède un effet postantibiotique prolongé (environ dix heures). À par d'autres infections que le *C difficile*, la fidaxomicine a une activité inhibitrice modérée contre les bactéries Gram positif et est un mauvais inhibiteur de la flore colique normale, y compris les anaérobies et les bacilles entériques Gram négatif. Après son administration par voie orale (200 mg deux fois par jour pendant dix jours), la fidaxomicine était peu concentrée dans le sérum, mais très concentrée dans les selles (moyenne d'environ 1 400 µg/g par selle). Des essais cliniques de phase 3 auprès d'adultes atteints d'une ICD a démontré qu'à la fin du traitement, la réponse clinique à la prise de 200 mg de fidaxomicine pendant dix jours n'était pas inférieure à celle de la prise de 125 mg de vancomycine par voie orale quatre fois par jour pendant dix jours. La fidaxomicine était toutefois supérieure à la vancomycine par voie orale pour réduire les ICD récurrentes et parvenir à une réponse clinique soutenue (évaluée le jour 28) chez les patients infectés par d'autres souches que les BI/NAP1/027.
CONCLUSION : La réponse clinique de la fidaxomicine n'était pas inférieure à celle de la vancomycine par voie orale à la fin du traitement de l'ICD. Il est démontré que la fidaxomicine est tout aussi sécuritaire que la vancomycine par voie orale, mais qu'elle est supérieure à cet antibiotique pour assurer une réponse clinique soutenue à l'ICD chez les patients infectés par d'autres souches que les BI/NAP1/027. Il faut faire preuve de prudence lorsqu'on utilise la monothérapie à la fidaxomicine pour traiter une IDC très complexe, car il existe peu de données sur le sujet. L'efficience de la fidaxomicine (en raison de son coût d'acquisition beaucoup plus élevé que celui de la vancomycine par voie orale) dépend de la volonté acceptable de payer un seuil par année de vie pondérée par la qualité

Until 2011, oral vancomycin was the only therapy approved by the United States (US) Food and Drug Administration to treat *Clostridium difficile* infections (CDIs), and is currently considered the gold standard comparator in clinical trials. The most recent US guidelines for treating CDIs, published by the Society for Healthcare and Epidemiology of America and the Infectious Disease Society of America,

[1]*Department of Medical Microbiology and Infectious Diseases, College of Medicine, University of Manitoba, Winnipeg, Manitoba*
Correspondence: Dr George G Zhanel, Clinical Microbiology, Health Sciences Centre, MS673-820 Sherbrook Street, Winnipeg, Manitoba R3A 1R9. e-mail ggzhanel@pcs.mb.ca

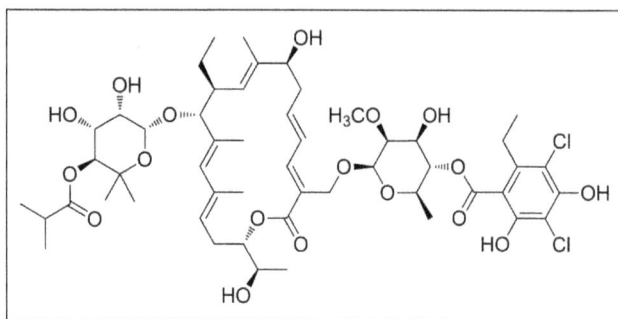

Figure 1) *Chemical structure of fidaxomicin*

recommends immediate cessation of antimicrobial treatment followed by therapy with oral metronidazole or oral vancomycin (1). Oral metronidazole at a dose of 500 mg three times daily for 10 to 14 days is preferred for a mild or moderate first episode. Oral vancomycin at 125 mg four times daily for 10 to 14 days is the agent of choice for a severe first episode. In severe, complicated CDI cases (presence of hypotension, ileus, shock or megacolon), oral vancomycin with or without intravenous metronidazole is recommended. First recurrent CDIs are to be treated similarly to an initial episode, while a tapered and/or pulse regimen of oral vancomycin is recommended for second and subsequent episodes.

Several limitations exist with current CDI therapies. While oral metronidazole is effective in treating mild to moderate CDIs (2), it has been demonstrated to be less effective than oral vancomycin for severe CDIs in two of three clinical trials (2-6). Oral vancomycin disrupts normal gut flora (7), and has a four times per day dosing regimen (1,8). Both oral vancomycin and oral metronidazole have been associated with colonization of vancomycin-resistant enterococci (VRE) (9-11). Recurrent infection occurs in approximately 20% to 30% of patients (12-14), with higher CDI recurrence rates observed in patients who have experienced multiple episodes (12) and in subgroups of high-risk patients (oncology, renal impairment, concomitant antibiotics, increased age, previous CDI episode) (15-19).

Fidaxomicin (previously known as OPT-80, PAR-101, tiacumicin B and difimicin) received Health Canada approval (Dificid, Merck and Co, USA) in June 2012 for the treatment of adults with a CDI (Dificid product monograph) (20). Fidaxomicin is marketed as a 200 mg tablet and is recommended to be administered orally twice daily for 10 days. The purpose of the present article was to review the available data on fidaxomicin regarding chemistry, mechanisms of action and resistance, in vitro activity, pharmacokinetic and pharmacodynamic properties, efficacy and safety in clinical trials, and place in therapy.

CHEMISTRY

Fidaxomicin is a first-in-class macrocyclic antibacterial agent for treatment of CDIs (21). It is an unsaturated, 18-membered macrocyclic lactone ring with a 7-carbon sugar constituent at carbon 12 and a 6-deoxy sugar at carbon 21 (Figure 1). Fidaxomicin is produced as a byproduct of fermentation by the actinomycete *Dactylosporangium aurantiacum* subspecies *hamdenesis* and has a molecular weight of 1056 g/mol. In vivo, fidaxomicin is primarily hydrolyzed at the fourth position isobutyryl ester by an unknown esterase to produce its main metabolite, OP-1118, which also provides resistance against C *difficile*.

MECHANISM OF ACTION

Fidaxomicin produces its antibacterial effects by inhibiting bacterial RNA polymerase at transcription initiation (22,23). Although fidaxomicin and rifamycins are both inhibitors of bacterial transcription, fidaxomicin acts at an earlier step in the transcription initiation pathway (24). Specifically, fidaxomicin binds to the DNA template-RNA polymerase complex and prevents the initial separation of DNA strands (ie, formation of the open DNA template-RNA polymerase

TABLE 1
In vitro activity of fidaxomicin against Gram-positive bacteria other than *Clostridium difficile*

Bacterium	Fidaxomicin MIC, µg/mL	Isolates tested, n
Aerococcus	0.5–16	10
Bacillus cereus	1	2
Bifidiobacterium	≤0.015–0.125	22
Bifidiobacterium longum	0.125	1
Clostridium perfringens	≤0.015–0.125	22
Clostridium innocuum	>32	20
Clostridium ramosum	>32	20
Eggerthella lenta	≤0.015–0.25	20
Enterococcus faecalis	0.5–4	63
Enterococcus faecium	1–8	64
Eubacterium limosum	16–>32	20
Finegoldia magna	0.5–2	21
Lactobacillus	≤0.015–>32	24
Lactobacillus acidophilus	>32	2
Lactobacillus casei	1–2	2
Lactobacillus rhamnosus	8–16	2
Micrococcus luteus	≤0.125	4
Micromonas micros	0.125	1
Parvimonas micra	≤0.015–2	20
Peptostreptococcus anaerobius	≤0.015–0.03	22
Peptostreptococcus (Peptoniphilus) asaccharolyticus	1	2
Peptococcus (Finegoldia) magna	0.5	1
Peptococcus (Micromonus) micros	0.125	1
Propionibacterium acnes	8	2
Staphylococcus aureus	2–16	100
Staphylococcus epidermidis	1–4	3
Staphylococcus intermedius	4	1
Staphylococcus, coagulase-negative	≤0.05–8	60
Streptococcus agalactiae	16–32	2
Streptococcus anginosus	4–>32	21
Streptococcus constellatus/intermedius	4–>32	26
Streptococcus pyogenes	4–16	23
Streptococcus pneumoniae	>32	2
Streptococcus sanguinis	32	1

Adapted from references 31, 34-41. MIC Minimum inhibitory concentration

complex), which precedes messenger RNA synthesis by inhibiting the σ subunit (23,25). Fidaxomicin's unique target site may explain its limited spectrum of antimicrobial activity because σ subunits differ among bacterial species (26). Isolates of C *difficile* resistant to rifamycins or to other antimicrobial classes (cephalosporins, fluoroquinolones, clindamycin) are not cross-resistant to fidaxomicin (23,24,27).

MECHANISM OF RESISTANCE

A study to determine the frequency of spontaneous (single step) resistance to fidaxomicin at four and eight times the minimum inhibitory concentration (MIC) in C *difficile* demonstrated low mutation rates ($<1.4 \times 10^{-9}$) (24). The resistant clones demonstrated stable reduced susceptibility (MICs of 2 µg/mL or 4 µg/mL) and carried mutations in either *rpoB* (Gln1074Lys or Val1143Phe) or *rpoC* (Asp237Tyr) genes, which cluster around the fidaxomicin binding site on RNA polymerase and did not demonstrate cross-resistance with other classes of antibiotics, including rifamycins (24). Another study using site-directed mutagenesis revealed that an isolate of C *difficile* with a Val1143Asp mutation demonstrated impaired fitness and delayed growth (28). Other reported laboratory-generated mutations included β' Arg89Gly, β Gln1074His, β Val1143Gln and β Val1143Asp (29).

TABLE 2
Minimum inhibitory concentration (MIC) determinations for fidaxomicin, OP-1118, vancomycin and metronidazole against toxin-positive clinical isolates of *Clostridium difficile*

Antimicrobial agent	Isolates tested, n	MIC range, µg/mL	MIC$_{50}$, µg/mL	MIC$_{90}$, µg/mL	Reference
Fidaxomicin	208	0.06–1	0.25	0.5	27
	110	0.015–0.25	0.125	0.125	42
	135	≤0.004–8	0.125	0.25	31
	38	≤0.008–0.25	0.125	0.125	43
	719	0.003–1	0.125	0.25	30
	114	0.008–0.125	0.06	0.125	44
	50	0.06–1	0.25	0.5	45
	50	0.03–0.5	0.25	0.5	41
OP-1118	135	0.25->128	4	8	31
Vancomycin	208	0.5–4	0.5	1	27
	719	0.25–8	1	2	30
	114	0.125–1	0.5	0.5	44
Metronidazole	208	0.25–4	0.5	1	27
	719	0.02–4	0.5	1	30
	114	0.125–2	0.5	1	44

MIC$_{50}$ MIC required to inhibit the growth of 50% of organisms; MIC$_{90}$ MIC required to inhibit the growth of 90% of organisms

TABLE 3
Stool and plasma concentrations of fidaxomicin and OP-1118 in patients with *Clostridium difficile* infection treated for 10 days with fidaxomicin

		Fecal concentrations, µg/g		Fidaxomicin and OP-1118 plasma concentrations, n								
					Fidaxomicin, ng/mL				OP-1118, ng/mL			
Fidaxomicin, mg/day	n	Fidaxomicin, mean ± SD	OP-1118, mean ± SD	Total, n	<5	5–20	20–100	>100	<5	5–20	20–100	>100
100	11	256±136	393±260	14	12	2	0	0	1	11	2	0
200	9	442±238	430±263	16	7	8	1	0	2	8	5	1
400	13	1433±975	760±373	16	3	11	2	0	0	7	9	1

Adapted from reference 46

Resistance to fidaxomicin did not develop during treatment in either phase 3 clinical study, although a single isolate from a cured patient (200 mg twice daily of fidaxomicin for 10 days) presented an elevated fidaxomicin MIC of 16 µg/mL at the time of recurrence (30). This isolate contained a single mutation in *rpoC* (Val1143Gly) (31).

Babakhani et al (32) and Leeds et al (33) generated stable (fidaxomicin MIC 1 µg/mL to 4 µg/mL) mutants by serial passage in the laboratory. Leeds et al (33) found mutations in *rpoB* and CD22120 (*marR* homologue), a mechanism outside of the RNA polymerase. Based on the available data, resistance to fidaxomicin is not expected; however, prospective collection of long-term surveillance data is prudent.

MICROBIOLOGY

Fidaxomicin is a narrow-spectrum agent that has been demonstrated to be selectively active against Gram-positive anaerobes (Table 1), including *Clostridium* (particularly *C difficile* and *Clostridium perfringens*) (31,34-41). It is less active against Gram-positive, nonspore-forming bacilli (eg, *Propionibacterium* and *Lactobacilli*) and *Peptostreptococci* (37), and is poorly active against anaerobic Gram-negative bacilli (38). Fidaxomicin MICs for most aerobic and anaerobic Gram-negative bacilli (eg, Enterobacteriaceae, *Pseudomonas*, *Campylobacter*, *Helicobacter*, *Haemophilus*, *Bacteroides*, *Fusobacterium*, *Porphyromonas*, *Prevotella* and *Veillonella*) exceed 32 µg/mL to 64 µg/mL (31). Fidaxomicin is inactive (MIC >64 µg/mL) against *Candida* species (31).

Table 2 summarizes the in vitro activities of fidaxomicin, OP-1118, metronidazole and vancomycin against *C difficile*, tested using the currently published Clinical and Laboratory Standards Institute method (27,30,31,41-45). Fidaxomicin possesses potent activity against *C difficile*, including MICs required to inhibit growth of 50% of organisms (MIC$_{50}$s) ranging from 0.06 µg/mL to 0.25 µg/mL and MICs required to inhibit growth of 90% of organisms (MIC$_{90}$s) ranging from 0.125 µg/mL to 0.5 µg/mL (27,30,31,41-45). Hecht et al (42) and Citron et al (43)

did not identify any difference in MIC related to restriction endonuclease analysis BI (NAP1/O27) group status. Goldstein et al (30) reported higher MICs for fidaxomicin, vancomycin, metronidazole and rifaximin for BI isolates than for non-BI isolates. Goldstein et al (30) and Louie et al (46) also reported that fidaxomicin susceptibility of baseline isolates did not predict clinical cure, failure or recurrence. In comparison with fidaxomicin, vancomycin and metronidazole, MIC$_{90}$s for *C difficile* were 0.5 µg/mL to 2 µg/mL and 1 µg/mL, respectively (Table 2). The antibacterial activity of OP-1118 (MIC$_{90}$, 8 µg/mL) was approximately eight to 16 times lower than the activity of fidaxomicin (31).

Fidaxomicin has been reported to have a low ecological impact on the intestinal microbiome (7,47). Babakhani et al (48) speculate, based on in vitro data, that the antibacterial activity of fidaxomicin should not be altered under physiological conditions in the human intestine.

PHARMACOKINETICS

When administered orally, fidaxomicin (similar to oral vancomycin) is minimally absorbed, being excreted almost entirely through the feces (46,49,50). Mean fecal concentration levels (on day 10 of dosing) of fidaxomicin and OP-1118 for patients with CDI who were treated for 10 days with 100 mg, 200 mg or 400 mg per day of fidaxomicin (50 mg, 100 mg and 200 mg twice daily) were 256 µg/g and 393 µg/g, 442 µg/g and 430 µg/g, and 1433 µg/g and 760 µg/g, respectively (46) (Table 3). If the MIC$_{90}$ for fidaxomicin versus *C difficile* is 0.5 µg/mL (Table 2) and the mean fecal fidaxomicin concentration is approximately 1400 µg/g, it indicates the mean fecal fidaxomicin concentrations are approximately 2800 times greater than the MIC$_{90}$ of *C difficile* (this compares with approximately 1000 times greater than the MIC$_{90}$ of *C difficile* for 125 mg oral vancomycin four times per day and approximately one to five times greater than the MIC$_{90}$ of *C difficile* for oral metronidazole 500 mg three times per day) (46).

TABLE 4
Summary of treatment outcomes for patients with *Clostridium difficile* infection treated with fidaxomicin (FDX) or vancomycin (VAN) from two phase 3 randomized double-blind clinical trials (modified intent to treat)

	Clinical response				Patients recurrence				Sustained response			
Study	FDX	VAN	Difference	P	FDX	VAN	Difference	P	FDX	VAN	Difference	P
OPT-80-003	88.2	85.8	2.4	NI	15.4	25.3	−9.9	0.005	74.6	64.1	10.5	0.006
OPT-80-004	87.7	86.8	0.9	NI	12.7	26.9	−14.2	<0.001	76.6	63.4	13.2	0.001

Data presented as % unless otherwise indicated. Study OPT-80-003: FDX n=287, VAN n=309; Study OPT-80-004: FDX n=253, VAN n=257. Adapted from references 13 and 14. NI Noninferior

In the same open-label dose-ranging trial (46), plasma concentration levels of fidaxomicin and OP-1118 (from patients who received fidaxomicin and had >1 plasma pharmacokinetic sample collected after the first dose) were below the limit of quantification (5 ng/mL) for 22 of 46 patients, and >90% of patients had plasma concentration levels <20 ng/mL (Table 3). In addition, Sears et al (49) demonstrated that fidaxomicin serum concentration levels did not increase compared with controls for patients with mild, moderate or severe renal impairment. Therefore, the majority of fidaxomicin and its active metabolite OP-1118 are not absorbed systemically, rather, they are primarily excreted in the feces following oral administration.

PHARMACODYNAMICS

Fidaxomicin and OP-1118 are bactericidal against *C difficile* in vitro (at four times the MIC, ≥ 3 $\log_{10}$ in 48 h), as well as against laboratory generated mutants with reduced susceptibility to fidaxomicin (MIC 1 µg/mL to 4 µg/mL) (32,51). The postantibiotic effect of fidaxomicin extends for approximately 10 h (range 5.5 h to 12.4 h), compared with vancomycin, which has a postantibiotic effect of 0 h to 1.5 h (51).

Fidaxomicin and OP-1118 have been demonstrated to inhibit toxin A and B production in *C difficile* in vitro (52). The ability of fidaxomicin and OP-1118 to inhibit expression of *C difficile* toxin A and B, and their gene products (*tcdA* and *tcdB*) was examined in vitro for two isolates; one isolate that demonstrated a high level of toxin expression and a second isolate that was a BI (NAP1/O27) strain (52). At ¼× the MIC, fidaxomicin and its metabolite reduced toxin expression by >60% for up to one week. Vancomycin and metronidazole (¼× the MIC) had no effect on toxin expression. At subinhibitory concentrations (¼× the MIC), both fidaxomicin and OP-1118 reduced toxin A-mediated enteritis in a mouse ileum model and cell rounding in human colonic CCD-18Co fibroblasts (53). In clinical trials, during the post-CDI treatment period, there was no difference among fidaxomicin and vancomycin treatment groups in *C difficile* colony forming units (CFUs) over time; however, toxin expression was reduced by 50% with fidaxomicin therapy (47).

Fidaxomicin, its metabolite OP-1118 and comparator drugs were assessed in vitro for their impact on new spore formation (54). At ¼× the MIC, fidaxomicin and OP-1118 inhibited spore production in both non-BI strains and in a BI strain (NAP1/O27). In contrast, vancomycin, metronidazole and rifaximin at sub-MIC drug concentrations failed to inhibit sporulation. In clinical trials, fecal spore counts (CFU count/g) for patients who had received fidaxomicin were 2.3 $\log_{10}$ lower at 21 to 28 days post-therapy than in patients who had received vancomycin (46). Inhibition of sporulation may provide, in part, a mechanism by which fidaxomicin improves sustained response and lowers the rate of recurrent infection, and may also be useful in decreasing *C difficile* shedding and transmission. Fidaxomicin and OP-1118 do not interfere with the initiation of spore germination, but rather inhibit outgrowth of vegetative cells from germinated spores (55).

Unlike oral vancomycin and oral metronidazole, fidaxomicin has minimal effects on the anaerobic colonic flora (7,37,38,46,47,56). Fecal samples from patients with CDI who were treated with oral fidaxomicin (200 mg twice per day) or oral vancomycin (125 mg four times per day) for 10 days showed sparing of major components of the anaerobic microflora (eg, *Bacteroides/Prevotella* group organisms as well as *Clostridium coccoides* and *Clostridium leptum*) with fidaxomicin, but

not with vancomycin. In the vancomycin treatment arm, there was a 2 $\log_{10}$ CFU/g to 4 $\log_{10}$ CFU/g reduction in anaerobes (*Bacteroides/Prevotella* group organisms), which persisted until day 28 of the study (47). The investigators concluded that whereas oral vancomycin and oral fidaxomicin were equally effective in resolving CDI symptoms, preservation of the normal colonic microflora by fidaxomicin was associated with a lower likelihood of CDI recurrence. Nerandzic et al (57) demonstrated that colonization with VRE and *Candida* were reduced by oral fidaxomicin compared with oral vancomycin in CDI patients who were negative for VRE and *Candida* before therapy. In patients with stool culture initially negative for VRE, 31% (n=160) of patients acquired VRE when treated with vancomycin versus only 7% (n=115) acquisition of VRE in fidaxomicin-treated patients (P=0.001) (57).

CLINICAL TRIALS

Two large, randomized, multicentre, double-blind phase 3 clinical trials examined the efficacy and safety of oral fidaxomicin versus oral vancomycin in adult patients with CDI (13,14). Study OPT-80-003 comprised 596 patients from the US and Canada (13), and study OPT-80-004 comprised 509 patients from the US, Europe and Canada (14). Patients with confirmed CDI who were ≥16 years of age and had no history or only one previous CDI episode in the past 90 days were eligible for inclusion. The presence of CDI was defined as diarrhea with >3 unformed stools 24 h before randomization and a positive toxin test for toxin A, B or both. Patients who were pregnant or breastfeeding, had previous fidaxomicin exposure, life-threatening or fulminant CDI, toxic megacolon, a history of ulcerative colitis or Crohn disease, or >1 CDI episode in the preceding three months were excluded. Patients were also excluded if they were presently taking other antibiotics for CDI, although they could have received up to four doses of oral vancomycin or oral metronidazole in the 24 h before randomization.

Patients were randomized to receive 200 mg of oral fidaxomicin twice daily or 125 mg of oral vancomycin four times daily for 10 days. The primary end point was clinical response (clinical cure). Clinical response was the resolution of diarrhea, defined as ≤3 unformed stools for two consecutive days that was maintained through the duration of therapy with no further CDI treatment required, assessed two days after the treatment period. Secondary end points were recurrence and sustained clinical response (global cure). CDI recurrence was assessed during the 28-day period after completion of therapy and defined as the reappearance of >3 unformed stools in any 24 h period, including a positive toxin test for toxin A, B or both and the need for CDI retreatment. Sustained response was the presence of clinical response and no recurrence or death during the 28-day follow-up period. The modified intent-to-treat (mITT) and per protocol populations were analyzed. The mITT analysis is presented in the present review. A one-sided lower 97.5% CI was used in analysis of the primary end point, with a noninferiority margin of −10% absolute difference. Secondary endpoints of recurrence and sustained clinical response were analyzed using two sided tests of population proportions, with α=0.05.

The treatment outcomes for study OPT-80-003 and OPT-80-004 are summarized in Table 4. In both clinical trials, oral fidaxomicin was noninferior to oral vancomycin for clinical response, with cure rates of approximately 87% in both treatment groups. Fidaxomicin demonstrated superiority to vancomycin for recurrence. The relative reduction in recurrence with fidaxomicin treatment was 39.1% and 52.8%

in study OPT-80-003 and OPT-80-004, respectively. Fidaxomicin was also superior for sustained clinical response, demonstrating higher global cure rates compared with vancomycin in the two trials. In study OPT-80-003 (13) (North America only), 38.1% of patients were infected with the BI/NAP1/027 strain. The lower CDI recurrence rate among patients treated with fidaxomicin relative to vancomycin was only observed for those infected with non-BI/NAP1/027 strains (13). Infection rates with the BI/NAP1/027 strain differed according to region in study OPT-80-004, with rates of 45.9% in the US and Canada, and 10.4% in Europe (14). In the OPT-80-004 study, CDI recurrence rates were numerically lower among fidaxomicin-treated patients infected with the BI/NAP1/027 and non-BI/NAP1/027 strains relative to those receiving vancomycin; however, the difference was statistically significant only for the non-BI/NAP1/027 subgroup (14).

Post hoc analysis of the data from the two phase 3 trials were performed for subgroups of patients at high risk for acquiring CDI and/or at increased risk for recurrent disease. These subgroups, described in separate publications, included patients of increased age, patients receiving concomitant antimicrobials, patients with a previous CDI episode, patients with cancer and patients with underlying renal dysfunction (15-19,58). The risk for recurrence among patients treated with oral fidaxomicin relative to oral vancomycin, stratified according to subgroup, is presented in Table 5. The effect of increasing age on the outcome of treatment for CDI with oral fidaxomicin in comparison with oral vancomycin was evaluated by Louie et al (18) using regression modelling. Study participants were stratified into age categories according to 10 year increments, with the lower category including patients from 18 to 40 years of age. The model predicted a 17% increased probability for CDI recurrence for each decade after age 40. Treatment with fidaxomicin was associated with a 60% lower risk for recurrence in multivariate analysis that included adjustment for patient age (18).

Mullane et al (17) evaluated the efficacy of oral fidaxomicin in comparison with oral vancomycin for the treatment of CDI among patients receiving concomitant antimicrobials. Topical antimicrobials, antimicrobials used for the treatment of CDI, and antifungal and antiviral agents with no antibacterial activity were excluded from the concomitant antimicrobial definition. Results of this analysis have been published only for the per protocol population. Among 999 patients, 275 (27.5%) received concomitant antimicrobials at some time during the study, with 192 (19.2%) receiving concomitant antimicrobials concurrent with the study medication. Clinical cure was significantly lower among patients who received concomitant antimicrobials concurrent with CDI treatment, relative to those that did not (84.4% versus 92.6%; 8.2% absolute difference 95% CI 3.0% to 13.9%). Among patients who received concomitant antimicrobials concurrent with the study medications, clinical cure was 90% for patients treated with oral fidaxomicin versus 79.4% for patients treated with oral vancomycin (P=0.04). Recurrence of CDI among patients who received concomitant antimicrobials at any time during the study was lower for those treated with fidaxomicin than those who received vancomycin (16.9% versus 29.2%; P=0.048) (17).

Cornely et al (19) compared treatment with oral fidaxomicin and oral vancomycin in a subset of patients with a first CDI recurrence. The published results for this subgroup analysis included 128 patients in the per protocol population who experienced an episode of CDI in the three months before randomization. Clinical cure for patients among this subpopulation was >90% for both fidaxomicin and vancomycin. However, a second recurrence was less frequent among patients who received fidaxomicin (19.7% versus 35.5% for vancomycin; P=0.045) (19).

Oral fidaxomicin compared with oral vancomycin for the treatment of CDI among patients with cancer was assessed by Cornely et al (15). Patients with solid tumours and/or hematological malignancies were identified according to system organ class and preferred term from active medical history entries of case report forms after coding by MedDRA version 10.0 (MedDRA, USA) according to indications for

TABLE 5
Recurrence in subpopulations of patients with *Clostridium difficile* infection treated with fidaxomicin or vancomycin in a post hoc analysis of two phase 3 randomized double-blind clinical trials

Subpopulation	Percentage of patients with recurrence			
	Fidaxomicin	Vancomycin	Difference	P
Concomitant antibiotics*	16.9	29.2	−12.3	0.048
Previous CDI episode*	19.7	35.5	−15.8	0.045
Cancer	13.5	29.6	−16.1	0.018
Renal impairment				
Stage 2	14.3	24.3	−10.0	0.040
Stage 3	21.4	33.0	−11.6	0.080
Stage 4 or higher	14.7	31.6	−16.9	0.092

Per protocol population; all other data represent the modified-intent-to-treat population. Adapted from references 15-19

concomitant medication entries and treatment-emergent adverse events. In total, 183 patients in the mITT population with active cancer were identified. The likelihood of CDI recurrence following treatment for patients with and without cancer was similar. Among patients with cancer, recurrence occurred in 13.5% of those treated with fidaxomicin versus 29.6% treated with vancomycin (P=0.018) (15). Recently, Esmaily-Fard et al (59) treated 22 cancer patients (lymphomas, leukemias and solid tumours) with CDI using fidaxomicin. Fidaxomicin was used in these patients because of recurrent CDI (16 of 22 [72%] patients) or failure of both oral metronidazole and oral vancomycin (six of 22 [28%] patients). Despite 19 of 22 (86%) patients receiving concomitant antimicrobials during CDI treatment, clinical response occurred in 91% of patients and overall sustained clinical response was observed in 82%. The researchers concluded that in cancer patients, fidaxomicin is an effective treatment for a first episode of CDI after failure of standard therapies and for treatment of recurrent CDI (59). However, in view of the small number of patients evaluated and the study design (retrospective case series) further data are required to support these conclusions.

Treatment of CDI with fidaxomicin in comparison with vancomycin among the subgroup of patients with renal impairment was evaluated by Mullane et al (16). Creatinine clearance (CrCl) was estimated using the Cockcroft-Gault equation with serum creatinine from a blood sample obtained on day 1 before the first dose of study medication. Patients were stratified according to renal function using criteria from the National Kidney Foundation Kidney Disease Outcomes Quality Initiative (60) as follows: normal (CrCl >90 mL/min/1.73 m²), stage 2 (CrCl 60 mL/min/1.73 m² to 89 mL/min/1.73 m²), stage 3 (CrCl 30 mL/min/1.73 m² to 59 mL/min/1.73 m²), stage 4 (CrCl 15 mL/min/1.73 m² to 30 mL/min/1.73 m²), stage 5 (CrCl <15 mL/min/1.73 m²). At baseline, 57.9% of patients in the mITT population with a CrCl estimate available had abnormal renal function. In a multivariate analysis, patients with stage 2 or higher chronic kidney disease were less likely to be cured of CDI (OR 0.53; P=0.03), and patients with stage 3 or greater chronic kidney disease were more likely to have a recurrence (OR 1.8; P=0.024). Oral fidaxomicin was associated with a lower risk for recurrent CDI relative to oral vancomycin, independent of renal function (16). The reader is cautioned about placing extensive weighting on data obtained from the subgroup analysis because the data obtained from these post hoc analyses were not as rigorous as those obtained from analyses of primary end point data.

REAL-WORLD EXPERIENCE
Several observational studies describing the real-world use of fidaxomicin have been published (61-65). Vargo et al (61) evaluated the clinical outcome of 61 patients treated for CDI with fidaxomicin at a single centre. Fifty-five (90.2%) patients received treatment for CDI in the preceding 30 days, concomitant antimicrobials were used by

60.7%, and severe infection was present in 31.1%. Slightly more than one-half of the patients received fidaxomicin in combination with another recognized treatment for CDI. Clinical cure was achieved in 72.1% of patients. Among patients who achieved clinical cure, recurrence was documented in 13.6%. Eiland et al (62) also assessed the clinical efficacy of fidaxomcin in a single centre, retrospective cohort study. Sixty patients were included in the analysis. Severe or severe-complicated disease was present in 45% of patients, concomitant antimicrobials were being administered to 55%, and 43.3% were being treated for a second or greater CDI episode. Overall, 96.7% of patients achieved clinical success, with recurrence documented in 10.3%. The difference in clinical efficacy reported between these two real-world evaluations and the phase 3 fidaxomicin clinical trials likely relates to differences among the patient populations studied (13,14,61,62).

Clutter et al (63) evaluated fidaxomicin for the treatment of CDI in recipients of a solid organ or hematopoietic stem cell transplant in comparison with conventional therapy (oral vancomycin and/or oral metronidazole). Fifty-nine transplant recipients were included in the analysis. Clinical cure was documented among 67% of patients (10 of 15) that received fidaxomicin versus 89% of patients (41 of 44) who received conventional therapy (P=0.06, not significant). Recurrence occurred in 7% of patients in both study groups. The non-randomized design of the study and small number of patients included make it difficult to draw significant conclusions concerning the efficacy of fidaxomicin relative to conventional therapy. Penziner et al (64) assessed the efficacy of fidaxomicin for the treatment of CDI among patients admitted to a critical care unit in comparison with patients treated on a general medicine ward. In total, 50 patients were included in the analysis, of whom 20 were receiving care in a critical care unit. Forty percent of patients treated in a critical care unit setting had severe-complicated disease as opposed to 10% of patients on a general medicine ward (P=0.031). Clinical cure was reported in 60% of patients treated in a critical care unit versus 67% of those treated on a general medicine ward (P=0.9). The response rate for patients having severe or severe-complicated CDI, irrespective of study location (critical care unit or medicine ward), was only 46%, in comparison with a response rate of 81% for patients with mild to moderate disease (P=0.02). Life-threatening or fulminant CDI was an exclusion criterion for the two large phase 3 fidaxomicin clinical trials (13,14). The results from Penziner et al (64) support caution with using fidaxomicin monotherapy to treat severe-complicated CDI until further data are available.

Novel fidaxomicin treatment regimens have also been assessed among patients with multiple CDI recurrences. Soriano et al (65) evaluated the efficacy of fidaxomicin administered as a 10-day chaser following a treatment course of oral vancomycin (n=8 patients). The study patients had between three and 10 CDI episodes. Five of the eight patients (62%) did not experience a further CDI recurrence following the fidaxomicin chaser. The same investigators also assessed a tapering regimen of fidaxomicin over 14 to 21 days following a 10-day fidaxomicin treatment course. The tapering regimen was evaluated in 11 patients who had between three and 11 CDI episodes. Nine patients (82%) did not experience a further recurrence of CDI. The reader is cautioned about placing extensive weighting on these real-world experience data because frequently these data are noncomparative and the studies include only a small number of patients treated.

ADVERSE EFFECTS

Fidaxomicin has been well tolerated in clinical trials. In the two phase 3 clinical studies (OPT-80-003 and OPT-80-004), adverse events were not significantly different among the fidaxomicin and vancomycin treatment groups (13,14,66). Adverse events possibly or definitely related to study treatment were primarily gastrointestinal in nature, and included nausea, vomiting, diarrhea, abdominal pain and constipation (13,14). Gastrointestinal adverse events requiring study discontinuation occurred in 2.3% of patients treated with fidaxomicin versus 1.4% of patients receiving vancomycin (P=0.24)

(66). At present, there are a lack of data regarding fidaxomicin use during pregnancy (66).

It should be noted that hypersensitivity reactions to fidaxomicin have been reported postmarketing. Iarikov et al (67) summarized data for 12 patients presenting with a hypersensitivity reaction in association with fidaxomicin use. Onset of symptoms occurred between 1 h and 7 days after starting fidaxomicin. The clinical presentation included facial, tongue or throat swelling, a burning sensation in the throat and rash. In two patients, symptoms recurred with re-exposure to fidaxomicin (67). The US Food and Drug Administration has added a warning about the possibility of hypersensitivity reactions to the fidaxomicin prescribing information (Dificid monograph). Hypersensitivity to fidaxomicin is listed as a contraindication to the use of this antimicrobial (Dificid monograph).

PHARMACOECONOMICS

Oral fidaxomicin has demonstrated superiority to oral vancomycin in achieving a sustained clinical response for CDI (in patients infected with non-BI/NAP1/027 strains), and this superiority is maintained in both severe and non-severe CDI, as well as in patients with a high risk for recurrent CDI (68). Whole-genome sequencing has recently demonstrated that this is due to fidaxomicin significantly reducing both the risk for relapse and reinfection (69). The increase in efficacy of oral fidaxomicin in preventing recurrent CDI relative to oral vancomycin should, however, be balanced with the increased cost of this antimicrobial. The acquisition cost of a 10-day course of fidaxomicin is significantly higher (five to >20 times) than the cost of a 10-day course of oral vancomycin (depending on the vancomycin formulation used). Wagner et al (70) developed a decision-tree model to determine the incremental cost per recurrence avoided by treating patients having severe CDI with oral fidaxomicin in comparison with oral vancomycin. This model considered patients treated in the Canadian health care system, and costs were presented in Canadian dollars. For a cohort of 1000 patients, the model predicted that treatment of severe CDI with fidaxomicin would result in an incremental cost of $13,202 per recurrence avoided. Furthermore, among 1000 patients with recurrent CDI, treatment with fidaxomicin would result in an incremental cost of $18,190 per second recurrence avoided. Overall, use of fidaxomicin for the treatment of patients with severe CDI was associated with a cost increase for the Canadian health care system (70).

Stranges et al (71) performed a cost utility analysis comparing oral fidaxomicin versus oral vancomycin for CDI treatment, using a decision analytic model from a third-party payer perspective (United States). These investigators reported an incremental cost-effectiveness ratio of USD$67,576/quality adjusted life-year (QALY) with fidaxomicin. Their analysis suggested that fidaxomicin may be cost effective in the US health care system based on a willingness to pay threshold of USD$100,000/QALY (71). Nathwani et al (72) used a one year time horizon Markov model with seven health states to analyze the cost-effectiveness of oral fidaxomicin versus oral vancomycin for the treatment of CDI from the perspective of Scottish public health care providers. This analysis was limited to patients with severe CDI or a first CDI recurrence. The main outcome was the incremental cost-effectiveness ratio expressed as a cost per QALY in British pounds, interpreted using a willingness to pay threshold of UK£20,000/QALY and UK£30,000/QALY. Fidaxomicin was found to be cost effective for severe CDI (incremental cost-effectiveness ratio = UK£16,529/QALY) and dominant (more effective and less costly) in patients who were treated for a first recurrence (72). A pharmacoeconomic analysis may be warranted for hospitals that are considering adding fidaxomicin to the formulary.

GUIDELINES/PLACE IN THERAPY

The European Society of Clinical Microbiology and Infectious Diseases recently published updated guidelines regarding the treatment of CDI (73). For treatment of an initial episode of nonsevere CDI, oral metronidazole is recommended, while oral fidaxomicin is considered a possible alternative therapy. For treatment of severe CDIs, oral vancomycin is recommended, with fidaxomicin again considered to be a potential alternative therapy. The guidelines further caution that there are no data currently available to support the use of fidaxomicin in life-threatening CDIs related to exclusion criteria in the two large phase 3 trials. Fidaxomicin is a recommended antimicrobial for treating patients with a first recurrence of CDI and for patients experiencing multiple recurrences (73). Public Health England also published guidelines in 2013 regarding therapy for CDI (74). These guidelines suggest consideration of fidaxomicin for patients with severe CDIs who are believed to be at high risk for recurrence, including elderly patients with multiple comorbidities and patients who are receiving concomitant antimicrobials. Fidaxomicin is further recommended by Public Health England as the preferred option for patients with recurrent CDI, regardless of disease severity (74). North American CDI treatment guidelines from the Society for Healthcare Epidemiology of America and the Infectious Diseases Society of America have not been updated since fidaxomicin received US Food and Drug Administration approval for CDI treatment (1).

SUMMARY

Fidaxomicin is noninferior to oral vancomycin in terms of clinical response at the end of CDI therapy. Fidaxomicin has been demonstrated to be as safe as oral vancomycin, but superior to vancomycin in achieving a sustained clinical response of CDI in patients infected with non-BI/NAP1/027 strains. Fidaxomicin superiority in patients infected with non-BI/NAP1/027 strains is maintained in both severe and nonsevere CDI, as well as in patients with a high risk for recurrent CDI. Caution should be exercised in using fidaxomicin monotherapy for treatment of severe complicated CDI because limited data are available. Whether fidaxomicin is cost effective (due to its significantly higher acquisition cost versus oral vancomycin) depends on the willingness to pay threshold per QALY as a measure of assessing cost effectiveness.

DISCLOSURES AND SOURCES OF FUNDING: GGZ has received research grants supported by Cubist US and Merck US. The remainder of the authors have no financial relationships or conflicts of interest to declare.

REFERENCES

1. Cohen SH, Gerding DN, Johnson S, et al. Clinical practice guidelines for Clostridium difficile infection in adults: 2010 update by the Society for Healthcare Epidemiology of America (SHEA) and the Infectious Diseases Society of America (IDSA). Infect Control Hosp Epidemiol 2010;31:413-55.
2. Zar FA, Bakkanagari SR, Moorthi KM, Davis MB. A comparison of vancomycin and metronidazole for the treatment of Clostridium difficile-associated diarrhea, stratified by disease severity. Clin Infect Dis 2007;45:302-7.
3. Louie TJ, Gerson M, Grimard D, et al. Results of a phase III trial clinical trial comparing tolevar, vancomycin and metronidazole in patient with Clostridium difficile-associated diarrhea (CDAD). 47th Annual Interscience Conference on Antimicrobial Agents and Chemotherapy (ICAAC). Chicago, September 17-20, 2007. (Abst K-425a).
4. Bouza E, Dryden M, Mohammed R, et al. Results of a phase III trial comparing tolevamer, vancomycin and metronidazole in patients with Clostridium difficile-associated diarrhoea. 18th European Congress of Clinical Microbiology and Infectious Diseases (ECCMID). Barcelona, April 19-22, 2008. (Abst O464).
5. Johnson S, Louie TJ, Gerding D, et al. Vancomycin metronidazole or tolevamer for Clostridium difficile infection: Results from two multinational randomized controlled trials. Clin Infect Dis 2014;59:345-54.
6. Wilcox MH. The trials and tribulations of treating Clostridium difficile infection – one step backward one step forward but still progress. Clin Infect Dis 2014;59:355-7.
7. Tannock GW, Munro K, Taylor C, et al. A new macrocyclic antibiotic, fidaxomicin (OPT-80), causes less alteration to the bowel microbiota of Clostridium difficile-infected patients than does vancomycin. Microbiol 2010;156:3354-9.
8. Venugopal AA, Johnson S. Fidaxomicin: A novel macrocyclic antibiotic approved for treatment of Clostridium difficile infection. Clin Infect Dis 2012;54:568-74.
9. Recommendations for preventing the spread of vancomycin resistance. Recommendations of the Hospital Infection Control Practices Advisory Committee (HICPAC). MMWR Recomm Rep 1995;44:1-13.
10. ASHP therapeutic position statement on the preferential use of metronidazole for the treatment of Clostridium difficile-associated disease. Am J Health Syst Pharm 1998;55:1407-11.
11. Al-Nassir WN, Sethi AK, Li Y, et al. Both oral metronidazole and oral vancomycin promote overgrowth of vancomycin-resistant enterococci during treatment of Clostridium difficile-associated disease. Antimicrob Agents Chemother 2008;52:2403-6.
12. Aslam S, Hamill RJ, Musher DM. Treatment of Clostridium difficile-associated disease: Old therapies and new strategies. Lancet Infect Dis 2005;5:549-57.
13. Louie TJ, Miller MA, Mullane KM, et al. Fidaxomicin versus vancomycin for Clostridium difficile infection. N Engl J Med 2011;364:422-31.
14. Cornely OA, Crook DW, Esposito R, et al. Fidaxomicin versus vancomycin for infection with Clostridium difficile in Europe, Canada, and the USA: A double-blind, non-inferiority, randomised controlled trial. Lancet Infect Dis 2012;12:281-9.
15. Cornely OA, Miller MA, Fantin B, et al. Resolution of Clostridium difficile-associated diarrhea in patients with cancer treated with fidaxomicin or vancomycin. J Clin Oncol 2013;31:2493-9.
16. Mullane KM, Cornely OA, Crook DW, et al. Renal impairment and clinical outcomes of Clostridium difficile infection in two randomized trials. Am J Nephrol 2013;38:1-11.
17. Mullane KM, Miller MA, Weiss K, et al. Efficacy of fidaxomicin versus vancomycin as therapy for Clostridium difficile infection in individuals taking concomitant antibiotics for other concurrent infections. Clin Infect Dis 2011;53:440-7.
18. Louie TJ, Miller MA, Crook DW, et al. Effect of age on treatment outcomes in Clostridium difficile infection. J Am Geriatr Soc 2013;61:222-30.
19. Cornely OA, Miller MA, Louie TJ, Crook DW, Gorbach SL. Treatment of first recurrence of Clostridium difficile infection: Fidaxomicin versus vancomycin. Clin Infect Dis 2012;55(S2):S154-61.
20. DIFICID® Product Monograph. Optimer Pharmaceuticals, Inc. 2013.
21. Johnson AP. Drug evaluation: OPT-80, a narrow-spectrum macrocyclic antibiotic. Curr Opin Investig Drugs 2007;8:168-73.
22. Osburne MS, Sonenshein AL. Inhibition by lipiarmycin of bacteriophage growth in Bacillus subtilis. J Virol 1980;33:945-53.
23. Artsimovitch I, Seddon J, Sears P. Fidaxomicin is an inhibitor of the initiation of bacterial RNA synthesis. Clin Infect Dis 2012;55(Suppl 2):S127-31.
24. Babakhani F, Seddon J, Sears P. Comparative microbiological studies of transcription inhibitors fidaxomicin and the rifamycins in Clostridium difficile. Antimicrob Agents Chemother 2014;58:2934-7.
25. Gualtieri M, Villain-Guillot P, Latouche J, et al. Mutation in the Bacillus subtilis RNA polymerase β' subunit confers resistance to lipiarmycin. Antimicrob Agents Chemother 2006;50:401-2.
26. Wostem MM. Eubacterial sigma-factors. FEMS Microbiol Rev 1998;22:127-50.
27. Karlowsky JA, Laing NM, Zhanel GG. In vitro activity of OPT-80 tested against clinical isolates of toxin-producing Clostridium difficile. Antimicrob Agents Chemother 2008;52:4163-5.
28. Kuehne SA, Dempster AW, Heeg D, et al. Use of allelic exchange to characterize the impact of rpoB/C mutations on fitness of Clostridium difficile and sensitivity to fidaxomicin. 23rd European Congress of Clincal Microbiology and Infectious Diseases (ECCMID). Berlin, April 27-30, 2013.
29. Seddon J, Babakhani F, Sears P. Mutant prevention concentration of fidaxomicin for Clostridium difficile. 52nd Annual Interscience Conference on Antimicrobial Agents and Chemotherapy (ICAAC). San Francisco, September 9-12, 2012. (Abstr A-1274).
30. Goldstein EJC, Citron DM, Sears P, et al. Comparative susceptibilities to fidaxomicin (OPT-80) of isolates collected at baseline, recurrence, and failure from patients in two phase III trials of fidaxomicin against Clostridium difficile infection. Antimicrob Agents Chemother 2011;55:5194-9.
31. Goldstein EJC, Babakhani F, Citron DM. Antimicrobial activities of fidaxomicin. Clin Infect Dis 2012;55(Suppl 2):S143-8.

32. Babakhani F, Gomez A, Robert N, Sears P. Postantibiotic effect of fidaxomicin and its major metabolite, OP-1118, against *Clostridium difficile*. Antimicrob Agents Chemother 2011a;55:4427-9.

33. Leeds JA, Sachdeva M, Mullin S, et al. in vitro selection via serial passage of *Clostridium difficile* mutants with reduced susceptibility to fidaximicin or vancomycin. J Antimicrob Chemother 2014;69:41-4.

34. Gerber M, Ackermann G. OPT-80 a macrocyclic antimicrobial agent for the treatment of *Clostridium difficile* infection: A review. Exp Opin Investig Drugs 2008;17:51-3.

35. Swanson RN, Hardy DJ, Shipkowitz NL, et al. In vitro and in vivo evaluation of tiacumicius B and C against *Clostridium difficile*. Antimicrob Agents Chemother 1991;35:1106-11.

36. Theriault RJ, Karwowski TP, Jackson M, et al. Tiacumicins a novel complex of 18-membered macrolide antibiotics. I. Taxonomy, fermentation and antibacterial activity. J Antibiotic (Tokyo) 1987;40:567-74.

37. Credito KL, Appelbaum PC. Activity of OPT-80, a novel macrocyclic, compared with those of eight other agents against selected anaerobic species. Antimicrob Agents Chemother 2004;48:4430-4.

38. Finegold SM, Molitoris D, Vaisanen ML, et al. In vitro activities of OPT-80 and comparator drugs against anaerobic bacteria. Antimicrob Agents Chemother 2004;48:4898-902.

39. Beidenbach DI, Ross JE, Putnam SD, Jones RN. In vitro activity of fidaxomicin (OPT80) tested against contemporary isolates of *Staphylococcus* spp. and *Enterococcus* spp. Antimicrobial Agents Chemother 2010;54:2273-5.

40. Babakhani F, Seddon J, Robert N, et al. Narrow spectrum activity and low fecal binding of OPT-80 and its major hydrolysis metabolite (OP-1118). 47th Annual Interscience Conference on Antimicrobial Agents and Chemotherapy (ICAAC). Chicago, September 17 to 20, 2007.

41. Citron DM, Tyrrell KL, Merriam V, Goldstein EJC. Comparative in vitro activities of LFF571 against *Clostridium difficile* and 630 other intestinal strains of aerobic and anaerobic bacteria. Antimicrob Agents Chemother 2012;56:2493-503.

42. Hecht DW, Galang MA, Sambol SP, et al. In vitro activities of 15 antimicrobial agents against 110 toxigenic *Clostridium difficile* clinical isolates collected from 1983 to 2004. Antimicrob Agents Chemother 2007;51:2716-9.

43. Citron DM, Babakhani F, Goldstein EJ, et al. Typing and susceptibility of bacterial isolates from the fidaxomicin (OPT-80) phase II study for C. *difficile* infection. Anaerobe 2009;15:234-6.

44. Rashid MU, Dalhoff A, Weintraub A, Nord CE. In vitro activity of MCB3681 against *Clostridium difficile* strains. Anaerobe 2014;28:216-9.

45. Goldstein EJC, Citron DM, Tyrrell KL, Merriam CV. Comparative in vitro activities of SMT19969, a new antimicrobial agent, against *Clostridium difficile* and 350 Gram-positive and Gram-negative aerobic and anaerobic intestinal flora isolates. Antimicrob Agents Chemother 2013;57:4872-6.

46. Louie T, Miller M, Donskey C, et al. Clinical outcomes, safety, and pharmacokinetics of OPT-80 in a phase 2 trial with patients with *Clostridium difficile* infection. Antimicrob Agents Chemother 2009;53:223-8.

47. Louie TJ, Cannon K, Byrne B, et al. Fidaxomicin preserves the intestinal microbiome during and after treatment of *Clostridium difficile* infection (CDI) and reduces both toxin reexpression and recurrence of CDI. Clin Infect Dis 2012;55(Suppl 2):S132-42.

48. Babakhani F, Seddon J, Robert N, et al. Effects of inoculum, pH, and cations on the in vitro activity of fidaxomicin (OPT-80, PAR-101) against *Clostridium difficile*. Antimicrob Agents Chemother 2010;54:2674-6.

49. Sears P, Crook DW, Louie TJ, Miller MA, Weiss K. Fidaxomicin attains high fecal concentrations with minimal plasma concentrations following oral administration in patients with *Clostridium difficile* infection. Clin Infect Dis 2012;55(Suppl 2):S116-20.

50. Seddon J, Babakhani F, Sears P. Mutant prevention concentration of fidaxomicin for *Clostridium difficile*. 52nd Annual Interscience Conference on Antimicrobial Agents and Chemotherapy (ICAAC). San Francisco, September 9-12, 2012. (Abstr. A-1274).

51. Babakhani F, Gomez A, Robert N, Sears P. Killing kinetics of fidaxomicin and its major metabolite, OP-1118, against *Clostridium difficile*. J Med Microbiol 2011;60:1213-7.

52. Babakhani F, Bouillaut L, Sears P, et al. Fidaxomicin inhibits toxin production in *Clostridium difficile*. J Antimicrob Chemother 2013;68:515-22.

53. Koon HW, Ho S, Hing TC, et al. Fidaxomicin inhibits *Clostridium difficile* toxin A-mediated enteritis in the mouse ileum. Antimicrob Agents Chemother 2014;58:4642-50.

54. Babakhani F, Bouillaut L, Gomez A, et al. Fidaxomicin inhibits spore production in *Clostridium difficile*. Clin Infect Dis 2012;55(Suppl 2):S162-9.

55. Allen CA, Babakhani F, Sears P, et al. Both fidaxomicin and vancomycin inhibit outgrowth of *Clostridium difficile* spores. Antimicrob Agents Chemother 2013;57:664-7.

56. Chilton CH, Crowther GS, Freeman J, et al. Successful treatment of simulated *Clostridium difficile* infection in a human gut model by fidaxomicin first line and after vancomycin or metronidazole failure. J Antimicrob Chemother 2014;69:451-62.

57. Nerandzic MM, Mullane K, Miller MA, et al. Reduced acquisition and overgrowth of vancomycin-resistant enterococci and *Candida* species in patients treated with fidaxomicin versus vancomycin for *Clostridium difficile* infection. Clin Infect Dis 2012;55(Suppl 2):S121-6.

58. Mullane KM. Fidaxomicin in *Clostridium difficile* infection: Latest evidence and clinical guidance. Ther Adv Chronic Dis 2014;5:69-84.

59. Esmaily-Fard A, Tverdek FP, Crowther, et al. The use of fidaxomicin for treatment of relapsed *Clostridium difficile* infections in patients with cancer. Pharmacother 2014;34:1220-5.

60. Levey AS, Coresh J, Balk E, et al. National Kidney Foundation practice guidelines for chronic kidney disease: Evaluation, classification, and stratification. Ann Intern Med 2003;139:137-47.

61. Vargo CA, Bauer KA, Mangino JE, Johnston JEW, Goff DA. An antimicrobial stewardship program's real-world experience with fidaxomicin for treatment of *Clostridium difficile* infection: A case series. Pharmacotherapy 2014;34:901-9.

62. Eiland EH, Sawyer AJ, Massie NL. Fidaxomicin use and clinical outcomes for *Clostridium difficile*-associated diarrhea. Infect Dis Clin Pract 2015;23:32-5.

63. Clutter DS, Dubrovskaya Y, Merl MY, Teperman L, Press R, Safdar A. Fidaxomicin versus conventional antimicrobial therapy in 59 recipients of solid organ and hematopoietic stem cell transplantation with *Clostridium difficile*-associated diarrhea. Antimicrob Agents Chemother 2013;57:4501-5.

64. Penziner S, Dubrovskaya Y, Press R, Safdar A. Fidaxomicin therapy in critically ill patients with *Clostridium difficile* infection. Antimicrob Agents Chemother 2015;59:1776-81.

65. Soriano MM, Danziger LH, Gerding DN, Johnson S. Novel fidaxomicin treatment regimens for patients with multiple *Clostridium difficile* infection recurrences that are refractory to standard therapies. Open Forum Infect Dis 2014 Aug 25;1:ofu069.

66. Weiss K, Allgren RL, Sellers S. Safety analysis of fidaxomicin in comparison with oral vancomycin for *Clostridium difficile* infection. Clin Infect Dis 2012;55(Suppl 2):S110-5.

67. Iarikov DE, Alexander J, Nambiar S. Hypersensitivity reactions associated with fidaxomicin use. Clin Infect Dis 2014;58:537-9.

68. Cornely OA, Nathwani D, Ivanescu C, et al. Clinical efficacy of fidaxomicin compared with vancomycin and metronidazole in *Clostridium difficile* infections: A meta-analysis and indirect treatment comparison. J Antimicrob Chemother 2014;69:2892-900.

69. Eyre DW, Babakhani F, Griffiths D, et al. Whole-genome sequencing demonstrates that fidaxomicin is superior to vancomycin for peventing reinfection and relapse of infection with *Clostridium difficile*. J Infect Dis 2014;209:1446-51.

70. Wagner M, Lavoie L, Goetghebeur M. Clinical and economic consequences of vancomycin and fidaxomicin for the treatment of *Clostridium difficile* infection in Canada. Can J Infect Dis Med Microbiol 2014;25:87-94.

71. Stranges PM, Hutton DW, Collins CD. Cost-effectiveness analysis evaluating fidaxomicin versus oral vancomycin for the treatment of *Clostridium difficile* infection in the United States. Value Health 2013;16:297-304.

72. Nathwani D, Cornely OA, Van Engen AK, Odufowora-Sita O, Retsa P, Odeyemi IAO. Cost-effectiveness analysis of fidaxomicin versus vancomycin in *Clostridium difficile* infection. J Antimicrob Chemother 2014;69:2901-12.

73. Debast SB, Bauer MP, Kuijper EJ, on behalf of the Committee. European Society of Clinical Microbiology and Infectious Diseases: Update on the treatment guidance document for *Clostridium difficile* infection. Clin Microbiol Infect 2014;20(Suppl 2):1-26.

74. Wilcox MH. Updated guidance on the management and treatment of *Clostridium difficile* infection. <www.his.org.uk> (Accessed September 17, 2014).

31

Avian influenza A (H5N1) infection with respiratory failure and meningoencephalitis in a Canadian traveller

Naheed Rajabali MD[1], Thomas Lim MD[2], Colleen Sokolowski MD[2], Jason D Prevost MD[2], Edward Z Lee MD[2]

N Rajabali, T Lim, C Sokolowski, JD Prevost, EZ Lee. Avian influenza A (H5N1) infection with respiratory failure and meningoencephalitis in a Canadian traveller. Can J Infect Dis Med Microbiol 2015;26(4):221-223.

In an urban centre in Alberta, an otherwise healthy 28-year-old woman presented to hospital with pleuritic chest and abdominal pain after returning from Beijing, China. After several days, this was followed by headache, confusion and, ultimately, respiratory failure, coma and death. Microbiology yielded influenza A subtype H5N1 from various body sites and neuroimaging was consistent with meningoencephalitis. While H5N1 infections in humans have been reported in Asia since 1997, this is the first documented case of H5N1 influenza in the Western Hemisphere. The present case demonstrated the typical manifestation of H5N1 influenza but, for the first time, also confirmed previous suggestions from human and animal studies that H5N1 is neurotropic and can manifest with neurological symptoms and meningoencephalitis.

Key Words: *Encephalitis; H5N1; Influenza A; Meningoencephalitis*

L'infection par la grippe aviaire A (H5N1) accompagnée d'une insuffisance respiratoire et d'une méningoencéphalite chez une voyageuse canadienne

Dans un centre urbain de l'Alberta, une femme auparavant en santé de 28 ans s'est rendue à l'hôpital en raison d'une douleur pleurétique et abdominale à son retour de Beijing, en Chine. Quelques jours plus tard, cette douleur a été suivie de céphalées et de confusion, puis la patiente a souffert d'une insuffisance respiratoire, d'un coma et est décédée. La microbiologie de divers sièges a révélé une grippe H5N1 de sous-type A, et la neuro-imagerie a corroboré la présence d'une méningoencéphalite. Des infections par la grippe H5N1 sont signalées chez les humains depuis 1997 en Asie, mais il s'agit du premier cas démontré dans l'hémisphère occidental. Ce cas présentait la forme classique de la grippe H5N1, mais pour la première fois, il confirmait également ce que laissaient entrevoir les études sur des humains et des animaux, soit que la grippe H5N1 est neurotrope et peut se manifester par des symptômes neurologiques et une méningoencéphalite.

In 1997, a poultry-originating influenza, H5N1 influenza virus, caused an outbreak in Hong Kong, China. This was the first time it had been isolated from a human patient. Since then, >600 people have been infected with the H5N1 virus worldwide in the past 10 years, with a mortality rate of approximately 61% (1). Human H5N1 virus infection generally manifests as severe pneumonia progressing to acute respiratory distress syndrome, but can also present with abdominal pain and diarrhea (1,2). It also demonstrates neurotropism, being isolated in the neurons of animals and asymptomatic individuals (3,4).

CASE PRESENTATION

A healthy 28-year-old woman presented to the Red Deer Regional Hospital (Red Deer, Alberta) emergency department December 28, 2013 with a two-day history of right-sided pleuritic chest pain, mild dyspnea, nausea, right upper quadrant abdominal pain, malaise and chills. Her symptoms began as isolated chest pain during her flight back to Canada after a three-week stay in Beijing, China, and she presented to the hospital the day after her return. Her history was negative for sick contacts, exposure to poultry or birds, and visits to outdoor markets or farms. Her temperature was 39.7°C with a heart rate of 125 beats/min and respiratory rate of 18 breaths/min. The rest of her vital signs were normal. Her physical examination was remarkable only for mild tenderness at the right upper abdominal quadrant. Bloodwork demonstrated an elevated leukocyte count of 12.6×10^9/L and was negative otherwise, including blood cultures.

An electrocardiogram showed sinus tachycardia with nonspecific T wave inversions in leads III and aVF. Her initial chest radiograph revealed a subtle rounded consolidation of the right lung apex. A subsequent computed tomography pulmonary angiogram of the chest ruled out pulmonary embolism, but identified a dense rounded consolidation of the right lung apex with surrounding ill-defined ground-glass attenuation. Chest pain was her predominant clinical symptom, and the patient was prescribed a five-day outpatient course of levofloxacin with a diagnosis of bacterial pneumonia.

She returned to the emergency department in the afternoon of January 1, 2014 with persistent shortness of breath and worsening right-sided chest pain, without cough. She had developed a frontal headache, lightheadedness, abdominal pain and several episodes of vomiting. This time, her respiratory rate was 22 breaths/min and she required supplemental oxygen at 2 L/min on nasal prongs to maintain an oxygen saturation of 92%. She had diminished breath sounds in the right lung zones. Her abdomen was diffusely tender, but more so in the right upper quadrant and epigastric region without guarding or distention.

Investigations again revealed leukocytosis at 10.2×10^9/L. A chest radiograph at 17:31 showed a small right pleural effusion and worsening of the right apical pneumonia. A chest tube was placed on the right, draining 300 mL of slightly cloudy, yellowish-tan pleural fluid. The patient's antimicrobial coverage was broadened to pipercillin-tazobactam and azithromycin for nonresolving pneumonia. The abdominal pain was attributed to the parapneumonic effusion because it resolved several hours following

[1]*University of Alberta, Edmonton;* [2]*Red Deer Regional Hospital, Red Deer, Alberta*
Correspondence: Dr Edward Z Lee, Red Deer Regional Hospital, 4312 54 Avenue, Red Deer, Alberta T4N 4M1. e-mail ezlee@gmail.com

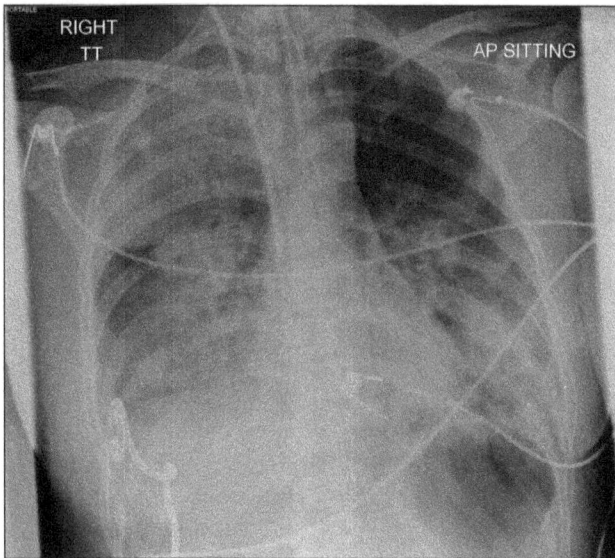

Figure 1) *Chest radiograph demonstrating right greater than left dense bilateral consolidation consistent with worsening pneumonia after the patient was transferred to the intensive care unit and intubated for respiratory failure*

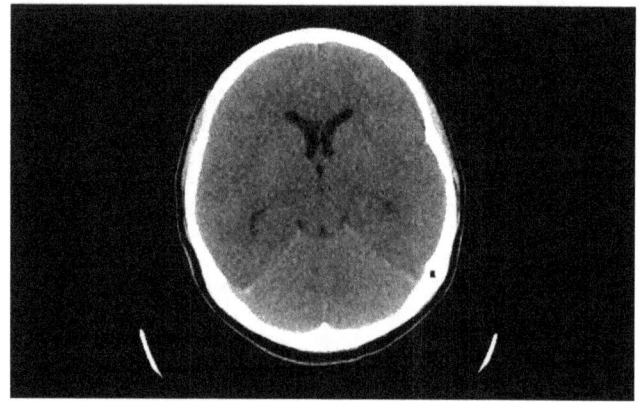

Figure 2) *Computed tomography scan of the head demonstrating generalized cerebral parenchymal swelling, diffuse sulcal space and cisternal space effacement suggestive of meningoencephalitis*

insertion of a chest tube. The pleural fluid was exudative using Light's criteria and pathology revealed scant benign mesothelial cells with reactive changes in the background of numerous neutrophils. No bacteria were seen on Gram stain and there was no growth on cultures. An abdominal ultrasound revealed two small liver hemangiomas and was otherwise unremarkable.

On the following morning, January 2, she felt worse overall and began to notice blood-tinged sputum with her cough. By the late evening, her oxygen requirements increased to 8 L/min. The chest radiograph demonstrated progressive bilateral lung consolidation. That evening, she had a transient loss of consciousness, with recovery, followed by blurred vision that then improved. She gave a history of intermittent neck pain. A neurological examination was performed, which revealed normal extraocular eye movements, no nystagmus, pupils that were equal and reactive to light symmetrically, normal facial nerves and normal trigeminal nerve sensation. The fundi were not visualized. At this point, the intensive care unit (ICU) was consulted.

In the evening, the patient complained of increasing dyspnea and persisting sharp, right-sided chest pain, again worse with inspiration. She was alert and oriented, denied having a headache, visual changes or neck stiffness. She also denied having a sore throat or abdominal pain.

On examination by the ICU, she showed signs of respiratory distress along with tachypnea at 24 breaths/min saturating at 96% on 8 L/min of oxygen by mask. She had normal vital signs otherwise and scored 15 on her Glasgow Coma Scale. She had an intermittent cough, productive of pink frothy sputum. She had diminished breath sounds bilaterally, but more severe throughout the right lung zones. Although alert, she was slow to answer questions and would occasionally stare away for several seconds requiring repeat prompting. She did not have other clinical features of seizure. Her responses were limited to two-word sentences. On one occasion, when she did not communicate verbally, she used a laptop computer. Although her typing motions appeared to be purposeful, the typed text was nonsensical. Otherwise, no gross neurological deficits were detected. She did not exhibit any facial droop or asymmetry, and she moved all four limbs spontaneously. She did not have meningismus.

Her diagnosis was believed to be worsening H1N1 influenza, given the recent regional H1N1 influenza outbreak. Repeat sputum cultures were sent, including samples for acid-fast bacteria and viral swabs. Oseltamivir was added at this time to the current antimicrobials.

Within 4 h, the patient's oxygen requirements increased to 12 L/min of oxygen by simple mask. She was alert, but markedly agitated, disoriented and confused. Again, no neck stiffness or discomfort were elicited.

She was transferred to the ICU where she was sedated and intubated. Her initial ventilator settings were pressure controlled ventilation 24 cmH$_2$0, positive end-expiratory pressure 12 cmH$_2$0, fraction of inspired oxygen 70%, peak pressure 39 cmH$_2$O, respiratory frequency and respiratory rate of 22 breaths/min, with volumes of 400 mL to 430 mL. Her postintubation arterial blood gases showed a pH 7.37, a partial pressure of carbon dioxide of 36 mmHg, a partial pressure of oxygen of 83 mmHg, a bicarbonate of 21 mmol/L, base deficit 4 and oxygen saturation of 93%.

The chest radiograph revealed right greater than left bilateral consolidation, consistent with worsening pneumonia (Figure 1).

At approximately 07:00 January 3, the patient became hemodynamically unstable. She was tachycardic with heart rates varying between 120 beats/min and 150 beats/min. Her blood pressure was labile, rising to 220/120 mmHg. Initially, it was believed that she was inadequately sedated and her midazolam and fentanyl infusions were increased. However, her tachycardia and hypertension persisted. When examined, the patient's pupils were dilated and unresponsive to light. At this point her midazolam and fentanyl infusions were discontinued. Her blood pressure initially normalized, then over the next 1 h to 2 h she became hypotensive requiring inotropic support. She was intravenously given mannitol 20% and furosemide, and hyperventilated to a partial pressure of carbon dioxide of 30 mmHg.

A neurological examination was completed at approximately 4 h and 8 h after sedating infusions were discontinued. She was unresponsive to painful stimuli, had absent cranial nerve responses and failed the apnea test.

A nonenhanced computed tomography scan of the head (Figure 2) demonstrated generalized cerebral parenchymal swelling, diffuse sulcal space and cisternal space effacement suggestive of meningoencephalitis.

A magnetic resonance examination of the brain (Figure 3) was obtained, confirming diffuse sulcal space and cisternal space effacement with diffusely increased signal of the extra-axial cerebrospinal fluid (CSF) spaces and ependyma of the lateral ventricles on fluid-attenuated inversion recovery imaging. The increased signal of the CSF spaces on fluid-attenuated inversion recovery imaging indicated proteinaceous debris within the CSF spaces and along the ependymal surface. Diffuse parenchymal swelling and slightly increased T2-weighted signal of the cortex of the temporal lobes, insular cortex and hippocampal regions was noted bilaterally, suggestive of encephalitis. Gadolinium-enhanced magnetic resonance angiography revealed markedly delayed intracranial arterial flow, with partial opacification of the anterior cerebral, middle cerebral and posterior cerebral arteries at 4 min postcontrast injection. Brisk flow to the scalp vessels was noted. Enhancement of the meninges was not observed, likely secondary to diminished intracranial blood flow.

The neurologist on call examined the patient 11 h after sedating medications had been discontinued. The abnormal findings of the earlier neurological examination were confirmed. The patient met the clinical criteria for brain death and was pronounced dead. A lumbar puncture was performed following brain death and before discontinuation of cardiorespiratory life support.

Samples from the nasopharyngeal swab, endotracheal aspirates and CSF tested positive for influenza A type H5N1. CSF showed 2+ white blood cells, 2+ red blood cells, without bacteria seen. Details of diagnostic specimen analysis and virological investigations were reported by Fonseca (5). Autoimmune serologies obtained later returned positive for perinuclear antineutrophil cytoplasmic antibody. Myeloperoxidase and antiglomerular basement membrane antibodies were both negative.

DISCUSSION

We report a fatal case of influenza A (H5N1) in a woman, 28 years of age, who presented in January 2014 with pleuritic chest pain, dyspnea and right upper quadrant abdominal pain due to pneumonia and a pleural effusion, followed by respiratory failure, agitation, confusion and coma, after a three-week visit to Beijing, China. She was diagnosed with acute respiratory distress syndrome, secondary to pneumonia and brain death due to meningoencephalitis. The diagnosis of H5N1 was established by isolating the virus from nasopharyngeal swabs, broncho-alveolar lavage and CSF.

Our patient's demographic is in keeping with what is commonly found in humans infected with H5N1. Most patients with influenza A (H5N1) virus infection have been previously healthy. The median age of patients with influenza A (H5N1) virus infection is approximately 18 years, with 90% of patients ≤40 years of age. Moreover, increases in human cases of influenza A (H5N1) have been observed during cooler months in association with increases in outbreaks among poultry (1,6-8).

Unique to our experience is that this is the first reported case of H5N1 influenza in the Western world because most cases remain endemic in Asia, the Middle East, Europe and Africa. Furthermore, until now, no cases of influenza A (H5N1) illness have been identified among short-term travellers visiting countries affected by outbreaks among poultry or wild birds (9).

Our patient's initial respiratory manifestation is a common finding in H5N1-infected humans, with the virus primarily affecting the lower respiratory tract causing respiratory failure. Diarrhea is also a common presenting feature of H5N1, occurring in up to 70% of patients. Besides these common presentations, patients have also been noted to complain of vomiting and abdominal pain. These symptoms correlate with findings of viral RNA in fecal samples and viral replication in intestines (1,2,4,10). Our patient complained of vomiting and crescendo-decrescendo abdominal pain, but did not have diarrhea.

Our patient also had mild intermittent headaches, confusion and demonstrated symptoms and a clinical course in keeping with

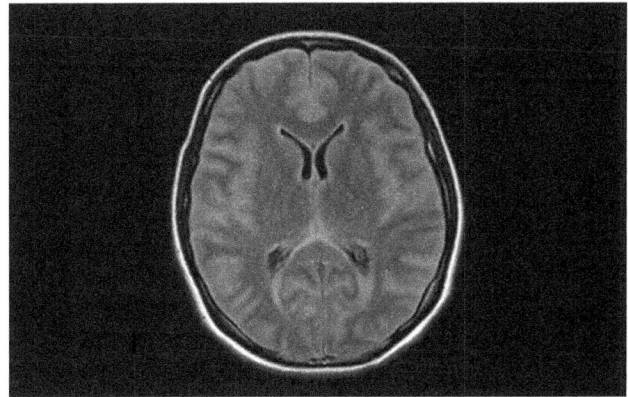

Figure 3) *Magnetic resonance examination of the brain revealing diffuse sulcal space and cisternal space effacement with diffusely increased signal of the extra-axial cerebrospinal fluid spaces and ependyma of the lateral ventricles on fluid-attenuated inversion recovery imaging. Diffuse parenchymal swelling and slightly increased T2-weighted signal of the cortex of the temporal lobes, insular cortex and hippocampal regions noted bilaterally suggests encephalitis*

meningoencephalitis. Encephalopathy and encephalitis in humans have been reported in cases associated with seasonal influenza A and B viruses (11,12,13). Only one case of human central nervous system involvement has been suggested by a patient who developed a coma from whom H5N1 was isolated from CSF (10) despite being noted in mammals such as ferrets, mice and felids (8). With respect to the child who developed a coma, imaging of the brain or histological analysis was not performed, and it is uncertain whether the patient experienced encephalopathy or true encephalitis. These reports suggest the H5N1 virus is becoming more neurologically virulent and adapting to mammals. Despite the trend in virulence, the mode of influenza virus transmission remains elusive to date. It is unclear how our patient acquired the H5N1 influenza infection because she did not have any known contact with any animals or poultry.

The nonspecific clinical presentation of H5N1 influenza virus has frequently led to underdiagnoses of subsequently confirmed cases (1). Infection with H5N1 influenza virus should be considered in the differential diagnosis for patients with epidemiological risk factors presenting with systemic manifestations, including the common respiratory and gastrointestinal symptoms, clusters of intermittent abdominal pain and headache, as well as signs of meningoencephalitis.

Having a high index of suspicion for H5N1 infection is essential to the appropriate management of the illness, because treatment with antiviral agents is likely to be beneficial only when it is started early in the course of illness (1,2,14).

REFERENCES

1. Abdel-Ghafar AN, Chotpitayasunondh T, Gao Z, et al. Update on avian influenza A (H5N1) virus infection in humans. N Engl J Med 2008;358:261-73.
2. Gambotto A, Barratt-Boyes S, de Jong M, et al. Human infection with highly pathogenic H5N1 influenza virus. Lancet 2007;371:1464-75.
3. Shinya K, Makino A, Hatta M, et al. Subclinical brain injury caused by H5N1 influenza virus infection. J Virol 2011;10:5202-7.
4. Gu J, Xie Z, Gao Z, et al. H5N1 infection of the respiratory tract and beyond: A molecular pathology study. Lancet 29;370:1137-45.
5. Fonseca K. Fatal avian influenza A(H5N1) infection in a Canadian traveler. Promed. <www.promedmail.org, archive no. 20140112.2167282> (Accessed on January 12, 2014.)
6. Park AW, Glass K. Dynamic patterns of avian and human influenza in east and southeast Asia. Lancet Infect Dis 2007;7:543-8.
7. Ortiz JR, Wallis TR, Katz MA, et al. No evidence of avian influenza A (H5N1) among returning US travelers. Emerg Infect Dis 2007;13:294-7.
8. Kaplan B, Webby R. The avian and mammalian host range of highly pathogenic avian H5N1 influenza. Virus Res 2013;178:3-11.
9. World Health Organization. Antigenic and genetic characteristics of zoonotic influenza viruses and development of candidate vaccine viruses for pandemic preparedness. Wkly Epidemiol Rec 2014; 89:105-16. <www.who.int/wer/2014/wer8911.pdf> (Accessed on March 16, 2014).
10. de Jong M, Van Cam B, Tu Qui P, et al. Fatal avian influenza A (H5N1) in a child presenting with diarrhea followed by coma. N Engl J Med 2005;352:686.
11. Morishima T, Togashi T, Yokota S, et al. Encephalitis and encephalopathy associatedwith an influenza epidemic in Japan. Clin Infect Dis 2002;35:512-7.
12. Steininger C, Popow-Kraupp T, Laferl H, et al. Acute encephalopathy associated with influenza A virus infection. Clin Infect Dis 2003;36:567-74.
13. Maricich SM, Neul JL, Lotze TE, et al. Neurologic complications associated with influenza A in children during the 2003-2004 influenza season in Houston, Texas. Pediatrics 2004;114:e626-e33.
14. Liu Q, Liu D, Yang Z, et al. Characteristics of human infection with avian influenza viruses and development of new antiviral agents. Acta Pharmacologica Sinica 2013;34:1257-69.

32

An unusual case of meningitis

Eric DR Pond BSc[1], Sameh El-Bailey MbChb DCP FRCPath[1,2], Duncan Webster MA MD FRCPC[3]

EDR Pond, S El-Bailey, D Webster. An unusual case of meningitis. Can J Infect Dis Med Microbiol 2015;26(3):e62-64.

Pasteurella multocida is a rare cause of bacterial meningitis. A 56-year-old man with several pets developed a profoundly decreased level of consciousness following left tympanomastoidectomy. Lumbar puncture produced cerebrospinal fluid with the typical findings of meningitis (low glucose, high protein, high leukocytes). Cultures from the cerebrospinal fluid and a swab of the left ear revealed Gram-negative coccobacillus identified as *P multocida*. The organism was sensitive to ceftriaxone, ampicillin and penicillin, and a 14-day course of intravenous penicillin was used as definitive treatment, resulting in full recovery. Although rare, *P multocida* should be considered as a potential cause of meningitis in patients with animal exposure, particularly in the setting of recent cranial surgery.

Key Words: Pasteurella multocida; *Meningitis*; *Tympanomoastoidectomy*; *Zoonosis*

Un cas inhabituel de méningite

Le *Pasteurella multocida* est une rare cause de méningite bactérienne. Un homme de 56 ans propriétaire de plusieurs animaux a présenté une importante diminution de son niveau de conscience après une tympanomastoïdectomie gauche. Le liquide céphalorachidien prélevé par ponction lombaire présentait les caractéristiques classiques de la méningite (glycémie basse, protéine élevée, leucocytes élevés). Les cultures du liquide céphalorachidien et un écouvillon de l'oreille gauche ont révélé un coccobacille à Gram négatif, le *P multocida*. L'organisme était sensible à la ceftriaxone, à l'ampicilline et à la pénicilline. Un traitement de pénicilline administré par voie intraveineuse pendant 14 jours a favorisé un rétablissement complet. Même si c'est rare, le *P multocida* doit être envisagé comme cause de méningite chez des patients exposés à des animaux, particulièrement après avoir subi une opération crânienne.

Pasteurella multocida is a Gram-negative coccobacillus. It is a small, encapsulated, nonmotile facultative anaerobe, commonly found as part of the commensal oral flora in animals. Carriage rates among domestic animals, such as cats and dogs, have been shown to be as high as 70% to 90% and 55%, respectively (1,2), and it is also carried by a variety of other domestic and wild animals (3). It is, therefore, an important zoonotic organism. *P multocida* has been reported to cause a variety of infections in humans including cellulitis, subcutaneous abscesses, septic arthritis, osteomyelitis, bacteremia, endocarditis, meningitis, and various oral and respiratory tract infections; however, skin manifestations are by far the most common (3).

The present article describes a rare case of *P multocida* meningitis in a patient following tympanomastoidectomy.

CASE PRESENTATION

A 56-year-old man developed chronic otorrhea related to left tympanic membrane perforation. He was admitted for an elective left typanomastoidectomy and removal of the incus and malleus with tympanoplasty. His medical history included hypertension, dyslipidemia, gout, polycystic kidney disease and gastroesophageal reflux disease. His surgical history was significant for previous left tympanoplasty and inguinal hernia repair. His medications at the time of admission were rosuvastatin, domperidone, esomeprazole, allopurinol, irbesartan/hydrochlorothiazide and labetalol.

On the first day postoperatively the patient experienced a sudden drop in his level of consciousness accompanied by marked agitation, and required intubation. His Glasgow Coma Scale score was 9 (eyes 3, verbal 3, motor 3). There were no focal neurological signs, his pupils were symmetrical but sluggish to react and the fundi appeared normal. His blood glucose level was 9.0 mmol/L. He was subsequently transferred to the intensive care unit. A computed tomography scan of the patient's head showed no structural abnormalities, no masses and no hematoma. Lumbar puncture was performed and revealed cloudy cerebrospinal fluid (CSF) with an elevated protein level (5.78 g/L), low glucose level (<1.0 mmol/L) and a leukocyte count of $11,974 \times 10^6$/L, with 95% neutrophils. Based on these findings, the patient was treated empirically for bacterial meningitis with intravenous (IV) vancomycin, ceftriaxone and dexamethasone pending culture results and sensitivities. Further blood work revealed a blood leukocyte count of 13.8×10^9/L, hemoglobin level of 123 g/L and platelet count of 154×10^9/L. His serum sodium level was 146 mmol/L, potassium level 3.6 mmol/L, chloride level 106 mmol/L, urea level 12.6 mmol/L and creatinine level 190 µmol/L.

Initial Gram stain of the CSF using the cytospin technique revealed abundant polymorphonuclear leukocytes and no organisms. Preliminary reports revealed growth of Gram-negative coccobacilli, and at this point metronidazole was also added to the treatment regime until an anaerobic cause was ruled out. Ultimately, the organism was identified from aerobic cultures as *P multocida* using the Vitek 2 identification system (bioMérieux, USA). Anaerobic cultures were negative. The isolate was sensitive to ceftriaxone, ampicillin and penicillin. Interestingly, a swab of the left ear performed on postoperative day 2 grew the same organism as that cultured from the CSF (growth on chocolate and blood agar; no growth on MacConkey's or inhibitory mold agar). The empirical antibiotics and dexamethasone were discontinued, and the patient was started on a 14-day course of IV penicillin G at a dose of 2,000,000 units every 4 h. The patient made a rapid recovery from his meningitis, and he was discharged on postoperative day 10 to continue treatment as an outpatient. On further questioning, it was revealed that the patient was the primary caregiver of several pet cats and a dog, although he reported no history of bites. The pets were allowed on the furniture, including his bed, and would occasionally lick his face.

[1]Dalhousie University; [2]Microbiology, Saint John Regional Hospital; [3]Internal Medicine/Medical Microbiology, Dalhousie University
Correspondence: Eric Pond, Medical Education 3 South, 400 University Avenue, Saint John, New Brunswick E2L 4L2 e-mail er513463@dal.ca

TABLE 1

A list of cases of *Pasteurella multocida* meningitis published in the English literature after 1999

Author (reference), year	Age, years (sex)	Predisposing factors	Animal exposure	Clinical findings	Treatment (duration)	Outcome
Brossier et al (13), 2010	46 (F)	Transethmoidal pituitary adenectomy	Contact with cats	Headache; fever; nuchal rigidity; epistaxis	Cefotaxime and ofloxacin (1 week)	Recovered
López et al (14), 2013	37 (M)	Chronic sinusitis; defect in lamina cribosa	Pig bite	Headache; vomiting; fever	Ceftriaxone	Recovered
Kawashima et al (15), 2010	44 (F)	None	Kissing her dog	Headache; fever; nausea; neck stiffness	Meropenem (1 week)	Recovered
Per et al (16), 2010	15 (M)	Kerion celci on head	Pet rabbit	Headache; weakness; confusion; lethargy; neck stiffness	Cefotaxime, cefazolin, penicillin	Recovered
Tjen et al (17), 2007	44 (F)	Otitis media	Face licked by pet dog	Headache; vomiting; fever; drowsy; neck stiffness; right-sided paralysis	Chloramphenicol	Recovered
Tattevin et al (18), 2005	60 (F)	Chronic mastoiditis	Cat bite	Fever; chills; rigors; nuchal rigidity; agitation; decreased responsiveness	Benzylpenicillin (2 weeks)	Recovered
Jordan et al (19), 2007	66 (M)	Otitis, alcoholism	Dog exposure	Not reported	Iv levofloxacin aztreonam (1 week); oral levofloxacin (18 days)	Recovered
O'Neill et al (20), 2005	72 (F)	None	Pet cat	Fever; jaundice; decreased level of consciousness; neck stiffness	Cefatoxime cefotaxime (14 days), penicillin (27 days)	Obstructive hydrocephalus requiring shunt and eventual recovery
Proulx et al (21), 2003	33 (F)	None	Dog scratch	Headache; neck pain; photo-phobia; fever; tachycardia	Penicillin (14 days)	Recovered
Armstrong et al (22), 2000	52 (M)	None	Pet dog, animal feces indoors	Found dead at home	–	Death

F Female; M Male

DISCUSSION

Meningitis is an uncommon outcome of *P multocida* infection (3), making *P multocida* a rare cause of adult bacterial meningitis. Two reviews spanning 1950 to 1999 report only 29 cases published in the English literature during that time period (4,5). Animal contact was a major risk factor, present in 89% of cases, and a history of a bite was much less common, occurring only 15% of the time (4). Previous cranial/facial surgery or skull fracture has been reported as a cause of *P multocida* meningitis (5-13). Table 1 summarizes adult cases of *P multocida* meningitis published in the English literature after 1999 (13-22). Animal contact was present in all cases, while only two (20%) reported a history of a bite. One patient had a history of cranial surgery (13).

The current report presents one of only a handful of cases of *P multocida* meningitis ever documented in the literature from a Canadian site (5,6,9,21,23). The patient developed a severely decreased level of consciousness after tympanomastoidectomy. The patient had the typical CSF findings of bacterial meningitis (low glucose, high protein, high leukocytes). Penicillin is the most commonly used antibiotic to treat *P multocida* meningitis (4,15), and our patient recovered fully with a course of IV penicillin G. Many of the more recent cases describe treating with third generation cephalosporins (Table 1).

P multocida meningitis has been reported following mastoidectomy (11,12), and the pathogenesis of infection is hypothesized to involve contiguous spread of the organism from a colonized ear canal. Supporting this theory, a swab of our patient's ear canal grew *P multocida*. Our patient had experienced chronic otorrhea. Local spread from an adjacent infected site has been proposed as an etiology (4) because chronic otitis media and otorrhea have been found in association with *P multocida* meningitis (4,19,24-27). Our patient showed no signs of clinical meningitis preoperatively; therefore, extension to the surgical site is the likely mechanism in this case. A preoperative ear swab has been proposed for patients having a mastoidectomy that have a history of exposure to animals (12), and may be supported by the present case.

ACKNOWLEDGEMENTS: The authors acknowledge the hard work and contribution of the technical staff of the Microbiology Division at the Saint John Regional Hospital (Saint John, New Brunswick).

REFERENCES

1. Owen CR, Buker EO, Bell JF, Jellison WL. *Pasteurella multocida* in animal mouths. Rocky Mountain Med J 1968;65:45-6.
2. Smith JE. Studies on *Pasteurella septica*. I. The occurrence in the nose and tonsils of dogs. J Comp Pathol Ther 1955;65:239-45.
3. Weber DJ, Wolfson JS, Swartz MN, Hooper DC. *Pasteurella multocida* infections. Report of 34 cases and review of the literature. Medicine (Baltimore) 1984;63:133-54.
4. Green BT, Ramsey KM, Nolan PE. *Pasteurella multocida* meningitis: Case report and review of last 11 y. Scand J Infect Dis 2002;34:213-74.
5. Kumar A, Devlin HR, Vellend H. *Pasteurella multocida* meningitis in an adult: Case report and a review. Rev Infect Dis 1990;12:440-8.
6. Goodman Y. Human *Pasteurella multocida* infections in Alberta. Can J Med Technol 1960;22:104-9.
7. Permezel JM, Smith CC, Flint E, Young HA. Opportunistic *Pasteurella multocida* meningitis. J Laryngol Otol 1984;98:939-40.
8. Roberts SR, Esther JW, Brewer JH. Post-traumatic *Pasteurella multocida* meningitis. South Med J 1988;81:675-6.
9. Dolman PJ, Ezzat S, Rootman J, Bowie WR. *Pasteurella multocida* meningitis following orbital exenteration. Am J Ophthalmol 1988;105:698-9.
10. Casolari C, Fabio U. Isolation of *Pasteurella multocida* from human clinical specimens: First report in Italy. Eur J Epidemiol 1988;4:389-90.
11. Parry CM, Cheesbrough JS, O'Sullivan G. Meningitis due to *Pasteurella multocida*. Rev Infect Dis 1991;13:187.
12. Dammeijer PF, McCombe AW. Meningitis from canine *Pasteurella multocida* following mastoidectomy. J Laryngol Otol 1991;105:571-2.
13. Brossier F, Clemenceau S, Lecso-Bornet M, Jarlier V, Sougakoff W. Two concomitant but unrelated cases of *Pasteurella multocida* infection, including meningitis secondary to pituitary adenoma microsurgery. Med Mal Infect 2010;40:590-2.

14. López C, Sanchez-Rubio P, Betrán A, Terré R. *Pasteurella multocida* bacterial meningitis caused by contact with pigs. Braz J Microbiol 2013;44:473-4.

15. Kawashima S, Matsukawa N, Ueki Y, Hattori M, Ojika K. *Pasteurella multocida* meningitis caused by kissing animals: A case report and review of the literature. J Neurol 2010;257:653-4.

16. Per H, Kumandaş S, Gümüş H, Oztürk MK, Coşkun A. Meningitis and subgaleal, subdural, epidural empyema due to *Pasteurella multocida*. J Emerg Med 2010;39:35-8.

17. Tjen C, Wyllie SA, Pinto A. *Pasteurella* meningo-encephalitis – a risk of household pets. J Infect 2007;55:479-80.

18. Tattevin P, Souala F, Gautier AL, et al. Diabetes in patients with pasteurellosis. Scand J Infect Dis 2005;37:731-3.

19. Jordan EF, Nye MB, Luque AE. Successful treatment of *Pasteurella multocida* meningitis with aztreonam. Scand J Infect Dis 2007;39:72-4.

20. O'Neill E, Moloney A, Hickey M. *Pasteurella multocida* meningitis: Case report and review of the literature. J Infect 2005;50:344-5.

21. Proulx NL, Freedman MS, Chan JW, Toye B, Code CC. Acute disseminated encephalomyelitis associated with *Pasteurella multocida* meningitis. Can J Neurol Sci 2003;30:155-8.

22. Armstrong GR, Sen RA, Wilkinson J. *Pasteurella multocida* meningitis in an adult: Case report. J Clin Pathol 2000;53:234-5.

23. Burdge DR, Scheifele D, Speert DP. Serious *Pasteurella multocida* infections from lion and tiger bites. JAMA 1985;253:3296-7.

24. McCue JD. *Pasteurella multocida* meningitis. J Maine Med Assoc 1979;70:461-2.

25. Smith FR. *Pasteurella multocida* meningitis. Postgrad Med J 1980;56:250-1.

26. Bruun B, Friis-Moller A. Meningitis and bacteremia caused by *Pasteurella multocida*. A case report. Acta Pathol Microbiol Immunol Scand 1983;91:329-331.

27. Godey B, Morandi X, Bourdiniere J, Heurtin C. Beware of dog licking ears. Lancet 1999;354:1267-8.

33

Seroprevalences of hepatitis B virus and hepatitis C virus among participants of an Asian health fair in the Lower Mainland, British Columbia

Stephen Ip MD[1], Jo-Ann Ford MSN[1], Kirby Lau BSc[1], Vladimir Marquez MDCM MSc[1], Marisa Guan MD[1], Carolyn Klassen MSN[1], Jessica Chan MD[2], WC Peter Kwan MD[1], Mel Krajden MD[3], Eric M Yoshida MD[1]

S Ip, J-A Ford, K Lau, et al. Seroprevalences of hepatitis B virus and hepatitis C virus among participants of an Asian health fair in the Lower Mainland, British Columbia. Can J Infect Dis Med Microbiol 2015;26(4):196-200.

BACKGROUND: The seroprevalences of hepatitis B virus (HBV) and hepatitis C virus (HCV) are 0.4% and 0.8%, respectively, in Canada, but varying rates have been reported in different populations. **OBJECTIVES:** To determine the seroprevalences of HBV and HCV among attendees of an Asian health fair in the Lower Mainland, British Columbia, as well as to correlate questionnaire answers regarding vaccination status to serological profiles. **METHODS:** Attendees at an Asian health fair were invited to participate in the present study on a voluntary basis. They provided answers to a questionnaire including ethnicity and vaccination status. Blood was then drawn for HBV and HCV serology. Active HBV was defined as HBV surface antigen (HBsAg) positive while HCV seroprevalence was defined as HCV antibody reactive. Previous exposure to HBV was defined as HBV core antibody (anti-HBc) positive and HBsAg negative. Nonimmunity was defined as anti-HBc negative and HBV surface antibody negative. Only those with correct demographic information matched to serological results were included in the study. **RESULTS:** There were 192 consenting attendees of the fair, of whom 112 were included in the study. Of the participants, 91% were Chinese. Active HBV infection was found in three participants (2.7% [95% CI 0.6% to 7.6%]) and HCV infection was found in two participants (1.8% [95% CI 0.2% to 6.3%]). More than 40% of participants had been previously exposed to HBV (42% [95% CI 33% to 51%]). Almost 20% demonstrated nonimmunity to HBV (19% [95% CI 12% to 27%]). There was significant discordance when questionnaire answers regarding vaccination status were compared with serological profiles. **CONCLUSION:** The seroprevalences of HBV and HCV in this cohort were 2.7% and 1.8%, respectively – higher than nationally reported rates. Our results highlight that the lack of knowledge of HBV infection and vaccination status remains a significant clinical issue in the Asian community of British Columbia.

Key Words: Hepatitis B, Hepatitis C, Seroprevalence

La séroprévalence des virus de l'hépatite B et de l'hépatite C chez les participants à une foire asiatique sur la santé du Lower Mainland, en Colombie-Britannique

HISTORIQUE : La séroprévalence des virus de l'hépatite B (VHB) et de l'hépatite C (VHC) s'élève à 0,4 % et à 0,8 %, respectivement, au Canada, mais les taux sont variables dans diverses populations. **OBJECTIFS :** Déterminer la séroprévalence du VHB et du VHC chez les participants à une foire asiatique sur la santé du Lower Mainland, en Colombie-Britannique, et lier les réponses au questionnaire sur le statut vaccinal avec les profils sérologiques. **MÉTHODOLOGIE :** Les participants à une foire asiatique sur la santé ont été invités à participer volontairement à l'étude. Ils ont répondu à un questionnaire contenant des questions sur l'ethnie et le statut vaccinal. Du sang a ensuite été prélevé en vue d'une sérologie du VHB et du VHC. Le VHB actif était défini comme un résultat positif à l'antigène de surface du VHB (AgHBs), tandis que la séroprévalence du VHC était définie comme une réaction aux anticorps anti-VHC. Une exposition passée au VHB était définie comme un résultat positif à l'antigène capsidique du VHB (anti-HBc) et négatif à l'AgHBs. La non-immunité était définie comme des résultats négatifs à l'anti-HBc et à l'anticorps de surface du VHB. Seulement ceux dont l'information démographique exacte correspondait aux résultats sérologiques ont participé à l'étude. **RÉSULTATS :** Au total, 192 participants consentants ont participé à la foire, dont 112 à l'étude. Des participants, 91 % étaient Chinois. Trois étaient atteints d'une infection active par le VHB (2,7 % [95 % IC 0,6 % à 7,6 %]) et deux, d'une infection par le VHC (1,8 % [95 % IC 0,2 % à 6,3 %]). Plus de 40 % des participants avaient déjà été exposés au VHB (42 % [95 % IC 33 % à 51 %]). Près de 20 % ont démontré une non immunité au VHB (19 % [95 % IC 12 % à 27 %]). On constatait une importante discordance entre les réponses au questionnaire sur le statut vaccinal et les profils sérologiques. **CONCLUSION :** La séroprévalence du VHB et le VHC de cette cohorte s'élevait à 2,7 % et à 1,8 %, respectivement, soit des résultats plus élevés que les taux nationaux. Ces résultats font ressortir que l'absence de connaissances sur l'infection par le VHB et le statut vaccinal demeure un problème clinique significatif dans la communauté asiatique de la Colombie-Britannique.

According to the Public Health Agency of Canada (1,2), the seroprevalences of hepatitis B virus (HBV) and hepatitis C virus (HCV) in Canada are estimated to be 0.4% and 0.8%, respectively; however, rates may vary significantly, with rates of chronic HBV as high as 5% to 15% being reported among Southeast Asian Canadians (Chinese and Vietnamese). Because at-risk populations for hepatitis (eg, certain ethnic groups) may be less likely to participate in epidemiological studies, HBV and HCV seroprevalences may be under-reported (1-3). Data regarding these populations are lacking in Canada. In a recent study at our centre (Vancouver General Hospital,

[1]*Department of Medicine, Division of Gastroenterology, University of British Columbia;* [2]*United Chinese Community Enrichment Services Society (SUCCESS);* [3]*BC Centre for Disease Control, Vancouver, British Columbia*
Correspondence: Dr Eric M Yoshida, Division of Gastroenterology, Vancouver General Hospital, University of British Columbia, 5th Floor, 2775 Laurel Street, Vancouver, British Columbia V5Z 1M9. e-mail eric.yoshida@vch.ca

Vancouver, British Columbia [BC]), the seroprevalences of HBV and HCV in admitted patients were higher than those in the general population (4). Therefore, we aimed to assess the seroprevalences of HBV and HCV in the community setting, among attendees at an Asian health fair. Given that this health fair was directed to the Asian community and provided both general medical and hepatitis information with discussions translated in both Cantonese and Mandarin, it would likely capture a population that may be under-represented in previous studies.

METHODS

The United Chinese Community Enrichment Services Society (SUCCESS), a nonprofit charitable organization in BC, holds an annual health fair in the Lower Mainland of BC. The present study was undertaken during one of these health fairs, held at a local community centre in September 2014. This health fair featured talks and discussions by physicians, including gastroenterologists, and other health care professionals, as well as display booths from various sponsors/supporters and private organizations. These lectures were translated in English, Cantonese and Mandarin. Advertisement for this event, including the availability of viral hepatitis testing, was circulated by radio, newspaper, the SUCCESS website and television announcements, as well as posters with full details posted throughout the community.

Attendees at this health fair who were interested in viral hepatitis testing presented to the viral hepatitis testing booth. These participants provided voluntary consent if they were interested in participating in the study. Volunteers were present to provide proper translation in English, Cantonese and Mandarin, if necessary. Study participants provided demographic information including age, ethnicity and years of residency in Canada. They also completed a questionnaire that documented whether they had been tested for hepatitis previously, were aware that they were a carrier or had chronic hepatitis, or had received vaccination(s) against hepatitis. If a family physician and/or specialist cared for the participant, this information was also recorded. Study participants allowed serological information (HBV and HCV serology) to be collected and compared with their questionnaire results.

If attendees were not interested in the study, they were allowed to have serology drawn nonetheless, but these serological results were not collected for the study and these individuals did not complete the questionnaire. Two individuals who presented to the booth for viral hepatitis testing did not wish to participate in the study. Their family doctor or a prearranged walk-in clinic followed up with their serological results.

Attendees were not asked to participate in the study when they entered the doors of the community hall, but they had the opportunity to present to the viral hepatitis testing booth (as well as other booths) and participate if interested. In general, the majority of attendees presented for viral testing; therefore, participants in the present study would be expected to be similar to other attendees.

Blood was drawn for HBV and HCV serology for evaluation by the BC Centre for Disease Control (BCCDC). Results were sent to participants' respective family physicians to ensure proper follow-up care. Those without a family physician had their results forwarded to a prearranged walk-in clinic. Only those with correct demographic information matched to results from the BCCDC were included in the study. The BCCDC required at least two personal identifying data to be correct (name, date of birth or provincial health number) for serological results to be released. The responses of participants from the questionnaires were then compared with their respective serological profiles.

Active HBV infection was defined as HBV surface antigen positive (HBsAg+). Previous HBV exposure was defined as HBV core antibody positive (anti-HBc+) and HBsAg negative (HBsAg−). Natural immunity was defined as previous HBV exposure with HBV surface antibody positivity (anti-HBc+ and anti-HBs+, ≥10 IU/mL) while HBV

TABLE 1
Results of the hepatitis questionnaire (n=112)

Questions	Yes	No	Unknown
Tested for hepatitis previously?	26 (23)	46 (41)	40 (36)
Told you were carrier or had chronic hepatitis?	7 (6)	74 (66)	31 (28)
Has physician for hepatitis?	3/7 (43)*	4/7 (57)	0/7 (0)
Been vaccinated for hepatitis previously?	32 (29)	21 (19)	59 (53)

Among those who stated they had been vaccinated previously, what vaccines did they receive? (n=32)	
Partial hepatitis A virus, partial hepatitis B virus†	5 (16)
Partial hepatitis A virus, complete hepatitis B virus	1 (3)
Partial hepatitis A virus	2 (6)
Partial hepatitis B virus	4 (13)
Complete hepatitis A virus	3 (10)
Complete hepatitis B virus	12 (38)
Complete hepatitis A virus and hepatitis B virus	5 (16)

*Data presented as n/n (%) or n (%). *Percentage calculated from seven participants; †Percentage calculated from 32 participants*

TABLE 2
Seroprevalence among participants (n=112)

Serology	n (%)	95% CI
Active HBV (HBsAg+)	3 (2.7)	(0.6–7.6)
HBV exposure (HBsAg−, anti-HBc+, anti-HBs+/anti-HBs−)	47 (42)	(33–51)
HBV natural immunity (anti-HBs+)*	41/47 (87)	(75–95)
HBV exposure but no immunity (anti-HBs−)	6/47 (13)	(5.3–25)
HBV immunity by vaccination (HBsAg−, anti-HBc- and anti-HBs+)	41 (37)	(28–46)
HBV nonimmunity (HBsAg−, anti-HBs− and anti-HBc−)	21 (19)	(12–27)
HCV seroprevalence (anti-HCV+)	2 (1.8)	(0.2–6.3)

Percentage calculated with respect to 47 participants. Anti-HBc (+/−) Anti-hepatitis B core total antibodies (positive or negative); Anti-HBs (+/−) Anti-hepatitis B surface antibody (positive or negative); Anti-HCV+ Anti-hepatitis C antibody positive; HBsAg (+/−) Hepatitis B surface antigen (positive or negative); HBV Hepatitis B virus; HCV Hepatitis C virus

immunity by vaccination was defined as anti-HBs+, HBsAg− and anti-HBc−. Nonimmunity to HBV was defined as HBV surface antibody negative (anti-HBs− <3 IU/mL), HBsAg− and anti-HBc−. HCV seroprevalence was defined as being HCV antibody reactive.

Comparisons among response groups were calculated using Fisher's exact test with GraphPad Prism (GraphPad Inc, USA); P<0.05 was considered to be statistically significant.

The present study was approved by the Clinical Research Ethics Board of the University of British Columbia (Vancouver, BC).

RESULTS

There were 192 participants who consented, of whom 112 (58%) were included in the study. The other participants were excluded because demographic information from the BCCDC did not completely match information collected from the health fair; thus, these data were considered to be inaccurate.

Among the 112 participants, the median age was 65 years (interquartile range 58 to 70 years). There was an approximately equal distribution with regard to sex. The majority (91%) of participants were Chinese, of whom 74% spoke Cantonese and 26% spoke Mandarin; the remaining 9% were Korean. These participants had resided in Canada for an average of 22 years. Almost all of the participants (97%) had a family physician.

TABLE 3
Correlation of questionnaire results and hepatitis B virus (HBV) serology

Have you ever been tested for hepatitis? (n=112)

	Yes	No	Unknown	P
Nonimmunity*	2/26 (7.7)	17/46 (37)	3/40 (7.5)	<0.01
Exposed to HBV[†]	15/26 (58)	18/46 (39)	18/40 (45)	0.42
Immune by vaccination[‡]	9/26 (35)	11/46 (24)	19/40 (48)	0.07

Have you ever been told you are a hepatitis carrier or have chronic hepatitis? (n=112)

	Yes	No	Unknown	P
Nonimmunity	0/7 (0)	19/74 (26)	2/31 (6.5)	<0.01
Exposed to HBV	7/7 (100)	28/74 (38)	15/31 (48)	<0.01
Immune by vaccination	0/7 (0)	27/74 (36)	14/31 (45)	<0.01

Have you had partial or complete vaccination to HBV?

	Complete (n=18)	Partial (n=9)	No (n=26)	Unknown (n=59)	P
Nonimmunity	4 (22)	0 (0)	7 (27)	10 (17)	0.34
Exposed to HBV	3 (17)	4 (44)	17 (65)	26 (44)	0.01
Immune by vaccination	11 (61)	5 (55)	2 (7.7)	24 (41)	<0.01

*Data presented as n/n (%) or n (%) unless otherwise indicated. *Nonimmunity was defined as anti-hepatitis B core total antibodies negative and anti-hepatitis B surface antibody negative; [†]Exposed to HBV was defined as anti-hepatitis B core total antibodies positive, anti-hepatitis B surface antibody negative and; and hepatitis B surface antigen (positive or negative); [‡]Immune by vaccination was defined as anti-hepatitis B core total antibodies negative and anti-hepatitis B surface antibody positive; HBV Hepatitis B virus*

Questionnaire results showed that 23% of the participants had been previously tested for hepatitis while 36% were unsure whether they had been tested (Table 1). A small percentage of participants (6%) had been told they were carriers or had chronic hepatitis, but only 43% of these individuals were being followed by their family physician or specialist with respect to their diagnosis. Nearly 30% of participants stated that they had been previously vaccinated for hepatitius A virus and/or HBV. Most commonly, they stated that they had complete vaccinations against HBV (38%).

Active HBV was found in three participants (2.7% [95% CI 0.6% to 7.6%]) and HCV infection was found in two participants (1.8% [95% CI 0.2% to 6.3%]) (Table 2). These cases of chronic hepatitis were previously known before testing, except for one new case of HCV. Only 60% of these individuals were followed by their family physician and/or specialist regarding their hepatitis. Surprisingly, 42% (95% CI 33% to 51%) of participants had been previously exposed to HBV, of whom six (13%) had no natural immunity (ie, anti-HBs−). More than one-third of participants (37% [95% CI 28% to 46%]) in the cohort had been vaccinated for HBV while 19% (95% CI 12% to 27%) had a serological panel consistent with no previous HBV vaccination or exposure to the virus (Table 2). Among participants who were anti-HBs+, the average level of these antibodies was 198 mIU/mL (95% CI 104 mIU/mL to 292 mIU/mL).

The correlation of questionnaire answers with serology results is presented in Table 3. The rate of nonimmunity to HBV was higher among participants who stated that they had never been tested for hepatitis compared with those who said they had been tested or that they did not know (37% versus 7.7% versus 7.5%, respectively; P<0.01). Otherwise, there were no other significant differences in the groups with respect to this question.

When participants were asked whether they had ever told that they were a hepatitis carrier or had chronic hepatitis, all seven individuals who answered "yes" had evidence of being previously exposed to HBV (four participants) or had active HBV (three participants) (Table 3). The study participant with known HCV was accounted for in the former group and was not followed by his family doctor and/or

specialist with respect to his positive anti-HCV result. The three participants with active HBV were followed by their family doctor and/or specialist with respect to their chronic hepatitis. Among the group who answered "no" or "unknown" to the same question, there were 28 (38%) and 15 (48%) individuals, respectively, who were exposed to HBV. Similarly, there were 19 (26%) and two (6.4%) individuals, respectively, who had no immunity to HBV.

When participants were asked regarding their previous vaccinations, interestingly, among the 19 individuals who stated that they had complete vaccinations to HBV, 22% actually had no immunity to HBV, 17% had natural immunity and 61% showed evidence of being vaccinated (Table 3). Nine individuals stated that they had been partially vaccinated to HBV (Table 3). Four (44%) of these individuals had natural immunity to HBV, while five (55%) had serological evidence of HBV vaccination. There were a significantly higher proportion of participants who were exposed to HBV who answered "no" or "unknown" when asked about previous HBV vaccination compared with the group who answered "yes" to complete HBV vaccinations (72% and 44% versus 17%, respectively; P<0.01).

DISCUSSION

In our study, the seroprevalences of HBV and HCV were 2.7% (95% CI 0.6% to 7.6%) and 1.8% (95% CI 0.2% to 6.3%), respectively – higher than nationally reported rates. These cases of hepatitis were known previously except for one new case of HCV. Surprisingly, >40% of participants had previously been exposed to HBV. Almost 20% were nonimmune to HBV. Collectively, our results suggest that viral hepatitis, especially HBV, remains an important issue in this Asian community in BC.

Previous studies have reported lower rates of HBV than in our cohort (1-3,5,6). In one study, Glasgow et al (5) demonstrated that the HBsAg seroprevalence among individuals 14 to 30 years of age was between 0.24% to 0.47% in a Northern Ontario town. Chiavetta et al (6) observed rates of 0.1% to 0.5% for HBV among first-time Canadian blood donors. Finally, Rotermann et al (3) examined the seroprevalences of HBV and HCV in 15 Canadian cities and collected survey information (conducted by Statistics Canada in collaboration with the Public Health Agency of Canada and Health Canada). These investigators reported the seroprevalence of HBV to be 0.4% for the entire population; however, the seroprevalence of HBV was 1.8% among nonwhite participants and 1.6% among the foreign-born population (11% were from Southeast Asian and Hong Kong).

Concerns about missing vulnerable populations (eg, ethnic groups) have been suggested in these previous studies (1-3). For example, the Public Health Agency of Canada reported much higher rates of HBV – as high as 5% to 15% – among Chinese and Vietnamese Canadians (1). A recent quality improvement project conducted in Vancouver also found higher rates of HBV and HCV among patients admitted at a tertiary hospital (4). Based on trends from Statistics Canada, Wong et al (7) estimated the prevalence of chronic HBV to be 5% among immigrants.

The seroprevalence of HBV in our study was consistent with these previous reports (1,4,7). Our rate may have been somewhat lower given the older population of our cohort (median age 65 years). In addition, the study participants have resided in Canada, on average, for >20 years. Therefore, our cohort may not be an accurate reflection of the higher burden of HBV among recent immigrants described in previous reports (4,7). The attendees who participated in this health fair may also be more health conscious and have taken preventive measures to avoid hepatitis. Although this would not affect the likelihood of vertical transmission of HBV, it may have been a factor with respect to horizontal transmission of HBV and HCV. Finally, given that universal screening of prenatal women with HBV vaccination of neonates was introduced in Canada in the late 1980s, followed by childhood vaccination in the 1990s and universal infant vaccination approximately 15 years ago (depending on the province), the participants in our study who were born outside of the country and of older age would not have been expected to have been vaccinated.

In fact, almost 20% of our cohort did not have immunity to HBV, suggesting that they had never received the HBV vaccination.

Our study also found that 42% of participants have been previously exposed to HBV. This proportion is substantially higher than the rate of 4.2% reported previously among all Canadians (3). The individuals in our cohort may have seroconverted their HBsAg spontaneously, given the large proportion of participants who were exposed to the virus (ie, anti-HBc+) but were HBsAg−. This may have occurred via acute HBV infection (eg, sexual relations with an HBV carrier or vertical transmission from mother to child) with immune clearance in which the patient was asymptomatic and/or did not seek medical attention. In a small minority of chronic HBV carriers, HBsAg sero-conversion may have also occur spontaneously after many decades. Although immunity may wane over five to 10 years, these individuals had no serological evidence of any protective antibodies. Occult HBV infection may also explain an isolated elevated anti-HBc level; however, HBV DNA or liver enzyme levels were not measured to help differentiate this entity.

In addition, our study demonstrated that approximately 40% of these individuals were unaware of their HBV exposure – these participants answered that they had not been tested for hepatitis or did not know their status. This previous exposure to HBV may lead to reactivation of HBV in the context of immunosuppression, causing severe or potentially fatal liver disease (8-10). Patients who will undergo chemotherapy, immunosuppression, or receive stem cell or solid organ transplantation should be screened for HBV (HBsAg and anti-HBc) (10).

Our study also found significant discordance between questionnaire answers regarding vaccination status and actual serological results (Table 3). For example, 22% of participants who stated they had complete vaccinations to HBV had no serological evidence of protective antibodies. In addition, there may be misunderstanding on the part of the study participants and/or misinformation by the family physician regarding vaccination status. Three study participants were told they had been a hepatitis carrier or had chronic hepatitis; however, they had only been exposed to HBV, with no evidence of active HBV. Our findings corroborate previous studies that have demonstrated that knowledge of HBV is limited in the Asian population (11), even among those with chronic HBV (12,13). The risk of social stigma has also been attributed to reduced HBV screening in the Asian community (14). Thus, continuing education of physicians and patients regarding viral hepatitis as well as encouragement of screening remain important issues in the Asian community in BC.

With regard to HCV, our seroprevalence rate was higher than previous reports (3,15). In a Canadian study examining 15 cities, the seroprevalence of HCV was reported to be 0.5% (3). Uhanova et al (15) reported the same rate from an administrative database of Manitoba from 1995 to 2002. The relatively higher HCV rate in our cohort was unexpected. This finding may relate to the older age of our population, which has been associated with HCV infection (3,15). Another possible explanation is unawareness of this disease among the

Asian community; in our study, one of the cases of HCV was newly diagnosed. Other risk factors for HCV, such as previous blood transfusions, intravenous drug use and sexual practices were not explored in our study.

Our study had several strengths. We were able to determine the true seroprevalence rates of an at-risk population. We were also able to correlate serological results with questionnaire answers. Our study may allow for generalizability to other similar cities in North America with a growing Asian and/or immigrant population.

Limitations of the present study include the significant loss of participants for analysis (42%) because of incorrect registration of data. Better coordination will be needed in the future between event organizers and the BCCDC to improve data collection. Our study also did not explore other important risk factors in our questionnaire (eg, sexual practices, intravenous drug use, etc). There was a selection bias in our study as well, given that the participants in our cohort voluntarily attended a health fair and may not accurately reflect the at-risk Asian population who may have limited knowledge of available resources or restricted access to health care. Furthermore, although we did identify four study participants with known hepatitis who wished to undergo hepatitis testing nonetheless, those with chronic liver disease may be less inclined to participate, given no potential gain in enrolling in the study as well as social stigma associated with testing. Recall bias was another potential limitation because participants were asked several questions that may be difficult to recollect such as vaccination status or years of residency in Canada.

We recognize that the attendees of a health fair are only a small sample of a much larger Asian community; therefore, the present study was hypothesis generating. Larger epidemiological studies, however, should be considered in this community to generate definitive conclusions. Future directions would include studies examining other factors related to HBV or HCV infection, such as socioeconomic status, among the Asian and/or immigrant populations. Local hepatitis screening programs aimed at this population will also be an important consideration for health care spending and resource allocation. Finally, ongoing education of HBV and HCV, such as the translated lectures and discussions at this Asian health fair, will be a critical aspect of ongoing medical care among this population. Further education of primary care physicians and counselling of patients will help promote knowledge of viral hepatitis and accurate dissemination of health information.

CONCLUSION
The seroprevalences of HBV and HCV found at an Asian health fair in the Lower Mainland of BC were 2.7% and 1.8%, respectively. Our results highlight that the lack of knowledge of HBV infection and vaccination status remains a significant clinical issue in the Asian community of BC.

ACKNOWLEDGEMENTS: The authors thank all participants in this study as well as the countless volunteers at this Asian health fair.

REFERENCES
1. Brief Report: Hepatitis B in Canada. Public Health Agency of Canada. 2011. <www.phac-aspc.gc.ca/id-mi/hepatitisBCan-hepatiteBCan-eng.php> (Accessed November 2014).
2. Hepatitis C in Canada: 2005-2010 Surveillance Report. Public Health Agency of Canada. 2012. <www.phac-aspc.gc.ca/sti-its-surv-epi/hepc/surv-eng.php> (Accessed November 2014).
3. Rotermann M, Langlois K, Andonov A, et al. Seroprevalence of hepatitis B and C virus infections: Results from the 2007 to 2009 and 2009 to 2011 Canadian Health Measures Survey. Health Rep 2013;24:3-13.
4. Kapleuto J, Kadatz M, Wormsbecker A. Screening, detecting and enhancing the yield of previously undiagnosed hepatitis B and C in patients with acute medical admissions to hospital: A pilot project undertaken at the Vancouver General Hospital. Can J Gastroenterol Hepatol 2014;28:315-8.
5. Glasgow KW, Schabas R, Williams DC, et al. A population-based hepatitis B seroprevalence and risk factor study in a northern Ontario town. Can J Public Health 1997;88:87-90.
6. Chiavetta JA, Escobar M, Newman A, et al. Incidence and estimated rates of residual risk for HIV, hepatitis C, hepatitis B and human T-cell lymphotropic viruses in blood donors in Canada, 1990-2000. CMAJ 2003;169:767-73.
7. Wong WW, Woo G, Jenny Heathcote E, et al. Cost effectiveness of screening immigrants for hepatitis B. Liver Int 2011;31:1179-90.
8. Law JK, Ho JK, Hoskins PJ, et al. Fatal reactivation of hepatitis B post-chemotherapy for lymphoma in a hepatitis B surface antigen-negative, hepatitis B core antibody positive patient: Potential implications for future prophylaxis recommendations. Leuk Lymphoma 2005;46:1085-9.

Seroprevalences of hepatitis B virus and hepatitis C virus among participants of an Asian health...

161

9. Yoshida EM, Ramji A, Erb SR, et al. De novo acute hepatitis B infection in a previously vaccinated liver transplant recipient due to a strain of HBV with a Met 133 Thr mutation in the "a" determinant. Liver 2000;20:411-4.

10. Di Bisceglie AM, Lok AS, Martin P, et al. Recent FDA warnings on hepatitis B reactivation with immune-suppressing and anti-cancer drugs: Just the tip of the iceberg? Hepatology 2015;61:703-11.

11. Cheung J, Lee TK, Teh CZ, et al. Cross-sectional study of hepatitis B awareness among Chinese and Southeast Asian Canadians in the Vancouver-Richmond community. Can J Gastroenterol 2005;19:245-9.

12. Kue J, Thorburn S. Hepatitis B knowledge, screening, and vaccination among Hmong Americans. J Health Care Poor Underserved 2013;24:566-78.

13. Tokes K, Quadri S, Cahill P, et al. Disease and treatment perceptions among Asian Americans diagnosed with chronic hepatitis B. J Gen Intern Med 2014;477-84.

14. Li D, Tang T, Patterson M, et al. The impact of hepatitis B knowledge and stigma on screening in Canadian Chinese population. Can J Gastroenterol 2012;26:597-602.

15. Uhanova J, Tate RB, Tataryn DJ, Minuk GY. A population-based study of the epidemiology of hepatitis C in a North American population. J Hepatol 2012;57:736-42.

34

Characterization of invasive *Neisseria meningitidis* from Atlantic Canada, 2009 to 2013: With special reference to the nonpolysaccharide vaccine targets (PorA, factor H binding protein, *Neisseria* heparin-binding antigen and *Neisseria* adhesin A)

Raymond SW Tsang MMedSc PhD[1], Dennis KS Law BA BSc[1], Rita R Gad MD DrPH[2], Tim Mailman MD FRCPC[3], Gregory German MD PhD FRCPC[4], Robert Needle MSc MLS (ASCP)[5]

RSW Tsang, DKS Law, RR Gad, T Mailman, G German, R Needle. Characterization of invasive *Neisseria meningitidis* from Atlantic Canada, 2009-2013: With special reference to the nonpolysaccharide vaccine targets (PorA, factor H binding protein, *Neisseria* heparin-binding antigen and *Neisseria* adhesin A). Can J Infect Dis Med Microbiol 2015;26(6):299-304.

BACKGROUND: Serogroup B *Neisseria meningitidis* (MenB) has always been a major cause of invasive meningococcal disease (IMD) in Canada. With the successful implementation of a meningitis C conjugate vaccine, the majority of IMD in Canada is now caused by MenB.
OBJECTIVE: To investigate IMD case isolates in Atlantic Canada from 2009 to 2013. Data were analyzed to determine the potential coverage of the newly licensed MenB vaccine.
METHODS: Serogroup, serotype and serosubtype antigens were determined from IMD case isolates. Clonal analysis was performed using multilocus sequence typing. The protein-based vaccine antigen genes were sequenced and the predicted peptides were investigated.
RESULTS: The majority of the IMD isolates were MenB (82.5%, 33 of 40) and, in particular, sequence type (ST)-154 B:4:P1.4 was responsible for 47.5% (19 of 40) of all IMD case isolates in Atlantic Canada. Isolates of this clone expressed the PorA antigen P1.4 and possessed the *nhba* genes encoding for *Neisseria* heparin-binding antigen peptide 2, which together matched exactly with two of the four components of the new four-component meningococcal B vaccine. Nineteen MenB isolates had two antigenic matches, another five MenB and one meningitis Y isolate had one antigenic match. This provided 75.8% (25 of 33) potential coverage for MenB, or a 62.5% (25 of 40) overall potential coverage for IMD.
CONCLUSION: From 2009 to 2013, IMD in Atlantic Canada was mainly caused by MenB and, in particular, the B:4:P1.4 ST-154 clone, which accounted for 47.5% of all IMD case isolates. The new four-component meningococcal B vaccine appeared to offer adequate coverage against MenB in Atlantic Canada.

Key Words: *Atlantic Canada; Invasive* Neisseria meningitidis*; MenB vaccine*

La caractérisation du *Neisseria meningitidis* invasif dans les Maritimes de 2009 à 2013, notamment les cibles du vaccin non polysaccharidique (porA, protéine de liaison au facteur H, antigène de liaison à l'héparine de *Neisseria* et adhésine A de *Neisseria*)

HISTORIQUE : Le *Neisseria meningitidis* du sérogroupe B (MenB) a toujours été une cause importante de méningococcie invasive (MI) au Canada. Depuis l'adoption d'un vaccin conjugué contre le méningocoque du groupe C, la majorité des MI au Canada sont désormais attribuables au MenB.
OBJECTIF : Examiner les isolats de cas de MI dans les Maritimes entre 2009 et 2013. Analyser les données pour déterminer la couverture potentielle du vaccin nouvellement homologué contre le MenB.
MÉTHODOLOGIE : Les chercheurs ont déterminé le sérogroupe, le sérotype et les antigènes des sous-types sérologiques des isolats de cas de MI. Ils ont effectué l'analyse clonale au moyen du typage génomique multilocus. Ils ont séquencé les gènes des antigènes du vaccin à base de protéines et examiné les peptides prédits.
RÉSULTATS : La majorité des isolats de MI étaient des MenB (82,5 %, 33 sur 40). Notamment, le type séquentiel (TS)-154 B:4:P1,4 était responsable de 47,5 % (19 sur 40) de tous les isolats de cas de MI dans les Maritimes. Les isolats de ce clone ont exprimé l'antigène porA P1.4 et étaient dotés des gènes *nhba* codant pour le peptide 2 de l'antigène de liaison à l'héparine de *Neisseria*. Ensemble, ces antigènes correspondaient exactement à deux des quatre composants du nouveau vaccin contre le méningocoque du groupe B à quatre composants. Dix-neuf isolats du MenB étaient dotés de deux correspondances antigéniques, tandis que cinq autres MenB et un isolat de la méningite Y étaient dotés d'une correspondance antigénique. Ces résultats assuraient une couverture potentielle du MenB de 72,7 % (24 sur 33) ou une couverture potentielle globale de la MI de 62,5 % (25 sur 40).
CONCLUSION : De 2009 à 2013, dans les Maritimes, la MI était surtout causée par le MenB, en particulier le clone B:4:P1.4 ST-154, responsable de 47,5 % de tous les isolats de cas de MI. Le nouveau vaccin contre le méningocoque du groupe B à quatre composants semble offrir une couverture pertinente contre le MenB dans cette région.

Invasive meningococcal disease (IMD) is a serious, nationally notifiable disease caused by the Gram-negative diplococcal bacterium *Neisseria meningitidis*. Invasive diseases caused by *N meningitidis* include meningitis, septicemia, pneumonia, septic arthritis and, occasionally, endocarditis, myocarditis and pericarditis, with an average case fatality rate of 10% (1). Six (A, B, C, W, X and Y) of the 12 recognized serogroups are

[1]*National Microbiology Laboratory, Public Health Agency of Canada, Winnipeg, Manitoba;* [2]*Communicable Disease Control Unit, Department of Health, Government of New Brunswick, Fredericton, New Brunswick;* [3]*Department of Pathology and Laboratory Medicine, IWK Health Centre, Halifax, Nova Scotia;* [4]*Department of Health, Government of Prince Edward Island, Charlottetown, Prince Edward Island;* [5]*Public Health Laboratory and Microbiology, Eastern Health, St John's, Newfoundland and Labrador*
Correspondence: Raymond SW Tsang, National Microbiology Laboratory, 1015 Arlington Street, Winnipeg, Manitoba R3E 3R2.
e-mail raymond.tsang@phac-aspc.gc.ca

TABLE 1
Distribution of serogroups* of invasive *Neisseria meningitidis* in Atlantic Canada from 2009 to 2013

| Year | Province | | | | |
	New Brunswick	Nova Scotia	Prince Edward Island	Newfoundland and Labrador	Atlantic Canada
2009	6 (4B, 1Y, 1W)	2 (1B, 1C)	1 (B)	4 (4B)	13 (10B, 1C, 1Y, 1W)
2010	6 (4B, 1Y, 1E)	2 (1B, 1Y)	0	2 (2B)	10 (7B, 2Y, 1E)
2011	3 (3B)	3 (2B, 1Y)	0	1 (1B)	7 (6B, 1Y)
2012	6 (6B)	1 (1B)	1 (1B)	0	8 (8B)
2013	2 (2B)	0	0	0	2 (2B)
2009 to 2013	23 (19B, 2Y, 1W, 1E)	8 (5B, 1C, 2Y)	2 (2B)	7 (7B)	40 (33B, 1C, 4Y, 1W, 1E)

Data presented as n (serogroup[s]). *At least 12 different serogroups are recognized by specific antisera: A, B, C, E, H, I, K, L, W, X, Y and Z

responsible for most of the invasive diseases, which occur globally (2,3). However, geographical differences in serogroup distribution is well known (4); and in Canada, most IMD in the past 20 years have been caused mainly by serogroups B (MenB) and C (MenC) and, to a lesser degree, by serogroups W (MenW) and Y (MenY) (5-10). Aside from the serogroup antigen, the *N meningitidis* major outer membrane proteins, PorB (serotype antigen) and PorA (serosubtype antigen) are also important surface markers for typing and characterization of strains. Traditionally, clonal analysis of *N meningitidis* strains were performed using multilocus enzyme electrophoresis, which grouped isolates into electrophoretic types. However, it is not a user-friendly method, and the results generated are not portable for comparison between different laboratories. Therefore, it has been replaced by the more objective method of multilocus sequence typing (MLST), with isolates grouped together into sequence types (STs). Related STs are grouped together into clonal complexes (CCs). Most IMDs, especially those found in teenagers, adolescents and young adults, as well as those occurring in clusters or in epidemic form, are caused by a few major CCs known as hypervirulent clones (11).

After the introduction of meningococcal A, C, W and Y conjugate vaccine programs in Canada (12), the incidence of MenC disease has decreased substantially, with only six culture-confirmed MenC cases identified in Canada in 2013 (13). MenB is now the only major serogroup of meningococci left to be controlled by the newer MenB vaccines, which have either been licensed recently in Canada (14), or are in advanced clinical trials and awaiting regulatory approval for licensure in Canada (15).

Unlike the capsule vaccine used for serogroups A, C, W and Y meningococci, a MenB capsule would be nonimmunogenic due to the presence of a self-antigen (16) and, therefore, not feasible. Noncapsule meningococcal vaccines developed in the past were based on the *porA* outer membrane protein (OMP) vesicles; however, such vaccines are strain specific, effective against strains displaying homologous PorA antigens to the OMP vesicle (OMV) vaccine. Nevertheless, they have been used successfully in the past to control epidemics of MenB IMD (17-20). Genome sequencing of microbial pathogens have renewed interest in the development of universal MenB vaccines. One such newer MenB vaccine (Bexsero, Novartis, Canada) recently licensed in Canada, has been developed using reverse vaccinology based on whole genome sequence information of meningococci (21). This four-component meningococcal B (4CMenB) recombinant vaccine comprises: factor H binding protein (fHbp) subfamily B or variant 1, peptide 1; *Neisseria* heparin binding antigen (NHBA) peptide 2; *Neisseria* adhesion A (NadA)-3.8; and the OMV vaccine used in New Zealand to control the MenB epidemic caused by the strain B:4:P1.4 (20). Another investigational MenB vaccine is based on a bivalent recombinant fHbp or lipoprotein 2086 (22).

fHbp is classified into three variants (1, 2 and 3) or two subfamilies, with subfamily A equivalent to variants 2 and 3, and subfamily B equivalent to variant 1. Because of amino acid sequence similarities between proteins in each subfamily of fHbp, cross-protection between proteins within a subfamily is possible, but not between subfamilies

(23). Similarly, cross-protection among multiple NHBA peptide types have been reported (24). With regard to NadA, cross-protection between peptides that belong to NadA-1 and NadA-2/3 have been reported (25).

In preparation for the introduction of the newer MenB vaccine in Canada, the National Microbiology Laboratory (NML; Winnipeg, Manitoba) in collaboration with provinces, has been expanding laboratory surveillance activities to include a more in-depth study of MenB strains (26,27), as well as characterization of the noncarbohydrate protein-based vaccine antigen genes in Canadian IMD isolates (28). The present study characterizes IMD case isolates submitted to the NML from Atlantic Canada over the period from January 1, 2009 to December 31, 2013. Characterization includes analysis of serogroup, serotype and serosubtype antigens, *porA* genotypes and nucleotide sequences of genes that encode for the protein-based vaccine targets, fHbp, NHBA and NadA.

METHODS

Individual IMD case isolates received at the NML between 2009 and 2013, from the Atlantic provinces of New Brunswick (NB), Nova Scotia (NS), Prince Edward Island (PEI), and Newfoundland and Labrador (NFLD) were included in the present study. All IMD case isolates were obtained from normally sterile body sites (such as blood, cerebrospinal fluid, synovial fluid, pleural fluid or pericardial fluid), as per the national case definition (http://dsol-smed.phac-aspc.gc.ca/dsol-smed/ndis/list-eng.php). In addition, the present study did not capture the polymerase chain reaction (PCR)-diagnosed culture-negative cases, including at least one such case identified in NB.

All isolates were tested for serogroup using bacterial agglutination and/or PCR methods using procedures previously described (26,27). Serotyping and serosubtyping were performed using a monoclonal antibody typing kit (Rijksinstitut voor Volksgezondheid en Milieu, Bilthoven, Netherlands) and indirect whole cell ELISA method (29). Monoclonal antibodies to serotypes 2c, 17, 19 and serosubtype P1.19 were provided by Dr Wendell Zollinger, Walter Reed Army Institute of Research, United States. Isolates were analyzed using multilocus sequence typing (MLST) according to Maiden et al (30) and ST/CC was assigned using tools available in the *Neisseria* MLST website (http://pubmlst.org/neisseria/). Variable regions of *porA* genes were determined using protocols described by Sacchi et al (31) and Clark et al (32), following the nomenclature given in the *N meningitidis porA* variable region database (http://pubmlst.org/neisseria/PorA/) and by de Filippis et al (33). The *fHbp*, *nhba* and *nadA* gene sequences were determined using PCR amplification and standard sequencing reactions, following the protocols described by Lucidarme et al (34); and their peptide types were determined using online tools available from the Neisseria.org website (http://pubmlst.org/neisseria/fHbp/ and http://pubmlst.org/neisseria/NHBA/ and http://pubmlst.org/neisseria/NadA/).

Patient age and sex, as well as specimen sources of the IMD isolates were obtained from specimen requisition forms. Population estimates were obtained from Statistic Canada's website (www.statcan.gc.ca/tables-tableaux/sum-som/l01/cst01/demo02a-eng.htm).

TABLE 2
Antigenic formula and *porA* genotypes of invasive *Neisseria meningitidis* in Atlantic Canada from 2009 to 2013

Antigenic formula	PorA genotype	Isolates, n
B:4:P1.4	P1.7-2,4,37	17
B:4:P1.4	P1.7-2,4,36	2
B:NT:P1.4	P1.7-2,4,37	1
B:4:P1.14	P1.22,14,36	2
B:4:P1.14	P1.22-1,14,38	1
B:4:P1.-	P1.12-6,13-4,35-1	1
B:4:P1.-	P1.22,14-6,36-2	1
B:15:P1.4	P1.7-2,4,37	1
B:15:P1.7,16	P1.7,16,35	1
B:17:P1.9	P1.22,9,35-1	1
B:17:P1.19	P1.19-1,15-11,36	2
B:1,19:P1.6	P1.18,25,38-1	1
B:1,19:P1.19	P1.19,13-1,36	1
B:1,19:P1.-	P1.18-1,34,38	1
C:2a:P1.-	P1.5,2,36-2	1
Y:2c:P1.5	P1.5-1,10-4,36-2	1
Y:15,19:P1.16	P1.21,16,37-1	1
Y:NT:P1.5	P1.5-1,10-4,36-2	1
Y:NT :P1.-	P1.18-1,3,38	1
W:NT:P1.-	P1.18-1,3,38	1
E:NT:P1.-	P1.22,14-6,36-2	1

TABLE 3
Predicted four-component menIngococcal B vaccine antigens present in invasive *Neisseria meningitidis* strains in Atlantic Canada from 2009 to 2013

Vaccine antigen type	Isolates, n (serogroup[s])
PorA antigen P1.4	21 (B)
Factor H-binding protein peptide	
1	1 (B)
4	20 (B)
13	2 (B)
14	1 (B)
16	3 (B; E; Y)
19	3 (B)
21	1 (Y)
22	2 (C, W)
23	1 (Y)
24	1 (Y)
47	1 (B)
106	1 (B)
110	1 (B)
414	1 (B)
626	1 (B)
Neisseria heparin-binding antigen peptide	
2	21 (B)
3	2 (B)
6	3 (2B, 1Y)
7	1 (B)
9	2 (Y)
17	1 (B)
20	2 (W, Y)
21	3 (B)
29	2 (B, C)
43	1 (B)
197	1 (B)
336	1 (E)
Nesseria adhesion A peptide	
1	1 (B)
3	1 (C)
8	1 (Y)

RESULTS

Temporal and geographical distribution of serogroups

Table 1 describes the serogroup distribution of invasive *N meningitidis* collected in Atlantic Canada from 2009 to 2013. Of the 40 invasive isolates collected, 33 (82.5%) belonged to MenB and 19 were submitted from NB.

Population biology of invasive *N meningitidis* in Atlantic Canada

Clonal analysis of the 33 MenB isolates revealed that 73% belonged to ST-41/44 CC, 9% to ST-269 CC and 6% to ST-32 CC, and the remaining 12% comprised one isolate each of ST-35 CC and ST-461 CC; two strains were not assigned to any known CC by the Neisseria.org MLST website (http://pubmlst.org/neisseria/).

Of the 24 isolates that belonged to ST-41/44 CC, 19 were ST-154 and the other five STs (ST-207, ST-340, ST-409, ST-7612, ST-9411) were each made up of only one isolate. The three MenB isolates that belonged to ST-269 CC were from NB (two isolates both typed as ST-8924) and NFLD (ST-1161). The two MenB isolates that belonged to ST-32 CC were from NFLD and were typed as ST-290 and ST-7814. The remaining four MenB isolates included one each of ST-8770 (ST-35 CC) from NB, ST-461 (ST-461 CC) from PEI, and two isolates of ST-5571 from NS (identified to belong to a new CC of MenB common in central and eastern Canada) (35).

The single MenC strain from NS belonged to ST-11 (ST-11/ ET-37 CC). Two of the four MenY isolates were from NB, and typed as ST-1466 (ST-174 CC) or ST-3923 (ST-167 CC). The other two MenY strains were from NS, and typed as ST-184 (ST-22 CC) or ST-8522 (not assigned to any known CC). The single MenW isolate from NB was typed as ST-1221 (ST-22 CC), and the MenE isolate also from NB was typed as ST-9856 (not assigned to any known CC).

ST-154 MenB

There were 19 individual MenB case isolates typed as ST-154 (ST-41/44 CC), which included 47.5% of all the invasive *N meningitidis* found in Atlantic Canada during the study period. Fifteen of the case isolates were from NB, two from NS and two from NFLD. These 19 ST-154 MenB cases involved 12 male and seven female patients, with ages ranging from one month to 92 years (median 11 years of age). Ten of the

isolates were recovered from blood cultures and the remaining nine were recovered from cerebrospinal fluid. Eighteen isolates were typed as B:4:P1.4 (serogroup B, serotype 4 and serosubtype P1.4), and one isolate was typed B:NT:P1.4 (nontypeable [NT]). The *porA* genotype for 17 isolates was P1.7-2,4,37 and two were typed as P1.7-2,4,36.

Characterization of noncarbohydrate protein-based meningococcal vaccine targets in MenB in Atlantic Canada

The antigenic formula (serotype and serosubtype antigens) expressed and the *porA* genotypes of the 40 invasive *N meningitidis* isolates are summarized in Table 2. Thirty-five isolates expressed seven different serotype antigens, and serotype 4 was the most commonly detected antigen in 24 isolates; five isolates did not express any detectable serotype antigens. Thirty-three isolates expressed eight different serosubtype antigens, including P1.4 detected in 21 isolates. Seven isolates did not express any detectable serosubtype antigens. There were 16 different *porA* genotypes found among the 40 isolates, and P1.7-2,4,37 was found in 19 of these (Table 2).

Aside from possessing the identical *porA* genotype of P1.7-2,4, all 19 ST-154 MenB isolates were found to have a *fHbp* gene allele predicted to encode for peptide 4 (variant 1 or subfamily B). Eighteen of the 19 isolates were found to have *nhba* genes predicted to encode for NHBA peptide 2 and the remaining isolate was predicted to encode NHBA peptide 7. None of the isolates possessed the *nadA* gene.

The remaining MenB isolates were more diverse in terms of their *porA*, *fHbp* and *nhba* gene sequences. From the 14 non-ST-154 MenB isolates, 11 different *fHbp* gene alleles were identified that encoded for peptides 1, 4, 13, 14, 16, 19, 47, 106, 110, 414 and 626. Eight NHBA peptide types (2, 3, 6, 17, 21, 29, 43 and 197) were also predicted to be encoded by the non-ST-154 MenB isolates based on their *nhba* gene sequences. Only two MenB isolates that belonged to the ST-32 CC were found to have the *nadA* genes: in one isolate, the *nadA* gene allele 1 was found, which encoded for NadA peptide 1; and the other isolate was found to have the *nadA* gene allele 85, not predicted to produce a NadA protein, due to a frame-shift mutation.

Overall, 21 of 33 MenB isolates were found to express the PorA antigen P1.4 and display the *porA* genotype of P1.7-2,4, which represented 87.5% of the MenB isolates that belonged to the ST-41/44 CC (n=24). Eleven fHbp peptide types were predicted from the 33 MenB isolates, with seven of them (peptides 1, 4, 13, 14, 110, 414 and 626) belonging to variant 1 or subfamily B; three peptide types (peptides 16, 19 and 106) belonged to variant 2 (subfamily A); and one peptide type (peptide 47) belonged to the variant 3 (also subfamily A). Twenty-seven (81.8%) of the 33 MenB isolates were predicted to encode variant 1 fHbp peptides; five isolates (15.2%) were predicted to encode variant 2 peptides; and one isolate (3.0%) predicted to encode variant 3 peptide.

Noncarbohydrate protein-based meningococcal vaccine targets in MenC, -Y, -W and -E isolates in Atlantic Canada

Five fHbp peptide types (peptides 16, 21, 22, 23 and 24) were found among the seven non-B meningococcal isolates; and only peptide 16 was found among the Atlantic Canada MenB isolates. In addition, five NHBA peptide types were found: peptides 6, 9, 20, 29 and 336; peptides 6 and 29 were also found among the MenB isolates in Atlantic Canada. Only two isolates were found to possess the *nadA* gene: in the MenC isolate, the *nadA* gene allele 3 encodes a *nadA-2/3* peptide 3, while a MenY isolate was found to have *nadA* allele 80, which encoded for a NadA-2/3 peptide 8.

Predicted 4CMenB (Bexsero) vaccine antigens present in invasive *Neisseria meningitidis* strains from Atlantic Canada

The variety of fHbp, NHBA and NadA peptide types found among invasive *N meningitidis* strains in Atlantic Canada is summarized in Table 3. No isolate was found to have all four antigens (PorA, fHbp, NHBA and NadA) displaying an exact match to the 4CMenB vaccine components. In addition, no isolate was found with three matching antigens to the 4CMenB vaccine. However, 19 isolates (all MenB) were found to have two antigens (PorA P1.4 and NHBA peptide 2) that displayed an exact match to the 4CMenB vaccine. An additional six isolates were found to have at least one antigen that matched with the 4CMenB vaccine (two MenB for PorA P1.4; two other MenB isolates with NHBA peptide 2; another MenB with fHbp peptide 1; and 1 MenY with a NadA peptide 8). Collectively, 25 isolates were found to have one or more antigens that matched the 4CMenB and, therefore, at least 62.5% of all invasive *N meningitidis* from Atlantic Canada in the period from 2009 to 2013, were predicted to be covered by the vaccine. However, the number of non-MenB strains studied was very small and, therefore, the prediction for these other serogroups would not be meaningful. The predicted coverage for MenB alone in Atlantic Canada was significantly higher (24 of 33 isolates [73%]) due to the predominant presence of the ST-154 clone, which shared two exact match antigens (PorA P1.4 and NHBA peptide 2) with the vaccine.

DISCUSSION

The present study provides a snap shot of the molecular epidemiology of IMD in Atlantic Canada from 2009 to 2013. A striking feature was the predominance of MenB (82.5%), as a cause of IMD in this region

of Canada. For the same period in western Canada, the overall abundance of MenB among all invasive *N meningitidis* case isolates was 42.9%, including 48.5% in British Columbia, 36.5% in Alberta, 39.1% in Saskatchewan and 45.0% in Manitoba (28). In Ontario, between 2001 and 2010, 39.1% of all invasive meningococcal case isolates were MenB (27). In Quebec, the percentage of MenB for the period of 2003 to 2010 was higher (71.1%) due to an increase in the B:17:P1.19 ST-269 clone, which emerged in 2003 (36) and persisted until at least 2010 (26).

Here, and in our previous studies, we have shown that the epidemiology of IMD in different parts of Canada may reveal both geographical and temporal differences. Clonal analysis of MenB in western Canada and Ontario reflected an endemic disease picture where no single clone or ST predominated (27,28). This was in contrast to the data from Quebec, where almost one-half (49%) of all MenB was typed as a single clone, ST-269, which accounted for 35% of all culture-confirmed IMD case isolates from 2003 to 2010 (26). In Atlantic Canada, most (57.6%) of the MenB isolates belonged to a strain characterized as ST-154 with the antigenic formula of B:4:P1.4. This strain was responsible for 47.5% of all culture-confirmed IMD cases in the region; however, the majority (15 of 19 [79%]) of the case isolates were identified in NB, including three to four culture-confirmed cases per year between 2009 and 2012. In 2013, only one culture-confirmed case was due to this strain. In contrast, for the same period, only five ST-154 MenB isolates were found among the culture-confirmed IMD cases in western Canada (28). The combined population in western Canada in 2012 was estimated to be 10.77 million, while in Atlantic Canada the combined population in 2012 was estimated to be 2.37 million. This MenB strain was also rare in Quebec (population estimated to be 7.9 million in 2010), with only two isolates found among 334 invasive MenB strains between 2003 and 2010 (26). In Ontario (population estimated to be 13.1 million in 2010), 10 such MenB strains were detected among 193 invasive MenB isolates between 2001 and 2010 (27). Sequence type 154 belongs to the ST-41/44 CC or lineage 3, a well-known hypervirulent clone. A strain characterized as B:4:P1.4 ST-154 or ST-42 was the cause of the MenB epidemic in New Zealand in the 1990s (37,38), which prompted the New Zealand government to commission production of a strain-specific OMV vaccine based on the PorA P1.4 OMP (20).

The percentage of MenB involving *fHbp* genes that encoded for variant 1 or subfamily B peptides was significantly higher in Atlantic Canada (82%) (the present study) than in western Canada (38%) (28), or in the Immunization Monitoring Program Active (IMPACT) study examining MenB isolates from 12 pediatric tertiary care centres across the country (64%) (39). The strain differences in these three studies were probably the reason for the observed difference in fHbp types reported. In western Canada, ST-213 CC was the second most common CC found, and most (92%) of the isolates from this CC were predicted to have fHbp peptide 45 (variant 3). In addition, the strains involved in MenB disease in western Canada were very diverse in terms of their antigens and ST, which presented a picture of endemic disease (28). In contrast, the IMPACT study was in some way skewed by the elevated incidence of MenB disease in Quebec over the past several years due to the ST-269 clone (26,40). Most ST-269 MenB were found to have the *fHbp* gene allele 15, predicted to synthesize variant 1 or subfamily B fHbp protein. In Atlantic Canada, the predominance of the ST-154 MenB strain, which uniformly have the *fHbp* gene allele 4, was predicted to synthesize variant 1 or subfamily B peptide. This contributed to the highest percentage of MenB found in Canada, predicted to be covered by the fHbp component present in the 4CMenB or the bivalent recombinant fHbp vaccine. A similar study from the United States revealed that 59% of MenB isolates were found to encode variant 1 or subfamily B fHbp peptides (41), while in Europe the percentage of MenB encoding for variant 1 or subfamily B fHbp differed according to country, and ranged from 65.2% to 76.7% (42).

Similar to the observation in western Canada, the *fHbp* genes in all seven non-MenB strains in Atlantic Canada encoded variant 2 or subfamily A fHbp proteins. None of the strains had the *nhba* gene, which predicts the synthesis of NHBA peptide 2. Only two non-MenB strains were found to have *nadA* genes that enable synthesis of NadA peptides, likely covered by the NadA component of the 4CMenB vaccine.

Overall, 25 (62.5%) of the 40 invasive strains found in Atlantic Canada had at least one antigen that matched exactly to the 4CMenB vaccine components. Additional coverage may be possible by the NHBA component of 4CMenB as cross-protection against different NHBA peptides that have been reported (24). Furthermore, components other than the *porA* P1.4 that are present in the OMV may also provide further protective immunity.

One limitation of the present study was the relatively small number of non-MenB strains examined and, therefore, the prediction for these other serogroups would not be meaningful. The predicted coverage for MenB alone in Atlantic Canada was significantly higher (24 of 33 [73%] isolates) due to the predominant presence of the ST-154 clone, which shared two exact match antigens (PorA P1.4 and NHBA peptide 2) with the vaccine. Second, we did not perform the meningococcal antigen typing system assay (43) to study the degree

of expression and cross-reactivity of antigens on clinical isolates with those in the 4CMenB vaccine. Regardless, true coverage may not be known unless the vaccine is used in a population because strains within a region may change over time. Furthermore, true vaccine coverage rates may change because the epidemiology of clones may shift over time and among regions (44-46).

ACKNOWLEDGEMENTS: The authors thank the staff of the National Microbiology Laboratory's DNA Core Facility for providing primers and assistance with DNA sequencing. They also thank Jianwei Zhou and Saul Deng for technical assistance, as well as the staff at the local and regional hospitals in the provinces of NB, NS, PEI and NFLD for providing the isolates for the study. This study made use of the Neisseria MLST website (http://pubmlst.org/neisseria/) developed by Keith Jolley and Man-Suen Chan, and located at the University of Oxford, United Kingdom. The development of the site has been funded by the Wellcome Trust and European Union.

DISCLOSURE: The authors have no financial relationships or conflicts of interest to declare.

REFERENCES

1. Rosenstein NE, Perkins BA, Stephens DS, Popovic T, Huges JM. Meningococcal disease. N Engl J Med 2001;344:1378-88.
2. Al-Tawfiq JA, Clark TA, Memish ZA. Meningococcal disease: The organism, clinical presentation, and worldwide epidemiology. J Trop Med 2010;17(Suppl):3-8.
3. Xie Q, Pollard AJ, Mueller JE, Norheim G. Emergence of serogroup X meningococcal disease in Africa: Need for a vaccine. Vaccine 2013;31:2852-61.
4. Harrison LH, Trotter CL, Ramsay ME. Global epidemiology of meningococcal disease. Vaccine 2009;27S:B51-63.
5. Deeks SL, Kertesz D, Ryan A, Johnson W, Ashton F. Surveillance of invasive meningococcal disease in Canada, 1995-1996. Can Commun Dis Rep 1997;23:121-5.
6. Squires SG, Pelletier L, Mungai M, Tsang R, Collins F, Stoltz J. Invasive meningococcal disease in Canada, 1 January 1997 to 31 December 1998. Can Commun Dis Rep 2000;26:177-82.
7. Squires SG, Deeks S, Tsang RSW. Enhanced surveillance of invasive meningococcal disease in Canada: 1 January 1998 through 31 December 2001. Can Commu Dis Rep 2004;30:17-28.
8. Watkins KM, Deeks SL, Medgaglia A, Tsang RSW. Enhanced surveillance of invasive meningococcal disease in Canada: 1 January 2002, through 31 December 2003. Can Commun Dis Rep 2006;32:97-107.
9. Navarro C, Deeks SL, Medagha A, Tsang RSW. Enhanced surveillance of invasive meningococcal disease in Canada: 1 January 2004, through 31 December, 2005. Can Commun Dis Rep 2007;33:1-15.
10. Li YA, Tsang R, Desai S, Deehan H. Enhanced surveillance of invasive meningococcal disease in Canada, 2006-2011. Can Communicable Dis Rep 2014;40:160-9.
11. Caugant DA. Population genetics and molecular epidemiology of *Neisseria meningitidis*. APMIS 1998;106:505-25.
12. National Advisory Committee on Immunization (NACI). An Advisory Committee Statement (ACS) update on the use of quadrivalent conjugate meningococcal vaccines. Can Commun Dis Rep 2013;39:1-40.
13. Tsang RSW, Hoang L, Tyrrell G, et al. Genetic and antigenic characterization of Canadian *Neisseria meningitidis* serogroup C (MenC) case isolates in the post-MenC conjugate vaccine era, 2009-2013. J Med Microbiol 2015;64:174-9.
14. Santolaya ME, O'Ryan ML, Valenzuela MT, et al. Immunogenicity and tolerability of a multicomponent meningococcal serogroup B (4CMenB) vaccine in healthy adolescents in Chile: A phase 2b/3 randomised, observer-blind, placebo-controlled study. Lancet 2012;379:617-24.
15. Richmond PC, Marshall HS, Nissan MD, et al. Safety, immunogenicity, and tolerability of meningococcal serogroup B

bivalent recombinant lipoprotein 2086 vaccine in healthy adolescents: A randomized, single-blind, placebo-controlled, phase 2 trial. Lancet Infect Dis 2012;12:597-607.
16. Finne J, Leinonen M, Makela PH. Antigenic similarities between brain components and bacteria causing meningitis. Implications for vaccine development and pathogenesis. Lancet 1983;322:355-7.
17. Bjune G, Hoiby EA, Gronnesby JK, et al. Effect of outer membrane vesicle vaccine against group B meningococcal disease in Norway. Lancet 1991;338:1093-6.
18. Sierra GVG, Campa HC, Varcacel NM, et al. Vaccine against group B *Neisseria meningitidis*: Protection trial and mass vaccination results in Cuba. NIPH Ann 1991;14:195-207.
19. de Moraes JC, Perkins BA, Camargo MC, et al. Protective efficacy of a serogroup B meningococcal vaccine in Sao Paulo, Brazil. Lancet 1992;340:1074-8.
20. Oster P, Lennon D, O'Hallahan, Mulholland K, Reid S, Martin D. MeNZB: A safe and highly immunogenic tailor-made vaccine against the New Zealand *Neisseria meningitidis* serogroup B disease epidemic strain. Vaccine 2005;23:2191-6.
21. Sette A, Rappuoli R. Reverse vaccinology: Developing vaccines in the era of genomics. Immunity 2010;33:530-41.
22. Pillai S, Howell A, Alexander K, et al. Outer membrane protein (OMP) based vaccine for *Neisseria meningitidis* serogroup B. Vaccine 2005;23:2206-9.
23. Masignani V, Comanducci M, Giuliani MM, et al. Vaccination against *Neisseria meningitidis* using three variants of the lipoprotein GNA1870. J Exp Med 2003;197:789-99.
24. Giuliani MM, Adu-Boble J, Comanducci M, et al. A universal vaccine for serogroup B meningococcus. Proc Natl Acad Sci USA 2006;103:10834-9.
25. Comanducci M, Bambini S, Brunelli B, et al. NadA, a novel vaccine candidate of *Neisseria meningitidis*. J Exp Med 2002;195:1445-54.
26. Zhou J, Lefebvre B, Deng S, et al. Invasive serogroup B *Neisseria meningitidis* in Quebec, Canada, 2003 to 2010: Persistence of the ST-269 clone since it first emerged in 2003. J Clin Microbiol 2012;50:1545-51.
27. Jamieson FB, Rawte P, Deeks, et al. Genetic and antigenic characterization of invasive endemic serogroup B *Neisseria meningitidis* from Ontario, Canada, in 2001-2010. J Med Microbiol 2013;62:46-55.
28. Law DKS, Zhou J, Deng S, et al. Determination of serotyping antigens, clonal analysis and genetic characterization of the 4CMenB vaccine antigen genes in invasive *Neisseria meningitidis* from Western Canada, 2009-2013. J Med Microbiol 2014;63:1490-9.
29. Abdillahi H, Poolman JT. Whole-cell ELISA for typing *Neisseria meningitidis* with monoclonal antibodies. FEMS Microbiol Lett 1987;48:367-71.

30. Maiden MCJ, Bygraves JA. Feil E, et al. Multilocus sequence typing: A portable approach to the identification of clones within populations of pathogenic microorganisms. Proc Natl Acad Sci USA 1998;95:3140-5.

31. Sacchi CT, Lemos AP, Brandt ME, et al. Proposed standardization of *Neisseria meningitidis* PorA variable-region typing nomemclature. Clin Diagn Lab Immunol 1998;5:845-55.

32. Clark SC, Diggle MA, Molling P, Unemo M, Olcen P. Analysis of PorA variable region 3 in menincococci: Implications for vaccine policy. Vaccine 2003;21:2468-73.

33. de Filippis I, Gopalan V, Huyen Y. PorA VR3 typing database: A web-based resource for the determination of PorA VR3 alleles of *Neisseria meningitidis*. Infect Gene Evol 2011;11:248-9.

34. Lucidarme J, Comanducci M, Findlow J, et al. Characterization of fHbp, nhba (gna2132), nadA, porA, and sequence type in group B meningococcal case isolates collected in England and Wales during January 2008 and potential coverage of an investigational group B meningococcal vaccine. Clin Vaccine Immunol 2010;17:919-29.

35. Tsang RSW, Lefebvre B, Jamieson FB, Gilca R, Deeks SL, Zhou J. Identification and proposal of a potentially new clonal complex that is a common cause of MenB disease in central and eastern Canada. Can J Microbiol 2012;58:1236-40.

36. Law DKS, Lorange M, Ringuette L, et al. Invasive meningococcal disease in Québec, Canada, due to an emerging clone of ST-269 serogroup B meningococci with serotype antigen 17 and serosubtype antigen P1.19 (B:17:P1.19). J Clin Microbiol 2006;44:2743-9.

37. Martin DR, Walker SJ, Baker MG, Lennon DR. New Zealand epidemic of meningococcal disease identified by a strain with phenotype B:4:P1.4. J Infect Dis 1998;177:497-500.

38. Dyet KH, Martin DR. Clonal analysis of the serogroup B meningococci causing New Zealand's epidemic. Epidemiol Infect 2006;134:377-83.

39. Bettinger JA, Scheifele DW, Halperin SA, et al. Diversity of Canadian meningococcal serogroup B isolates and estimated coverage by an investigational meningococcal serogroup B vaccine (4CMenB). Vaccine 2014;32:124-30.

40. Gilca R, Deceuninck G, Lefebvre B, et al. The changing epidemiology of meningococcal disease in Québec, Canada, 1991-2011: Potential implications of emergence of new strains. PloS One 2012;7:1-9.

41. Wang X, Cohn A, Comanducci M, et al. Prevalence and genetic diversity of candidate vaccine antigens among invasive *Neisseria meningitidis* isolates in the United States. Vaccine 2011;29:4739-44.

42. Murphy E, Andrew L, Lee KL, et al. Sequence diversity of the factor H binding protein vaccine candidate in epidemiologically relevant strains of serogtoup B *Neisseria meningitidis*. J Infect Dis 2009;200:379-89.

43. Plikaytis BD, Stella M, Boccadifuoco G, et al. Interlaboratory standardization of the sandwich enzyme-linked immunosorbent assay designed for MATS, a rapid, reproducible method for estimating the strain coverage of investigational vaccines. Clin Vaccine Immunol 2012;19:1609-17.

44. Perez-Trallero E, Esnal O, Marimon JM. Progressive decrease in the potential usefulness of meningococcal serogroup B vaccine (4CMenB, Bexsero®) in Gipuzkoa, Northern Spain. PLoS One 2014;9:e116024.

45. Tzanakaki G, Hong E, Kesanopoulos K, et al. Diversity of Greek meningococcal serogroup B isolates and estimated coverage of the 4CMenB meningococcal vaccine. BMC Microbiol 2014;14:111.

46. Vogel U, Taha MK, Vazquez JA, et al. Predicated strain coverage of a meningococcal multicomponent vaccine (4CMenB) in Europe: A qualitative and quantitative assessment. Lancet Infect Dis 2013;13:416-25.

35

A family cluster of Chagas disease detected through selective screening of blood donors: A case report and brief review

Guillaume Mongeau-Martin DCS[1], Momar Ndao DVM PhD[1,2], Michael Libman MDCM[1],
Gilles Delage MD[3], Brian J Ward MSc, MDCM [1,2]

G Mongeau-Martin, M Ndao, M Libman, G Delage, BJ Ward. A family cluster of Chagas disease detected through selective screening of blood donors: Case report and brief review. Can J Infect Dis Med Microbiol 2015;26(3):157-161.

Chagas disease (CD) is a protozoan infection caused by *Trypanosoma cruzi*, which is transmitted by triatomine insect vectors in parts of Latin America. In a nonendemic country, such as Canada, spread can still occur via vertical transmission, and infected blood or organ donations. The Canadian Blood Services and Héma-Québec have both implemented selective screening of blood donors for CD based on risk factors. In 2011, Héma-Québec identified two seropositive 'at-risk' Chilean siblings who had donated blood in Montreal, Quebec. They were referred to the JD MacLean Centre for Tropical Diseases (Montreal, Quebec) for confirmatory testing (*T cruzi* excreted-secreted antigen ELISA, polymerase chain reaction and/or radioimmunoprecipitation assay) and follow-up. Screening of the rest of the family revealed two other seropositive family members (the mother and sister). While their geographical history in Chile suggests vectorial transmission, this family cluster of CD raises the possibility of vertical transmission. Congenital infection should always be considered among CD-positive mothers and pregnant women. With blood donor screening, Canadian physicians will increasingly see patients with CD and should know how to manage them appropriately. In addition to the case presentation, the authors review the transmission, screening and clinical management of CD in a nonendemic context.

Key Words: *Blood donor screening; Chagas disease; ELISA; PCR; RIPA; Vertical transmission*

Une grappe familiale de maladie de Chagas décelée grâce au dépistage sélectif des donneurs de sang : rapport de cas et brève analyse

La maladie de Chagas (MC) est une infection protozoaire causée par le *Trypanosoma cruzi*, transmis par des vecteurs d'insectes du genre triatomine dans certaines régions d'Amérique latine. Dans un pays non endémique comme le Canada, la propagation est possible par transmission verticale et par les dons de sang ou d'organes infectés. La Société canadienne du sang et Héma-Québec ont tous deux adopté le dépistage sélectif des donneurs de sang pour déceler la MC en fonction des facteurs de risque. En 2011, Héma-Québec a repéré deux membres d'une fratrie chilienne séropositifs « à risque » qui avaient donné du sang à Montréal, au Québec. Ils ont été orientés vers le Centre des maladies tropicales JD MacLean de Montréal pour subir les tests de confirmation (test ELISA des antigènes excrétés-sécrétés par *T cruzi*, réaction en chaîne de la polymérase ou test de radio-immunoprécipitation) et profiter d'un suivi. Le dépistage du reste de la famille a révélé deux autres membres séropositifs (la mère et la sœur). Étant donné leur origine géographique, on pourrait subodorer une transmission vectorielle, mais la grappe familiale de MC soulève la possibilité d'une transmission verticale. L'infection congénitale devrait toujours être envisagée chez les mères et les femmes enceintes positives à la MC. Grâce au dépistage des donneurs de sang, les médecins canadiens verront de plus en plus de patients atteints de la MC. Ils devraient donc savoir comment la prendre en charge correctement. En plus de la présentation de cas, les auteurs passent en revue la transmission, le dépistage et la prise en charge clinique de la MC dans un contexte non endémique.

Chagas disease (CD) is a zoonotic disease caused by *Trypanosoma cruzi*, a protozoan parasite that is endemic in parts of Mexico, Central and South America (1). It is transmitted by triatomine insect vectors, members of the *Reduviidae* family. CD can also be spread by congenital transmission from mother to fetus, by blood transfusion or organ transplantation and, more rarely, by consumption of food contaminated with *T cruzi* (2).

Most individuals infected by *T cruzi* experience a nonspecific acute phase with influenza-like symptoms. After one to two months, infected individuals typically enter an asymptomatic, chronic phase referred to as the indeterminate form of CD (3). While most infected individuals remain asymptomatic their entire lives, 20% to 30% develop cardiac or gastrointestinal (GI) complications over the course of several decades (2). Acute CD is relatively simple to diagnose by microscopy of whole anticoagulated blood or polymerase chain reaction (PCR) to detect the presence of *T cruzi* DNA in the blood. During the chronic phase, the parasitemia is low and intermittent, and diagnosis relies on serological methods (eg, ELISA, indirect fluorescent antibody test, radioimmunoprecipitation assay [RIPA]) (4,5).

In nonendemic countries such as Canada, CD is mainly diagnosed among Latin American migrants (6). Based on the large Latin American immigrant population in the United States, it is estimated that >300,000 Americans have CD (7). In Canada, the demographics are very different, with an estimated 5553 infected immigrants residing in the country in 2010 (6). Limited spread of CD can still

[1]*JD MacLean Tropical Diseases Centre;* [2]*National Reference Centre for Parasitology, Research Institute of the McGill University Health Centre, Montreal;* [3]*Héma-Québec Inc, Ville Saint-Laurent, Quebec*

Correspondence: Dr Brian J Ward, Tropical Diseases Centre, Montreal General Hospital, 1650 Cedar Avenue, Room L10-509, Montreal, Quebec H3G 1A4.e-mail brian.ward@mcgill.ca

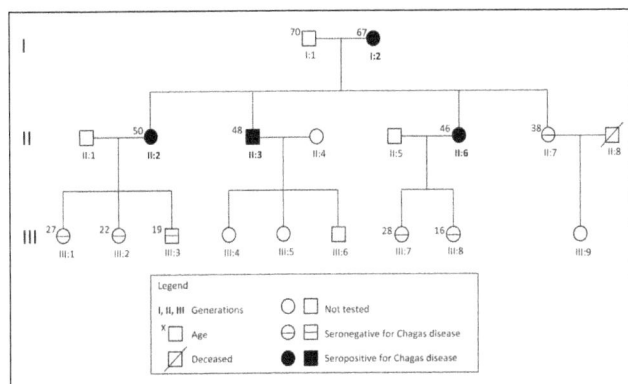

Figure 1) *Genogram of the family*

TABLE 1
Test results for first and second generations

Family member	Serological testing	PCR	Electrocardiogram	Echo-cardiogram
I:2	NRCP TESA +	−	Abnormal: right bundle branch block, prolonged QRS and incomplete left posterior fascicular block	Normal
II:2	NRCP TESA +	−	Rightward axis, otherwise normal	Normal
II:3	Abbott PRISM® + NRCP TESA + RIPA +	−	Sinus bradycardia, otherwise normal	Normal
II:6	Abbott PRISM® + NRCP TESA + RIPA +	−	Abnormal: sinus bradycardia and nonspecific T wave abnormality	Normal
II:7	NRCP TESA −	−	Normal	Normal

+ Positive; − Negative; NRCP National Reference Centre for Parasitology; PCR Polymerase chain reaction; RIPA Radioimmunoprecipitation assay; TESA Trypanosoma cruzi excreted-secreted antigens

occur in nonendemic countries through congenital transmission and via infected blood and organ donations. Although only a small number of cases of blood-transmitted CD have been reported in North America over the past 26 years (two in Canada [8,9]), these documented cases are likely to represent the tip of the iceberg because most such infections would be asymptomatic and go undiagnosed.

In May 2010, the Canadian Blood Services (CBS), which provides transfusion services for all provinces except Quebec, implemented selective screening of blood donors for CD using the Abbott PRISM Chagas Assay (a chemiluminescent immunoassay; Abbott Laboratories, USA) (10). Details of this screening program have been described recently (11). As of early 2013, CBS had screened >27,000 'at-risk' donors (based on travel, residence and maternal ancestry) and >80,000 'no risk' donors, and identified 14 seropositive subjects in the first group (0.05%) and one seropositive subject in the second group (0.001%) (12). A similar program had been implemented in March 2009 by Héma-Québec, the provider of transfusion services in that province (13) (www.hema-quebec.qc.ca). As of October 2013, 11,730 at-risk donors have been tested by Héma-Québec, and four confirmed positive donors have been found (Dr Gilles Delage, Héma-Québec, personal communication). In July 2011, this program identified two seropositive 'at-risk' Chilean siblings who had donated blood in Montreal, Quebec. These siblings are part of the family of Chilean immigrants that is the focus of the present article.

CASE PRESENTATION

In 2011, the two siblings, II:3 and II:6 (48 and 46 years of age, respectively [Figure 1]), donated blood at a Héma-Québec clinic. On their donor questionnaires, they both answered affirmatively to all three of the CD 'at-risk' questions: they were born in Chile to a Chilean mother and had lived in Chile for many years (17 and 15 years, respectively, before emigrating to Canada). Initial screening by Héma-Québec (PRISM Chagas Assay, Abbott) suggested that they were both seropositive, and their status was confirmed by repeat testing using the same assay. They were referred to the JD MacLean Centre for Tropical Diseases at the McGill University Health Centre (Montreal, Quebec) for assessment. Blood was drawn for confirmatory serological testing using a *T cruzi* excreted-secreted antigen ELISA (TESA-ELISA) (14,15) and PCR by the National Reference Centre for Parasitology (NRCP) in Montreal. Some samples were also tested using RIPA by Quest Diagnostics (USA). Neither had any cardiac nor GI symptoms, and physical examinations were normal. The brother's (II:3) electrocardiogram (ECG) showed sinus bradycardia, but was otherwise normal. His sister (II:6) had an abnormal ECG with sinus bradycardia and nonspecific T wave changes. Their echocardiograms were both normal. They were asked to bring their parents (I:1, I:2) and their two other sisters (II:2, II:7) to the clinic to be tested for CD.

Their mother (I:2, 67 years of age) and sisters (II:2 and II:7, 50 and 38 years of age, respectively) were tested using TESA-ELISA and PCR at the NRCP. The father (I:1, 70 years of age) declined to be tested. The eldest daughter (II:2) had no cardiac symptoms, although she had noted mild, intermittent diarrhea and abdominal cramps for the past three years. Neither the mother (I:2) nor the youngest sister (II:7) had any cardiac or GI complaints and their physical examinations were entirely normal. The mother's ECG was abnormal, with a right bundle branch block, a prolonged QRS and incomplete left posterior fascicular block. The eldest sister (II:2) had rightward axis deviation with an otherwise normal ECG. The youngest sister's (II:7) ECG was normal. Cardiac ultrasounds for these three members of the family (I:1, II:2 and II:7) were all essentially normal.

A summary of test results for the first and second generations is presented in Table 1. Four of the five family members tested were found to be positive by ≥1 of the serological assays. Only the youngest sister (II:7) was found to be seronegative for CD. PCR testing was negative for all four of the seropositive family members.

Because CD can be transmitted congenitally, the two CD-positive sisters (II:2, II:6) were advised to bring their five children to the Tropical Diseases Centre for testing (III:1-3 and III:7-8). All were found to be seronegative.

DISCUSSION

A family with four CD-positive individuals is a rare finding in a nonendemic country such as Canada. However, with the introduction of a screening program for blood donors, Canadian physicians will likely encounter an increasing number of newly diagnosed CD patients and will have to educate and manage these patients appropriately. The present case provides a good opportunity to review and discuss issues related to CD diagnosis and treatment.

Transmission
This family cluster raises important questions about when and how they became infected. Individual infection (via the triatomine vector), congenital infection, oral infection (eg, contaminated food) and transfusion/transplantation all need to be considered. In these cases, none of those infected had a history of either transfusion or organ transplant.

The fact that the mother (I:2) of three of the CD-positive children (II:2, II:3, II:6) was seropositive raises the possibility of congenital transmission. Because maternal-fetal transmission rates are only 5% to 6% (16,17), it is unlikely that all three were vertically infected. However, the degree to which the parasite is controlled by the mother can have a powerful influence on the likelihood of transmission through

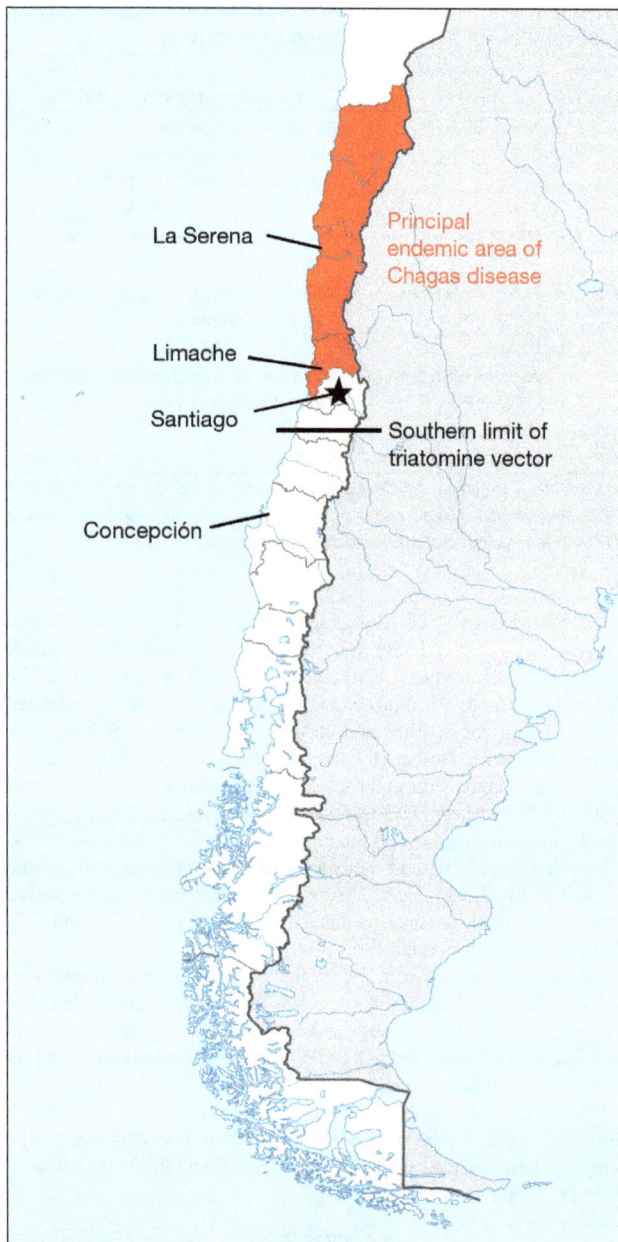

La Serena

Principal
endemic area of
Chagas disease

Limache

Santiago

Southern limit of
triatomine vector

Concepción

Figure 2) *Chile: Principal endemic area of Chagas disease in the middle of the 20th century (19,21). Produced using a blank map found on Wikimedia Commons (http://commons.wikimedia.org/wiki/File:Chile_location_map.svg).*

the placenta (17). Family clusters of congenital infection have been reported in the Southern Cone region of South America (18). Although the matriarch in the family cluster (I:2) was PCR-negative at 67 years of age, we do not know the level of parasitemia during each of her pregnancies.

This family's geographical history is useful in determining the relative risk of individual versus congenital infection (Figure 2). The parents (I:1, I:2) and their children (II:2, II:3, II:6, II:7) were all born in Chile. The mother (I:2) was born in 1944 in Limache, a small town north of Santiago. The father (I:1) was born in 1941 in La Serena, and moved to Limache when he married I:2 in 1960. Their first two children (II:2, II:3) were born in Limache in 1961 and 1962, respectively. In 1964, the family moved to Concepción, a larger city south of Santiago, where the two youngest children (II:6, II:7) were born (1964 and 1973, respectively). After the Chilean political turmoil in 1973,

the family was separated: the oldest siblings (II:2, II:3) moved north to La Serena, the mother (I:2) left for Santiago with her youngest daughter (II:7), and her other daughter (II:6) moved to Limache. Finally, in 1979, the entire family emigrated to the province of Quebec, where they currently reside.

Based on this history, it is plausible that the matriarch (I:2) and the three positive children (II:2, II:3, II:6) contracted CD by vectorial transmission in Limache, which was a small municipality in Valparaíso, one of the principal CD-endemic regions of Chile in the mid-20th century (19) (Figure 2). Housing quality is an important risk factor for triatomine infestation (eg, cane/thatch roofs, adobe/stone walls, poor ventilation) (20) and the family described their home as a rudimentary 'country house'. However, these three children lived in Limache for only short periods of time (<3 years for II:2 and II:3 and six years for II:6), which narrows the time frame for vectorial transmission. Vectorial infection in La Serena is another possibility for II:2 and II:3, who lived in this small town for six years after the 1973 political crisis. In both of these smaller, rural communities, oral infection by contaminated food, juice or water may also have occurred. The only uninfected child in the second generation (II:7) was born in Concepción, which is below the southern limit of the geographical distribution of the triatomine vector in Chile (21), and lived only in Concepción and Santiago.

Screening

This family cluster illustrates the potential impact of screening programs for *T cruzi* infection. Not only did it prevent the introduction of potentially contaminated blood into the blood pool, it also led to the diagnosis of CD in two additional family members (I:2, II:2). At the time of writing, the CBS selective screening program had identified 15 *T cruzi* antibody-positive donors in the first three years of operation (12). Whether selective screening based on risk factors is sufficient to prevent the introduction of blood products contaminated with *T cruzi* into the blood pool is a legitimate concern. Alternative and more comprehensive approaches include universal testing (every donor, every donation) and screening at the first interaction with blood services (so-called 'screening in') with subsequent rescreening based on new risks (eg, travel or residence in CD-endemic areas). A recent serosurvey involving >84,000 subjects who answered 'no' to all of the 'risk questions' found only one CD-positive individual (12,22), demonstrating that selective screening programs will only miss a very small number of cases in Canada. Vertical transmission of CD in nonendemic countries, such as Canada (11), Switzerland (23) and Spain (24), can occur and be undetected in the absence of selective prenatal screening. Although a screening program for pregnant women could theoretically identify candidates for serological screening, such a program would be cumbersome and very low yield. However, such a program would permit newborns of seropositive mothers to be tested at birth by PCR and/or microscopy of cord/venous blood (25) or by serology at eight to 10 months of age, after maternal antibodies are no longer present (26). CD can usually be successfully treated in infants (refer to Treatment section). Fortunately, none of the five children in the third generation of our family cluster were found to be CD positive.

Evaluation of patients diagnosed with CD

Subjects identified in screening programs (eg, blood bank, possibly prenatal care) first need to have the diagnosis confirmed using one or more reference tests (eg, TESA-ELISA, RIPA, PCR). Although there is no 'gold standard' assay, several such tests are available through the NRCP (www.nrcp.ca) in Canada or through other reference laboratories (eg, Centers for Disease Control and Prevention, www.cdc.gov). It is generally appropriate to screen the siblings and parents of any CD-positive subject as well as the children of infected mothers. A complete medical history and a physical examination should be performed, with a focus on signs and symptoms suggestive of cardiac or GI manifestations. Recommended testing includes a 12-lead ECG in all CD-positive patients (27). An echocardiogram can also be performed, especially if there are worrisome cardiac symptoms (eg, palpitations, chest pain) or conduction defects. CD-positive subjects with GI complaints can be assessed with barium studies and/or endoscopy. Asymptomatic patients should be followed up on an annual basis to identify new symptoms and to repeat an ECG and/or echocardiogram. At the time of writing, the four CD-positive subjects in this family cluster have been followed for approximately three years with no evidence of new or progressive cardiac or GI symptoms/abnormalities.

Treatment

Benznidazole and nifurtimox are currently the only antitrypanosomal drugs used to treat CD. Both are reasonably effective in acute (≥60%) and congenital infections (approximately 100%) (25,28,29). However, both are associated with significant side effects (30). Although success rates fall dramatically after one year of age in congenital disease, treatment with one of these drugs is still recommended for all individuals <18 years of age in the chronic phase (27). While there is no compelling evidence for treatment in adults between 18 and 50 years of age with chronic CD, the results of several small observational studies (reviewed in Viotti et al [31]) suggest that benznidazole can slow the progression of cardiac disease. As a result, a consensus is growing that treatment should at least be offered to all CD patients between 18 and 50 years of age (32). The question of whether benznidazole can slow or prevent progression of CD cardiomyopathy is currently being evaluated in a large, randomized,

multinational study, Benznidazole Evaluation for Interrupting Trypanosomiasis (BENEFIT) (33). Results from this trial should be available sometime in 2015. Because toxicity with either benznidazole or nifurtimox can be severe and tends to increase in older individuals (30), the risk:benefit ratio of treatment worsens with age (27,31,32). As a result, there are no clear treatment guidelines for any of the 46- to 67-year-old adult patients in our family cluster, particularly for subjects I:2 and II:6, who have abnormal ECGs but normal echocardiograms. After discussion of the pros and cons of therapy, all four decided not to initiate treatment until the results of the BENEFIT trial are known. Although there was considerable optimism that posaconazole may be a less toxic alternative therapy, the results of a recent randomized, controlled trial versus benznidazole are not encouraging (34). New drugs with greater efficacy in the chronic phase of CD are urgently needed.

CONCLUSION

The present report describes an unusual family cluster of CD and illustrates the importance of screening 'at-risk' blood donors. Not only did this program prevent the entry of contaminated blood into the blood system, it also led to the diagnosis of CD in two other members of this family. Vertical transmission should always be considered when dealing with CD-positive mothers and, especially, pregnant women, because at-risk newborns and infants can be tested and successfully treated if found to be positive.

REFERENCES

1. Coura JR, Borges-Pereira J. Chagas disease: 100 years after its discovery. A systemic review. Acta Trop 2010;115:5-13.
2. Shikanai-Yasuda MA, Carvalho NB. Oral transmission of Chagas disease. Clin Infect Dis 2012;54:845-52.
3. Andrade JP, Marin Neto JA, et al. I Latin American Guidelines for the diagnosis and treatment of Chagas' heart disease: Executive summary. Arq Bras Cardiol 2011;96:434-42.
4. WHO Expert Committee. Control of Chagas disease. Brasilia: World Health Organization, 2002. World Health Organ Tech Rep Ser 905.
5. Otani MM, Vinelli E, Kirchhoff LV, et al. WHO comparative evaluation of serologic assays for Chagas disease. Transfusion 2009;49:1076-82.
6. Schmunis GA, Yadon ZE. Chagas disease: A Latin American health problem becoming a world health problem. Acta Trop 2010;115:14-21.
7. Bern C, Montgomery SP. An estimate of the burden of Chagas disease in the United States. Clin Infect Dis 2009;49:e52-4.
8. Nickerson P, Orr P, Schroeder ML, Sekla L, Johnston JB. Transfusion-associated Trypanosoma cruzi infection in a non-endemic area. Ann Intern Med 1989;111:851-3.
9. Lane DJ, Sher G, Ward B, Ndao M, Leiby D, Hewlett B. Investigation of the second case of transfusion transmitted Chagas' disease in Canada. San Francisco: 42nd Annual Meeting of the American Society of Hematology, December 1 to 5, 2000.
10. Canadian Blood Services. Implementation of selective Chagas disease (Trypanosoma cruzi) antibody testing for at-risk blood donors. <http://www.transfusionmedicine.ca/sites/transfusionmedicine/files/news/2010_Notice_CMAJ.pdf> (Accessed October 20, 2013).
11. O'Brien SF, Scalia V, Goldman M, et al. Selective testing for Trypanosoma cruzi: The first year after implementation at Canadian Blood Services. Transfusion 2013;53:1706-13.
12. O'Brien SF, Scalia V, Goldman M, et al. Evaluation of selective screening of donors for antibody to Trypanosoma cruzi: seroprevalence of donors who answer "no" to risk questions. Transfusion 2014;54:863-9.
13. Hema-Québec. Chagas Disease – New selection criterion concerning Chagas disease. <www.hema-quebec.qc.ca/donner/don-de-sang/qui-peut-donner-du-sang/maladie-de-chagas.en.html> (Accessed October 20, 2013).
14. Ndao M, Spithill TW, Caffrey R, et al. Identification of novel diagnostic serum biomarkers for Chagas' disease in asymptomatic subjects by mass spectrometric profiling. J Clin Microbiol 2010;48:1139-49.

15. Berrizbeitia M, Figueroa M, Ward BJ, et al. Development and application of an ELISA assay using excretion/secretion proteins from epimastigote forms of T. cruzi (ESEA antigens) for the diagnosis of Chagas disease. J Trop Med 2012;2012:875909.
16. Torrico F, Alonso-Vega C, Suarez E, et al. Maternal Trypanosoma cruzi infection, pregnancy outcome, morbidity, and mortality of congenitally infected and non-infected newborns in Bolivia. Am J Trop Med Hyg 2004;70:201-9.
17. Apt W, Zulantay I, Arnello M, et al. Congenital infection by Trypanosoma cruzi in an endemic area of Chile: A multidisciplinary study. Trans R Soc Trop Med Hyg 2013;107:98-104.
18. Sánchez Negrette O, Mora MC, Basombrío MA. High prevalence of congenital Trypanosoma cruzi infection and family clustering in Salta, Argentina. Pediatrics 2005;115:e668-72.
19. Schofield CJ, Apt W, Miles MA. The ecology of Chagas disease in Chile. Ecol Dis 1982;1:117-29.
20. Schenone H, Villarroel F, Alfaro E. [Epidemiology of Chagas disease in Chile. Housing conditions related to the presence of Triatoma infestans and the rate of humans and animals infected by Trypanosoma cruzi]. Bol Chil Parasitol 1978;33:2-7.
21. Schenone H, Carrasco J, Dedios F, et al. [Determination of the southern limit of dispersion of domiciliary Triatoma infestation and trypanosomal infection in Chile]. Bol Chil Parasitol 1961;16:59-62.
22. Fearon MA, Scalia V, Huang M, Dines I, Ndao M, Lagacé-Wiens P. A case of vertical transmission of Chagas disease contracted via blood transfusion in Canada. Can J Infect Dis Med Microbiol 2013;24:32-4.
23. Jackson Y, Myers C, Diana A, et al. Congenital transmission of Chagas disease in Latin American immigrants in Switzerland. Emerg Infect Dis 2009;15:601-3.
24. Munoz J, Coll O, Juncosa T, et al. Prevalence and vertical transmission of Trypanosoma cruzi infection among pregnant Latin American women attending 2 maternity clinics in Barcelona, Spain. Clin Infect Dis 2009;48:1736-40.
25. Revista da Sociedade Brasileira de Medicina Tropical – International Colloquium. Congenital infection with Trypanosoma cruzi: From mechanisms of transmission to strategies for diagnosis and control. Rev Soc Bras Med Trop 2003;36:767-71.
26. Carlier Y, Torrico F, Sosa-Estani S, et al. Congenital Chagas disease: Recommendations for diagnosis, treatment and control of newborns, siblings and pregnant women. PLoS Negl Trop Dis 2011;5:e1250.
27. Bern C MSPHBL, Montgomery SP, Herwaldt BL, et al. Evaluation and treatment of Chagas disease in the United States: A systematic review. JAMA 2007;298:2171-81.

28. Rodriques Coura J, de Castro SL. A critical review on Chagas disease chemotherapy. Mem Inst Oswaldo Cruz 2002;97:3-24.

29. Altcheh J, Biancardi M, Lapena Λ, Ballering G, Freilij H. [Congenital Chagas disease: Experience in the Hospital de Ninos, Ricardo Gutierrez, Buenos Aires, Argentina]. Rev Soc Bras Med Trop 2005;38 Suppl 2:41-5.30.

30. Bern C. Antitrypanosomal therapy for chronic Chagas disease. N Engl J Med. 2011;364:2527-34.

31. Viotti R, Alarcón de Noya B, Araujo-Jorge T, et al; Latin American Network for Chagas Disease, NHEPACHA. Towards a paradigm shift in the treatment of chronic Chagas disease. Antimicrob Agents Chemother 2014;58:635-9.

32. Rassi A Jr, Rassi A, Marin-Neto JA. Chagas disease. Lancet 2010;375:1388-402.

33. Marin-Neto JA, Rassi A Jr, Avezum A Jr, et al. The BENEFIT trial: Testing the hypothesis that trypanocidal therapy is beneficial for patients with chronic Chagas heart disease. Mem Inst Oswaldo Cruz 2009;104(Suppl 1):319-24.

34. Molina I, Gómez i Prat J, Salvador F, et al. Randomized trial of posaconazole and benznidazole for chronic Chagas' disease. N Engl J Med 2014;370:1899-908.

Pasteurella species peritoneal dialysis-associated peritonitis: Household pets as a risk factor

Philippe Guillaume Poliquin MD FRCPC[1], Philippe Lagacé-Wiens MD FRCPC[2,3], Mauro Verrelli MD FRCPC[4], David W Allen MD[5], John M Embil MD FRCPC[2,6]

PG Poliquin, P Lagacé-Wiens, M Verrelli, DW Allen, JM Embil. *Pasteurella* species peritoneal dialysis-associated peritonitis: Household pets as a risk factor. Can J Infect Dis Med Microbiol 2015;26(1):52-55.

BACKGROUND: *Pasteurella* species are Gram-negative coccobacilli that are a part of the normal oropharyngeal flora of numerous domestic animals. They have been recognized as a rare but significant cause of peritonitis in patients undergoing peritoneal dialysis (PD). A consensus about management strategies for PD-associated peritonitis caused by *Pasteurella* species currently does not exist.
METHODS: The microbiological database serving the Manitoba Renal Program was searched from 1997 to 2013 for cases of *Pasteurella* species PD-associated peritonitis, and charts were reviewed. PubMed was searched for case reports and data were abstracted.
RESULTS: Seven new local cases and 30 previously reported cases were analyzed. This infection is clinically similar to other forms of PD peritonitis, with household pet exposure appearing to be the strongest risk factor. Cats are the most commonly implicated pet. Direct contact between the pet and the equipment was commonly reported (25 of 37 patients) but was not necessary for infection to develop. The mean duration of treatment was 15 days. Complication rates were low, with only 11% of patients requiring PD catheter removal. There was no mortality reported.
CONCLUSION: *Pasteurella* species are a rare cause of PD-associated peritonitis that can be successfully treated with a two-week course of intraperitoneal antibiotics with a high likelihood of catheter salvage.

Key Words: *Cat*; Pasteurella multocida; Pasteurella *species*; *Peritoneal dialysis*; *Peritonitis*

La péritonite associée à la dialyse péritonéale causée par des espèces de *Pasteurella* : les animaux domestiques sont un facteur de risque

HISTORIQUE : Les espèces de *Pasteurella* sont des coccobacilles à Gram négatif qui font partie de la flore oropharyngée normale de nombreux animaux domestiques. Ils constituent une cause de péritonite rare, mais importante, chez les patients sous dialyse péritonéale (DP). Il n'y a pas de consensus quant aux stratégies de prise en charge de la péritonite associée à la dialyse péritonéale causée par les espèces de *Pasteurella*.
MÉTHODOLOGIE : Les chercheurs ont exploré la base de données microbiologiques du Programme de lutte contre la maladie du rein du Manitoba de 1997 à 2013 pour déceler les cas de péritonite associée à la DP causée par les espèces de *Pasteurella* et ont examiné leur dossier. Ils ont fouillé PubMed pour trouver des rapports de cas et en ont extrait des données.
RÉSULTATS : Les chercheurs ont analysé sept nouveaux cas locaux et 30 anciens cas. Cette infection est similaire sur le plan clinique à d'autres formes de péritonite associée à la DP, dont le principal facteur de risque semble être l'exposition à un animal domestique. Les chats sont les plus en cause. On signale souvent un contact direct entre l'animal et le matériel (25 patients sur 37), mais il n'est pas nécessaire pour provoquer l'infection. Le traitement durait en moyenne 15 jours. Le taux de complications était faible, puisque seulement 11 % des patients ont dû faire retirer leur cathéter de DP. Aucun décès n'a été signalé.
CONCLUSION : Les espèces de *Pasteurella* sont de rares causes de péritonite associée à la DP qu'on peut soigner par un traitement de deux semaines aux antibiotiques intrapéritonéaux. Ce traitement s'associe à une forte probabilité de sauvegarder le cathéter.

*P*asteurella multocida is a Gram-negative coccobacillus first identified in 1878 in diseased birds (1). Since then, *P multocida* has become associated primarily with skin and soft tissue infections following animal bites. The organism is known to colonize the upper respiratory tract of 90% of cats and 66% of dogs (2). Contamination with *P multocida* may result in a wide range of infections including pneumonia, endocarditis and meningitis (1).

Among more unusual sites, *P multocida* has been found to cause peritonitis in individuals undergoing peritoneal dialysis (PD) for renal replacement (3). Patients undergoing PD consider it to be a convenient alternative to hemodialysis that is associated with a reduced impact on their quality of life (4). One of the major drawbacks of PD, however, is the risk for peritonitis due to frequent manipulation of the catheter and PD equipment (5). Despite improvement in infection rates due to better equipment and a focus on hand hygiene, an event rate of 0.5 episodes/patient/year is average (6).

Over the past 15 years, eight cases of *P multocida* PD peritonitis have been observed within the Manitoba Renal Program (Winnipeg, Manitoba), which currently provides care to 280 PD patients. In the present article, we briefly describe seven of these cases; the eighth case was previously reported in the *Canadian Journal of Infectious Diseases & Medical Microbiology* (7) due to its unique features as a polymicrobial zoonosis. In addition, we reviewed and analyzed the available published case reports of *Pasteurella* species PD-associated peritonitis (2,3,7-30). While the burden of such infections is small in comparison with the usual microbiology, both the prevalence of chronic renal disease (31) and pet ownership are increasing (32). As a result, we anticipate that there will be an increase in cases of PD peritonitis

[1]*Section of Paediatric Infectious Diseases, Department of Paediatrics and Child Health;* [2]*Department of Medical Microbiology and Infectious Diseases, University of Manitoba;* [3]*Department of Clinical Microbiology, St Boniface General Hospital;* [4]*Section of Nephrology, Department of Internal Medicine, University of Manitoba, and Manitoba Renal Program;* [5]*Section of Cardiology;* [6]*Section of Infectious Diseases, Department of Internal Medicine, University of Manitoba, Winnipeg, Manitoba*
Correspondence: Dr John M Embil, Infection Prevention and Control Unit, Health Sciences Centre, MS673, 820 Sherbrook Street, Winnipeg, Manitoba R3A 1R9. e-mail jembil@hsc.mb.ca

caused by *Pasteurella* species. Collectively, analysis of the 37 available cases enabled the creation of meaningful recommendations to guide future therapy.

METHODS

Identification of local cases

The electronic microbiology laboratory database that serves the Manitoba Renal Program was searched for *P multocida* or *Pasteurella* species isolated from peritoneal fluid from January 1, 1997 to June 30, 2013. Patient charts were abstracted for the following: age, sex, co-morbidities, PD history, animal exposure and symptoms. Laboratory data, including white blood cell (WBC) counts from peripheral blood and peritoneal fluid as well as Gram stain and culture results, were collected.

Review of published reports

The PubMed database was searched from 1966 to June 1, 2013 using the MeSH terms ("Pasteurella"[Mesh] OR "Pasteurella pneumotropica"[Mesh] OR "Pasteurella multocida"[Mesh] OR "Pasteurella Infections"[Mesh]) AND ("Peritoneal Dialysis"[Mesh] OR "Peritoneal Dialysis, Continuous Ambulatory"[Mesh] OR "Peritonitis"[Mesh]). This search returned 64 citations. Cases describing a PD-associated episode of peritonitis caused by *Pasteurella* species were included. Bibliographies were reviewed for additional cases. Individual reports were abstracted for the same information as the local cases.

Local case series

All of the cases included in the present series ultimately yielded *P multocida* from culture of the PD fluid obtained at the time of presentation. None of these local patients experienced a relapse of PD peritonitis caused by *Pasteurella* species. All patients were initially treated using the PD program's standing protocol for the empirical treatment of PD peritonitis – specifically, once-daily intraperitoneal (IP) cefazolin (or vancomycin for beta-lactam allergic patients) and tobramycin. Table 1 demonstrates dosing guidelines used at the authors' institution.

Case 1: A 28-year-old woman with a history of tetralogy of Fallot, hypertension and congenital solitary kidney developed end-stage renal disease (ESRD) managed by continuous ambulatory peritoneal dialysis (CAPD). She had been on CAPD for one month and presented with a 5 h history of severe abdominal pain and chills. Her cat had chewed on her dialysate line earlier that day. She was started on IP cefazolin and tobramycin for 48 h. Treatment was tailored to IP ceftazidime for an additional 12 days, with clinical improvement within 24 h.

Case 2: A 37-year-old man who had been on CAPD for 15 months for ESRD secondary to diabetic nephropathy sought medical attention for a one-day history of abdominal pain, fever and chills. His cat had bitten the dialysate line the day before, although a puncture was not observed. He was started on IP cefazolin and tobramycin, and experienced prompt recovery. The tobramycin was discontinued after five days and he completed 14 total days of IP cefazolin.

Case 3: A 41-year-old man who had been on CAPD for ESRD secondary to diabetic and hypertensive nephropathy for the past 18 months sought medical attention for a 4 h history of abdominal pain, fever, chills, nausea, vomiting and diarrhea. The patient noted that his dialysate fluid had been cloudy that morning. He was the owner of three cats that were allowed into the PD area, and reported that one may have bitten the tubing. He demonstrated rapid improvement after initiation of IP cefazolin and tobramycin. Tobramycin was discontinued on day 5 and he completed 14 days of IP cefazolin.

Case 4: A 51-year-old woman who had been on CAPD for the past seven months for ESRD secondary to hypertension sought medical attention for a 5 h history of abdominal pain, fever, nausea and vomiting. She indicated that her dialysate fluid was cloudy during her most recent session. Although she owned a cat, she reported that it was not permitted within the PD area. The patient was treated with three days of IP cefazolin and tobramycin, with marked improvement within 24 h

TABLE 1
Intraperitoneal antibiotic dosing

Antibiotic	Dose
Cefazolin	1.5 g intraperitoneal once daily if ≥50 kg
	1 g intraperitoneal once daily if <50 kg
Ceftazidime	1.5 g intraperitoneal once daily
Vancomycin	If no residual renal function:
	2 g intraperitoneal every 7 days if ≥50 kg
	1 g intraperitoneal every 7 days if <50 kg
	If patient has residual renal function with urine output >100 mL/day:
	Same empirical doses as above; however, dosing is adjusted after vancomycin level is obtained four to five days after initial dose
Tobramycin	60 mg intraperitoneal once daily if ≥50 kg
	40 mg intraperitoneal once daily if <50 kg

of therapy. IP antibiotics were discontinued and patient completed 14 days of amoxicillin-clavulanic acid orally.

Case 5: A 37-year-old woman who had been on CAPD for 11 years for ESRD secondary to chronic interstitial nephropathy sought medical attention for a 10 h history of abdominal pain, chills and diarrhea. She had regular contact with a domestic cat but not in the vicinity of her PD equipment. She was treated with IP cefazolin and ceftazidime for five days but had ongoing cloudy dialysate and abdominal pain. The PD catheter was removed, and she completed her therapy with three days of ceftriaxone and one week of oral amoxicillin.

Case 6: A 59-year-old woman who had been on CAPD for the past three years for ESRD secondary to diabetic nephropathy sought medical attention for a four-day history of nausea and vomiting and a one-day history of abdominal pain. The woman had regular contact with a domestic cat in her home, but no documented contact with PD equipment or tubing. She received a five-day course of IP cefazolin and tobramycin followed by IP ceftazidime for 14 days with complete recovery.

Case 7: A 69-year-old woman with an underlying history of diabetes mellitus, hypertension, thalassemia and diabetic nephropathy was started on CAPD. She presented three days later with cloudy dialysate and subjective fever. She reported abdominal pain with her latest fluid exchange. Concern was raised that her cat may have bitten the cycler line. She was discharged from the emergency department with reassurance but was asked to return because *P multocida* was recovered in the PD fluid culture. She was successfully treated as an outpatient with two days of IP cefazolin and tobramycin followed by seven days of IP ceftazidime and seven days of oral amoxicillin-clavulanic acid.

RESULTS

The local database search revealed the seven cases described above. An additional published case from our centre (7) was added to 29 published cases identified using the search strategy described above. This resulted in a total of 37 cases for analysis. The vast majority (33 of 37) of cases were secondary to *P multocida*, with one each of *P aerogenes*, *P canis*, *P dagmatis* and *P pneumotropica* accounting for the remainder.

Demographics

The mean (± SD) patient age was 44.4±17.6 years (range eight to 75 years), with a male-to-female ratio of 1:1. There were three pediatric patients. Cases were heterogeneous regarding the underlying reason for renal failure, including both congenital as well as acquired causes. PD modality varied, with 43% using continuous cycling PD, 41% using CAPD and 16% being unspecified. The mean length of time on PD was 24.1 months, with a wide range (three days to 11 years).

Clinical and laboratory features at presentation

The median time to presentation was 18.5 h (range 1 h to 168 h). Information on clinical presentation was available for 34 of 37 patients. Abdominal pain was most commonly reported (91%). Other signs and

TABLE 2
Management approaches for patients with *Pasteurella* peritoneal dialysis-associated peritonitis

	Proportion of patients receiving specified treatment
Initial management	
Intraperitoneal antibiotics only	27/37 (73)
Intravenous antibiotics only	4/37 (11)
Combination intravenous/intraperitoneal/oral	3/37 (8)
No therapy	2/37 (5)
Definitive therapy	
Intraperitoneal antibiotics only	19/34 (56)
Intravenous antibiotics only	6/34 (18)
Combination intraperitoneal/oral	3/34 (9)
Oral antibiotics only	6/34 (18)
Duration of therapy, days, mean ± SD (range)	15.2±4.1 (7–24)
Duration of therapy, days, median	14

Data presented as n/total n (%) unless otherwise indicated

symptoms included: nausea and vomiting (65%), cloudy dialysate fluid (50%), fever (38%), chills (29%) and diarrhea (12%). No patients were asymptomatic. A tunnel site infection was diagnosed in one of 37 patients.

The peripheral WBC count was available for 26 of 36 patients, with an average WBC count of $10.8×10^9$/L ($3.7×10^9$/L to $20.7×10^9$/L). Numerically, the WBC was abnormal in only 54% of cases (as per the reported normal range for individual institutions). The peritoneal fluid cell count was universally abnormal, with an average of $6621×10^6$/L (range $210×10^6$/L to $25,879×10^6$/L; normal $<100×10^6$/L). The Gram stain was not reliably helpful, demonstrating Gram-negative rods in only six of 33 cases. Blood cultures were not routinely drawn; two patients had *P multocida* bacteremia, one asymptomatically and one with a shock-like syndrome.

Animal type and degree of contact

Cats were the most commonly implicated animal, accounting for 83% (31 of 37) of cases. Exposure to animals other than cats occurred conclusively in four cases. This appeared to be more common in the few pediatric patients (two of three nonfeline exposure) and resulted in non-*P multocida* infections. Direct contact between the animal and the equipment was documented in 25 of 37 cases, of which 10 of 25 confirmed a puncture of the line or fluid bags. An additional 10 cases reported no contact between the animal and PD equipment or treatment area. There was no association between type of exposure and PD modality (P=0.304). There was a significant difference in time from symptom onset to presentation between patients with a bite or puncture of the PD catheter tubing compared with patients with non-specific contact (15 h versus 44 h; P=0.04).

Management and outcomes

The approach to management of these infections was highly variable within the reported literature in terms of both route of delivery and length of therapy (Table 2). Outcomes were generally favourable. Two patients experienced a septic shock-like syndrome requiring admission to the intensive care unit. One patient experienced a recurrence four weeks after discontinuation of therapy. The PD catheter was removed in 11% (four of 37) of patients. There was no discernible association between a particular therapeutic regimen and a poor outcome. No mortality was reported.

DISCUSSION

Since the first case of *P multocida* peritonitis was described in 1987, this organism has become recognized as an infrequent but clinically significant cause of PD-associated peritonitis (3). The seven cases from our centre represent the largest series reported to date. Together with the existing 30 published reports, important trends emerge (2,3,7-30).

Overall, patients with *Pasteurella* species PD-associated peritonitis have a very similar symptom constellation to other forms of infectious peritonitis. When our patients were compared with patients from a recent case series of PD-associated peritonitis (5), rates of abdominal pain (91% versus 88%), nausea and vomiting (65% versus 51%) and fever (38% versus 29%) were similar. Observation of a cloudy effluent was less common in infections caused by *Pasteurella* species (50%) compared with other organisms (84%). This may be due to the relatively rapid median time to presentation for care of 18.5 h. Given that cases occurred in PD recipients with both lengthy (11 years) and limited (third day of PD) experience, it is evident that ongoing education regarding the risk of PD-associated peritonitis in the presence of household pets is critical.

Exposure to a colonized animal is a prerequisite of infection; however, the degree of contact necessary for infection appeared to be limited. Direct contact between the animal and the equipment was documented in 25 of 37 cases, of which 10 of 25 confirmed a puncture of the line or fluid bags. More intriguing were the 10 cases that reported only casual contact between the owner and the animal. While a surreptitious contact event cannot be excluded, the observation that animal breeders can acquire oropharyngeal colonization with *Pasteurella* species raises the possibility that self-inoculation from the patient's own flora may underlie some of these infections (33). Furthermore, it has been demonstrated using pulsed-field electrophoresis that *Pasteurella* species oropharyngeal colonization with the same organism can occur in both patient and pet (24).

The most recent recommendations of the International Society for Peritoneal Dialysis recommend a three-week course of antimicrobial therapy for Gram-negative peritonitis (34). Based on previously published reports and our case series, it appears that, when compared with infection caused by other Gram-negative microorganisms, patients with PD-associated peritonitis caused by *Pasteurella* species experienced fewer recurrences and catheter loss events. The vast majority of these patients were successfully treated with a 14-day course of antimicrobial therapy, primarily delivered intraperitoneally. The one recurrence occurred in a patient treated for three weeks (11). Shorter courses of therapy (as short as seven days) have provided equivalent outcomes but the data are insufficient to allow definitive conclusions about shorter duration of therapy. Catheter loss was uncommon (four of 37). This compared favourably with a previously reported rate of 23% in non-*Enterobacteriaceae* Gram-negative-induced peritonitis (5). As such, a 14-day course of IP antibiotic therapy aimed at catheter salvage appears to be warranted for PD-associated peritonitis caused by *Pasteurella* species. On average, substantial clinical improvement occurred within 48 h to 72 h of initiation of therapy. The lack of mortality is reassuring, especially given that *P multocida* bacteremia typically carries a 30% mortality rate (22).

Given the heterogeneity of antibiotic choices, it is difficult to draw definitive conclusions about optimal antimicrobial choice. In general, however, penicillin- or ampicillin-based regimens are preferred for non-β-lactamase-producing isolates (1). Third-generation cephalosporins are believed to have equivalent activity to penicillin and ampicillin. Oral fluoroquinolone monotherapy was successfully used in five of 33 patients. Aminoglycoside IP monotherapy was used in three patients (3,11,17), one of whom (11) experienced the only recurrence following three weeks of therapy. This event, together with the unreliable activity of aminoglycosides against *Pasteurella* species described in the literature (35), suggests that aminoglycoside monotherapy in *Pasteurella* species peritonitis should be avoided.

There are several limitations inherent to retrospective review of isolated case reports. Those most pertinent to the present report include: patient recall bias, specifically with regard to animal exposure; inconsistent reporting/documentation of risk factors (such as type and extent of animal exposure) leading to infection; publication bias; differences in practice patterns within and between centres; and reliable laboratory identification of rare microorganisms. Recognizing the limits of this type of study, we believe that sufficient points of commonality have emerged to allow these trends to be reported.

CONCLUSION

The present case series and review of published reports is the largest and most complete to date, and provides a clear picture of PD-associated peritonitis caused by *Pasteurella* species. This infection is indistinguishable from other forms of PD peritonitis except for a tendency toward rapid (<24 h of symptoms) presentation for care. These organisms should be suspected as an etiological agent if there is a pet at home, even if direct contact between the pet and the equipment was not observed. Moreover, a history of a puncturing animal bite to PD tubing or fluid bags should raise the index of suspicion. Gram stain and WBC counts from both peripheral blood and peritoneal fluid are not helpful in distinguishing *Pasteurella* species from other infectious agents causing PD-associated peritonitis. This infection can occur in both novel and experienced PD users. As a result, PD patients should be regularly asked about pet ownership. Periodic reminders of infection control procedures should be stressed in routine follow-up appointments of PD patients with household pets.

The suggestion in the International Society for Peritoneal Dialysis guideline of empirical Gram-positive and Gram-negative therapy for PD-associated peritonitis is appropriate even if *Pasteurella* species are suspected (34). If *Pasteurella* species are recovered from PD fluid culture, we suggest a 14-day course of IP therapy guided by antimicrobial susceptibilities; aminoglycoside monotherapy should be avoided. Antibiotic-based PD catheter salvage therapy is an appropriate goal given that this approach was successful in 90% of published cases.

DISCLOSURES: The authors have no conflicts of interest to declare.

ACKNOWLEDGEMENTS: There were no study sponsors or funding sources.

ETHICS APPROVAL: Ethics approval was not required for this study.

REFERENCES

1. Zurlo JJ. *Pasteurella* species. In: Mandell GL, Bennett JE, Dolin R, editors. Mandell, Douglas, and Bennett's Principles and Practice of Infectious Diseases, Seventh Edition. Philadelphia: Elsevier, 2010:2939-42.
2. Sillery J, Heargreaves J, Kuznia C, Abbe C. *Pasteurella multocida* peritonitis: Another risk of animal-assisted therapy. Infect Control Hosp Epidemiol 2004;25:5-6.
3. Paul RV, Rostand G. Cat bite peritonitis: *Pasteurella multocida* peritonitis following feline contamination of peritoneal dialysis tubing. Am J Kid Dis 1987;10:318-9.
4. Juergensen E, Wuerth D, Finkelstein SH, Juergensen PH, Bekui A, Finkelstein FO. Hemodialysis and peritoneal dialysis: Patients' assessment of their satisfaction with therapy and the impact of the therapy on their lives. Clin J Am Soc Nephrol 2006;1:1191-6.
5. Oliveira LG, Luengo J, Caramori JC, Montelli AC, Cunha Mde L, Barretti P. Peritonitis in recent years: Clinical findings and predictors of treatment response of 170 episodes at a single Brazilian center. Int Urol Nephrol 2012;44:1529-37.
6. Troidle L, Finkelstein F. Treatment and outcome of CPD-associated peritonitis. Ann Clin Microbiol Antimicrob 2006;5:6.
7. Al-fifi Y, Sathianathan C, Murray B-L, Alfa M. Pets are 'risky business' for patients undergoing continuous ambulatory peritoneal dialysis. Can J Infect Dis Med Microbiol 2013;24:e96-8.
8. Antony SJ, Oglesby KA. Peritonitis associated with *Pasteurella multocida* in peritoneal dialysis patients – case report and review of the literature. Clin Nephrol 2007;1:52-6.
9. Campos A, Taylor JH, Campbell M. Hamster bite peritonitis: *Pasteurella pneumotropica* peritonitis in a dialysis patient. Pediatr Nephrol 2000;15:31-2.
10. Castellan I, Marín JP, Gallego S, et al. *Pasteurella canis* peritonitis in a peritoneal dialysis patient. Perit Dial Int 2011;31:503-4.
11. Cooke FJ, Kodjo A, Clutterbuck EJ, Bamford KB. A case of *Pasteurella multocida* peritoneal dialysis-associated peritonitis and review of the literature. Int J Infect Dis 2004;8:171-4.
12. Frankel AH, Cassidy MJD. *Pasteurella multocida* peritonitis in CAPD: Beware of the cats. Perit Dial Int 1991;11:84-5.
13. Freeman AF, Zheng XT, Lane JC, Shulman ST. *Pasteurella aerogenes* hamster bite peritonitis. Pediatr Infect Dis J 2004;23:368-70.
14. Iwashima K, Tsujimoto Y, Tabata T, et al. Two case reports of *Pasteurella* peritonitis in peritoneal dialysis. Nihon Toseki Igakkai Zasshi 2008;41:213-18.
15. Joh J, Padmanabhan R, Bastani B. *Pasteurella multocida* peritonitis following cat bite of peritoneal dialysis tubing. Am J Nephrol 1998;18:258.
16. Kanaan N, Gavage P, Janssens M, Avesani V, Gigi J, Goffin E. *Pasteurella multocida* in peritoneal dialysis: A rare cause of peritonitis associated with exposure to domestic cats. Acta Clinica Belgica 2002;57:254-6.
17. Loghman-Adham M. *Pasteurella multocida* peritonitis in patients underdoing peritoneal dialysis. Pediatr Nephrol 1997;11:353-4.
18. Mackay K, Brown L, Hudson F. *Pasteurella multocida* peritonitis in peritoneal dialysis patients: Beware of the cat. Perit Dial Int 1997;17:608-10.
19. Malik A, al Aly Z, Mailey KS, Bastani B. *Pasteurella multocida* peritoneal dialysis-associated peritonitis: A report of two cases and review of the literature. J Nephrol 2005;18:791-3.
20. Mat O, Moenens F, Beauwens R, Rossi C, Muniz-Martinez M-C. Indolent *Pasteurella multocida* peritonitis in a CCPD patient. 25 years of "cat-bite peritonitis": A review. Perit Dial Int 2005;25:88-90.
21. Mugambi SM, Ullian ME. Bacteremia, sepsis, and peritonitis with *Pasteurella multocida* in a peritoneal dialysis patient. Perit Dial Int 2010;30:381-3.
22. Musio F, Tiu A. *Pasteurella multocida* peritonitis in peritoneal dialysis. Clin Nephrol 1998;1998:258-61.
23. Rondon-Berrios H, Trevejo-Nunez GJ. Pets or pest: Peritoneal dialysis-related peritonitis due to *Pasteurella multocida*. J Microbiol Immunol Infect 2010;43:155-8.
24. Satomura A, Yanai M, Fujita T, et al. Peritonitis associated with *Pasteurella multocida*: Molecular evidence of zoonotic etiology. Ther Apher Dial 2010;14:373-6.
25. Uribarri J, Bottone EJ, London RD. *Pasteurella multocida* peritonitis: Are peritoneal dialysis patients on cyclers at increased risk? Perit Dial Int 1996;16:648.
26. van Langenhove G, Daelemans R, Zachee P, Lins RL. *Pasteurella multocida* as a rare cause of peritonitis in peritoneal dialysis. Nephron 2000;85:282-4.
27. Wallet F, Toure F, Devalckenaere A, Pagniez D, Courcol RJ. Molecular identification of *Pasteurella dagmatis* peritonitis in a patient undergoing peritoneal dialysis. J Clin Microbiol 2000;38:4681-2.
28. Weiss GA, Panesar M. *Pasteurella multocida* peritonitis with bacteremia on initiation of peritoneal dialysis. Perit Dial Int 2012;32:363-4.
29. Hamai K, Imai H, Ohtani H, et al. Repeated cat-associated peritonitis in a patient on automated noctornal intermittent peritoneal dialysis. Clin Exp Nephrol 1999;1:51-61.
30. Makin AJ, Cartwright KA, Banks RA. Keeping the cat out of the bag: A hazard in continuous ambulatory peritoneal dialysis. BMJ 1991;303:1610-1.
31. Arora P, Vasa P, Brenner D, et al. Prevalence estimates of chronic kidney disease in Canada: Results of a nationally representative survey. CMAJ 2013;185:E417-23.
32. Perrin T. The business of urban animals survey: The facts and statistics on companion animals in Canada. Can Vet J 2009;50:48-52.
33. Donnio P, LeGoff C, Avril J, Pouedras P, Gras-Rouzet S. *Pasteurella multocida*: Oropharyngeal carriage and antibody response in breeders. Vet Res 1994;25:8-15.
34. Li P, Szeto C, Piraino B, et al. Peritoneal dialysis-related infections recommendations: 2010 Update. Perit Dial Int 2010;30:393-423.
35. Stevens D, Higbee J, Oberhoffer T, Everett E. Antibiotics susceptibilities of human isolates of *Pasteurella multocida*. Antimicrob Agents Chemother 1979;16:322-4.

An educational forum to engage infectious diseases and microbiology residents in resource stewardship modelled after the Choosing Wisely campaign

Derek R MacFadden MD[1], Wayne L Gold MD[1], Ibrahim Al-Busaidi MD[1], Jeffrey D Craig MD[1], Dan Petrescu MD[1], Ilana S Saltzman MD[1], Jerome A Leis MD, MSc[1,2]

DR MacFadden, WL Gold, I Al-Busaidi, et al. An educational forum to engage infectious diseases and microbiology residents in resource stewardship modelled after the Choosing Wisely campaign. Can J Infect Dis Med Microbiol 2015;26(5):231-233.

BACKGROUND: Rising costs present a major threat to the sustainability of health care delivery. Resource stewardship is increasingly becoming an expected competency of physicians. The Choosing Wisely framework was used to introduce resource stewardship at a national educational retreat for infectious disease and microbiology residents.

METHODS: During the 2014 Annual Canadian Infectious Disease and Microbiology Resident Retreat in Toronto, Ontario, infectious disease (n=50) and microbiology (n=17) residents representing 11 Canadian universities from six provinces, were invited to participate in a modified Delphi panel. Participants were asked, in advance of the retreat, to submit up to five practices that infectious disease and microbiology specialists should not routinely perform due to lack of proven benefit(s) and/or potential harm to patients. Submissions were discussed in small and large group forums using an iterative approach involving electronic polling until consensus was reached for five practices. A finalized list was created for both educational purposes and for residents to consider enacting; however, it was not intended to replace formal society-endorsed statements. A follow-up survey at two-months was conducted.

RESULTS: Consensus was reached by the residents regarding five low-value practices within the purview of infectious diseases and microbiology physicians. After the retreat, 20 participants (32%) completed the follow-up survey. The majority of respondents (75%) believed that the session was at least as relevant as other sessions they attended at the retreat, including 95% indicating that at least some of the material discussed was new to them. Since returning to their home institutions, nine (45%) respondents have incorporated what they learned into their daily practice; four (20%) reported that they have considered initiating a project related to the session; and one (5%) reported having initiated a project.

CONCLUSIONS: The present educational forum demonstrated that trainees can become actively engaged in the identification and discussion of low-value practices. Embedding residence training programs with resource stewardship education will be necessary to improve the value of care offered by the future members of our profession.

Key Words: *Choosing Wisely; Health care resources; Health care value; Resource stewardship,*

Un forum d'éducation pour que les résidents en infectiologie et en microbiologie s'investissent dans la gestion des ressources conformément à la campagne *Choosing Wisely*

HISTORIQUE : Les coûts croissants représentent une menace importante pour la pérennité des soins de santé. De plus en plus, on s'attend que les médecins aient les compétences nécessaires pour gérer les ressources. Lors d'une journée de réflexion nationale pour les résidents en infectiologie et en microbiologie, la gestion des ressources a été abordée conformément au cadre *Choosing Wisely*.

MÉTHODOLOGIE : Pendant la journée de réflexion canadienne annuelle de 2014 pour les résidents en infectiologie et en microbiologie tenue à Toronto, en Ontario, des résidents en infectiologie (n=50) et en microbiologie (n=17) représentant 11 universités canadiennes réparties dans six provinces ont été invités à participer à un groupe Delphi modifié. Avant la journée de réflexion, ils ont été invités à soumettre jusqu'à cinq pratiques que les spécialistes de l'infectiologie ou de la microbiologie ne devraient pas effectuer systématiquement parce que leurs avantages ne sont pas démontrés ou qu'elles comportent des risques potentiels pour les patients. Ils ont examiné ces pratiques lors de forums en petits et grands groupes selon une méthode itérative par sondage électronique, jusqu'à atteindre un consensus pour cinq pratiques. Une liste définitive a été créée pour des besoins d'éducation et pour que les résidents envisagent de la respecter. Cette liste ne visait toutefois pas à remplacer les documents officiels approuvés par la Société. Un sondage de suivi a été effectué au bout de deux mois.

RÉSULTATS : Les résidents sont parvenus à un consensus sur cinq pratiques de faible valeur qui relèvent des médecins en infectiologie et en microbiologie. Après la journée de réflexion, 20 participants (32 %) ont rempli le sondage de suivi. La majorité d'entre eux (75 %) trouvaient que cette séance était au moins aussi pertinente que les autres séances auxquelles ils avaient assisté pendant la journée de réflexion, et 95 % ont indiqué qu'au moins une partie de ce qui avait été abordé était nouveau pour eux. Depuis leur retour au sein de leur établissement, neuf (45 %) répondants avaient intégré ce qu'ils avaient appris à leur pratique, quatre (20 %) ont déclaré avoir envisagé un projet lié à la séance et un (5 %) a affirmé avoir lancé un projet.

CONCLUSIONS : Le présent forum d'éducation a démontré que les résidents peuvent s'investir pour cerner les pratiques de faible valeur et en discuter. Il faudra intégrer la gérance de l'éducation aux programmes de résidence pour améliorer la valeur des soins offerts par les futurs membres de notre profession.

The rising cost of health care is one of the greatest threats to the sustainability and advancement of medical practice (1). Recognizing that some medical practices lack supporting evidence and may be harmful to patients, the American Board of Internal Medicine launched the Choosing Wisely campaign in 2012, which sought to empower both medical practitioners and patients to make clinical decisions that promote high-value care (2). This initiative has been adopted and adapted throughout the United States and Canada,

[1]*Division of Infectious Diseases, Department of Medicine, University of Toronto;* [2]*Centre for Quality Improvement and Patient Safety, University of Toronto, Toronto, Ontario*

Correspondence: Dr Jerome A Leis, Sunnybrook Health Sciences Centre, Room H463, 2075 Bayview Avenue, Toronto, Ontario M4N 3M5. e-mail jerome.leis@sunnybrook.ca

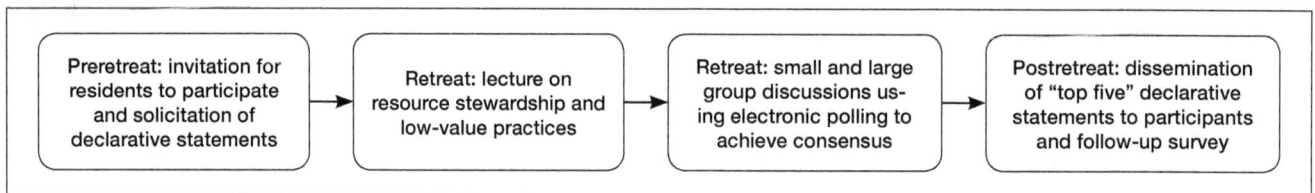

Figure 1) *Flow diagram of the educational formats and process to generate the 'top five' declarative statements*

TABLE 1

"Five things physicians and patients should question" regarding low-value practices in infectious diseases and microbiology as developed by residents in infectious diseases and microbiology

Do not routinely repeat CD4 measurements in patients with HIV infection who are stable on antiretroviral therapy with suppressed viral loads for >2 years.

In prospective trials, among patients who have responded to antiretroviral therapy with HIV-1 RNA below 50 copies/mL and rises in CD4 cell count >200 cells/µL, there was little clinical benefit from continued measurement of CD4 cell count. The 2014 recommendations of the International Antiviral Society – United States Panel state that measurement of CD4 is optional (7).

Do not perform tuberculin skin testing for diagnostic purposes in cases of suspected active tuberculosis in adults.

Tuberculin skin tests in adult patients with suspected active tuberculosis is not recommended by current guidelines because positive results may lead to unnecessary multidrug treatment when they occur in cases of latent tuberculosis, or to erroneous exclusion of tuberculosis in patients with false-negative tests (8).

Do not routinely perform repeat magnetic resonance imaging for uncomplicated bacterial vertebral osteomyelitis following clinical improvement using appropriate antimicrobial therapy.

In patients who are clinically improving, unless a large epidural abscess was present on initial imaging, observational studies suggest that repeat spinal imaging generally does not alter management and may lead to unnecessary prolongation of antimicrobial therapy (9).

Do not routinely prescribe intravenous forms of highly bioavailable antimicrobial agents for patients who can reliably receive and absorb medications via the enteral route.

Among patients who can reliably receive and absorb medications via the enteral route, there is no additional benefit of using intravenous formulations of clindamycin, fluoroquinlones, linezolid, metronidazole, tetracyclines or trimethoprim/sulfamethoxazole (10). Oral administration may permit more timely hospital discharge and reduce the use of intravascular catheters in both inpatient and outpatient settings.

Do not routinely request transesophageal echocardiography in patients with uncomplicated *Staphylococcus aureus* bacteremia.

Transesophageal echocardiography may be safely avoided in patients with *S aureus* bacteremia who lack several infective endocarditis risk factors. These include absence of a permanent intracardiac device, sterile follow-up blood cultures within four days after the initial set, no hemodialysis dependence, nosocomial acquisition of *S aureus* bacteremia, absence of secondary foci of infection and no clinical signs of infective endocarditis (negative predictive value 93% to 100%) (11).

spreading beyond internal medicine to other medical specialties. There are presently >70 societies participating in the United States and at least 30 in Canada (3). These societies have engaged members to create lists of "five things that physicians and patients should question" to begin discussions about ways to improve the value of health care (3).

While physicians must take ownership and achieve competence in the area of resource stewardship, this important aspect of physician competence has not traditionally been incorporated into medical school

curricula and residency training (4). Traditionally, infectious disease specialists and microbiologists have played important roles in infection prevention and control, and antimicrobial stewardship; however, broader training and involvement in resource stewardship has generally been lacking. Extending the scope of infectious diseases and microbiology practice to include resource stewardship should be viewed as being complimentary to these existing roles.

The practice patterns of attending physicians, encountered early by learners, can have a lasting impact on the future practices of trainees (5). We believe that engaging residents in active reflection regarding the consequences of their clinical decisions and actions may have lasting effects on their future patterns of practice (5). Therefore, we sought to engage infectious diseases and microbiology residents from across Canada in developing their own statements, modelled after the Choosing Wisely campaign, to facilitate reflection and education regarding resource stewardship in infectious diseases and microbiology training and, in doing so, demonstrate a method of consensus building through facilitated discussion. It was not our intent to replace a formal Choosing Wisely initiative in infectious diseases and microbiology with official support of societies, but rather to introduce the concept at the trainee level with the hope that they would apply this knowledge to their own practices.

METHODS

During the 2014 Annual Canadian Infectious Diseases and Microbiology Resident Retreat held from August 11 to 14, 2014, in Toronto, Ontario, infectious diseases and microbiology trainees (representing 11 Canadian universities and all six provinces with training programs in infectious diseases and microbiology [British Columbia, Alberta, Manitoba, Ontario, Quebec and Nova Scotia]) who enrolled in the retreat, were asked to participate in a modified Delphi panel (6) modelled after the Choosing Wisely initiative (Figure 1). Participants included 50 residents in infectious diseases (adult infectious diseases [n=35], pediatric infectious diseases [n=15] and microbiology [n=17]). The retreat was an educational forum organized by residents in the Adult Infectious Diseases program at the University of Toronto (Toronto, Ontario), who determined the curriculum and teaching formats for the sessions.

In advance of the retreat, attendees were asked to participate in this session beginning with reflection of both personal practice patterns and those of their attending physicians, to identify unnecessary tests or procedures falling within their own scopes of practice that could be eliminated (3). These practices were defined as those lacking proven benefit or posing potential harm to patients. A brief description of the format of the session was provided, including examples of appropriate and inappropriate submissions in the form of declarative statements (3). An example of an inappropriate recommendation included "do not routinely order urine cultures to assess patients with changes in mental status who do not have signs or symptoms of urinary tract infection", because infectious disease physicians and microbiologists are not typically the individuals who assess these patients and order this test.

Of 67 participants from 11 Canadian universities, 18 (27%) provided submissions in advance of the session. These were formatted into 15 declarative statements by three of the authors (DRM, WLG, JAL) and were accompanied by supporting evidence. The statements were then circulated to all participants before the retreat. The 90 min session included several educational formats. A collaborative approach to this exercise was emphasized. To begin, a lecture introduced the concepts of high- and low-value health care, resource stewardship, the Choosing Wisely campaign and included a review of the list of declarative statements. The overall goal of the session was for the participants to apply the knowledge learned from the large group lecture to finalize a list of statements, which they determined to be actionable and through implementation, may improve the value of care provided. Following the large group lecture, participants were divided into small groups (eight to 10 participants per group); residents in the Adult Infectious Diseases program at the University of Toronto were responsible for facilitating discussions to arrive at consensus within each group regarding their 'top five list', which they presented to the group at large. The rationales for their choices were recorded. All participants were then polled in real-time using interactive polling software (www.polleverywhere.com) and a 'top 10 list' was created. Using a modified Delphi method (6), polling and open discussion continued through three additional rounds, until consensus was reached. This was defined as two consecutive polls without change in rank of the statements. Final statements were formalized and disseminated to all participants to both ensure integrity of the statements, and to encourage engagement of faculty and residents at their own institutions in further discussions. Two months following the retreat, participants were surveyed to obtain quantitative feedback on the impact of this session. Research ethics board approval was obtained.

RESULTS

Participants achieved consensus regarding "five things physicians and patients should question" (3) related to infectious diseases practice (Table 1). Each statement pertains to a test or procedure encountered in infectious diseases or microbiology practice for which there is an evidence base to support reducing or eliminating its use (7-11). Twenty participants (32%) completed the survey. Eighty percent of responders agreed/strongly agreed that an effective presentation style was used (55% somewhat agree; 25% strongly agree). The majority of participants (75%) believed that the session was at least as relevant as other sessions at the retreat (as relevant 55% ; somewhat more relevant 15%; more relevant 5%), with 95% indicating that at least some of the material discussed was new to them (80% somewhat new to respondent; 15% new to respondent). After returning to their home institutions, nine respondents (45%) reported they have incorporated what they learned into their daily practice. Four respondents (20%) reported that they have considered initiating a project related to the session and one respondent (5%) reported having initiated a project.

DISCUSSION

Through this national educational forum, we demonstrated feasibility of introducing the concept of high-value health care delivery into the curriculum of infectious diseases and microbiology trainees, through the generation of individual and peer-developed statements modelled after the Choosing Wisely campaign. The items, identified by the residents, have not been rigorously scrutinized for official endorsement by any professional society, but represent the opinions of infectious diseases and microbiology trainees who have not yet completed their training. With additional years of training and practice, other declarative statements may have been included and some excluded.

However, the primary objective of this session was to facilitate reflection and education regarding resource stewardship at the trainee level. Despite a low response rate to our postretreat survey, we demonstrated that participants who replied are contemplating or have initiated projects related to this project, which was a goal of the session.

We conclude that an interactive, educational forum modelled after the Choosing Wisely campaign was an effective way of introducing the concepts of resource stewardship to subspecialty trainees. Embedding resource stewardship in residency training curricula, as highlighted at our retreat, represents one approach that may improve the value of care offered by the future members of our profession (4).

ACKNOWLEDGEMENTS: The authors acknowledge Dr Wendy Levinson of Choosing Wisely Canada for her review of the manuscript and her advice on this initiative. They thank the participants of the 2014 Canadian Infectious Diseases and Microbiology Resident Retreat for their participation in the conference, and for their thoughtful submissions and discussions relating to resource stewardship in infectious diseases and microbiology.

DISCLOSURES: The authors have no financial relationships or conflicts of interest to declare.

REFERENCES

1. Curfman G, Morrissey S, Drazen J. High-value health care – a sustainable proposition. N Engl JMed 2013 September 17 [Epub ahead of print].
2. Caasel C, Guest J. Choosing Wisely – helping physicians and patients make smart decisions about their care. JAMA 2012;307:1801-2.
3. Levinson W, Huynh T. Engaging physicians and patients in conversations about unnecessary tests and procedures: Choosing Wisely Canada. CMAJ 2014;186:325-6.
4. McMillan J, Ziegelstein R. Implementing a graduate medical education campaign to reduce or eliminate potentially wasteful tests or procedures. JAMA Intern Med 2014;174:1693.
5. Detsky A, Verma A. A new model for medical education: Celebrating restraint. JAMA 2012;308:329-30.
6. Dalkey N, Helmer O. An experimental application of the Delphi method to the use of experts. Manage Sci 1963;9:458-67.
7. Gunthard H, Aberg J, Eron J, et al. Antiretroviral treatment of adult HIV infection: 2014 recommendations of the International Antiviral Society – USA panel. JAMA 2014;312:410-25.
8. Pai M, Minion J, Jamieson F, Wolfe J, Behr M. Diagnosis of active tuberculosis and drug resistance. In: Canadian Tuberculosis Standards, 7th edn. Ottawa: Public Health Agency of Canada 2014:43-61.
9. Zarrouk V, Feydy A, Salles F, et al. Imaging does not predict the clinical outcome of bacterial vertebral osteomyelitis. Rheumatology 2007;46:292-5.
10. Centers for Disease Control. Core Elements of Hospital Antibiotic Stewardship Programs. Atlanta: US Department of Health and Human Services, CDC; 2014. <www.cdc.gov/getsmart/healthcare/pdfs/core-elements.pdf> (Accessed August 29, 2014).
11. Holland TL, Arnold C, Fowler VG Jr. Clinical management of *Staphylococcus aureus* bacteremia: A review. JAMA 2014;312:1330-41.

Staphylococcus pettenkoferi bacteremia: A case report and review of the literature

Abdulaziz Ahmed Hashi MD[1], Johannes Andries Delport MBChB MMed[2],
Sameer Elsayed MD FRCPC FACP[2,3], Michael Seth Silverman MD FRCPC FACP[3]

AA Hashi, JA Delport, S Elsayed, MS Silverman. *Staphylococcus pettenkoferi* bacteremia: A case report and review of the literature. Can J Infect Dis Med Microbiol 2015;26(6):319-322.

Staphylococcus pettenkoferi is a relatively recently described coagulase-negative staphylococci species first described in 2002. Since then, nine additional cases of infection caused by this species have been reported in various countries around the world, including Germany, Belgium, France, South Korea, Italy, Brazil and Mexico. The present report describes a case of S *pettenkoferi* peripheral line-associated bacteremia. To our knowledge, the present report is the first description of human infection caused by S *pettenkoferi* in Canada. The present report also provides an overview of the laboratory detection of uncommon coagulase-negative staphylococci.

Key Words: *Bacteremia; Coagulase negative; MALDI-ToF; Staphylococcus pettenkoferi*

La bactériémie à *Staphylococcus pettenkoferi* : rapport de cas et analyse bibliographique

Le *Staphylococcus pettenkoferi* est une espèce de staphylocoque à coagulase négative qui a été décrit pour la première fois en 2002. Depuis, neuf autres cas d'infections causées par cette espèce ont été signalés dans divers pays du monde, y compris l'Allemagne, la Belgique, la France, la Corée du Sud, l'Italie, le Brésil et le Mexique. Le présent rapport décrit un cas de bactériémie à S *pettenkoferi* associée à un cathéter périphérique. En autant que les auteurs le sachent, il s'agit du premier rapport d'infection humaine à S *pettenkoferi* au Canada, qui donne également un aperçu de la détection en laboratoire de staphylocoques à coagulase négative rares.

CASE PRESENTATION

A 75-year-old woman presented to the emergency department after experiencing an unwitnessed fall at home. She had been experiencing symptoms consistent with vertigo for a few days before presentation. Her medical history was significant for hypertension, type 2 diabetes mellitus, psoriasis, dyslipidemia, a seizure disorder and right knee arthroplasty. Collateral history revealed that she had been assessed one week before for a planned total left knee arthroplasty, which had subsequently been postponed after the patient had been found to have a truncal rash that had been present for two weeks.

Her physical examination was significant for a petechial maculo-papular rash on her chest, arms and legs, as well as a positive Dix-Hallpike test. Vitals signs were within normal parameters and she was afebrile. Initial laboratory investigations (electrolytes, urea, creatinine, glucose) were unremarkable. She had a hemoglobin level of 138 g/L, white blood cell count of 9.0×10^9 cells/L and a platelet count of 176×10^9/L. While in the emergency department, a peripheral intravenous (IV) catheter was placed at the dorsum of her left hand for administration of fluids.

The patient was admitted for further assessment and evaluation. Twelve hours later, she became febrile, but was otherwise asymptomatic. Two blood samples were drawn from separate venipuncture sites and sent for culture. Both sets of blood cultures were positive for Gram-positive cocci in clusters. She was then administered empirical IV vancomycin (1 g every 12 h).

Staphylococcus pettenkoferi was isolated in both blood cultures using a 3 h short-incubation matrix-assisted laser desorption/ionization time-of-flight (MALDI-ToF) identification protocol. It was approximately 36 h from

TABLE 1
Susceptibilities for isolated *Staphylococcus pettenkoferi* performed using AST-GP67 cards on the Vitek 2* system

Drug	S pettenkoferi	
	VMICINT	VMICDIL, mg/L
Clindamycin	Susceptible	≤0.25
Erythromycin	Susceptible	0.5
Oxacillin/cloxacillin	Susceptible	2
Trimethoprim/sulfamethaoxazole	Susceptible	≤10
Vancomycin	Susceptible	1

*BioMerieux, France. VMICDIL Vitek mean inhibitory dilution interpretation; VMICINT Vitek mean inhibitory concentration interpretation

the time of blood culture draws until preliminary results demonstrated coagulase-negative staphylococci, and 51 h for the final culture result of S *pettenkoferi*. The positive blood cultures were subcultured onto a Columbia blood-agar plate (Oxoid, Thermo Fisher Scientific Inc, USA) and incubated at 35°C in 5% CO_2 for 3 h. Identification of the isolates was performed using the Microflex LT with FlexControl version 3.4 software (Bruker Corporation, USA) for the automatic acquisition of mass spectra in the linear positive mode within a range of 2 kDa to 20 kDa. Automated analysis of the raw spectral data was performed using the MALDI BioTyper automation version 3.1 software (Bruker Corporation, USA).

The isolate was identified as S *pettenkoferi* (score 1.904); the top four choices were all strains of S *pettenkoferi*. *Staphylococcus parauberis* (score 1.250) was considered to be the next most likely identification.

[1]*Department of Medicine;* [2]*Department of Pathology and Laboratory Medicine;* [3]*Department of Medicine, Division of Infectious Diseases, The University of Western Ontario, London, Ontario*
Correspondence: Dr Abdulaziz Ahmed Hashi, Department of Medicine, Victoria Hospital, Room E6-117, London, Ontario N6A 5A5. e-mail ahashi2@uwo.ca

TABLE 2
Patient demographics, mode of diagnosis and treatment

Study	Age, years/sex	Comorbidities	Presentation	Culture	Biochemistry/diagnosis	Treatment	Outcome
Trülzsch et al (1), 2002; Germany (strain B3117 [index strain])	25/unknown	Extrapulmonary TB	Fever of unknown origin, weight loss; found to have TB	Blood culture	Biochemistry: API/ID32 Staph* initially suggested *Kocuria rosea* or *Staphylococcus capitis*. Diagnosis: confirmed using 16S rRNA gene sequencing followed by genomic DNA preparation and pulsed-field gel electrophoresis.	Rifampin, pyrazinamide, ethambutol. Specific treatment of *S pettenkoferi* not mentioned.	Successful (recovered)
Loiez et al (3), 2007; France	63/male	Diabetes, chronic diabetic foot infection	Osteomyelitis displayed in x-ray findings following worsening pain, redness and wound exudate	Bone biopsy (4 of 6 specimens produced bacteria)	Biochemistry: API/ID32 Staph initially suggested *K rosea* and *Micrococcus lylae*; a second API/ID32 Staph strip using a larger inoculum and incubation period suggested *S capitis* or *Staphylococcus auricularis*. Diagnosis: confirmed using MicroSeq 500† DNA sequencing of 16S rRNA genes with subsequent homology search on NCBI GenBank compared with entry strain B3117 from 2002.	Transtarsal amputation, then pristinamycin ×14 weeks	Successful (recovered)
Trülzsch et al (2), 2007; Germany (strain K6999)	Unknown	Unknown	Unknown	Blood culture	Biochemistry: API/ID32 Staph initially suggested *S capitis* or *S auricularis*. Diagnosis: confirmed using 16S rRNA gene sequencing (one base pair difference), partial *rpoB* gene sequencing (99.8% similarity), 100% DNA–DNA hybridization and RiboPrint‡ analysis (nearly identical) compared with strain B3117 from 2002.	Unknown	Unknown
Trülzsch et al (2), 2007; Belgium (isolate 229)	Unknown	Unknown	Unknown	Blood culture	Biochemistry: API/ID32 Staph initially suggested *S capitis* or *S auricularis*. Diagnosis: Confirmed using 16S rRNA gene sequencing (identical), partial *rpoB* gene sequencing (99.8% similarity) and RiboPrint analysis (nearly identical) compared with strain B3117 from 2002.	Unknown	Unknown
Trülzsch et al (2), 2007; Belgium (isolate 230)	Unknown	Unknown	Unknown	Blood culture	Biochemistry: API/ID32 Staph initially suggested *S capitis* or *S auricularis*. Diagnosis: confirmed using 16S rRNA gene sequencing (identical), partial *rpoB* gene sequencing (99.8% similarity) and RiboPrint analysis (nearly identical) compared with strain B3117 from 2002.	Unknown	Unknown
Song et al (4), 2009; South Korea	76/male	Recurrent pulmonary TB	Admitted for recurrent pulmonary TB. Developed Stevens-Johnson syndrome. Became febrile while being treated for both; found to have bloodstream infection	Blood cultures from different lumens of a central line	Biochemistry: MicroScan WalkAway Pos Combo Panel§ suggested *Staphylococcus hominis* (92%) or *S auricularis* (99%); VITEK 2 Gram Positive Identification system suggested *S auricularis* (70%), *S capitis* (50%), or *Staphylococcus wrneri* (50%); API/ID32 Staph V4 1 Kit suggested *S capitis* (61.5%) or *Kocuria varians/K rosea* (27.8%). Gene sequencing: gene sequencing of 16S rRNA using the MicroSeq Microbial Identification System¶ and a consensus sequence of 495 base pairs suggested *Staphylococcus caprae* (99.36%), *Staphylococcus hyicus* (96.94%), or *Staphylococcus cohnii* (97.08%). Diagnosis: using a larger sequence of 1533 base pairs and sending the data to GenBank suggested *S pettenkoferi*. Phylogenetic tree confirmed isolate to be most consistent with *S pettenkoferi*.	Vancomycin 2 g IV every 24 h ×1 week	Successful (negative blood cultures; patient then treated for TB)
d'Azevedo et al (5), 2010; Brazil	56/unknown	Unknown	Unknown	Blood cultures	Biochemistry: VITEK 2* identification system suggested *K varians*. Diagnosis: confirmed using DNA sequencing of 16S rRNA and *sodA* genes with subsequent homology search on GenBank matching *S pettenkoferi*.	Unknown	Unknown

Continued on next page

TABLE 2 – CONTINUED

Study	Age, sex	Comorbidities	Presentation	Culture	Biochemistry/diagnosis	Treatment	Outcome
Mammina et al (6), 2011; Italy	49/male	Post-traumatic hydrocephalus	Surgical treatment of hydrocephalus. Underwent placement of ventriculo-peritoneal drain, replaced by external ventricular drain 10 days later due to occlusion of internal device. External drain became infected. Treated, but developed shock 10 days later	Blood cultures (source of sepsis suspected of being bloodstream)	Biochemistry: VITEK 2 suggested S capitis; API/ID32 Staph suggested S capitis. Diagnosis: confirmed using DNA sequencing of 16S rRNA genes with homology search on GenBank (100% similarity to strains B3117 and A6664).	Daptocycin 8 mg/kg and Pip-Tazo 4.5 g × 4 doses, then daptomycin alone	Unsuccessful (died)
Morfin-Otero, et al (7), 2012; Mexico	Newborn/male	Premature (33 weeks)	Fever	Blood cultures (1 of 3)	Biochemistry: API/ID 32 Staph suggested K varians; Sensititre did not identify isolate. Diagnosis: confirmed using DNA sequencing of 16S rRNA, sodA and tuf genes with subsequent homology search on GenBank matching S pettenkoferi.	Ampicillin ×4 days, amikacin ×4 days, then ampicillin ×10 days	Successful (recovered)
Morfin-Otero, et al (7), 2012; Mexico	45/male	AIDS, herpes zoster, hepatitis C	Cerebral toxoplasmosis	Blood cultures (2 of 2)	Biochemistry: API/ID32 Staph suggested K varians; Sensititre suggested Staphylococcus cohnii epidermidis. Diagnosis: confirmed using DNA sequencing of 16S rRNA, sodA and tuf genes with subsequent homology search on GenBank matching S pettenkoferi.	Clindamycin ×8 days, trimethoprim/ sulfamethoxazole ×8 days, azithromycin ×8 days, amphotericin B ×8 days	Unsuccessful (died)

*BioMerieux, France; †Applied Biosystems, USA; ‡DuPont, USA; §Beckman Coulter, USA; ¶Life Technologies, USA. IV Intravenous; NCBI National Center for Biotechnology Information; rRNA Ribosomal RNA; TB Tuberculosis

A score >1.700 and a differential spread of 0.654 (being greater than the recommended 0.200 spread) helped secure the identification of this organism to genus and species.

The isolate was catalase positive, with a Gram-stain consistent with a Staphylococcus species, differentiating it from the next available genus identification of Streptococcus. As part of the routine processing of positive blood cultures with Gram stain suggestive of staphylococci species, polymerase chain reaction was performed for detection of methicillin resistance and to differentiate the strain from Staphylococcus aureus. Neither the nuc nor mecA genes were detected, therefore, confirming that this was a coagulase-negative methicillin-susceptible staphylococcal strain.

Susceptibility testing was performed using AST-GP67 cards on the Vitek 2 (BioMerieux, France) microbial identification system. The isolate had a minimum inhibitory concentration of 2 mg/L for oxacillin indicating that it was susceptible. Susceptibilities are listed in Table 1.

The patient developed erythema and mild tenderness at the site of her peripheral intravenous catheter, and was diagnosed with catheter-associated bacteremia. The IV catheter was removed and her antibiotic therapy was changed to 2 g IV cloxacillin every 6 h, after having received two days of IV vancomycin. A transthoracic echocardiogram demonstrated no evidence of valvular heart disease or vegetations. Consideration was initially given to conducting a skin biopsy to better delineate the cause of the patient's rash; however, the rash resolved spontaneously. Her vertigo improved with the use of particle repositioning manoeuvres. The patient was given a prescription to complete a seven-day course of 500 mg oral cloxacillin every 6 h for six days because she had completed one day of IV cloxacillin in hospital. She was then discharged home. Repeat blood cultures taken five days after completion of antibiotic therapy were negative.

DISCUSSION

S pettenkoferi is a coagulase-negative Staphylococcus. S pettenkoferi was first described by Trülzsch et al (1) in 2002. While the authors initially reported two cases of infection with this organism (strains B3117 and A6664), subsequent investigations revealed that only one of the isolates (B3117) was S pettenkoferi (2); that strain was recovered from a blood culture sample in a patient with extra pulmonary tuberculosis. Since then, nine cases have been documented in the literature (Table 2). Trülzsch et al (2) described three more isolates of S pettenkoferi in Germany and Belgium (strain K699, isolate 229 and isolate 230) all from blood cultures, and all displaying 100% DNA-DNA homology with strain B3117 from their 2002 study. Also in 2007, the first case of S pettenkoferi osteomyelitis was described by Loïez et al (3) in France in a 63-year old diabetic man using bone biopsy cultures. Song et al (4) described the first case of S pettenkoferi in Asia in 2008 from central line blood cultures in a 76-year old man in South Korea with tuberculosis and Stevens-Johnson syndrome who developed bacteremia. The first South American case of S pettenkoferi was described by d'Azevedo et al (5) using blood cultures from a patient in Brazil. Other cases have also been reported including one case in Italy (6) using blood cultures and two cases in Mexico (an adult with HIV and a premature infant) using blood cultures, which were the first reported cases in North America (7).

To our knowledge, this is the first case of *S pettenkoferi* reported in Canada. While our patient did have a history of a maculopapular rash, the rash was deemed unlikely to be related to her infection, particularly because it preceded her IV catheter insertion. We were unable to perform convalescent serology for infectious causes of rash because the patient was subsequently lost to follow-up.

It is known that coagulase-negative staphylococci are associated with infections of indwelling and implanted devices (8). This is possibly consistent with the present patient's presentation, although a peripheral IV site was believed to be involved in her case. With regard to antibiotic choice, different agents have been used (see Table 2). To the best of our knowledge, our patient was the first to be treated successfully with cloxacillin, albeit having previously received a short course of vancomycin (Table 1).

We suspect that *S pettenkoferi* is significantly more commonly encountered than the above reports would suggest. Laboratory identification can be challenging because biochemical tests may result in misidentification of *S pettenkoferi* as *Staphylococcus hominis*, *Staphylococcus auricularis*, *Staphylococcus capitis* and *Kocuria varians* (Table 2). In several situations, the correct identity of the bacterium was not made until molecular tests, such as 16S ribosomal RNA (rRNA) gene sequencing were performed. Notwithstanding, while genetic sequencing of 16S rRNA has been the most commonly used method to confirm the diagnosis of *S pettenkoferi*, strain A6664, one of the two originally described *S pettenkoferi* isolates, has a slightly different *rpoB* gene sequence and does not have 100% DNA-DNA homology with the other strains described in 2007 by Trülzsch et al (2) compared to strain B31117. This suggests that it is a different species altogether and, therefore, 16S rRNA gene sequencing may not be sufficiently robust to definitively diagnose the presence of *S pettenkoferi*.

A limitation of our study is the lack of sequencing data because the isolate is no longer available. Nevertheless, we believe that in the present case the species diagnosis is confirmed. Our laboratory uses MALDI-ToF mass spectrometry. MALDI-ToF has been used to correctly identify other coagulase-negative staphylococci that have been under-reported in the past, such as *Staphylococcus lugdunensis* (9). The use of MALDI-ToF may result in increased reports of *S pettenkoferi* infection. In studies performed at our institution, the Bruker MALDI-ToF correctly identified 485 of 485 coagulase-negative staphylococci to the species level. Included in these were 117 isolates of *S capitis* and *S hominis* species that were all identified correctly by the MALDI-ToF with none being identified as *S pettenkoferi* (10,11).

DISCLOSURES: The authors have no financial relationships or conflicts of interest to declare.

REFERENCES

1. Trülzsch K, Rinder H, Trcek J, et al. 'Staphylococcus pettenkoferi', a novel staphylococcal species isolated from clinical specimens. Diagn Microbiol Infect Dis 2002;43:175-82.
2. Trülzsch K, Grabein B, Schumann P, et al. *Staphylococcus pettenkoferi* sp. nov., a novel coagulase-negative staphylococcal species isolated from human clinical specimens. Int J Syst Evol Microbiol 2007;57:1543-8.
3. Loïez C, Wallet F, Pischedda P, et al. First case of osteomyelitis caused by 'Staphylococcus pettenkoferi'. J Clinical Microbiol 2007;45:1069-71.
4. Song SH, Park JS, Kwon HR, et al. Human bloodstream infection caused by *Staphylococcus pettenkoferi*. J Med Microbiol 2009;58:270-2.
5. d'Azevedo PA, Comin G, Cantarelli V. Characterization of a new coagulase-negative *Staphylococcus* species (*Staphylococcus pettenkoferi*) isolated from blood cultures from a hospitalized patient in Porto Alegre, Brazil. Rev Soc Bras Med Trop 2010;43:331-2.
6. Mammina C, Bonura C, Verde MS, et al. A fatal bloodstream infection by *Staphylococcus pettenkoferi* in an intensive care unit patient. Case Rep Crit Care 2011;2011:612732.
7. Morfin-Otero R, Martínez-Vasquez MA, López D, et al. Isolation of rare coagulase-negative isolates in immunocompromised patients: *Staphylococcus gallinarum*, *Staphylococcus pettenkoferi*, and *Staphylococcus pasteuri*. Ann Clin Lab Sci 2012;42:182-5.
8. Huebner J, Goldmann DA. Coagulase-negative *Staphylococci*: Role as pathogens. Annu Rev Med 1999;50:223-36.
9. Szabados F, Anders A, Kaase M, et al. Late periprosthetic joint infection due to *Staphylococcus lugdunensis* identified by matrix-assisted laser desorption/ionisation time of fight mass spectrometry: A case report and review of the literature. Case Rep Med 2011;2011:1-4.
10. Delport J, Peters G, John M, et al. Coagulase-negative *Staphylococci*: Comparing MALDI-TOF to VITEK 2 and MIDI gas liquid chromatography. 2013 June 28th International Congress of Chemotherapy and Infections, Yokohama, Japan. June 5 to 8, 2013.
11. Delport J, Peters G, John M, et al. Bruker MALDI-TOF: Identification of coagulase negative staphylococci. 2013 October ID Week 2013, San Francisco, California, USA. October 2 to 6, 2013.

39

Cost effectiveness of 'on demand' HIV pre-exposure prophylaxis for non-injection drug-using men who have sex with men in Canada

Estelle Ouellet MPA MD(c), Madeleine Durand MD MSc FRCPC, Jason R Guertin MSc PhD(c),
Jacques LeLorier MD PhD FRCPC FISPE, Cécile L Tremblay MD FRCPC

E Ouellet, M Durand, JR Guertin, J LeLorier, CL Tremblay. Cost-effectiveness of 'on demand' HIV pre-exposure prophylaxis for non-injection drug-using men who have sex with men in Canada. Can J Infect Dis Med Microbiol 2015;26(1):23-29.

BACKGROUND: Recent trials report the efficacy of continuous tenofovir-based pre-exposure prophylaxis (PrEP) for prevention of HIV infection. The cost effectiveness of 'on demand' PrEP for non-injection drug-using men who have sex with men at high risk of HIV acquisition has not been evaluated.

OBJECTIVE: To conduct an economic evaluation of the societal costs of HIV in Canada and evaluate the potential benefits of this PrEP strategy.

METHODS: Direct HIV costs comprised outpatient, inpatient and emergency department costs, psychosocial costs and antiretroviral costs. Resource consumption estimates were derived from the *Centre Hospitalier de l'Université de Montréal* HIV cohort. Estimates of indirect costs included employment rate and work absenteeism. Costs for 'on demand' PrEP were modelled after an ongoing clinical trial. Cost-effectiveness analysis compared costs of 'on demand' PrEP to prevent one infection with lifetime costs of one HIV infection. Benefits were presented in terms of life-years and quality-adjusted life-years.

RESULTS: The average annual direct cost of one HIV infection was $16,109 in the least expensive antiretroviral regimen scenario and $24,056 in the most expensive scenario. The total indirect cost was $11,550 per year. Total costs for the first year of HIV infection ranged from $27,410 to $35,358. Undiscounted lifetime costs ranged from $1,439,984 ($662,295 discounted at 3% and $448,901 at 5%) to $1,482,502 ($690,075 at 3% and $485,806 at 5%). The annual cost of PrEP was $12,001 per participant, and $621,390 per infection prevented. The PrEP strategy was cost-saving in all scenarios for undiscounted and 3% discounting rates. At 5% discounting rates, the strategy is largely cost-effective: according to least and most expensive scenarios, incremental cost-effectiveness ratios ranged from $60,311 to $47,407 per quality-adjusted life-year.

CONCLUSION: This 'on demand' PrEP strategy ranges from cost-saving to largely cost-effective. The authors believe it represents an important public health strategy for the prevention of HIV transmission.

Key Words: *Cost effectiveness; HIV; Prophylaxis*

La rentabilité de la prophylaxie préexposition du VIH sur demande au Canada pour les hommes qui ne consomment pas de drogues injectables, mais qui ont des relations sexuelles avec d'autres hommes

HISTORIQUE : De récents essais rendent compte de l'efficacité d'une prophylaxie préexposition continue à base de ténofovir (PrEP) pour prévenir l'infection par le VIH. La rentabilité de la PrEP sur demande n'a pas été évaluée chez les hommes qui ne consomment pas de drogues injectables, mais qui ont des relations sexuelles avec d'autres hommes très susceptibles de contracter le VIH.

OBJECTIF : Réaliser une évaluation économique des coûts du VIH pour la société au Canada et évaluer les avantages potentiels de cette stratégie de PrEP.

MÉTHODOLOGIE : Les coûts directs du VIH incluaient les coûts des rendez-vous ambulatoires, des séjours hospitaliers et des visites à l'urgence, les coûts psychosociaux et les coûts des antirétroviraux. L'évaluation de la consommation des ressources était dérivée de la cohorte de VIH du Centre hospitalier de l'Université de Montréal. Les évaluations des coûts indirects incluaient le taux d'emploi et l'absentéisme au travail. Les coûts de la PrEP sur demande reprenaient le modèle d'un essai clinique en cours. L'analyse de rentabilité reposait sur une comparaison des coûts de la PrEP sur demande pour prévenir une infection avec les coûts de traitement à vie d'une infection par le VIH. Les avantages étaient présentés d'après les années de vie et les années de vie pondérées par la qualité.

RÉSULTATS : Le coût direct annuel moyen d'une infection par le VIH s'élevait à 16 109 $ d'après le scénario de posologie antirétrovirale le moins coûteux, et à 24 056 $ d'après le scénario le plus coûteux. Le coût indirect total s'élevait à 11 550 $ par année. Les coûts totaux pour la première année d'infection par le VIH oscillaient entre 27 410 $ et 35 358 $. Les coûts de traitement à vie non actualisés variaient entre 1 439 984 $ (662 295 $ actualisés à 3 % et 448 901 $, à 5 %) et 1 482 502 $ (690 075 $ à 3 % et 485 806 $ à 5 %). Le coût annuel de la PrEP était de 12 001 $ par participant, et de 621 390 $ par infection prévenue. La stratégie de PrEP était économique dans tous les scénarios non actualisés et actualisés à 3 %. Dans les scénarios actualisés à 5 %, la stratégie était largement rentable. En effet, selon les scénarios le moins et le plus coûteux, le rapport coût-efficacité différentiel se situait entre 60 311 $ et 47 407 $ par année de vie pondérée par la qualité.

CONCLUSION : Cette stratégie de PrEP sur demande se situe quelque part entre la production d'économies et une rentabilité substantielle. Les auteurs sont d'avis qu'elle représente une importante stratégie de santé publique pour prévenir la transmission du VIH.

Although there has been a decrease in new HIV infections worldwide, increases in new HIV infections among non-injection drug-using (IDU) men who have sex with men (MSM) are concerning (1), and show the limitations of our current prevention strategies. In Canada, the proportion of new HIV infections among MSM in 2011 was higher than in 2008. Of the 73,000 individuals living with HIV

Centre de Recherche du Centre Hospitalier de l'Université de Montréal, Montréal, Québec
Correspondence and reprints: Dr Cécile Tremblay, Laboratoire de santé publique du Québec, Institut national de santé publique du Québec, 20045 chemin Sainte-Marie, Sainte-Anne-de-Bellevue, Quebec H9X 3R5. e-mail c.tremblay@umontreal.ca

in Canada, almost one-half (46.7%) are MSM (2). Continuous pre-exposure prophylaxis (PrEP) is a promising approach for the prevention of HIV infection in combination with other prevention strategies. Recent clinical trials have shown that such PrEP, administered continuously on a daily basis, can reduce the risk of infection, although results vary according to the patient population studied and adherence to treatment (3-7).

In an effort to improve PrEP efficacy (treatment adherence and limit exposure to drugs), researchers have developed PrEP strategies other than administering them on a daily basis. One of these strategies is 'on demand' PrEP administration. An *Agence Nationale de Recherche sur le SIDA*-sponsored, randomized, double-blinded, placebo-controlled PrEP clinical trial that targets non-IDU MSM at high risk for HIV acquisition evaluated this strategy (8). The 'on demand' protocol entails taking the drug 24 h before the first sexual encounter, every 24 h during the sexual activity and 24 h after the last sexual encounter. It may require more planning than administration on a daily basis, but could lead to inferior drug consumption per month depending on the level of sexual activity of the participant. This drug-based intervention, referred to as *Intervention Préventive de l'Exposition aux Risques avec et pour les hommes Gays* (IPERGAY), is accompanied by intense counselling on safe sex as well as condom distribution. IPERGAY is the first trial aiming to establish the efficacy of 'on demand' PrEP. While the clinical trial is underway both in France and in Canada, our objective is to provide an economic evaluation from a societal perspective of costs of HIV in Canada because health care costs vary according to jurisdictions, and to evaluate the potential benefits of this 'on demand' PrEP strategy (if it is effective).

METHODS

Microcosting methods similar to those used in other HIV prevention studies (9,10) were applied. All costs are reported in 2012 Canadian dollars (USD$0.98, €0.77). The cost of preventing one infection was compared with the lifetime cost of one HIV infection. This approach is recommended by the Centers for Disease Control and Prevention (CDC; Georgia, USA): "The lifetime treatment cost of an HIV infection can be used as a conservative threshold value for the cost of averting one infection" (11).

Costs of HIV infection

To model the costs of HIV infections, an inventory of all health care inputs consumed during the course of HIV disease was created. The *Centre Hospitalier de l'Université de Montréal* (CHUM) HIV cohort database was used, for which administrative as well as clinical data are collected on all individuals on a per-visit basis. These patients were treated according to Quebec guidelines (12). Data from all HIV-infected homosexual male non-IDUs were included in the present study because high-risk non-IDU MSM is the population targeted by the 'on demand' PrEP intervention of interest.

Direct medical costs: Direct HIV patient care costs comprised five broad categories: outpatient care, inpatient care, emergency department care, psychosocial care and antiretroviral therapy (ART). For outpatient care, subcategories included personnel costs, laboratory testing and overhead costs. For personnel costs, time spent and wages for nursing services were included (13), as well as fee-for-service billing from doctors (14). During the first visit, laboratory testing included complete blood count, CD4 count, viral load, viral genotyping, HLA-B5701 genotype, lipid profile, kidney and liver function tests, urine test, blood glucose test, sexually transmitted disease (syphilis, chlamydia, gonorrhoea) tests, hepatitis, varicella and toxoplasmosis serology, as well as tuberculosis testing (15). Follow-up visits included complete blood count, CD4 count, kidney and liver function tests, and viral load. For the inpatient and emergency department categories, average physician fee-for-service (14) and operating cost were included (16). For the psychosocial care, the hourly wages of social workers and psychologists were included (16). For ART, drug costs and pharmacist dispensing fees were included (17).

Primary data on the number and type of resources consumed were collected from the CHUM database (722 patients). Resource utilization was first measured by calculating the annual average visits (or hospitalization days) per patient. This resource utilization indicator was multiplied by unit costs to obtain the total annual average resource costs per patient. This procedure was performed for the first four direct HIV patient care costs categories. For ART, the costs of antiretrovirals and pharmacist dispensing fee were summed. The total cost was presented as the average annual cost of ART per patient. The costs of different therapy lines was taken into consideration in the cost-effectiveness analysis. From a drug-acquisition perspective, the least expensive scenario was established with Atripla™ (Gilead Sciences Inc, USA) (the least expensive first-line therapy) and the most expensive scenario with the combination of Prezista™ (Janssen Therapeutics, USA), Norvir™ (Abbvie Inc, USA) and Truvada™ (Gilead Sciences Inc, USA) (the most expensive first-line therapy). Due to suggestions in recent literature, it was assumed that after one year of ART, the efficiency of a first-line regimen is compromised due to nonadherence and the development of drug resistance (18). Therefore, the introduction of second-line therapy (Isentress™ (Merck & Co, Inc, USA), Intelence™ (Janssen Therapeutics, USA), Norvir and Prezista) was initiated at year 1 after diagnosis. At year 1, 20% of patients failed the first-line regimen; at year 2, 25% cessed first-line; and starting at year 3, incremental declines of 10% per year were estimated until year 10, when 100% of patients had made the switch to second-line therapy.

Indirect costs: Indirect HIV infection costs comprised two categories: lost revenue due to employment rate gap; and work absenteeism.

The gap in employment rate was estimated by using the difference in employment rate between the general male population in Quebec (19) and the HIV-positive homosexual male population in Ontario (A Burchell, personal communication, April 30, 2013). This was believed to be a good approximation of the gap between the male homosexual and HIV-positive male homosexual population because the literature indicates that there is no difference in the employment rate in Canada between the general male population and the homosexual male population (20). Ontario data for employment rate (21) were used because the employment rate for HIV-positive homosexual males in Quebec was unavailable. The employment rate has been systematically lower in Quebec than in Ontario since 1976 (except for the 15- to 24-year-old age group, but this comprises only 7% of the HIV-positive population in Quebec) (21,22). Thus, using the Ontario data gives a conservative estimate of productivity losses in Quebec. To calculate lost revenue, the age structure for both employment rate and wages (Quebec data) were taken into consideration (19).

In terms of work absenteeism, it was assumed that each outpatient/psychosocial visit necessitates 4 h and inpatient/emergency care visit leads to 8 h of missed work per day. The annual average hours of missed work per patient in the CHUM cohort was multiplied by the average hourly wage for three age groups (15 to 24 years, 25 to 54 years and ≥55 years) (23).

Costs of the intervention: 'on demand' PrEP

To model the costs of 'on demand' PrEP, the intervention proposed in the IPERGAY clinical trial protocol was used (8).

Direct costs: The costs of IPERGAY PrEP strategy includes six outpatient visits per year, including nursing costs, laboratory testing and overhead costs, as described above. The annual cost of Truvada (17), the prophylactic drug provided, was added to the total costs, as well as the cost of condoms supplied at each visit. The most expensive scenario of the 'on demand' Truvada was used in the present analysis. This scenario entails a level of sexual activity that requires drug administration on a daily basis.

Indirect costs: For the indirect costs, it was estimated that 4 h of work would be missed for each outpatient visit. These 24 h of work missed per year were then multiplied by the average hourly wage (23) weighted by the age distribution of male workers and their employment rate (19) to obtain the average annual indirect cost per patient for participating to the 'on demand' PrEP intervention.

TABLE 1
Annual cost of HIV infection per patient (2012 $)

Direct cost	Average annual costs per patient*	Reference
Outpatient: first visit	$683	MSSS (16)
Outpatient: follow-up	$272	MSSS (16)
Outpatient total	$934	MSSS (16)
Emergency department visits	$116	MSSS (16), CHUM database
Social worker	$14	MSSS (16), CHUM database
Psychologist	$39	MSSS (16), CHUM database
HIV medication (least/most expensive)	$14,093/$22,040	RAMQ (17)
Hospitalization	$913	MSSS (16),CHUM database
Total direct cost (least/most expensive)	$16,109/$24,056	
Indirect cost	**Average annual costs per patient†**	**Reference**
Average annual salary losses due to unemployement, weighted according to age distribution	$10,925	A Burchell (personal communication, April 30, 2013), INSPQ (22), CANSIM (23)
Average annual productivity cost due to medical follow-up, weighted according to age distribution	$625	CANSIM (19), INSPQ (22)
Total indirect costs	$11,550	
Total costs (least/most expensive)	$27,659/$35,606	

*Calculated by multiplying the average annual visits distributed on sample by unit cost. See Supplementary Tables 1 and 3 for more details; †See Supplementary Tables 2, 3 and 5 for more details. MSSS Ministère de la santé et services sociaux du Québec; RAMQ Régie de l'assurance maladie du Québec; INSPQ Institut national de santé publique du Québec; CANSIM Statistics Canada socioeconomic database

Cost to prevent one infection

The cost of preventing one infection reflects the annual average cost of the 'on demand' PrEP intervention required to avert one infection. This annual average cost is proportional to the number of participants of the 'on demand' PrEP intervention needed to prevent one infection. To estimate this number of participants, it was hypothesized that the number needed to treat (NNT) derived from the clinical trial conducted by Grant et al (4) would be equivalent to the NNT in the IPERGAY trial. The Grant et al (4) clinical trial tested continuous Truvada PrEP for high-risk homosexual males. It was anticipated that PrEP efficacy would be improved by increasing treatment adherence and limiting exposure to drugs with the 'on demand' PrEP strategy. In this context, it was believed to be appropriate to assume a NNT equivalent to, if not lower than the one derived from the Grant et al (4) trial. This NNT of 51.78 was based on the event rate of the control group (5%) and of the PrEP group (3%), and was adjusted for the length of the Grant et al (4) clinical trial (1.2 years). The cost of preventing one infection is obtained by multiplying the annual cost per participant of the 'on demand' PrEP intervention by the NNT.

Cost-effectiveness analysis

The cost-effectiveness analysis guidelines suggested by the CDC (11) were followed to provide an economic understanding of the societal costs of HIV in Canada and the potential benefits of this 'on demand' PrEP strategy. The annual cost of the 'on demand' PrEP intervention to prevent one infection was first compared (using the NNT) with the total cost of an HIV infection. The total cost of HIV infection was the annual societal cost of an HIV infection multiplied by the life expectancy of HIV-positive individuals diagnosed at 30 years of age. Thirty years of age is the median age group with the highest rates of new diagnosis in the past five years in Quebec (22). Life expectancy for an individual diagnosed at this age is 35.2 years, according to a collaborative analysis of 14 cohort studies (24).

The benefits were also presented in terms of life-years and quality-adjusted life years (QALY). Using the concept of utilities, life-years were adjusted to the asymptomatic HIV health state. A meta-analysis by Tengs and Lin (25) indicates that one year of life for an asymptomatic HIV patient is equivalent to 0.94 of one year of life for a healthy individual. The lifetime societal cost of an HIV infection and benefits (life-years and QALY) was presented as undiscounted, and discounted at 3% and 5%, in accordance with the Canadian guidelines for the

TABLE 2
Annual costs of 'on demand' PrEP strategy per participant (2012 $)

	Cost	Reference
Outpatient visits	$2,041*	MSSS (16)
Medication (tenofovir/ emtricitabine)	$9,505*	RAMQ (17)
Condoms	$48	
Work absenteeism	$408†	CANSIM (19)‡, INSPQ (22)
Costs per participant	$12,001	
Costs per infection prevented	$621,390	Grant et al (4)

*See Supplementary Table 1 for more details; †See Supplementary Table 4 for more details; ‡Statistics Canada socioeconomic database; INSPQ Institut national de santé publique du Québec; MSSS Ministère de la santé et services sociaux du Québec; RAMQ Régie de l'assurance maladie du Québec

economic evaluation of health interventions (26). Because all costs incurred with the 'on demand' PrEP intervention are limited to the first year of follow-up, no discounting is required. As such, both discounted and undiscounted amounts will remain the same.

RESULTS

Direct and indirect costs of an HIV infection

Table 1 presents the annual cost of an HIV infection. The average annual direct cost of an HIV infection was $16,109 in the least expensive scenario and $24,056 in the most expensive scenario (most expensive first-line ART). The total indirect cost was $11,550. The average annual salary loss due to unemployment, weighted by age distribution, was $10,925, representing 95% of the indirect cost of an HIV infection. Indirect costs calculation details are presented in the supplementary data. In the least expensive scenario, the total cost for the first year of HIV infection was $27,659. In the most expensive scenario, the cost was $35,606. With the second-line therapy introduced fully at year 10 of infection, the cost of HIV infection increased to $42,197.

When multiplied by life expectancy at 30 years of age, the least expensive scenario with undiscounted lifetime costs was $1,439,984 ($662,295 discounted at 3% and $448,901 at 5%), and the most expensive scenario with undiscounted lifetime costs was $1,482,502 ($690,075 at 3% and $485,806 at 5%).

TABLE 3
Cost-effectiveness analysis for prevention of an infection acquired at 30 years of age (2012 $)

Costs	Undiscounted lifetime		Discounted at 3%		Discounted at 5%		Reference
	Least expensive	Most expensive	Least expensive	Most expensive	Least expensive	Most expensive	
PrEP-related strategy	$621,390	$621,390	$621,390	$621,390	$621,390	$621,390	See Table 2
HIV infection*	$1,439,984	$1,482,502	$662,295	$690,075	$448,901	$485,806	Collaboration (24)
Incremental cost†	−$818,594	−$861,112	−$40,905	−$68,684	$172,489	$135,584	
Benefits, life-years	Undiscounted lifetime		Discounted at 3%		Discounted at 5%		Reference
PrEP-strategy	50.08		25.73		18.26		CHMD (52)
HIV infection	35.20		21.49		16.37		Collaboration (24)
Incremental benefits	14.88		4.24		1.88		
Benefits (QALY)	Undiscounted lifetime		Discounted at 3%		Discounted at 5%		Reference
PrEP-strategy	50.08		25.73		18.26		CHMD (52)
Asymptomatic HIV infection (0.94 QALY)	33.09		20.21		15.39		Teng (25), Collaboration (24)
Incremental benefits	16.99		5.53		2.86		
Incremental cost-effectiveness ratio	Cost-saving	Cost-saving	Cost-saving	Cost-saving	$60,223	$47,338	

Total costs from Table 1 are multiplied by four years (estimated length of first-line therapy). Cost of second-line therapy is multiplied by life expectancy at 30 years of age, minus four years (31.2 years). The sum of the results is calculated. Costs and years are discounted as appropriate; †Calculated by substracting cost of HIV infection to cost of pre-exposure prophylaxis (PrEP)-related strategy. CHMD Canadian Human Mortality Database; QALY Quality-adjusted life-years

Cost of 'on demand' PrEP intervention

As shown in Table 2, the annual cost of 'on demand' PrEP intervention as defined in the IPERGAY clinical trial was $12,001 per participant, and $621,390 per infection prevented.

Cost-effectiveness analysis

Table 3 presents the results of the cost-effectiveness analysis of the least and most expensive costing scenarios. At $621,390, the cost per infection prevented was lower than the undiscounted lifetime costs of an HIV infection by −$818,594 (−$40,905 at 3% and +$172,489 at 5%) in the least expensive scenario. In the most expensive scenario, the cost per infection prevented was lower than the undiscounted lifetime costs of an HIV infection by −$861,112 (−$68,684 at 3% and +$135,584 at 5%). The undiscounted benefits of preventing an infection were of almost 15 life-years gained (4.24 at 3% and 1.88 at 5%). When adjusted for the quality of life, the undiscounted benefits of preventing an infection were of almost 17 QALY (5.53 at 3% and 2.86 at 5%). The IPERGAY strategy was cost-saving in all scenarios, except when discounted at 5%, when the incremental cost effectiveness ratio was $60,223 and $47,338 per QALY in the least and most expensive scenarios, respectively.

Sensitivity analysis

The analysis of the efficiency of a first-line regimen was also performed based on a different assumption. Second-line therapy for 100% of patients was introduced at year 4 after diagnosis. The number derived from this assumption lead to results similar to those presented in Table 3. At $621,390, the cost per infection prevented was lower than the undiscounted lifetime costs of an HIV infection by −$406,977 (−$20,575 at 3% and +$193,231 at 5%) in the least expensive scenario. In the most expensive scenario, the cost per infection prevented was lower than the undiscounted lifetime costs of an HIV infection by −$438,766 (−$51,001 at 3% and +$163,641 at 5%).

Table 3 presents the cost-effectiveness analysis of infections prevented at 30 years of age. Analysis of infections prevented at 20 and 40 years of age was also performed. The rate of new diagnosis among the 15 to 24 years of age group is significantly higher than the rate among the 35 to 44 years of age group. However, the latter age group has historically had the highest new diagnosis rate (22). Life expectancy for individuals diagnosed at 20 years of age is 43.1 years, and is 28.3 years for a diagnosis made at 40 years of age (24). At 20 years of age, the cost per infection prevented in the least expensive scenario was lower than the

undiscounted lifetime costs of a HIV infection by −$651,050 (−$40,641 discounted at 3% and +$176,511 at 5%). In the most expensive scenario, the cost per infection prevented was lower than the undiscounted lifetime costs of a HIV infection by −$682,839 (−$71,068 at 3% and +$146,922 at 5%). At 40 years of age, the cost per infection prevented in the least expensive scenario was lower than the undiscounted lifetime costs of a HIV infection by −$193,800 (+$143,256 discounted at 3% and +$211,641 at 5%). In the most expensive scenario, the cost per infection prevented was lower than the undiscounted lifetime costs of an HIV infection by −$225,589 (+$112,829 at 3% and +$182,052 at 5%).

DISCUSSION

Antiretroviral drugs can be used to prevent HIV transmission. Universal HIV testing to enhance the identification of HIV-positive individuals followed by immediate treatment of all HIV-positive individuals can yield substantial benefits to individuals and affect the dynamics of HIV transmission (27,28). However, the deployment of such a program, with its extensive breadth and depth, presents a formidable challenge (29). ART can also be used to protect uninfected individuals both before and after exposure to HIV infection. Several public health authorities have recommended the use of PrEP as part of a comprehensive prevention package to decrease HIV transmission (30,31). Although some studies have shown the PrEP could be cost-effective in certain settings, particularly in high-risk individuals, it is important to estimate the impact of such strategies in a universal health care setting, where allocation of scarce resources needs to target the most effective strategies. In this context, 'on demand' PrEP compared with continuous PrEP may be an interesting approach, limiting the use and cost of drugs with the potential of preventing similar numbers of infections. This strategy is being evaluated in France and in Canada, and we aimed to evaluate its potential cost effectiveness in our universal health care system.

Very few studies have estimated the cost of HIV infection in Canada (32,33). Our costing estimates are in agreement with these studies. Krentz et al (32) estimated the 2006 total direct costs of an HIV infection to be $13,908 per patient. The Canadian AIDS society estimated the 2009 lifetime costs of an HIV infection to be $1.3 million per person (33). In the United States, the most recent estimates cited by the CDC come from a 2006 study by Schackman et al (34). Schackman et al estimated the undiscounted lifetime direct HIV treatment costs to be $618,900 in 2004. In 2012, our undiscounted lifetime direct HIV treatment costs estimate was $1,028,367. Our data suggest that 'on demand' PrEP, modelled assuming the same level of success as the IPERGAY trial, can be cost-saving because the net benefits (life-years and QALY) of the intervention are greater than current standards of care, and the cost of the intervention is less than the lifetime cost of an infection undiscounted and discounted at a 3% rate (11). The incremental cost-effectiveness ratio of the lifetime costs of an infection discounted at a 5% rate was largely cost effective. There is some consensus in discounting practice in health economics evaluations: both public and health professional tend to choose lower discount rates in health-related comparisons than in finance-related comparisons (35). We followed the Panel on Cost-Effectiveness in Health and Medicine recommendation and use the 3% discount rate in the reference case (36,37), but we also present the 5% discount rate. Moreover, our results are consistent with the majority of previous modelling work on the cost-effectiveness of PrEP interventions among MSM. Most authors found PrEP to be cost-effective when targeting high-risk MSM (6,38-41). However, the models used and costing of HIV infection/PrEP interventions vary considerably among authors.

One could argue that the first dimension of our cost-effectiveness analysis is not consistent in terms of time frame, presenting the costs for one year of 'on demand' PrEP versus 35.2 years of infection. We chose to analyze our results this way because we could not predict how many years a participant would use the program. However, once an individual is infected, he becomes HIV-positive for the rest of his life. We were comfortable presenting the results in this manner because in a risk-management perspective, the IPERGAY strategy has fixed and, thus, predictable costs over a certain period of time, whereas HIV infection costs are harder to estimate over time because they are and will be variable. Moreover, the CDC states that "the lifetime treatment cost of an HIV infection can be used as a conservative threshold value for the cost of averting one infection" (11). Furthermore, we considered a Markov chain model not feasible, given that transition probabilities for the current situation are not available in the published literature.

The possibility that PrEP could result in increased risk-taking behaviour (ie, increased unprotected sex, number of partners, etc) with accompanying increases in health care costs was not factored into our analysis. Although the literature does not provide a definite consensus on behavioral changes (42-50), the importance of behavioral interventions to accompany any wide-scale provision of PrEP to high-risk populations is underscored. In the IPERGAY trial, intensive counselling on the importance of safe sex and condom distribution is provided. Moreover, the participants are selected assuming that they do not use condoms consistently and have multiple partners. The cost of emerging resistance to Truvada was not included in our analysis because recent clinical trials failed to show any cases, suggesting that the percentage of emerging drug resistant cases would be negligible (3-5,49,50).

The main limitation of our costing methodology relies in our estimates of indirect costs. We focused on the impact of morbidity on productivity losses instead of mortality because of the prolonged life expectancy since the arrival of highly active ART. Nevertheless, some authors still chose to measure the income foregone because of mortality (33,51). Also, the impact of morbidity on productivity could have been better estimated by a presenteeism indicator and by taking into account volunteer time and patient/family leisure time. It would have been preferable to control for variables that influence wages (ie, level of education, type of employer, years of experience, geographical location, etc.) to estimate costs related to productivity losses, but such comprehensive datasets were not available. However, we are confident that these estimates present a more accurate picture of HIV costs to society than if we had not included them (9). Another limitation of the present study is that we were unable to estimate the non-ART drugs costs, although according to the Krentz and Gill (32) study, they should be considered to be negligible. The out-of-pocket expenses (ie, copayment) for which we could not provide any estimates should be evaluated. Even if the database from medical sites outside Montréal were not accessible, we are confident that the CHUM sample is representative of health care

resource utilization in the province of Quebec because the majority (62.1%) of declared cases within the MSM population since 2002 are Montreal residents (22). Although CHUM's non-IDU MSM HIV-positive patients database may be biased toward sicker patients, it captures the entire spectrum of health services that may be used during the course of an HIV infection, which would not be the case if we used databases from community HIV clinics.

In the context of an eventual wider implementation of the program following CDC/WHO guidelines (30,31), health care resource utilization may have slightly been underestimated because the MSM-IDU HIV-positive population was excluded from our analysis to abide by the IPERGAY protocol. The results of this cost-effectiveness analysis should not be generalized to other populations such as IDU or serodiscordant couples for whom PrEP is recommended by the CDC/WHO, given that the rates of HIV acquisition are lower than for the MSM group (2,22).

SUPPLEMENTARY TABLE 1
Direct cost, 2012 $

Cost inputs	Unit cost	Reference
Outpatient care		
Overhead costs	$40.92 per visit	Annexe à la circu-laire 2013-028 (16)
Physician, general practicioner	$55.00 per visit	RAMQ (14)
Physician, specialist	$80.00 per visit	RAMQ (14)
Nurse, first visit*	$32.63 per visit	FIQ (13)
Nurse, follow-up†	$8.16 per visit	FIQ (13)
Laboratory testing, first visit	$529.20 per visit	Belval (15)
Laboratory testing, follow-up	$142.60 per visit	Belval (15)
Total first visit	$683	
Total follow-up	$272	
ED		
Overhead costs	$215.17 per visit	Annexe à la circu-laire 2013-028 (16)
Physician, general practicioner‡	$65.75 per visit	RAMQ (14)
Physician, specialist§	$139.85 per visit	RAMQ (14)
Total	$421	
Inpatient care		
Overhead costs	$1112.00 per day	Annexe à la circu-laire 2013-028 (16)
Physician, general practitioner ED‡	$65.75 per visit	RAMQ (14)
Physician, specialist ED§	$139.85 per visit	RAMQ (14)
Physician, specialist hospitalization¶	$62.66 per day	RAMQ (14)
Total	$1,407	
Social worker	$64.68 per hour	Annexe à la circu-laire 2013-028 (16)
Psychologist	$86.60 per hour	Annexe à la circu-laire 2013-028 (16)
Antiretroviral therapy		
Pharmacist dispensing fee	$9.00 per prescription	
Atripla	$1,165 per month	RAMQ (17)
Prezista	$855 per month	RAMQ (17)
Norvir	$172 per month	RAMQ (17)
Truvada	$783 per month	RAMQ (17)
Intelence	$654 per month	RAMQ (17)
Isentress	$690 per month	RAMQ (17)

*Average hourly wage of clinical nurse, specialized nurse practitioner, nurse practitioner candidate and nurse; †Calculated by dividing average hourly wage by average duration of follow-up visit (approximately 15 min); ‡Average fee of a simple visit and an elaborate visit; §Average fee of an internist, a cardiologist, a pneumologist and a microbiologist consult at the emergency department (ED); ¶Average fee of an internist, a cardiologist, a pneumologist and a microbiologist consult during hospitalization. RAMQ Régie de l'assurance maladie du Québec; FIQ Fédération interprofessionnelle de la santé du Québec

In summary, there are many potential benefits of 'on demand' PrEP-related strategy for non-IDU MSM at high risk for HIV acquisition, including its favourable cost-effectiveness ratio and its reasonably predictable long-term costs. Within the next few years, the first results of the IPERGAY clinical trial will become available. It will be interesting to find out if the 'on demand' strategy results in greater adherence to the prophylactic preexposure drug, increased number of averted infections and its subsequent economic impact.

DISCLOSURES: MD is a postdoctoral fellow from the CIHR HIV Clinical Trial Network. JRG is recipient of a CIHR Frederick Banting and Charles Best Doctoral Award and of a Pfizer Post-Doctoral Mentorship Award. CT is a scholar from *Fonds de la Recherche du Québec en Santé*. CT is the Pfizer/University of Montréal Chair on HIV translational Research.

SOURCE OF SUPPORT: Grant from *Réseau SIDA et Maladies Infectieuses du Fonds de la Recherche du Québec en Santé*.

SUPPLEMENTARY TABLE 2
Indirect cost: Average hourly wage weighted by age distribution of HIV infections*, 2012 $

	Age, years			
	15–24	25–54	≥55	Reference
Average hourly wage, $	13.57	25.29	25.08	CANSIM (23)
Proportion of HIV infections, %	0.07	0.82	0.11	INSPQ (22)
Average hourly wage, weighted by age distribution of HIV infections				$24.44

Calculated by multiplying the proportion of HIV infections by the average hourly wage per age group. The results are then summed. CANSIM Statistics Canada socioeconomic database; INSPQ Institut national de santé publique du Québec

SUPPLEMENTARY TABLE 3
Indirect cost: Salary losses per HIV infection due to work absenteeism, 2012 $

	Hours missed per day of work*	Average annual visits distributed on sample†	Annual salary losses per patient
Outpatient	4	4‡	$391.10
Emergency department	8	0.28	$53.86
Social worker	4	0.21	$43.92
Psychologist	4	0.45	$20.94
Inpatient	8	0.59	$115.22
Total salary losses, $		$625.05	

Assumptions; †Calculated by multiplying average annual visits by average annual patients using the service and then by dividing this results by total number of patients; ‡Recommended number of follow-up visits per year; §Calculated by multiplying the average hourly wage weighted by age distribution ($24.44) by the number of hours missed per day of work

SUPPLEMENTARY TABLE 4
Indirect cost: Salary losses per IPERGAY participant due to work absenteeism, 2012 $

	Average hourly wage, $	Proportion of workers, %	General population employment rate, 2012	Average hourly wage, weighted by employment rate and proportion of workers	Wage losses, $
Age, years					
15–24	13.57	0.13	0.556	0.98	23.54
25–54	25.29	0.68	0.838	14.41	345.87
≥55	25.08	0.18	0.352	1.59	38.14
Total salary losses					407.55
Reference	CANSIM (23)	CANSIM (19)			

CANSIM Statistics Canada socioeconomic database

SUPPLEMENTARY TABLE 5
Indirect cost: Salary losses per HIV infection due to employment rate gap, 2012 $

	HIV age distribution	HIV-positive MSM employment rate, 2010	General population employment rate, 2010	Employment rate gap	Average annual salary, $	Annual salary losses per patient, $
Age, years						
15–24	0.07	43.80	56.90	0.13	20,566	189
25–54	0.82	56.10	82.80	0.27	48,546	10,655
≥55	0.11	33.20	34.80	0.02	46,681	80
Total salary losses						10,925*
Reference	INSPQ (22)	A Burchell (personal communication, April 30, 2013)	CANSIM (19)			CANSIM (23)

*Calculated by multiplying the employment rate gap by the proportion of HIV infections by the average annual salary per age group. The results are then summed.
CANSIM Statistics Canada socioeconomic database; INSPQ Institut national de santé publique du Québec; MSM Men who have sex with men*

REFERENCES

1. Sullivan PS, Hamouda O, Delpech V, et al. Reemergence of the HIV epidemic among men who have sex with men in North America, Western Europe, and Australia, 1996-2005. Ann Epidemiol 2009;19:423-31.
2. Public Health Agency Canada. Summary: Estimates of HIV prevalence and incidence in Canada, 2011. Centre for Communicable Diseases and Infection Control: 2012;9.
3. Van Damme L, Corneli A, Ahmed K, et al. Preexposure prophylaxis for HIV infection among African women. N Engl J Med 2012;367:411-22.
4. Grant RM, Lama JR, Anderson PL, et al. Preexposure chemoprophylaxis for HIV prevention in men who have sex with men. N Engl J Med 2010;363:2587-99.
5. Thigpen MC, Kebaabetswe PM, Paxton LA, et al. Antiretroviral preexposure prophylaxis for heterosexual HIV transmission in Botswana. New Engl J Med 2012;367:423-34.
6. Paltiel AD, Freedberg KA, Scott CA, et al. HIV preexposure prophylaxis in the United States: Impact on lifetime infection risk, clinical outcomes, and cost-effectiveness. Clin Infect Dis 2009;48:806-15.

7. Walensky RP, Ross EL, Kumarasamy N, et al. Cost-effectiveness of HIV treatment as prevention in serodiscordant couples. N Engl J Med 2013;369:1715-25.

8. U.S. National Institutes of Health. On demand antiretroviral pre-exposure prophylaxis for HIV infection in men who have sex with men (IPERGAY). U.S. National Institutes of Health. <http://clinicaltrials.gov/ct2/show/NCT01473472?term=Ipergay&rank=1> (Accessed July 2014).

9. Drummond MF, Sculpher MJ, Torrance GW, O'Brien BJ, Stoddart GL. Methods for the Economic Evaluation of Health Care Programs, 3rdedn. New York: Oxford University Press, 2005.

10. Schackman BR, Metsch LR, Colfax GN, et al. The cost-effectiveness of rapid HIV testing in substance abuse treatment: Results of a randomized trial. Drug Alcohol Depend 2013;128:90-7.

11. CDC. [Internet] HIV Cost-Effectiveness. Center for Disease Control and Prevention (CDC). <www.cdc.gov/hiv/topics/preventionprograms/ce/index.htm> (Accessed July 2014).

12. La Direction des Communications du ministère de la Santé et des Services sociaux. L'examen médical de l'adulte vivant avec le virus de l'immunodéficience acquise (VIH). Gouvernement du Québec; 2013;139.

13. FIQ. Convention collective. Fédération Interprofessionnelle de la Santé du Québec (FIQ) 20 mars 2011-31 mars 2015. p. 258.

14. Régie de l'assurance maladie du Québec. Manuel des médecins spécialistes. 2013;178.

15. Belval M. Laboratoires regroupés du CHUM. Centre Hospitalier de l'Université de Montréal; April 2013.

16. MSSS. Liste des taux applicables au 1er mai 2013. Annexe à la circulaire 2013-028 (03014219): Ministère de la santé et services sociaux du Québec (MSSS); May 2013;12

17. Régie de l'assurance maladie du Québec. Liste des médicaments. November 2013;909.

18. Lee FJ, Amin J, Carr A. Efficacy of initial antiretroviral therapy for HIV-1 infection in adults: A systematic review and meta analysis of 114 studies with up to 144 weeks' follow-up. PLoS One 2014;9:e97482.

19. CANSIM. Table 282-0002- Labour force survey estimates (LFS), 2010 and 2012 employment and employment rate by sex and age group, annual. Statistics Canada. <www5.statcan.gc.ca/cansim/> (Accessed July 2014).

20. Carpenter CS. Sexual orientation, work, and income in Canada. Can J Econ 2008;41:1239-61.

21. ISQ. Taux d'emploi des hommes selon certains groupes d'âge, Québec, Ontario, Canada, 1976 à 2011: Institut de la statistique du Québec (ISQ). <www.stat.gouv.qc.ca/donstat/societe/march_travl_remnr/parnt_etudn_march_travl/pop_active/b006_1976-2011.htm> (Accessed May 2013).

22. Institut national de santé publique du Québec. Programme de surveillance de l'infection par le virus de l'immunodéficience humaine (VIH) au Québec : cas cumulatifs 2002-2012. Laboratoire de santé publique du Québec; 2013;69.

23. CANSIM. [Internet] Table 282-0072 – Labour force survey estimates (LFS), wages of employees by sex and age group, annual. 2012. Québec. Statistics Canada. <www5.statcan.gc.ca/cansim/a26> (Accessed May 2013).

24. Antiretroviral Therapy Cohort Collaboration. Life expectancy of individuals on combination antiretroviral therapy in high-income countries: A collaborative analysis of 14 cohort studies. Lancet 2008;372:293-9.

25. Tengs TO, Lin TH. A meta-analysis of utility estimates for HIV/AIDS. Med Decis Making 2002;22:475-81.

26. CADTH. Guidelines for the economic evaluation of health technologies: Canada, 3rd edn. Ottawa: Canadian Agency for Drugs and Technologies in Health, 2006.

27. Walensky RP, Paltiel AD, Losina E, et al. Test and Treat DC: Forecasting the impact of a comprehensive strategy in Washington, DC. CID2010;51:392-400.

28. Weber J, Tatoud R, Fidler S. Postexposure prohylaxis, preexposure prophylaxis of universal test and treat: The strategic use of antiretroviral drugs to prevent HIV acquisition and transmission. AIDS 2010;24(Suppl 4):S27-S39.

29. Gardner EM, McLees MP, Steiner JF, et al. The spectrum of engagement in HIV care and its relevance to test-and-treat strategies for prevention of HIV infection. Clin Infect Dis 2011;52:793-800.

30. CDC. PrEP: A New Tool for HIV Prevention. <www.cdc.gov/hiv/pdf/prevention_PrEP_factsheet.pdf> (Accessed April 2013).

31. WHO. Consolidated guidelines on HIV prevention, diagnosis, treatment and care for key populations. Switzerland: World Health Organization, 2014.

32. Krentz HB, Gill MJ. Cost of medical care for HIV-infected patients within a regional population from 1997 to 2006. HIV Med 2008;9:721-30.

33. Kingston-Riechers J. The Economic Cost of HIV/AIDS in Canada. Canadian AIDS Society; 2011;17.

34. Schackman BR, Gebo KA, Walensky RP, et al. The lifetime cost of current human immunodeficiency virus care in the United States. Med Care 2006;44:990-7.

35. West RR, McNabb R, Thompson AG, Sheldon TA, Grimley EJ. Estimating implied rates of discount in healthcare decision-making. Health Technol Assess 2003;7:1-60.

36. Weinstein MC, Siegel JE, Gold MR, Kamlet MS, Russell LB. Recommendations of the Panel on Cost-Effectiveness in Health and Medecine. JAMA 1996;276:1253-8.

37. Walensky RP, Freedberg KA, Weinstein MC, Paltiel AD. Cost-effectiveness of HIV testing and treatment in the United States. Clin Infect Dis 2007;45(Suppl 4):S248-S254.

38. Gomez GB, Borquez A, Caceres CF, et al. The potential impact of pre-exposure prophylaxis for HIV prevention among men who have sex with men and transwomen in Lima, Peru: A mathematical modelling study. PLoS Med 2012;9:e1001323.

39. Desai K, Sansom SL, Ackers ML, et al. Modeling the impact of HIV chemoprophylaxis strategies among men who have sex with men in the United States: HIV infections prevented and costeffectiveness. AIDS 2008;22:1829-39.

40. Koppenhaver RT, Sorensen SW, Farnham PG, Sansom SL. The costeffectiveness of pre-exposure prophylaxis in men who have sex with men in the United States: An epidemic model. J Acquir Immune Defic Syndr 2011;58:e51-e52.

41. Juusola JL, Brandeau ML, Owens DK, Bendavid E. The cost-effectiveness of preexposure prophylaxis for HIV prevention in the United States in men who have sex with men. Ann Intern Med 2012;156:541-50.

42. Golub S, Kowalczyk W, Weinberger C, Parsons JT. Preexposure prophylaxis and predicted condom use among high-risk men who have sex with men. J Acquir Immune Defic Syndr 2010;54:548-55.

43. Eaton L, Kalichman SC. Risk compensation in HIV prevention: Implications for vaccines, microbicides, and other biomedical HIV prevention technologies. Curr HIV/AIDS Rep 2007;4:165-72.

44. Martin JN, Roland ME, Neilands T, et al. Use of postexposure prophylaxis against HIV infection following sexual exposure does not lead to increases in high-risk behavior. AIDS 2004;18:787-92.

45. Crepaz N, Hart TA, Marks G. Highly active antiretroviral therapy and sexual risk behavior: A meta-analytic review. JAMA 2004;292:224-36.

46. Liu AY, Vittinghoff E, Chillag K, et al. Sexual risk behavior among HIV-uninfected men who have sex with men participating in a tenofovir preexposure prophylaxis randomized trial in the United States. J Acquir Immune Defic Syndr 2013;64:87-94.

47. Thng C, Thorpe S, Schembri G, et al. Acceptability of HIV pre-exposure prophylaxis (PrEP) and associated risk compensation in men who have sex with men (MSM) accessing GU services. HIV Med 2012;13:84.

48. Baeten JM, Donnell D, Ndase P, et al. Antiretroviral prophylaxis for HIV prevention in heterosexual men and women. N Engl J Med 2012;367:399-410

49. Buchbinder SP, Liu AY. CROI 2014: New tools to track the epidemic and prevent HIV infections. Top Antivir Med 2014;22:579-93.

50. Brooks RA, Landovitz RJ, Kaplan RL, Lieber E, Lee SJ, Barkley TW. Sexual risk behaviors and acceptability of HIV pre-exposure prophylaxis among HIV-negative gay and bisexual men in serodiscordant relationships: A mixed methods study. AIDS Patient Care STDs 2012;26:87-94.

51. Hutchinson AB, Farnham PG, Dean HD, et al. The economic burden of HIV in the United States in the era of highly active antiretroviral therapy: Evidence of continuing racial and ethnic differences. J Acquir Immune Defic Syndr 2006;43:451-7.

52. CHMD. [Internet] Life tables – Male. Canadian Human Mortality Database (CHMD). <www.bdlc.umontreal.ca/chmd/prov/que/que.htm> (Accessed April 2013).

40

The role of pediatricians as key stakeholders in influencing immunization policy decisions for the introduction of meningitis B vaccine in Canada: The Ontario perspective

Hirotaka Yamashiro MD FRCP C FAAP, Nora Cutcliffe MSc PhD, Simon Dobson MD FRCP C,
David Fisman MD MPH FRCP C, Ronald Gold MD MPH

H Yamashiro, N Cutcliffe, S Dobson, D Fisman, R Gold. The role of pediatricians as key stakeholders in influencing immunization policy decisions for the introduction of meningitis B vaccine in Canada: The Ontario perspective. Can J Infect Dis Med Microbiol 2015;26(4):183-190.

As key stakeholders in immunization policy decisions, the Pediatricians of Ontario held an accredited conference on January 18, 2014, to discuss prevention of invasive meningococcal disease. Five key recommendations were put forth regarding immunization strategies to protect children from meningococcal serogroup B disease. The recently approved four-component meningococcal B (4CMenB) vaccine should be recommended and funded as part of Ontario's routine immunization schedule and should also be mandated for school attendance. Public funding for 4CMenB immunization is justified based on current MenB epidemiology, vaccine coverage, cost effectiveness and acceptability, as well as legal, political and ethical considerations related to 4CMenB immunization, particularly because routine recommendations and funding are currently in place for vaccination against meningococcal serogroups that cause significantly less disease in Canada than MenB. Broadly, the goals are to assist individual practitioners in advocating the benefits of 4CMenB vaccination to parents, and to counterbalance recommendations from the National Advisory Committee on Immunization and the Canadian Paediatric Society.

Key Words: *4CMenB vaccine; Immunization policy; Invasive meningococcal disease (IMD); Pediatricians; Preventive care; Serogroup B*

Le rôle des pédiatres comme principaux intervenants pour influencer les décisions relatives aux politiques sur l'introduction du vaccin contre la méningite du sérogroupe B au Canada : le point de vue de l'Ontario

À titre de principaux intervenants à l'égard des décisions relatives aux politiques de vaccination, les *Pediatricians of Ontario* a organisé un colloque agréé le 18 janvier 2014 pour discuter de la prévention des méningococcies invasives. Il a formulé cinq grandes recommandations sur les stratégies de vaccination pour protéger les enfants des méningococcies du sérogroupe B (MenB). Le vaccin contre le méningocoque de sérogroupe B (4CMenB) qui a récemment été approuvé devrait être recommandé et financé dans le cadre du calendrier de vaccination systématique de l'Ontario et être exigé pour pouvoir fréquenter l'école. Le financement public du vaccin 4CMenB est justifié compte tenu de l'épidémiologie actuelle de la MenB, de la couverture vaccinale, de l'efficience et de l'acceptabilité, de même que des considérations juridiques, politiques et éthiques liées au vaccin 4CMenB, particulièrement parce que les recommandations et le financement de la vaccination systématique sont déjà en place au Canada contre des sérogroupes du méningocoque qui sont beaucoup moins graves que le MenB. En général, le regroupement vise ainsi à aider les praticiens à préconiser les avantages du vaccin 4CMenB auprès des parents et à compenser les recommandations du Comité consultatif national d'immunisation et de la Société canadienne de pédiatrie.

In Canada, the list of 'licensed but unfunded' vaccines, which are approved by Health Canada but unfunded by provincial health authorities, continues to expand. New professional guidance is required to clarify the optimal use and benefits of such vaccines, including educational campaigns developed according to public health departments, physicians, pharmacists, manufacturers and professional associations (1). Professional medical associations play a particularly important role in advocating for licensed vaccines (both funded and unfunded), not only because the public values expert medical advice that is independent of government or industry, but because individuals typically trust physicians and related professional bodies (2).

UNIQUE CONTRIBUTION OF THE PEDIATRICIANS OF ONTARIO IN SHAPING IMMUNIZATION POLICY

In Ontario, the Pediatrics Section of the Ontario Medical Association and the Pediatricians Alliance of Ontario act jointly as the 'Pediatricians of Ontario' to represent Ontario's 1200 pediatricians, and to advocate for the delivery of excellent children's health care (3,4). As a bold step toward advancing childhood immunization, the Pediatricians of Ontario held a conference, accredited by the Maintenance of Certification program of the Royal College of Physicians and Surgeons of Canada, on January 18, 2014, in Toronto, to discuss the prevention of invasive meningococcal disease (IMD) in

Pediatrics Section, Ontario Medical Association (PSOMA) and Pediatricians Alliance of Ontario (PAO); 'Pediatricians of Ontario'
Correspondence: Dr Ronald Gold, University of Toronto, 46 Waverley Road, Toronto, Ontario M4L 3T1.
e-mail rongold16@gmail.com

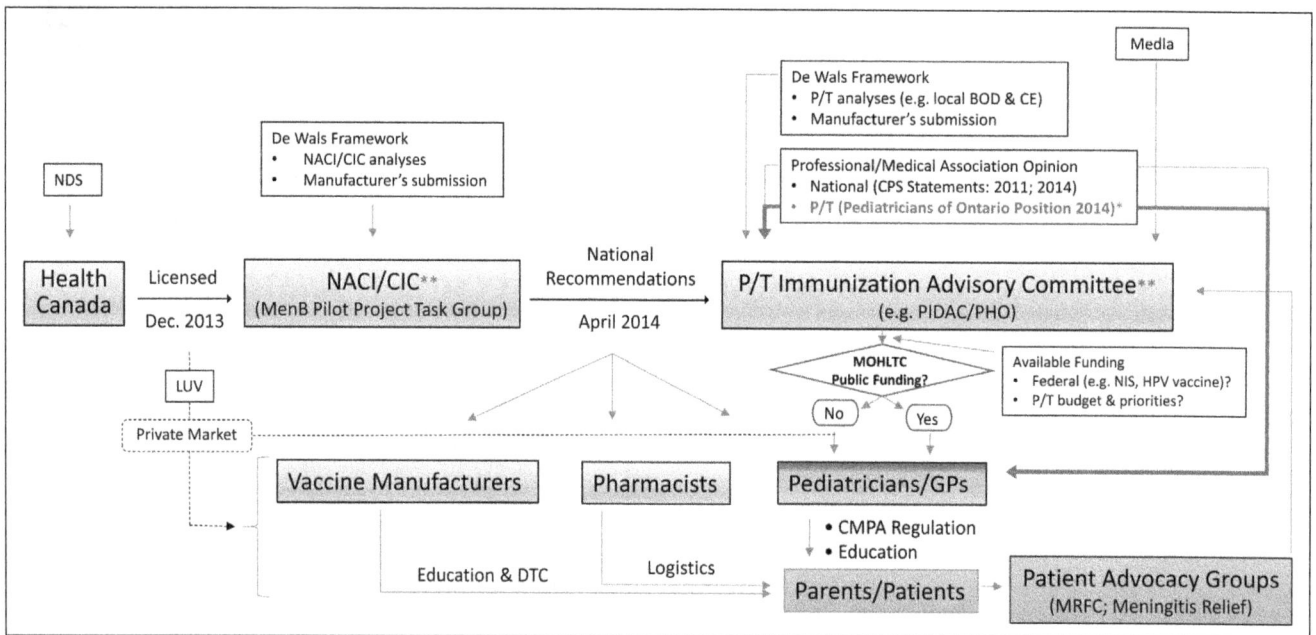

Figure 1) *Role of the Pediatricians of Ontario in influencing immunization policy and funding decisions (eg, four-component meningococcal B vaccine). *Pediatricians of Ontario contribute a critical voice in informing provincial immunization policy decisions (and informing GPs) regarding 4CMenB vaccination; **Pediatricians of Ontario also seeking increased opportunities for direct contribution as key stakeholders on national and jurisdictional immunization advisory committees. BOD Burden of disease; CE Cost effectiveness; CIC Canadian Immunization Committee; CMPA Canadian Medical Protective Association; CPS Canadian Paediatric Society; Dec December; DTC Direct to consumer; GPs General practitioners; HPV Human papillomavirus; LUV Licensed but unfunded; MOHLTC Ministry of Health and Long-Term Care (Ontario); MRFC Meningitis Research Foundation of Canada; NACI National Advisory Committee on Immunization; NDS New drug submission; NIS National Immunization Strategy; PHO Public Health Ontario; PIDAC Provincial Infectious Disease Advisory Committee; P/T Provincial/territorial*

Ontario. This meeting included participation of 41 members (19 onsite, 22 by live broadcast webinar) and is archived at www.pedsontario.com, Members Section. Our goal is to ensure that Ontario pediatricians play an integral role as key stakeholders in influencing immunization policy and funding decisions, particularly related to the introduction of the newly approved four-component meningococcal B (4CMenB) vaccine (5).

The Pediatricians of Ontario position is intended to provide medical opinion, in addition to statements issued by the National Advisory Committee on Immunization (NACI) (6,7) and/or Canadian Immunization Committee, and the Canadian Paediatric Society (8,9). In advocating the benefits of 4CMenB immunization to public health policy makers and to Ontario pediatricians in frontline practice, the present position paper should broaden the use of the 4CMenB vaccine (Figure 1; bold arrows).

MENINGITIS B EPIDEMIOLOGY

IMD is a rapidly progressing, life-threatening infection caused by *Neisseria meningitidis*. According to data extracted from the enhanced IMD surveillance system (10), between 154 and 229 cases of IMD were reported per year in Canada (2006 to 2011), with a mean annual incidence rate of 0.58 per 100,000. Four serogroups (B, C, W-135 and Y) accounted for 91% of reported cases. The introduction of the meningococcal C conjugate vaccine across Canada from 2002 to 2005 led to reduced incidence of IMD due to serogroup C (MenC), with serogroup B (MenB) now being the most common cause of IMD. From 2006 to 2011, MenB accounted for 50% to 62% of all IMD cases in Canada. The incidence of MenB is highest in the pediatric population, with national age-specific incidence rates (cases per 100,000) reported to be 5.8, 1.4 and 0.7, respectively, for children younger than one year of age; one to four years of age; and 15 to 19 years of age, in 2011 (6). Notably, 84% of all IMD cases in Canadian infants were caused by MenB (11).

In Ontario, the annual incidence of MenB from 2000 to 2010 ranged from 0.11 to 0.27 per 100,000 (12). Of key importance, the incidence of IMD due to MenC was 0.27 per 100,000 in 2001, at the peak of the

outbreak, and was 0.10 per 100,000 at the time of introducing the MenC conjugate vaccine in 2005 (Figure 2) (13). It should be emphasized that MenB incidence was higher than that of MenC in 2005 (0.15 per 100,000) and has remained above this level (ranging from 0.11 to 0.27 per 100,000 from 2005 to 2010) (12). The same trends have been observed nationally, with MenB incidence exceeding that of MenC every year between 2002 to 2009 (14). These incidence data, combined with the frequency of death and disabling sequelae, provide a strong rationale to extend IMD prevention by introducing routine immunizing programs to protect against serogroup B.

RECOMMENDATIONS OF THE PEDIATRICIANS OF ONTARIO FOR IMMUNIZATION AND PREVENTION OF MenB

Despite aggressive and timely treatment efforts, MenB can kill or cause serious life-long disabilities within 24 h of onset (15). Vaccination is, therefore, the best defense against this devastating disease. While MenA, MenC and quadrivalent (MenACWY) vaccines have been available for several years (16), the new 4CMenB vaccine was first licensed in 2013 (5,17-19), filling a final critical gap in IMD prevention. In Canada, the 4CMenB vaccine is approved for children and adolescents two months to 17 years of age (5). During the January 18, 2014 meeting of the Pediatricians of Ontario, draft recommendations were proposed by panel speakers, and five key recommendations (R1 to R5) regarding immunization policy were put forth following discussion by all meeting participants, with a primary focus on 4CMenB vaccination for children.

The Pediatricians of Ontario:

Recommendation (R) 1: Support the routine use of the newly licensed 4CMenB vaccine for children;

R2: Recommend that Ontario funds the newly licensed 4CMenB vaccine as part of its public immunization program (ie, as a critical priority among other 'licensed but unfunded' vaccines) to ensure vaccine access for all Ontario families;

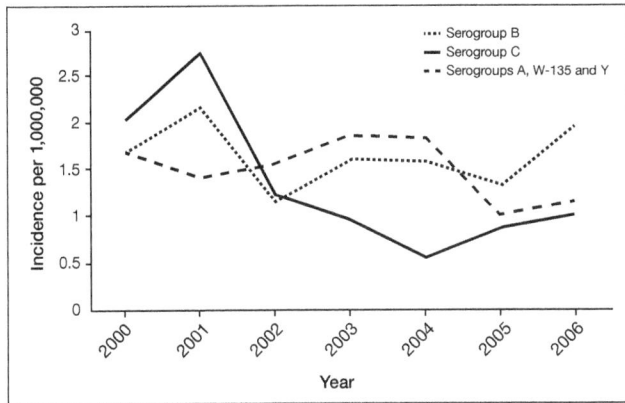

Figure 2) *Annual incidence of invasive meningococcal disease according to serogroup in Ontario, 2000 to 2006*

TABLE 1
Pediatricians of Ontario member survey responses to recommendations

Extent of agreement/ disagreement	Recommendation				
	1	2	3	4	5
Strongly agree	64 (53.33)	64 (53.78)	65 (54.62)	75 (63.03)	73 (61.34)
Agree	44 (36.67)	43 (36.13)	41 (34.45)	39 (32.77)	37 (31.09)
Neutral	7 (5.83)	7 (5.88)	9 (7.56)	5 (4.2)	8 (6.72)
Disagree	3 (2.50)	2 (1.68)	2 (1.68)	0 (0)	0 (0)
Strongly disagree	2 (1.67)	3 (2.52)	2 (1.68)	0 (0)	1 (0.84)
Total respondents	120 (100)	119 (100)	119 (100)	119 (100)	119 (100)

Data presented as n (%)

R3: Support public funding for other 'licensed but unfunded' vaccines, including vaccines targeting hepatitis A and B (administered together), human papillomavirus (HPV) for males and MenACWY for infants;

R4: Recommend ongoing review and alignment of legally mandated vaccines (as specified under the Immunization of School Pupils Act [ISPA]) with those recommended by NACI and with publicly funded vaccines and;

R5: Recommend that pediatricians secure increased membership on national (ie, NACI and/or Canadian Immunization Committee) and jurisdictional (ie, Provincial Infectious Disease Advisory Committee or Public Health Ontario) immunization advisory committees, to ensure direct contribution to key policy/funding decisions.

To evaluate the extent of agreement with these recommendations, a follow-up survey was conducted online to canvass all members of the Pediatricians of Ontario between April 1 (following the release of the NACI statement regarding the use of the 4CMenB vaccine [6]) and April 24, 2014. During the survey period, 120 responses were received, corresponding to a response rate of 10%. While the response rate was low, respondents confirmed broad agreement with proposed recommendations (Table 1). Specifically, >89% strongly agreed or agreed with all five recommendations, with 53% to 63% in strong agreement. These data are consistent with significant member interest in advocating for pediatric immunization, reinforcing our support for publicly funding of 4CMenB and other 'licensed but unfunded' vaccines.

STATUS OF 4CMenB IMMUNIZATION RECOMMENDATIONS AND PUBLIC PROGRAMS

The provincial recommendations proposed by the Pediatricians of Ontario (R1 and R2) stand in contrast with current NACI recommendations, which state that, given the current available information regarding the burden of IMD in Canada, as well as the lack of evidence and range of uncertainty of underlying assumptions (particularly concerning the predicted level of strain susceptibility, duration of protection, impact on meningococcal carriage and herd immunity and potential adverse effects of vaccination at the population level), a recommendation for implementing a routine immunization program for MenB in Canada cannot be made at the present time (6). However, the vaccine may be considered (permissively) on an individual basis, for individuals ≥2 months of age. The NACI recommendations also offer impractical guidance for vaccine use in the management of outbreaks and travel, ie, by advising that laboratory testing (which may be inaccessible) be conducted before vaccine administration.

Notably, the recommendations of the Pediatricians of Ontario are in alignment with current recommendations of the Joint Committee on Immunisation in the United Kingdom (20) and the Australian Technical Advisory Group on Immunisation in Australia (18), which recommend routine 4CMenB immunization of infants. The Pediatricians of Ontario position is also consistent with previously published NACI (21,22) and Canadian Paediatric Society (23) statements, identifying the need to develop a MenB vaccine.

At the regional level in Canada, the Ministry of Health and Social Services of Quebec announced, in April 2014, its plan to fund a local, targeted 4CMenB vaccination campaign in the Saguenay–Lac-Saint-Jean region. The decision was made due to the high incidence of MenB infection in this region (24). The campaign, which ran from May 5, 2014, to December 31, 2014, represented the first Canadian 4CMenB vaccination program, and was also the most comprehensive program globally, because it encompasses all individuals two months to 20 years of age, and province-wide coverage of high-risk groups (25). In February 2015, a publicly funded MenB vaccination program was also implemented at Nova Scotia's Acadia University, in response to an institutional outbreak (two MenB cases), targeting all students and faculty/staff with certain medical conditions (26).

PEDIATRICIANS OF ONTARIO OPINION – SUPPORTING 4CMenB VACCINATION

Because the primary responsibility of frontline pediatricians is to protect individual children, the Pediatricians of Ontario presented arguments to support routine use (R1) and funding (R2) of the 4CMenB vaccine in Ontario. Given the periodic and sporadic nature of surges in incidence of group B meningococcus, we advocate for proactive prevention of MenB disease, rather than waiting for outbreaks, before implementing targeted or outbreak control strategies. The Pediatricians of Ontario position is consistent with past public health guidance regarding IMD vaccine recommendations. Our arguments address the burden of MenB disease, vaccine coverage, cost effectiveness (as primary concerns raised by policy-makers), as well as acceptability, and legal, political and ethical considerations related to 4CMenB vaccine introduction. In particular, we submit that currently available estimates are conservative in terms of describing MenB incidence and vaccine coverage of MenB strains, as well as the economic attractiveness of 4CMenB vaccination. By providing more accurate assessments, we aim to assist practitioners in communicating effectively with parents regarding MenB disease and 4CMenB immunization and, more broadly, to inform policy decision makers and help justify vaccine program implementation in Ontario.

Technical limitations result in conservative estimation of MenB disease burden

Although IMD caused by MenB is rare, currently available data inevitably underestimate actual MenB incidence, due to limitations in case ascertainment. Notably, laboratory confirmation is a necessary part of case reporting. Early treatment with antibiotics can limit the ability to detect *N meningitidis* using culture methods alone, producing 'culture-negative' results. In addition, increased use of polymerase chain reaction (PCR) testing would increase identification of the causal serogroup by 30% to 50% (27). However, PCR testing was introduced only in 2009, and of the cases identified nationally and in Ontario, only 10% and 7% were confirmed by PCR, respectively (10,13). While active surveillance systems, such as the Canadian Immunization

Monitoring Program, ACTive (28) and the Toronto Invasive Bacterial Disease Network (29), offer improvements over passive surveillance (via notifiable disease reports), underdetection of MenB cases may still occur, due to the uncommon usage of PCR testing in Canada. Hence, in general, current incidence data for MenB are conservative.

Predicted strain coverage by 4CMenB vaccine is conservative

Although significant challenges have hindered the development of a vaccine against MenB disease due to the lack of an immunogenic capsule (30,31), the ground-breaking reverse vaccinology approach has enabled identification of several subcapsular, surface-expressed protein antigens that are both highly conserved among MenB strains and able to induce bactericidal antibodies (32). This research laid the foundation for developing the current 4CMenB vaccine, comprised of three purified recombinant protein antigens, along with an outer membrane vesicle component (containing the PorA protein subtype 1.4) (33). The immunogenicity, safety and tolerability of this newly approved 4CMenB vaccine has been demonstrated in clinical trials in >8000 subjects to date (27). Specifically, the vaccine has been shown to elicit a strong immune response in infants, toddlers and adolescents (34-36) based on the serum bactericidal assay (SBA), an established correlate of protection for MenB (37).

The 4CMenB vaccine will not be expected to provide protection against all circulating MenB strains, however, because not all strains express antigens contained in the vaccine. Hence, evaluation of strain coverage is necessary (18). To estimate potential coverage of the vaccine, a new assay has been developed, referred to as the Meningococcal Antigen Typing System (MATS) (38). Using small sera volumes, the high throughput-MATS assay can quantify and characterize the protein concentration of vaccine antigens expressed on MenB strains, and will estimate the proportion of circulating strains that may be expected to be killed by antibodies induced by the 4CMenB vaccine (27). For MATS calculations, individual strain killing is predicted when at least one recombinant protein antigen concentration equals or exceeds its validated positive bactericidal threshold value (or the presence of the dominant PorA 1.4 variant is detected) (33), thus making the strain susceptible to killing by vaccine-induced antibodies. In essence, MATS testing can assess the degree to which the vaccine antigens match the surface proteins of a diverse panel of disease-causing MenB strains. This approach has been used to assess vaccine coverage of strains representing specific geographical areas (39).

In Canada, the potential of the 4CMenB vaccine to cover circulating strains from 2006 to 2009 has been tested; 157 isolates were recently characterized using MATS. The predicted strain coverage of the 4CMenB vaccine was 66% (40). However, MATS estimates are believed to be conservative. A recent study from the United Kingdom tested a representative sample from all MenB disease isolates collected in England and Wales in 2007 to 2008 against pooled sera from infant and adolescent vaccines, using both human SBA and MATS assays (33). While MATS predictions and human SBA results were significantly associated (P=0.022), MATS predicted 4CMenB vaccine coverage of 70%, whereas human SBA results indicated 88% killing. Because fully 66% of strains predicted 'not covered' by MATS were killed in the human SBA assay (and thus represented false negatives by MATS), it was suggested that possible bactericidal synergy may occur for antibodies raised against multiple antigens, even when MATS results indicate that individual antigen levels fall below their respective positive bacterial thresholds. In addition, in the Canadian study, it was also suggested that because expression of one of the protein antigens is repressed in in vitro (but not in in vivo) conditions, MATS may underestimate the contribution of that antigen to vaccine strain coverage (40). Overall, researchers have concurred that MATS is a conservative predictor of 4CMenB strain coverage (27,33,38,40).

It should be noted that because all four protein antigens of the 4CMenB vaccine may be present in the outer membrane of non-B serogroups, antibodies induced by the vaccine may also have bactericidal activity against other serotypes of IMD (35). Hence, while the vaccine is anticipated to outperform the MATS estimate of protection against 66% of MenB strains (as argued above), the vaccine's effectiveness may also extend to non-B strains (8,15). In this context, the innovative research that has led to the revolutionary development of the 4CMenB vaccine may indeed be considered to be the first step toward universal strain coverage across all IMD serogroups (41).

Current economic assessments underestimate the attractiveness of 4CMenB immunization

It is critically important that the assessment of vaccine cost effectiveness be evaluated in accordance with current best practice guidelines for the economic evaluation of communicable disease control interventions (42). For 4CMenB vaccination, cost-effectiveness models (eg, estimating cost per quality-adjusted life year [QALY] [cost/QALY] and number needed to vaccinate [NNV]) should assume dynamic disease transmission, with direct vaccine impact on vaccinated individuals, as well as indirect impact on unvaccinated individuals. First, the use of an early outer membrane vesicle vaccine targeting MenB, a single component preparation of the current 4CMenB vaccine, has led to successful control of an epidemic of group B meningococcal disease in New Zealand (43,44). Second, herd immunity effects associated with indirect protection have been profoundly underestimated before the widespread utilization of other recently introduced vaccines, including Haemophilus influenzae type b vaccine (45); conjugate pneumococcal vaccines (46); HPV vaccine (47,48); rotavirus vaccines (49); and group C conjugate meningococcal vaccine (13), also strengthening the rationale for dynamic cost-effectiveness modelling approaches for 4CMenB immunization.

Moreover, while the impact of 4CMenB vaccine on MenB carriage dynamics is not yet known, there is reasonable expectation of vaccine efficacy against meningococcal B carriage rates (and hence broader herd immunity impact), based on available literature to date (20,50). Indirect effects will be evaluated in the near term in global surveillance and phase IV studies. In the interim, however, as post-implementation phase data are awaited, available models for 4CMenB vaccination have unfortunately focused primarily on static analyses (including Markov models and decision trees), assuming only direct protection of vaccines, to calculate cost/QALY (6) and NNV (8,12). As a result, cost/QALY and NNV results from 'static risk' modelling are likely misestimated. Notably, for static models estimating NNV, the magnitude of distortion is projected to be greatest with partially effective vaccines and those against diseases with lower reproductive numbers, such as meningococcal infection, in which even modest reductions in carriage may lead to collapse of disease in a population (51). In general, although static risk estimates have been used by policy makers in the economic evaluation of routine 4CMenB immunization, vaccine benefits are likely to extend beyond those vaccinated. Hence, there is need for significant caution in accepting conclusions from static modelling studies that suggest 4CMenB immunization programs may not be cost effective.

Given the wide range of clinical sequelae that can result from IMD, including amputation, cognitive delay, requirement for multiple corrective surgeries and future loss of productivity (52,53), it is important that the full range of sequelae be included in economic evaluations of vaccination. Failure to do so will result in analyses that are biased against vaccine economic attractiveness.

Another key concept to consider is that cost effectiveness of immunization needs to be estimated against the costs and consequences of nonadoption of routine 4CMenB immunization programs (or by targeting selective at-risk populations), which may culminate in the need to implement reactive outbreak control strategies. Because MenB is highly unpredictable, outbreak control can be extremely disruptive from a public health standpoint, requiring extensive resources to manage, ie, in terms of organizing vaccine supply and delivery, setting up local clinics, and swiftly developing effective educational programs, as reported during the 2013 to 2014 United States college outbreak campaigns (54). Significant expenses will inevitably be incurred in treating additional patients who are infected before clinic mobilization, and to provide prophylactic antimicrobials and vaccines to exposed contacts (55).

Finally, it must be emphasized that cost effectiveness is one of several drivers of the decision to adopt a novel vaccine (56); ethical, political, and disease dynamic considerations are also important. Other vaccines, even against IMD, have been funded in Ontario, despite having high costs per health outcome; most notably, the MenC immunization program was implemented for public health reasons beyond merely cost analyses, and is now considered to be highly effective – in fact, a public health triumph. In essence, society has accepted vaccination against MenC because prevention of such a rare, but serious disease is deemed a worthwhile public health goal (57).

Public funding is critical for vaccine acceptance

Parental acceptance of meningococcal vaccines is very high in Canada (58). To assess parental acceptability of 4CMenB vaccine, a national study was conducted with parents presenting infants two to six months of age for vaccination (59). Parents were given a short description of meningitis and the new vaccine, and then were surveyed as to their intention to vaccinate. Results demonstrated that the majority (84.7%) of parents intended to vaccinate their infants with MenB vaccine when it was free of charge as a publicly funded vaccine. Intention to vaccinate decreased to 63% (at $50 per dose) and 46.8% (at $100 per dose). Yearly income was explanatory only at the extreme income levels (>$80,000 versus <$40,000). To explore this heuristic further, parents were surveyed regarding their beliefs about public funding. Specifically, absence of public funding had a substantial impact regarding beliefs about MenB vaccine: 82% of parents agreed that if MenB 'was really an important threat to infants'; if the vaccine was 'really effective (81%); and if the vaccine was 'safe' (74%), then Public Health would fund the MenB vaccine. Hence, public funding adds validity to the importance and value of immunization. In contrast, unfunded vaccines may be perceived as targeting diseases that are less severe, may be viewed as unsafe and are particularly vulnerable to anti-vaccination sentiment (1). Overall, public funding is believed necessary to convey a deep societal commitment to the extraordinary value of childhood immunization in Canada (60), and is anticipated to be a critical factor in influencing acceptance of the 4CMenB vaccine.

Legal issues: ISPA and Canadian Medical Protective Association regulations support immunization against IMD

Recent amendments have been made to Ontario's ISPA to strengthen the protection of school children from vaccine-preventable diseases. Effective July 1, 2014, meningococcal disease, pertussis and varicella have been added as designated diseases requiring proof of immunization for school attendance (or parental request for exemption) (61). The Pediatricians of Ontario support this new ISPA legislation, which clearly demonstrates the Ontario government's commitment to meningitis prevention through vaccination. Specifically, the amendment requires immunization with meningococcal conjugate-C vaccine (no earlier than one year of age), and meningococcal conjugate-ACWY at 12 years of age (grade 7 or above) (62). While 4CMenB immunization has not yet been explicitly legislated, it should be noted that the ISPA was amended in October 2013, before vaccine licensure in December 2013.

In general, the recent ISPA amendments represent tangible progress in terms of ongoing review and alignment of legally mandated vaccines with those routinely recommended by NACI and funded in Ontario (as called for in R4). Interestingly, the Pediatricians of Ontario survey results (Table 1) indicate that R4 had the highest percentage (>95%) of member agreement (ie, 63% strongly agreed; 33% agreed), versus other recommendations ranging from 89% to 92% agreement, suggesting that R4 resonated most deeply with Ontario pediatricians, likely due to challenges in managing questions regarding vaccine requirements, and the accompanying paperwork for school expulsion and re-entry. Furthermore, because the Pediatricians of Ontario position is that the 4CMenB vaccine should be routinely recommended (R1) and publicly funded (R2), we also urge that the vaccine should be added to the list of immunizations

required for school entry (as part of a continuous review and amendment process, R4), to extend protection against future outbreaks of meningococcal disease.

Under current ISPA regulation, parents are likely to be confused about which meningococcal vaccines (ie, against specific serogroups) are included. Moreover, given that the 4CMenB vaccine targets the most prevalent IMD serogroup in Ontario, the rationale for 4CMenB's exclusion from current ISPA regulation will be difficult to explain and, potentially, to legally defend. In addition to recommending that 4CMenB vaccination be legislated, the Pediatricians of Ontario also advocate for public funding of other vaccines in Ontario (R3), including those against hepatitis A and B (administered together); HPV for males; and MenACWY for infants, and similarly, for the inclusion of these immunizations on the list designated under the ISPA.

Another key legal issue is that the Canadian Medical Protective Assoiciation (CMPA) (63) has advised physicians on their obligation to inform parents about new vaccines that are licensed but not publicly funded. If the issue were to come before the courts, 'standard of care' is determined by factors such as: medical publications, common practice of other physicians, and recommendations from governments or professional bodies. CMPA specifies that if a risk is rare, but the potential outcome is severe, there is an obligation to discuss this with patients (63). Hence, a routine recommendation for the 4CMenB vaccine (as called for by the Pediatricians of Ontario; R1) would satisfy one of these conditions. The presence of Ontario legislation mandating vaccination against less prevalent serogroups of IMD may be argued to be another (62). Previous NACI statements identifying the need for a MenB vaccine may also weigh as relevant evidence (21,22). Therefore, even while the vaccine is not yet included in routine vaccination programs, it remains the responsibility of pediatricians, general practitioners and public health officials to educate and advise parents about the vaccine, enabling them to make informed decisions regarding immunization of their children (11). Pediatricians in particular are in a position to recommend 4CMenB vaccination, because infants are at the highest risk.

Political considerations anticipated to be paramount

Given the unpredictability and high media profile surrounding MenB disease, political issues are anticipated to be paramount in determining the priority of 4CMenB vaccine funding in jurisdictional immunization programs. Notably, the WHO has recently issued a guidance document outlining key principles for introducing a new vaccine into publicly funded programs (64). This report indicates that certain diseases, including meningitis (and dengue), may not cause high mortality, but because of the fear they engender among the public and clinicians (due to difficulties with diagnosis and inadequate treatments), as well as the great disruptions caused by outbreaks, such diseases are often ranked as top priorities by political leaders, the medical community and the public. In Canada, there is strong public perception that IMD prevention is a priority. It will be difficult for politicians to resist the plea to introduce 4CMenB vaccine programs to prevent this disease in children and adolescents, especially when vaccine programs already exist for less prevalent serogroups. Indeed, powerful public appeal processes are already in place, as evidenced by the formation of politically active patient advocacy groups, comprised mainly of families affected by meningitis (65,66).

Ethical considerations raised

A number of ethical questions must be raised in the context of introducing the new 4CMenB vaccine. First and foremost, given that IMD is not limited to serogroups A,C,W and Y, for which vaccines are currently available (and funded across many Canadian jurisdictions) (67), is it ethically responsible to not extend protection by implementing routine immunization programs for a vaccine targeting MenB, which is the most common cause of IMD? Second, if a sophisticated breakthrough vaccine against devastating MenB disease has been developed and gained approval as the new standard of care in Canada, does it not follow from an ethics perspective that appropriate immunization programs should be implemented and funded, to avoid future morbidity and mortality in the pediatric population? Finally, from a public health equity standpoint, if access to funded 4CMenB immunization is denied, is it fair to offer vaccination only to wealthy Canadians?

CONCLUSION

The arguments presented herein are intended to assist practicing clinicians in advocating the benefits of 4CMenB vaccination, facilitating recommendations for individual children. However, in addressing the broader public health perspective, the primary intent of the present article is to inform policy and funding decisions, and provide counterbalance to current NACI opinion, surrounding 4CMenB immunization, particularly in targeting Ontario's immunization advisory bodies (eg, Provincial Infectious Disease Advisory Committee/Public Health Ontario). In putting forth R5, we also recommend that pediatricians should seek increased opportunities for direct participation on national (NACI) and jurisdictional immunization advisory committees, to contribute the pediatricians' view as a critical voice in formulating policies regarding IMD immunization and public funding programs.

Ultimately, the Pediatricians of Ontario position underscores the urgent medical need for MenB prevention in reducing childhood mortality and morbidity; we advocate that the new 4CMenB vaccine should be included in Ontario's routine immunization schedule. While we emphasize that the decision to introduce the 4CMenB vaccine should be based on up-to-date, accurate estimates (primarily including local disease epidemiology, vaccine strain coverage and cost effectiveness), we submit that assumptions and/or estimates used in these areas have been conservative in evaluations to date, thus underestimating the true value of 4CMenB immunization. Our view is that public funding for 4CMenB immunization is justified, particularly because routine recommendations and funding are currently in place for meningococcal serogroups that cause significantly less disease in Canada. We propose that Ontario (and other Canadian jurisdictions) must continue to invest in childhood immunization, based not only on past successes, as observed with the MenC vaccine, but also to minimize future disease burden by extending immunization coverage as the most efficient strategy for IMD prevention. Overall, within the context of the rapidly advancing Canadian vaccine landscape, the Pediatricians of Ontario aim to spark discussion and build consensus, particularly regarding funding for vaccines targeting IMD, across a wide audience of policy-makers in the fields of pediatrics, infectious disease, public health and family medicine.

GRANT FUNDING: The January 18, 2014 meeting and publication were funded by an American Academy of Pediatrics Educational Grant, Ontario Chapter (Pediatricians Alliance of Ontario), supported by Novartis.

ACKNOWLEDGEMENTS: From the Educational Grant described above, Dr Cutcliffe received funding for medical writing and manuscript preparation, and Dr Dobson and Dr Gold received honoraria for their presentations at the January 18, 2014 meeting of the Pediatrics Section of the Ontario Medical Association/Pediatricians Alliance of Ontario. The authors gratefully thank Robyn Neville-Kett, Executive Director, Pediatrics Section of the Ontario Medical Association/Pediatricians Alliance of Ontario, for overseeing the grant application process, disbursement of all grant funds, and for her assistance with compiling survey data. They also thank Maria Major, Medical Science Liaison – Vaccines, Novartis Pharmaceuticals Canada Inc, for her contribution to the literature search, including key epidemiology data and figures, in preparing the manuscript.

REFERENCES

1. Scheifele DW, Ward BJ, Halperin SA, McNeil SA, Crowcroft NS, Bjornson G. Approved but non-funded vaccines: Accessing individual protection. Vaccine 2014;32:766-70.
2. Freed GL, Clark SJ, Butchart AT, Singer DC, Davis MM. Sources and perceived credibility of vaccine-safety information for parents. Pediatrics 2011;127(Suppl 1):S107-S12.
3. Pediatrics Section of the Ontario Medical Association (PSOMA). <www.pedsontario.com/about/> (Accessed February 27, 2015).
4. Pediatricians Alliance of Ontario (PAO). <http://pao.tracmed.com/pediatricians-alliance-of-ontario/> (Accessed February 27, 2015).
5. Novartis Press Release. Health Canada approves Bexsero*, the first vaccine available to prevent meningococcal serogroup B (MenB). December 9, 2013. <www.novartis.ca/cs/www.novartis.ca-v2/downloads/en/News/FINAL_Press_Release_Bexsero_12-06-13_E.pdf> (Accessed February 27, 2015).
6. Meningococcal B pilot project task group. The recommended use of the multicomponent meningococcal B (4CMenB) vaccine in Canada: Common guidance statement. March 26, 2014. 1-76.
7. National Advisory Committee on Immunization (NACI), Advice for the use of the multicomponent meningococcal serogroup B (4CMenB) vaccine. April 2014. 1-41. ISBN 978-1-100-23516-5. <http://publications.gc.ca/site/eng/463960/publication.html> (Accessed February 27, 2015).
8. Robinson JL. Immunization for meningococcal serogroup B: What does the practitioner need to know? Paediatr Child Health 2014;19:91-4.
9. Robinson J. What is new from the Canadian Paediatric Society Committee on Infectious Diseases and Immunization? Can J Infect Dis Med Microbiol 2014;25:130-2.
10. Li YA, Tsang R, Desai S, Deehan H. Enhanced surveillance of invasive meningococcal disease in Canada, 2006-2011. Public Health Agency of Canada CCDR 2014;40:160-9. <www.phac-aspc.gc.ca/publicat/ccdr-rmtc/14vol40/dr-rm40-09/dr-rm40-09-surv-eng.php> (Accessed February 27, 2015).
11. Sadarangani M, Bettinger JA, Scheifele DW. How best to describe the risk of meningococcal B infection? Paediatr Child Health 2013;18:543.
12. Dang V, Jamieson F, Wilson S, et al. Epidemiology of serogroup B invasive meningococcal disease in Ontario, Canada, 2000 to 2010. BMC Infect Dis 2012;12:202.
13. Kinlin LM, Jamieson F, Brown EM, et al. Rapid identification of herd effects with the introduction of serogroup C meningococcal conjugate vaccine in Ontario, Canada, 2000–2006. Vaccine 2009;27:1735-40.
14. Bettinger JA, Scheifele DW, Le Saux N, et al. The disease burden of invasive meningococcal serogroup B disease in Canada. Pediatr Infect Dis J 2013;32:e20-e25.
15. World Health Organization. Bacterial Meningitis. <http://apps.who.int/nuvi/meningitis/en/> (Accessed February 27, 2015).
16. World Health Organization. Meningococcal Meningitis. Fact sheet 141. November 2012. <www.who.int/mediacentre/factsheets/fs141/en/index.html> (Accessed February 27, 2015).
17. Joint Committee on Immunisation. JCVI interim position statement on use of Bexsero® meningococcal B vaccine in the UK. July 2013. <www.gov.uk/government/uploads/system/uploads/attachment_data/file/224896/JCVI_interim_statement_on_meningococcal_B_vaccination_for_web.pdf> (Accessed February 27, 2015).
18. Australian Technical Advisory Group on Immunisation (ATAGI) Statement. Advice for immunisation providers regarding the use of Bexsero® – a recombinant multicomponent meningococcal B vaccine (4CMenB). March 2014. <www.immunise.health.gov.au/internet/immunise/publishing.nsf/Content/atagi-advice-bexsero> (Accessed February 27, 2015).
19. FDA News Release. FDA approves a second vaccine to prevent serogroup B meningococcal disease. Jan. 23, 2015. <www.fda.gov/NewsEvents/Newsroom/PressAnnouncements/ucm431370.htm> (Accessed February 27, 2015).
20. Joint Committee on Immunisation. JCVI position statement on use of Bexsero® meningococcal B vaccine in the UK. March 2014. <www.gov.uk/government/uploads/system/uploads/attachment_data/file/294245/JCVI_Statement_on_MenB.pdf> (Accessed February 27, 2015).

21. National Advisory Committee on Immunization (NACI). Statement on recommended use of meningococcal vaccines. CCDR 2001;27(ACS-6):2-36.

22. National Advisory Committee on Immunization (NACI). Update on the Invasive Meningococcal Disease and Meningococcal Vaccine Conjugate Recommendations. CCDR April 2009;35(ACS-3):1-40.

23. Salvadori M, Bortolussi R. Meningococcal vaccines in Canada: An update. Paediatr Child Health 2011;16:485.

24. Agence de la santé et des services sociaux du Saguenay–Lac-Saint-Jean. Communiqué. Campagne de vaccination ciblée contre le méningocoque dans la région du Saguenay–Lac-Saint-Jean. April 22, 2014. <http://santesaglac.com/medias/Vaccination_mening_B/Communique-Meningo-Saglac-22-avril-16h_FINAL.pdf> (Accessed February 27, 2015).

25. Agence de la santé et des services sociaux Québec. Targeted Meningococcal Serogroup B Vaccination Campaign in the Saguenay–Lac-Saint-Jean Region. April 2014. <www.msss.gouv.qc.ca/sujets/santepub/vaccination/index.php?accueil_en> (Accessed February 27, 2015).

26. Acadia University students line up for meningitis vaccinations. CBC News. February 18, 2015. <www.cbc.ca/news/canada/nova-scotia/acadia-university-students-line-up-for-meningitis-vaccinations-1.2961246> (Accessed February 27, 2015).

27. Major M, Moss S, Gold R. From genes to vaccine: A breakthrough in the prevention of meningococcal group B disease. Paediatr Child Health 2011;16:e61.

28. IMPACT. Canadian Immunization Monitoring Program, ACTive. Surveillance. What is IMPACT? <www.cps.ca/en/impact> (Accessed February 27, 2015).

29. Toronto Invasive Bacterial Diseases Network (TIBDN). Surveillance for invasive infection due to Neisseria meningitidis. <http://tibdn.ca/studies/surveillance-meningitidis> (Accessed February 27, 2015).

30. Finne J, Leinonen M, Mäkelä PH. Antigenic similarities between brain components and bacteria causing meningitis: Implications for vaccine development and pathogenesis. Lancet 1983;322:355-7.

31. Bai X, Borrow R. Genetic shifts of Neisseria meningitidis serogroup B antigens and the quest for a broadly cross-protective vaccine. Expert Rev Vaccines 2010;9:1203-17.

32. Rappuoli R. Reverse vaccinology. Curr Opin Microbiol 2000;3:445-50.

33. Frosi G, Biolchi A, Sapio ML, et al. Bactericidal antibody against a representative epidemiological meningococcal serogroup B panel confirms that MATS underestimates 4CMenB vaccine strain coverage. Vaccine 2013;31:4968-74. <www.sciencedirect.com/science/article/pii/S0264410X13010906> (Accessed February 27, 2015).

34. Gossger N, Snape MD, Yu LM, et al. Immunogenicity and tolerability of recombinant serogroup B meningococcal vaccine administered with or without routine infant vaccinations according to different immunization schedules: A randomized controlled trial. JAMA 2012;307:573-82.

35. Vesikari T, Esposito S, Prymula R, al. Immunogenicity and safety of an investigational multicomponent, recombinant, meningococcal serogroup B vaccine (4CMenB) administered concomitantly with routine infant and child vaccinations: Results of two randomised trials. Lancet 2013;381:825-35.

36. Santolaya ME, O'Ryan ML, Valenzuela MT, et al. Immunogenicity and tolerability of a multicomponent meningococcal serogroup B (4CMenB) vaccine in healthy adolescents in Chile: A phase 2b/3 randomised, observer-blind, placebo-controlled study. Lancet 2012;379:617-24.

37. Frasch CE, Borrow R, Donnelly J. Bactericidal antibody is the immunologic surrogate of protection against meningococcal disease. Vaccine 2009;27(Suppl 2):B112-6.

38. Donnelly J, Medini D, Boccadifuoco G, et al. Qualitative and quantitative assessment of meningococcal antigens to evaluate the potential strain coverage of protein-based vaccines. Proc Natl Acad Sci USA 2010;107:19490-5.

39. Australian Government. Department of Health. Therapeutic Goods Administration. AusPAR Attachment 2. Extract from the Clinical Evaluation Report for Multi-Component Meningococcal B vaccine. May 3, 2013.

40. Bettinger JA, Scheifele DW, Halperin SA, et al. Diversity of Canadian meningococcal serogroup B isolates and estimated coverage by an investigational meningococcal serogroup B vaccine (4CMenB). Vaccine 2013;32:124-30.

41. Rappuoli R. The challenge of developing universal vaccines. F1000 Med Rep 2011;3:16.

42. Pitman R, Fisman D, Zaric GS, et al. Dynamic transmission modeling: A report of the ISPOR-SMDM modeling good research practices task force-5. Value Health 2012;15:828-34. <www.ispor.org/workpaper/modeling_methods/dynamic_transmission_modeling-5.pdf> (Accessed February 27, 2015).

43. Delbos V, Lemée L, Bénichou J, et al. Impact of MenBvac, an outer membrane vesicle (OMV) vaccine, on the meningococcal carriage. Vaccine 2013;31:4416-20.

44. Holmes J, Martin D, Ramsay C, Ypma E, Oster P. Combined administration of serogroup B meningococcal vaccine and conjugated serogroup C meningococcal vaccine is safe and immunogenic in college students. Epidemiol Infect 2008;136:790-9.

45. Schuchat A, Messonnier NR. From pandemic suspect to the postvaccine era: The Haemophilus influenzae story. Clin Infect Dis 2007;44:817-9.

46. Kellner JD, Scheifele D, Vanderkooi OG, MacDonald J, Church DL, Tyrrell GJ. Effects of routine infant vaccination with the 7-valent pneumococcal conjugate vaccine on nasopharyngeal colonization with Streptococcus pneumoniae in children in Calgary, Canada. Pediatr Infect Dis J 2008;27:526-32.

47. Fairley CK, Hocking JS, Gurrin LC, Chen MY, Donovan B, Bradshaw C. Rapid decline in presentations of genital warts after the implementation of a national quadrivalent human papillomavirus vaccination programme for young women. Sex Transm Infect 2009;85:499-502.

48. Ali H, Donovan B, Wand H, et al. Genital warts in young Australians five years into national human papillomavirus vaccination programme: National surveillance data. BMJ 2013;346.

49. Glass RI, Patel M, Parashar U. Lessons from the US rotavirus vaccination program. JAMA 2011;306:1701-2.

50. Read R, Baxter D, Chadwick D, et al. Impact of quadrivalent conjugate (MenACWY-CRM) and serogroup B (4CMenB) meningococcal vaccines on meningococcal carriage in English university students (Abst). Meningitis and septicemia in children and adults 2013; London, England. November 2013.

51. Tuite AR, Fisman DN. Number-needed-to-vaccinate calculations: Fallacies associated with exclusion of transmission. Vaccine 2013;31:973-8. <http://dx.doi.org/10.1016/j.vaccine.2012.11.097> (Accessed February 27, 2015).

52. Sanchez IR, Meltzer MI, Shepard C, et al. Economics of an adolescent meningococcal conjugate vaccination catch-up campaign in the United States. Clin Infect Dis 2008;46:1-13.

53. Shepard CW, Ortega-Sanchez IR, Scott RD, Rosenstein NE, the ABCs Team. Cost-effectiveness of conjugate meningococcal vaccination strategies in the United States. Pediatrics 2005;115:1220-32.

54. Centers for Disease Control and Prevention. Serogroup B Meningococcal Vaccine and Outbreaks. <www.cdc.gov/meningococcal/outbreaks/vaccine-serogroupB.html> (Accessed February 27, 2015).

55. Ontario Ministry of Health. Infectious Diseases Protocol. Appendix A: Disease-Specific Chapters. Chapter: Meningococcal disease, invasive. Revised January 2014. <www.health.gov.on.ca/en/pro/programs/publichealth/oph_standards/docs/meningococcal_chapter.pdf> (Accessed February 27, 2015).

56. Erickson L, De Wals P, Farand L. An analytical framework for immunization programs in Canada. Vaccine 2005;23:2470-6.

57. Stanley M. Perspective: Vaccinate boys too. Nature 2012;488:S10.

58. Public Health Agency of Canada. Survey of Parents on Key Issues Related to Immunization. EKOS Research Associates Inc. September 2011. <http://resources.cpha.ca/immunize.ca/data/1792e.pdf> (Accessed February 27, 2015).

59. Fisher W, Bettinger J, Gilca V, et al. Understanding the impact of approved but unfunded vaccine status on parental acceptance of a novel meningococcal sergroup B vaccine for infants (Abst 0351). 32nd Meeting of the European Society for Paediatric Infectious Diseases (ESPID); Dublin, Ireland. May 8, 2014.

60. Scheifele DW, Halperin SA, Bettinger JA. Childhood immunization rates in Canada are too low: UNICEF. Pediatr Child Health 2014;19:237-8.

61. Toronto Public Health Communique. May 2014. Issue 32. <http://www1.toronto.ca/City%20Of%20Toronto/Toronto%20 Public%20Health/Health%20Professionals/Files/pdf/C/ CommuniqueMay2014Web.pdf> CommuniqueMay2014Web.pdf> (Accessed February 27, 2015).

62. Government of Ontario. Immunization of School Pupils Act. R.R.O. 1990. REGULATION 645. <www.e-laws.gov.on.ca/html/ regs/english/elaws_regs_900645_e.htm> (Accessed February 27, 2015).

63. Canadian Medical Protective Association (CMPA). January 2009 (IS0887-E). New vaccines – What are your obligations? An article for physicians by physicians. <www.cmpa-acpm.ca/safety/-/asset_ publisher/N6oEDMrzRbCC/content/new-vaccines-what-are-your-obligations> (Accessed February 27, 2015).

64. World Health Organization. Principles and considerations for adding a vaccine to a national immunization programme – from decision to implementation and monitoring. April 2014. <www.who.int/immunization/documents/general/ ISBN_978_92_4_15068_92/en/> (Accessed February 27, 2015).

65. Meningitis Research Foundation of Canada. <www.meningitis.ca/ en/Home.aspx> (Accessed February 27, 2015).

66. Meningitis Relief. <www.meningitisrelief.com/home.html> (Accessed February 27, 2015).

67. National Advisory Committee on Immunization (NACI). Update on the use of quadrivalent conjugate meningococcal vaccines. CCDR. January 2013;39(ACS-1):1-40. <www.phac-aspc.gc.ca/ publicat/ccdr-rmtc/13vol39/acs-dcc-1/index-eng.php> (Accessed February 27, 2015).

41

Urinary tract infection diagnosis and response to therapy in long-term care: A prospective observational study

Peter Daley MD MSc FRCPC DTM+H[1], Carla Penney BSc[1], Susan Wakeham BSc[1], Glenda Compton MN RN[2], Aaron McKim MD CCFP[2], Judy O'Keefe MSW RSW[2], Brendan Barrett MD FRCPC[1], Lindsay Nicolle MD FRCPC[3]

P Daley, C Penney, S Wakeham, et al. Urinary tract infection diagnosis and response to therapy in long-term care: A prospective observational study. Can J Infect Dis Med Microbiol 2015;26(3):133-136.

BACKGROUND: The prevalence of asymptomatic bacteriuria among residents of long-term care (LTC) facilities is high, and is a source of inappropriate antibiotic prescription.
OBJECTIVE: To establish symptoms and signs associated with a positive urine culture, and to determine whether antibiotic therapy is associated with functional improvement.
METHODS: A total of 101 LTC patients were prospectively observed after submission of urine for culture.
RESULTS: The culture positivity rate was consistent with the expected asymptomatic bacteriuria rate. Change in mental status and male sex were associated with culture positivity. Treatment decisions were not consistent with culture results. Treatment did not lead to improvement in activities of daily living scores at two days or seven days.
DISCUSSION: Significant growth cannot be well predicted based on clinical variables; thus, the decision to submit urine is somewhat arbitrary. Because urine culture testing and treatment does not lead to functional improvement, restricting access to the test may be reasonable.
CONCLUSION: Urine culture testing in LTC facilities does not lead to functional improvement.

Key Words: *Antibiotic stewardship; Asymptomatic bacteriuria; Diagnosis; Long-term care; Urinary tract infection*

Le diagnostic d'infection urinaire et la réponse au traitement en soins de longue durée : une étude d'observation prospective

HISTORIQUE : La prévalence de bactériuries asymptomatiques est élevée chez les résidents d'établissements de soins de longue durée (SLD). Elle suscite la prescription inappropriée d'antibiotiques.
OBJECTIF : Déterminer les signes et symptômes associés à une culture d'urine positive et établir si l'antibiothérapie favorise une amélioration fonctionnelle.
MÉTHODOLOGIE : Au total, 101 patients en SLD ont fait l'objet d'une observation prospective après l'envoi d'un prélèvement d'urine pour culture.
RÉSULTATS : Le taux de cultures positives était conforme au taux prévu de bactériuries asymptomatiques. La détérioration de l'état mental et le sexe masculin s'associaient à des cultures positives. Les décisions thérapeutiques n'étaient pas en accord avec les résultats des cultures. Le traitement ne suscitait pas d'amélioration à l'indice d'activités de la vie quotidienne au bout de deux ou sept jours.
EXPOSÉ : Les variables cliniques ne permettent pas de prévoir une croissance importante. Ainsi, la décision de faire une culture d'urine est quelque peu arbitraire. Puisque les cultures d'urine et le traitement n'assurent pas d'amélioration fonctionnelle, il est peut-être raisonnable de restreindre l'accès aux analyses.
CONCLUSION : Dans les établissements de SLD, les analyses d'urine ne favorisent pas d'amélioration fonctionnelle.

Urinary tract infection (UTI) is a common diagnosis among residents in long-term care (LTC) settings, and a common reason to prescribe antibiotics. The annual prevalence of antibiotic use in LTC is high – between 47% and 79% (1), or 5.9% of all residents on a given day (2). The rate of antibiotic use without adequate clinical rationale has been reported to be as high as 38% in 42 facilities (3) and 42% in one facility (4).

Attention to antimicrobial stewardship through appropriate antibiotic use can reduce drug costs (5), and can reduce *Clostridium difficile* diarrhea rates in LTC (6). For these reasons, LTC is an appropriate population in which to study antibiotic stewardship and to intervene to improve use. A cluster randomized study has shown that implementing consensus treatment guidelines for UTI in LTC can reduce antibiotic consumption for UTI (7).

Residents of LTC facilities without indwelling urinary catheters have a prevalence of asymptomatic bacteriuria (>10^8 colony-forming units/L) of approximately 40% (8). Screening for or treatment of asymptomatic bacteriuria is not associated with reduction in mortality (8-10), and may contribute to inappropriate antibiotic use, which drives the selection of antibiotic resistance among bacteria in the patient's resident flora (11).

Among LTC residents with a change in clinical status, positive urine culture is often interpreted as the cause, leading to overdiagnosis of UTI. In a recent prospective study involving 399 clinically suspected UTI episodes, there was very poor correlation among symptoms, urine culture results and the decision to use antibiotics (12). A multivariate logistic regression for factors associated with bacteriuria and pyuria revealed that dysuria, change in character of urine and change in mental status were statistically associated with bacteriuria and pyuria, although associations were weak (RR 1.38 to 1.58). Clearly, the diagnosis and treatment of UTI in LTC is not simple or consistent, and evidence to guide the decision to collect urine culture is not available.

[1]*Memorial University;* [2]*Long-Term Care, Eastern Health, St John's, Newfoundland and Labrador;* [3]*University of Manitoba, Winnipeg, Manitoba*
Correspondence: Dr Peter Daley, Room 1J421, Health Sciences Center, 300 Prince Phillip Drive, Saint John's, Newfoundland and Labrador A1B 3V6. e-mail pkd336@mun.ca

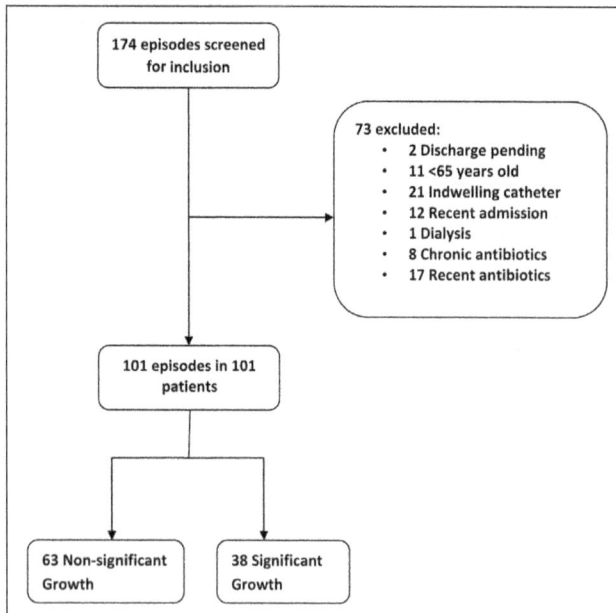

Figure 1) *Participant recruitment*

TABLE 1
Demographic characteristics

Characteristic (n=101)	
Age, years, mean ± SD	84.0±8.6
Female sex, %	79.2
Number of comorbidities, mean ± SD	1.8±1.0
Dementia	58 (57.4)
Stroke	13 (12.9)
Liver disease	1 (1.0)
Depression	41 (40.6)
Kidney disease	12 (11.9)
Diabetes	25 (24.8)
Cancer	9 (8.9)
Chronic obstructive pulmonary disease	15 (14.9)
Baseline ADL score, mean ± SD (independent = 0, total dependence = 28)	11.9±8.7
Mental status in past seven days	
Disorganized speech	12 (11.9)
Altered perception	19 (18.8)
Unresponsiveness	1 (1.0)
Lethargy	19 (18.8)

Data presented as n (%) unless otherwise indicated. ADL Activities of daily living

Confounding the assessment of the relationship between these three clinical variables and positive laboratory results is the fact that clinical decline, for various reasons, can lead to dehydration, causing a change in character of urine and change in mental status. These signs are often considered to be the result of a UTI (rather than dehydration) and treated as such. Residents with cognitive impairment are more likely to have positive urine cultures (8) and are also more vulnerable to delirium, which frequently leads clinicians to interpret a causal relationship between changes in mentation and bacteriuria. To date, no study has considered the clinical outcome after antibiotic therapy to validate the diagnostic criteria. We performed a prospective observational efficacy study to identify symptoms associated with a positive urine culture, and assessed clinical response to antibiotic therapy.

METHODS

Six LTC facilities in St John's, Newfoundland and Labrador, ranging from 40 beds to 377 beds, were selected for inclusion based on their high urine culture submission rates. Consecutive urine samples received in the central microbiology laboratory from these LTC facilities between June 24 and July 17, 2013 and between January 20 and March 20, 2014 were identified, and a research associate visited the relevant facility on the day of submission. Receipt of urine for culture was considered to be evidence that nursing staff suspected UTI. Exclusion criteria were applied as follows:

- Not anticipated to remain in the nursing home for LTC (ie, short-term residents or pending discharge);
- Anticipated life expectancy <4 weeks as assessed by nursing staff;
- <65 years of age;
- Indwelling catheter or surgical urinary collection device;
- Current renal dialysis;
- Current anti-infective therapy for any reason;
- Resided in the nursing home for <4 weeks (providers did not have adequate time to determine resident's baseline functional status).

The study was approved by local health research ethics authority to approach nursing staff for consent to participate. Consent forms and study information sheets were circulated to LTC facilities before the study. The nurse (or delegate) who collected the urine specimen was identified and interviewed on the day of collection, and again after two days and five to seven days. Patient information, including

comorbidity and baseline functional capacity (28-point activities of daily living [ADL] scale including mobility in bed, transfers, locomotion, dressing, toileting, personal hygiene and feeding, and four-point mental status scale [12]), was collected from the nurse. The patient, the family, the caregivers and the attending physician were not interviewed. Urine culture was performed quantitatively, according to laboratory protocol.

Univariate logistic regression was performed using SPSS version 20.0 (IBM Corporation, USA) to determine whether nurse-reported clinical symptoms were associated with the primary outcome: growth of at least 10^8 colony-forming units/L of uropathogenic bacteria in urine culture. Symptoms and functional status were described over time. Change in ADL score over time was analyzed using a paired-samples t test (two-sided).

Variable(s) considered to be potentially predictive of significant growth included demographic characteristics (age, sex, LTC facility, total comorbidities), reasons for collection (change in mental status, change in behaviour, change in character of urine, fever, change in gait or fall, change in voiding pattern, flank pain, patient or family request, abnormal laboratory test result, dysuria, change in functional status, previous UTI, malaise), baseline functional capabilities (ADL score, disorganized speech in the past seven days, altered perception in the past seven days, unresponsive episodes in the past seven days and lethargy in the past seven days), and nurse-reported symptoms (fever, change in behaviour, change in mental status, diarrhea, abdominal pain, shortness of breath, weakness, dysuria, change in character of urine, change in frequency of urination and flank pain). Variables with ≤2 positive responses were removed (change in functional status, change in gait or fall, results of other workup performed, other concurrent infection, dehydration, shortness of breath, syncope, diarrhea, baseline unresponsiveness, cough).

RESULTS

A total of 174 urine specimens were considered, and 101 episodes from 101 patients were observed (Figure 1). Thirty-eight (37.6%) of 101 episodes demonstrated significant growth of bacteria in urine. In 36.6% of episodes, the nurse making the decision to collect urine was interviewed; in other episodes, alternate nurses also familiar with the patient were interviewed. Patient demographics are summarized in Table 1. The mean (± SD) age was 84.0±8.6 years, 79.2% were women and there were a mean of 1.8±1.0 comorbidities per patient. Baseline

TABLE 2
Reasons for urine culture collection (n=101)

Clinical reason	n (%)
Change in behaviour	35 (34.7)
Dysuria	31 (30.7)
Change in character of urine	30 (29.7)
Change in mental status	26 (25.7)
Change in voiding pattern	21 (20.8)
Other reason	14 (13.9)
Patient or family request	11 (10.9)
Previous urinary tract infection	11 (10.9)
Flank pain	8 (7.9)
Malaise	6 (5.9)
Fever or chills	5 (5.0)
Abnormal laboratory test result	4 (4.0)
Change in gait or fall	3 (3.0)
Change in functional status	1 (1.0)

ADL score was 11.9±8.7, with zero representing total independence and 28 representing total dependence.

Predefined reasons for urine collection ranged from one to seven reasons (mean 2.0 reasons), and are listed in descending order of frequency in Table 2. The previously described significant clinical predictors (dysuria, change in character of urine and change in mental status) were among the most common reasons. Other reasons for collection included pyuria (n=4 patients), hyperglycemia (n=2), test of cure (n=1), urine retention (n=1), hematuria (n=1), "routine checkup" (n=1), abdominal pain (n=1), previous sample mixed growth (n=1) and doctor's request (n=1).

Most episodes did not have adequate record of vital signs or blood testing performed to apply published diagnostic criteria. Body temperature was measured for eight (7.9%) episodes, blood pressure was measured for six (5.9%) episodes, a dipstick test was performed for 25 (24.8%) episodes and a complete blood count was obtained for 16 (15.8%) episodes. Among 38 urine specimens with significant growth, 25 (65.8%) grew *Escherichia coli*, five (10.5%) grew *Proteus* species, four (13.2%) grew *Klebsiella* species, three (7.9%) grew *Enterococcus* species and one (2.6%) grew yeast.

Using univariate regression, there were two predictors that were significantly associated with the outcome (male sex, RR 5.58 [95% CI 1.23 to 25.43]; and change in mental status, RR 13.83 [95% CI 1.81 to 105.81]). Change in character of urine approached significance (RR 14.51 [95% CI 0.66 to 320.71]) (Table 3).

Antibiotic treatment was given in 48 of 101 (47.5%) episodes (Table 4). Treatment decision did not correlate well with significant growth (kappa = 0.44). Nineteen (40%) of 48 of antibiotic prescriptions were given to patients without significant growth, and nine (17.0%) of 53 episodes with significant growth were not treated. Using univariate regression, no clinical or demographic variables were associated with the decision to treat. Significant growth was predictive of the decision to treat (RR 40.01 [95% CI 4.00 to 401.53]). Mean time between collection and treatment was 1.44 days (range eight days before collection to 10 days after collection). In 21 (43.8%) of 48 cases treated, treatment was given before preliminary culture results were provided. Among episodes with significant growth that were treated, four (14.3%) of 28 patients were given an antibiotic to which the bacteria was reported to be resistant.

ADL score at baseline (before decompensation prompting urine collection) was compared with ADL score at 48 h (the time period required for culture results to become available), and ADL score at five days (resolution of episode), in groups based on significant growth and treatment (Table 5). There was no significant difference observed in any group between baseline and 48 h, or between 48 h and five to seven days.

TABLE 3
Univariate correlation of predictors with significant growth (n=38 of 101 episodes)

Characteristic	n	RR	95% CI	P
Age	101	0.99	0.93–1.06	0.79
Male sex	21	5.58	1.23–25.43	0.026
Total comorbidities	101	0.87	0.53–1.47	0.61
Long-term care facility	101	1.39	0.95–2.02	0.087
Stated reason for urine collection				
Fever	5	0.00		1.0
Change in voiding pattern	21	16.70	0.16–1754.36	0.24
Patient or family request	11	0.12	0.007–1.91	0.13
Abnormal laboratory test result	4	2.85	0.16–51.27	0.48
Previous urinary tract infection	11	1.28	0.19–8.48	0.80
Baseline functional capacity				
Baseline ADL score	101	1.03	0.97–1.10	0.38
Baseline disorganized speech	12	1.02	0.14–7.59	0.97
Baseline altered perception	19	0.36	0.05–2.60	0.31
Baseline periods of lethargy	19	4.20	0.91–19.37	0.065
New symptoms				
Change in behaviour	32	3.41	0.11–104.90	0.48
Change in mental status	37	13.83	1.81–105.81	0.011
Abdominal pain	10	0.68	0.083–5.60	0.72
Weakness	10	0.90	0.026–30.91	0.95
Worsening in ADL score	4	0.00		1.0
Dysuria	32	2.10	0.14–32.13	0.60
Change in character of urine	30	14.51	0.66–320.71	0.090
Flank pain	9	infinity		1.0
Change in frequency of urination	23	0.079	0.002–2.62	0.16

ADL Activities of daily living

TABLE 4
Treatment decision

	Growth		
Treatment decision	Significant	Nonsignificant	Total
Antibiotic prescribed	29 (60)	19 (40)*	48
Antibiotic not prescribed	9 (17)*	44 (83)	53
Total	38	63	101

*Data presented as n or n (%). *Inappropriate treatment decision*

DISCUSSION

The objective of the present study was to identify the symptoms or signs associated with the nurse's (or delegate's) decision to submit urine for culture, and to assess the clinical response to antibiotic therapy. We found two predictors of significant growth (male sex and change in mental status). Most examined clinical indicators were not significantly predictive of positive culture. A sex difference may have been related to a cleaner urine collection among males, leading to less mixed growth, or reflect patterns of urine collection among nurses.

Our study had significant limitations. Because of the small sample size, CIs for RRs were very wide. We considered input from nurses only, and family or physicians may have had different perceptions of clinical symptoms and signs. However, nurses in LTC make the decision to collect urine specimens. We were not able to interview the nurse who collected the specimen in many cases because that individual had finished the work shift. Nurses working on the next shift may not have completely understood the reasons for urine collection.

Our study demonstrates that the application of surveillance diagnostic criteria developed for LTC may be difficult, due to the lack of patient investigation performed in the LTC setting.

Consistent with previous studies (13), the observed rate of significant growth among patients with urine collected (38%) closely matches published rates of asymptomatic bacteriuria in this population

TABLE 5
Change in activities of daily living (ADL) score*

Group	n	Mean ADL, baseline	Mean ADL, 48 h	P, baseline to 48 h	Mean ADL, 5–7 days	P, 48 h to 5–7 days
Culture positive, treated	28	11.5	12.2	0.30	12.2	No difference
Culture positive, not treated	9	17.6	16.4	0.35	16.4	No difference
Culture negative, treated	18	12.1	12.1	No difference	12.1	No difference
Culture negative, not treated	44	10.9	11.2	0.29	11.3	0.34

Zero represents total independence, 28 represents total dependence

(40% [8]), indicating that clinical suspicion has no predictive capacity. Pretest probability in the symptomatic patient equals pretest probability in the asymptomatic patient, meaning the clinical suspicion of the diagnosis of UTI is not contributory. The present study did not include patients with indwelling catheters, among whom the rate of bacteriuria would be expected to be higher.

Urine culture results did not influence physician prescription decisions because physicians chose to treat culture-negative patients, to not treat culture-positive patients, to treat before culture results, and to use antibiotics to which the laboratory reported the organisms to be resistant.

Furthermore, we observed no functional improvement from antibiotic treatment. ADL scores did not change over two days or seven days in any treatment group. Using this functional status outcome, neither the test result nor the therapy led to clinical benefit. Without a randomized design, culture-positive and culture-negative patients may have been different before the study began; thus, this estimate may be biased. Culture-positive patients who were not treated had worse ADL scores at baseline, suggesting that lower functioning patients may be selected for no treatment because of a poor prognosis. Although predictors for significant growth may be defined by observational studies, if treatment of significant growth does not lead to clinical improvement, then significant growth is not a suitable outcome. Further research should define UTI diagnostic criteria based on clinical benefit following successful treatment.

The present study was the first to observe clinical outcomes as a measure of effectiveness of diagnosis and treatment for UTI in LTC.

An editorial has suggested that there is adequate equipoise to propose a randomized trial comparing delayed antibiotic therapy with immediate antibiotic therapy, or comparing hydration to antibiotic therapy (14). A further suggestion to randomly assign LTC patients to management with urine culture or no urine culture appears to be reasonable. Further research regarding clinical outcomes is needed, including the effect of urine culture testing on mortality.

A laboratory policy to provide urine culture testing services only to selected LTC patients may reduce antibiotic consumption, although if physicians treat without culture results, this reduction would not be achieved. Requiring physicians to call the laboratory to receive urine culture reports reduced inappropriate treatment for asymptomatic bacteriuria among inpatients by 36% (15), suggesting that laboratory policy interventions may influence antimicrobial use significantly. At the same time, investigations such as blood culture could be encouraged. Blood culture results have greater specificity for infection and influence therapy more directly.

AUTHOR CONTRIBUTIONS: PD: proposal, ethics, analysis, manuscript; CP: data collection, analysis; SW: data collection; BB: manuscript editing; LN: manuscript editing.

REFERENCES

1. van Buul LW, van der Steen JT, Veenhuizen RB, et al. Antibiotic use and resistance in long term care facilities. J Am Med Dir Assoc 2012;13:568.e1-13.
2. Daneman N, Gruneir A, Newman A, et al. Antibiotic use in long-term care facilities. J Antimicrobial Chemother 2011;66:2856-63.
3. Zimmer JG, Bentley DW, Valenti WM, Watson NM. Systemic antibiotic use in nursing homes. A quality assessment. J Am Geriatr Soc 1986;34:703-10.
4. Peron EP, Hirsch AA, Jury LA, Jump RL, Donskey CJ. Another setting for stewardship: High rate of unnecessary antimicrobial use in a veterans affairs long-term care facility. J Am Geriatr Soc 2013;61:289-90.
5. Goff DA. Antimicrobial stewardship: Bridging the gap between quality care and cost. Curr Opin Infect Dis 2011;24(Suppl 1):S11-20.
6. Brakovich B, Bonham E, Vanbrackle L. War on the spore: *Clostridium difficile* disease among patients in a long-term acute care hospital. J Healthc Qual 2013;35:15-21
7. Loeb M, Brazil K, Lohfeld L, et al. Effect of a multifaceted intervention on number of antimicrobial prescriptions for suspected urinary tract infections in residents of nursing homes: Cluster randomised controlled trial. BMJ 2005;331:669.
8. Nicolle LE. Asymptomatic bacteriuria in the elderly. Infect Dis Clin North Am 1997;11:647-62.

9. Nicolle LE, Bjornson J, Harding GK, MacDonell JA. Bacteriuria in elderly institutionalized men. N Engl J Med 1983;309:1420-5.
10. Abrutyn E, Mossey J, Berlin JA, et al. Does asymptomatic bacteriuria predict mortality and does antimicrobial treatment reduce mortality in elderly ambulatory women? Ann Intern Med 1994;120:827-33.
11. Loeb M, Bentley DW, Bradley S, et al. Development of minimum criteria for the initiation of antibiotics in residents of long-term-care facilities: Results of a consensus conference. Infect Control Hosp Epidemiol 2001;22:120-4.
12. Juthani-Mehta M, Quagliarello V, Perrelli E, Towle V, Van Ness PH, Tinetti M. Clinical features to identify urinary tract infection in nursing home residents: A cohort study. J Am Geriatr Soc 2009;57:963-70.
13. Juthani-Mehta M, Tinetti M, Perrelli E, Towle V, Van Ness PH, Quagliarello V. Diagnostic accuracy of criteria for urinary tract infection in a cohort of nursing home residents. J Am Geriatr Soc 2007;55:1072-7.
14. Nicolle LE. Symptomatic urinary tract infection in nursing home residents. J Am Geriatr Soc 2009;57:1113-4.
15. Leis JA, Rebick GW, Daneman N, et al. Reducing antimicrobial therapy for asymptomatic bacteriuria among noncatheterized inpatients: A proof-of-concept study. Clin Infect Dis 2014;58:980-3.

42

Exogenous endophthalmitis caused by *Enterococcus casseliflavus*: A case report and discussion regarding treatment of intraocular infection with vancomycin-resistant enterococci

Byron M Berenger MD[1,2], Shobhana Kulkarni MD[3,4], Brad J Hinz MD[5], Sarah E Forgie MD[1,6]

BM Berenger, S Kulkarni, BJ Hinz, SE Forgie. Exogenous endophthalmitis caused by *Enterococcus casseliflavus*: A case report and discussion regarding treatment of intraocular infection with vancomycin-resistant enterococci. Can J Infect Dis Med Microbiol 2015;26(6):330-332.

BACKGROUND: Endophthalmitis caused by enterococci is rare, and cases involving vancomycin-resistant enterococci are even more so. Due to the poor bioavailability of many antibiotics in the vitreous chamber, special considerations are required when choosing antibiotics to treat these infections. The authors report the first case of exogenous endophthalmitis caused by *Enterococcus casseliflavus* via the unique mechanism of high-velocity water stream trauma from a toy water gun.

A previously healthy four-year old boy presented with endophthalmitis of the left eye after injury from a water gun. Empirical treatment for endophthalmitis was started on presentation to the ophthalmologist. After the identification of the pathogen and a review of the literature, the antibiotic regimen was changed to include intravitreal ampicillin and amikacin with systemic linezolid.

Endophthalmitis caused by *E casseliflavus* and other vancomycin-resistant enterococci are challenging to treat. Rapid identification of vancomycin-resistant enterococcal endophthalmitis is important to guide appropriate antibiotic therapy. Systemic linezolid achieves excellent intravitreal concentrations, and should be used in combination with intravitreal and topical antibiotics.

Key Words: *Endophthalmitis*; Enterococcus; Enterococcus casseliflavus; Vancomycin-resistant

L'endophtalmie exogène attribuable à l'*Enterococcus casseliflavus* : rapport de cas et exposé sur le traitement de l'infection intra-oculaire par des entérocoques résistant à la vancomycine

HISTORIQUE : L'endophtalmie est rarement attribuable aux entérocoques, et les cas découlant d'entérocoques résistant à la vancomycine le sont encore plus. Étant donné la piètre biodisponibilité de nombreux antibiotiques dans la cavité vitréenne, il faut tenir compte de facteurs particuliers lors de la sélection du traitement de ces infections. Les auteurs présentent le premier cas d'endophtalmie exogène causée par une *Enterococcus casseliflavus* contractée après un traumatisme imputable au mécanisme unique de jet d'eau à grande vitesse propulsé par un pistolet à eau.

Un garçon de quatre ans auparavant en santé a consulté à cause d'une endophtalmie de l'œil gauche après une blessure contractée par un pistolet à eau. L'ophtalmologiste a prescrit un traitement empirique dès la consultation. Après avoir confirmé l'agent pathogène et analysé les publications, il a modifié la posologie antibiotique pour inclure de l'ampicilline intravitréenne et de l'amikacine combinée à de la linézolide systémique.

L'endophtalmie causée par l'*E casseliflavus* et d'autres entérocoques résistant à la vancomycine est difficile à traiter. Il est important de déceler rapidement l'endophtalmie par entérocoque résistant à la vancomycine pour orienter l'antibiothérapie. La linézolide systémique, qui assure d'excellentes concentrations intravitréennes, devrait être combinée à des antibiotiques intravitréens et topiques.

Endophthalmitis is caused by the introduction of a pathogen into the intraocular space via trauma, ocular surgery, or direct extension of a superficial eye infection (exogenous endophthalmitis) or hematogenously (endogenous endophthalmitis). Endophthalmitis caused by vancomycin-resistant enterococci (VRE) is rare, described in only a few published case reports. One type of VRE, *Enterococcus casseliflavus* is inherently resistant to vancomycin due to the chromosomally encoded *vanC* gene, and has been reported once as a cause of endogenous endophthalmitis (1,2). We report the first case of exogenous endophthalmitis caused by *E casseliflavus* via the unique mechanism of high-velocity water stream trauma from a toy water gun.

For VRE infections, ampicillin or amoxicillin are reasonable antibiotic choices if the isolate is susceptible. In the absence of high-level aminoglycoside resistance, ampicillin may be combined with an aminoglycoside for a synergistic effect (3). Other clinically available antibiotics with activity against VRE include: linezolid, daptomycin and tigecycline (4,5).

Treatment of bacterial endophthalmitis is difficult due to the severe and rapid retinal damage that occurs as a result of bacterial growth and inflammatory response, and it involves a combination of intravitreal and systemic antibiotics with vitrectomy (6). Although there is a lack of strong evidence supporting an added benefit of systemic antibiotics, they are recommended in severe cases of endophthalmitis and routinely for exogenous endophthalmitis (6,7). Poor penetration of systemic or topical antibiotics into the vitreous chamber makes administration of antibiotics to prevent further bacterial growth challenging, especially in the context of resistant organisms such as VRE.

CASE PRESENTATION

A previously healthy, fully immunized, four-year-old boy, with no previous visual issues, presented with endophthalmitis of the left eye. He and his siblings had been playing with water guns several hours before presentation, and water was squirted into his eye. The water was from

---

[1]Department of Medical Microbiology and Immunology, University of Alberta; [2]Alberta Provincial Laboratory for Public Health; [3] DynaLIFE[Dx] Diagnostic Laboratory Services; [4]Department of Laboratory Medicine and Pathology; [5]Department of Ophthamology; [6]Department of Pediatrics, University of Alberta, Edmonton, Alberta
Correspondence: Dr Sarah Forgie, Department of Pediatrics, Edmonton Clinic Health Academy, 3-558D 11405 87 Avenue, Edmonton, Alberta T6G 2J3. e-mail s.forgie@ualberta.ca

a wading pool that had been filled with tap water the same day. The child experienced acute onset of pain and, approximately 2 h later, reported 'white dots' obscuring his vision. Six hours after the initial insult, his mother noticed that his left cornea was cloudy and his conjunctiva was red. He was immediately taken to his local hospital and assessed promptly by the local ophthalmologist. His pupils were asymmetric, his conjunctiva was injected on the left and there was corneal opacity. The remainder of his physical examination was unremarkable. Given the mechanism of the injury, the diagnosis was not clear, and the ophthalmologist transferred him to a tertiary eye care centre 5 h away for further management. The child presented to the tertiary care centre with severe anterior chamber inflammation, miosis and inferior hypopyon. The vitreous cavity was filled with purulent debris with no view of the fundus. B-scan ultrasonography revealed vitritis with no foreign body. Given the unusual mechanism of injury, it was not clear whether this was endophthalmitis or a severe inflammatory response to trauma. The Retina Service was consulted and, after assessment, the child was scheduled for surgery

Approximately 26 h after the injury, the child underwent anterior chamber exploration and pars plana vitrectomy. Vitrectomy allowed visualization of white retinal infiltrates and the absence of a foreign body. After vitrectomy wash out, the vitreous chamber was injected with 1 mg vancomycin, 2.25 mg ceftazidime and 1 mg dexamethasone (routine drugs administered for exogenous endophthalmitis) (8). Topical and systemic medications were also administered including: one drop 0.5% moxifloxacin hourly, one drop 1% prednisolone daily, one drop 2% homatropine every 12 h, 30 mg/kg/day oral ciprofloxacin divided every 12 h and 60 mg/kg/day intravenous vancomycin divided every 6 h.

Gram stain of the vitreous fluid revealed >25 polymorphonuclear leukocytes and >25 Gram-positive cocci in pairs and chains (intracellular and extracellular) per 1000× field. After 18 h of incubation on blood agar, there was growth of yellow-pigmented, alpha-hemolytic colonies, which were Gram-positive cocci in pairs and chains. Mass spectrometry (Vitek MS BioMérieux, France) identified the organism as *E casseliflavus* (99.9% certainty) within 45 min. The medical microbiologist was immediately alerted of the identification of this intrinsically vancomycin-resistant organism and treatment options were discussed with the pediatric infectious disease and ophthalmology physicians.

The discussion prompted an immediate return to the operating room for additional intravitreal antibiotics and a repeat vitreous washout. Using the local antibiogram for this organism, published susceptibilities and the experience of Hillier et al (9,10) treating an *E gallinarum* endophthalmitis secondary to a metallic foreign body, the treatment plan consisted of intravitreal ampicillin (50 mg) and amikacin (400 mg), as well as intravenous ampicillin (300 mg/kg/day divided every 6 h). Topical treatment consisted of 0.3% gentamicin (one drop four times per day) and 1% prednisolone (one drop four times per day). Twelve hours after the antibiotic change to ampicillin, linezolid (30 mg/kg/day divided every 8 h) was added. Systemic and topical antimicrobials were continued for 14 days. Table 1 summarized the antibiotic susceptibilities.

The patient was closely monitored in the ophthalmology clinic. The hypopyon did not recur and the vitreous cavity remained opaque with no view of the fundus at 10 days after the initial anterior chamber washout with vitrectomy. The visual acuity began to decrease three weeks postincident; however, clinical examination did not support repeat infection and it was likely due to development of outer cortical vitreous separation causing vitreous debris. Over time, the vitreous cavity and anterior segment cleared, and vision improved to 20/400 at seven weeks, 20/400 at 17 weeks and 20/70 at 16 months postincident.

DISCUSSION

The present case highlights the importance of interdisciplinary medical care, and the effective use of laboratory technology to assure early and appropriate antimicrobial treatment. Rapid identification of this isolate was achieved using mass spectrometry, a process that previously would take 8 h to 12 h. In addition, effective communication between the

TABLE 1

Susceptibilities of the *Enterococcus casseliflavus* isolate compared with EUCAST and CLSI breakpoints

Antibiotic	Isolate MIC	Interpretation	EUCAST[†]	CLSI[‡]
Ampicillin	≤2	Sensitive	≤4	≤8
Vancomycin	4	Resistant*	≤4	≤4
Gentamicin synergy	N/A	Sensitive	≤128	≤500
Linezolid	2	Sensitive	≤4	≤2

*Data presented as µg/mL. Minimum inhibitory concentrations (MICs) were determined using the Vitek 2, GP 67 card (BioMérieux, France). Vitek 2 reports gentamicin synergy as sensitive or resistant without an MIC. *Vancomycin was reported resistant due to the intrinsic carriage of VanC in E casseliflavus. †Data adapted from reference 7. ‡Data adapted from reference 6. CLSI Clinical Laboratory Standards Institute; EUCAST European Committee on Antimicrobial Susceptibility Testing; N/A Not available*

medical microbiologist and the clinical team allowed prompt treatment changes. This stresses the importance of interdisciplinary teams in the health care environment, especially when dealing with challenging infections such as VRE endophthalmitis.

Early vitrectomy is an important component for treating severe endogenous or postsurgical endophthalmitis, and is routinely performed for exogenous endophthalmitis because it improves outcomes and enhances clearance of bacteria, inflammatory cells and debris (6,8). During vitrectomy, iatrogenic complications such as retinal detachment may occur; therefore, repeat vitrectomy is avoided unless intravitreal debris persist (8,11). In our case, vitrectomy was performed in an acceptable time frame given that the child came from a rural area and the initial diagnosis was initially ambiguous. Repeat vitreous washout and the administration of additional intravitreal antibiotics was performed because VRE was isolated and it was resistant to the initial intravitreal antibiotic regimen.

In exogenous endophthalmitis, vision is restored to 20/40 or better in 15% to 40% of cases and, in acute postoperative endophthalmitis, approximately 50% have visual acuity of 20/40 or better and 15% to 36% have visual acuity of 20/200 (6). Therefore, the outcome in the present case (visual acuity of 20/70) is acceptable given that the treatment of VRE is challenging, especially when the infection is in the vitreous chamber where there is poor penetration of systemic or topical antibiotics.

There are no published data regarding the penetration of ampicillin into the human vitreous chamber. Animal data reveal that when administered intravenously, levels of ampicillin in the vitreous fluid were approximately 2-log less than in the serum (12), and when administered orally, amoxicillin levels in the vitreous fluid were approximately 1.5- to 2-log less effective at killing *Micrococcus luteus* than levels in serum (13). Therefore, extrapolating from animal data, there is poor penetration of ampicillin and amoxicillin into the vitreous fluid.

Gentamicin also has poor penetration into the vitreous fluid. Human studies reveal no detectable gentamicin in the vitreous fluid when doses were administered intramuscularly (1.6 mg/kg) or subconjunctivally (40 mg) (14). These data are supported with animal studies (15). Furthermore, intravitreal gentamicin has been linked to macular infarction; however, intravitreal amikacin has a lower incidence of macular infarction (16).

Linezolid resistance in *Enterococcus* is rare and there is evidence that it penetrates the vitreous chamber. Administration of two doses of oral linezolid (600 mg every 12 h) in noninflamed eyes, achieved a mean (±SD) concentration in the vitreous fluid of 5.7±2.7 µg/mL (versus 10.3±4.1 µg/mL in the serum) 6 h postdose (see Table 1 for susceptibility breakpoints). Using the same linezolid regimen, Horcadjada et al (17) found concentrations in the vitreous fluid to be higher than 4 µg/mL in the majority of patients studied, 12 h after the second dose. When only one dose was administered, it was difficult to achieve levels higher than 2 µg/mL (17-19). Unlike systemic linezolid, topical administration of linezolid in animal studies revealed negligible penetration into the vitreous fluid (20). Therefore, when administered orally or intravenously, linezolid concentrations in the vitreous chamber are above the minimum inhibitory concentration for most *Enterococci*.

Daptomycin is another alternative for treatment of VRE; however, there are limited data regarding its penetration into the vitreous chamber. One case of endogenous endophthalmitis caused by methicillin-resistant *Staphylococcus aureus* bacteremia, refractory to vancomycin and linezolid treatment in a patient experiencing chronic renal failure demonstrated vitreous fluid levels three times the Clinical and Laboratory Standards Institute susceptible breakpoint of ≤4 µg/mL 42 h after one dose of intravenous daptomycin (21).

Tigecycline is a potential antibiotic to use for VRE infections; however, topical or systemic use of tigecycline for eye infections has not been investigated. Tigecycline also has an unfavourable side effect profile and a United States Food and Drug Administration black box warning against its intravenous use (22).

In the present case, no source of the endophthalmitis other than the water stream trauma from the toy water gun was identified. Water toys and squirt guns are capable of generating pressurized water streams that pose a risk for increased intraocular pressure and ocular injury (23). While *Enterococci* are not typically associated with water, we speculate that the wading pool (that was used to fill the water guns) may have been contaminated with fecal matter. Given the timing of the insult, the clinical presentation and the lack of another identifiable source, the present case is likely one of *E casseliflavus* exogenous endophthalmitis caused by high-velocity water stream trauma from a toy water gun.

CONCLUSION

Endophthalmitis caused by *E casseliflavus* and other VRE are challenging to treat, due to reduced antimicrobial options and the poor penetration of topical and systemic antibiotics into the vitreal space. Therefore, rapid identification of the organism and knowledge of antimicrobial penetration into the vitreal space is important to guide therapy. Systemic linezolid alone may achieve intravitreal concentrations above the minimum inhibitory concentration for VRE; however, based on the literature, a combination of antibiotics delivered via intravitreal injection, systemic and topical routes should be used to treat VRE endophthalmitis.

DISCLOSURES: The authors have no financial relationships or conflicts of interest to declare.

AUTHOR CONTRIBUTIONS: All authors read and approved the final manuscript. BMB was involved in the clinical management of the patient, performed literature review and drafted the manuscript. SF was the pediatric infectious disease consultant in the present case. BH was the opthalmologist involved in the case and obtained consent from the patient's parents. SK was the medical microbiologist in the present case. All authors were involved in critical appraisal and revision of the manuscript.

ACKNOWLEDGEMENTS: The authors are grateful to the staff in the Department of Microbiology at DynaLIFEDx for the laboratory work performed for the present case.

REFERENCES

1. Cetinkaya Y, Falk P, Mayhall CG. Vancomycin-resistant *Enterococci*. Clin Microbiol Rev 2000;13:686-707.
2. Sambhav K, Mathai A, Reddy AK, Reddy BV, Bhatia K, Balne PK. Endogenous endophthalmitis caused by *Enterococcus casseliflavus*. J Med Microbiol 2011;60:670-2.
3. Habib G, Hoen B, Tornos P, et al. Guidelines on the prevention, diagnosis, and treatment of infective endocarditis (new version 2009): The Task Force on the Prevention, Diagnosis, and Treatment of Infective Endocarditis of the European Society of Cardiology (ESC). Endorsed by the European Society of Clinical Microbiology and Infectious Diseases (ESCMID) and the International Society of Chemotherapy (ISC) for Infection and Cancer. Eur Heart J 2009;2369-413.
4. Clinical Laboratory Standards Institute: Performance Standards for Antimicrobial Susceptibility Testing; Twenty-Third Informational Supplement. Clinical and Laboratory Standards Institute 2013, CLSI Document M100-S23.
5. European Committee on Antimicrobial Testing: Breakpoint tables for interpretation of MICs and zone diameters. 2013, version 3.1.
6. Vaziri K, Schwartz SG, Kishor K, Flynn HW. Endophthalmitis: State of the art. Clin Ophthalmol 2015;9:95-108.
7. Flynn HW, Scott IU. Legacy of the endophthalmitis vitrectomy study. Arch Ophthalmol 2008;126:559-61.
8. Callegan MC, Engelbert M, Parke DW, Jett BD, Gilmore MS. Bacterial endophthalmitis: Epidemiology, therapeutics, and bacterium-host interactions. Clin Microbiol Rev 2002;15:111-24.
9. Choi S-H, Lee S-O, Kim TH, et al. Clinical features and outcomes of bacteremia caused by *Enterococcus casseliflavus* and *Enterococcus gallinarum*: Analysis of 56 cases. Clin Infect Dis 2004;38:53-61.
10. Hillier RJ, Arjmand P, Rebick G, Ostrowski M, Muni RH. Post-traumatic vancomycin-resistant enterococcal endophthalmitis. J Ophthalmic Inflamm Infect 2013;3:42.
11. Kuhn F, Gini G. Ten years after... are findings of the Endophthalmitis Vitrectomy Study still relevant today? Albrecht von Graefes Arch Klin Ophthalmol 2005;243:1197-9.
12. Röber H, Göring W, Sous H, Reim M. Concentration of ampicillin in the vitreous after cryocoagulation. Albrecht v Graefes Arch klin exp Ophthal 1977;204:275-80.
13. Faigenbaum SJ, Boyle GL, Prywes AS, Abel RJ, Leopold IH. Intraocular penetrating of amoxicillin. Am J Ophthalmol 1976;82:598-603.

14. Rubinstein E, Goldfarb J, Keren G, Blumenthal M, Treister G. The penetration of gentamicin into the vitreous humor in man. Invest Ophthalmol Vis Sci 1983;24:637-9.
15. Verbraeken H, Verstraete A, Van de Velde E, Verschraegen G. Penetration of gentamicin and ofloxacin in human vitreous after systemic administration. Graefes Arch Clin Exp Ophthalmol 1996;234(Suppl 1):S59-65.
16. D'Amico DJ, Caspers-Velu L, Libert J, et al. Comparative toxicity of intravitreal aminoglycoside antibiotics. Am J Ophthalmol 1985;100:264-75.
17. Horcajada JP, Atienza R, Sarasa M, Soy D, Adan A, Mensa J. Pharmacokinetics of linezolid in human non-inflamed vitreous after systemic administration. J Antimicrob Chemother 2009;63:550-2.
18. Fiscella RG, Lai WW, Buerk B, et al. Aqueous and vitreous penetration of linezolid (Zyvox) after oral administration. Ophthalmol 2004;111:1191-5.
19. Ciulla TA, Comer GM, Peloquin C, Wheeler J. Human vitreous distribution of linezolid after a single oral dose. Retina 2005;25:619-24.
20. Saleh M, Jehl F, Dory A, et al. Ocular penetration of topically applied linezolid in a rabbit model. J Cataract Refract Surg 2010;36:488-92.
21. Sheridan KR, Potoski BA, Shields RK. Presence of adequate intravitreal concentrations of daptomycin after systemic intravenous administration in a patient with endogenous endophthalmitis. J Human Pharmacol Drug Ther 2010;30:1247-51.
22. Center for Drug Evaluation, Research: Drug Safety and Availability – FDA Drug Safety Communication: FDA warns of increased risk of death with IV antibacterial Tygacil (tigecycline) and approves new Boxed Warning. US Food and Drug Administration 2013. <www.fda.gov/Drugs/DrugSafety/ucm369580.htm> (Accessed September 3, 2015).
23. Duma SM, Bisplinghoff JA, Senge DM, McNally C, Alphonse VD. Eye injury risk from water stream impact: Biomechanically based design parameters for water toy and park design. Curr Eye Res 2012;37:279-85.

Permissions

All chapters in this book were first published in CJIDMM by Hindawi Publishing Corporation; hereby published with permission under the Creative Commons Attribution License or equivalent. Every chapter published in this book has been scrutinized by our experts. Their significance has been extensively debated. The topics covered herein carry significant findings which will fuel the growth of the discipline. They may even be implemented as practical applications or may be referred to as a beginning point for another development.

The contributors of this book come from diverse backgrounds, making this book a truly international effort. This book will bring forth new frontiers with its revolutionizing research information and detailed analysis of the nascent developments around the world.

We would like to thank all the contributing authors for lending their expertise to make the book truly unique. They have played a crucial role in the development of this book. Without their invaluable contributions this book wouldn't have been possible. They have made vital efforts to compile up to date information on the varied aspects of this subject to make this book a valuable addition to the collection of many professionals and students.

This book was conceptualized with the vision of imparting up-to-date information and advanced data in this field. To ensure the same, a matchless editorial board was set up. Every individual on the board went through rigorous rounds of assessment to prove their worth. After which they invested a large part of their time researching and compiling the most relevant data for our readers.

The editorial board has been involved in producing this book since its inception. They have spent rigorous hours researching and exploring the diverse topics which have resulted in the successful publishing of this book. They have passed on their knowledge of decades through this book. To expedite this challenging task, the publisher supported the team at every step. A small team of assistant editors was also appointed to further simplify the editing procedure and attain best results for the readers.

Apart from the editorial board, the designing team has also invested a significant amount of their time in understanding the subject and creating the most relevant covers. They scrutinized every image to scout for the most suitable representation of the subject and create an appropriate cover for the book.

The publishing team has been an ardent support to the editorial, designing and production team. Their endless efforts to recruit the best for this project, has resulted in the accomplishment of this book. They are a veteran in the field of academics and their pool of knowledge is as vast as their experience in printing. Their expertise and guidance has proved useful at every step. Their uncompromising quality standards have made this book an exceptional effort. Their encouragement from time to time has been an inspiration for everyone.

The publisher and the editorial board hope that this book will prove to be a valuable piece of knowledge for researchers, students, practitioners and scholars across the globe.

List of Contributors

Kelsey Hunt MSc, Stephanie Konrad MSc and Hyun J Lim PhD
Department of Community Health and Epidemiology

Prosanta Mondal MSc
School of Public Health

Stuart Skinner MD MSc and Kali Gartner BSc
Department of Medicine, University of Saskatchewan, Saskatoon, Saskatchewan

Shauna McQuarrie MD
Manitoba HIV Program

Ken Kasper MD and Yoav Keynan MD PhD
Manitoba HIV Program
Department of Internal Medicine, University of Manitoba

Dana C Moffatt MD
Department of Internal Medicine, University of Manitoba

Daniel Marko MD
Diagnostic Services of Manitoba, Winnipeg, Manitoba

Weidong Mu PhD and Qiang Zuo MSc
Department of Orthopedics, Provincial Hospital Affiliated to Shandong University, Jinan, Shandong Province

Qiang Zuo MSc and Lele Dong BD
Department of Orthopedics, the First Affiliated Hospital of Baotou Medical College, Baotou, Inner Mongolia

Lingyun Zhou MSc
International Education College, Jiang Xi University of Traditional Chinese Medicine, Nanchang, Jiangxi Province

Tongping Hu MSc
Clinical Laboratory, the First Affiliated Hospital of Baotou Medical College

Hua Zhang MSc
Department of Oncology, the Third Affiliated Hospital of Inner Mongolia Medical College, Baotou, Inner Mongolia, People's Republic of China

Jacqueline Willmore MPH, Brenda MacLean RN BScN MEd, Isra Levy MD MSc Lise Labrecque MHSc BSW and Cameron McDermaid MHSc
Ottawa Public Health

Vera Etches MD MHSc
Ottawa Public Health
University of Ottawa, Ottawa, Ontario

Edward Ellis MD MPH
Public Health and Preventive Medicine Consultant
University of Ottawa, Ottawa, Ontario

Carla Osiowy PhD and Anton Andonov MD PhD
National Microbiology Laboratory, Public Health Agency of Canada
University of Manitoba, Winnipeg, Manitoba

Anna Majury DVM PhD
Public Health Ontario
Queen's University, Kingston

Camille Achonu MHSc
Public Health Ontario, Toronto

Maurica Maher MD
Health Canada, Ottawa, Ontario

H D'Angelo-Scott PhD and J Cutler MHSc
Canadian Field Epidemiology Program, Public Health Agency of Canada

D Friedman PhD and A Hendriks MPH
City of Ottawa Public Health, Centre for Communicable Disease and Infection Control

AM Jolly PhD
University of Ottawa, Ottawa, Ontario

Ontario HIV Treatment Network Cohort Study Team
Michael Manno MSc
Ontario HIV Treatment Network

Ann N Burchell PhD and Sandra L Gardner PhD
Ontario HIV Treatment Network
Dalla Lana School of Public Health, University of Toronto

Peggy Millson MD
Dalla Lana School of Public Health, University of Toronto

Robert S Remis MD MPH
Dalla Lana School of Public Health, University of Toronto
Public Health Laboratories, Public Health Ontario

Janet Raboud PhD
Dalla Lana School of Public Health, University of Toronto
Toronto General Research Institute, University Health Network

Vanessa G Allen MD
Public Health Laboratories, Public Health Ontario

Tony Mazzulli MD
Public Health Laboratories, Public Health Ontario
Department of Microbiology, Mount Sinai Hospital
Department of Laboratory Medicine and Pathobiology, University of Toronto

Ahmed M Bayoumi MD MSc
Centre for Research on Inner City Health, The Keenan Research Centre in the Li KaShing Knowledge Institute, St Michael's Hospital
Institute of Health Policy, Management and Evaluation, University of Toronto
Department of Medicine, University of Toronto

Rupert Kaul MD PhD
Department of Medicine, University of Toronto

Frank McGee
AIDS Bureau, Ontario Ministry of Health and Long-Term Care

Wendy Wobeser MD MSc
Hotel Dieu Hospital
Queen's University, Kingston

Curtis Cooper MD
Ottawa Hospital
University of Ottawa, Ottawa

Sean B Rourke PhD
Ontario HIV Treatment Network
Centre for Research on Inner City Health, The Keenan Research Centre in the Li KaShing Knowledge Institute, St Michael's Hospital
Department of Psychiatry, University of Toronto

The Canadian Nosocomial Infection Surveillance Program

Geoffrey Taylor MD and Lynora Saxinger MD
University of Alberta Hospital, Edmonton, Alberta

Denise Gravel MSc
Centre for Communicable Diseases and Infection Control, Public Health Agency of Canada, Ottawa, Ontario

Kathryn Bush MSc
Alberta Health Services, Calgary

Kimberley Simmonds MSc
Alberta Health, Edmonton, Alberta

Anne Matlow MD
The Hospital for Sick Children, Toronto, Ontario

Joanne Embree MD and John Embil MD
Health Sciences Centre, Winnipeg, Manitoba

Nicole Le Saux MD
The Children's Hospital of Eastern Ontario, Ottawa, Ontario

Lynn Johnston MD
Queen Elizabeth II Health Sciences Centre, Halifax, Nova Scotia

Virginia Roth MD and Kathryn N Suh MD
The Ottawa Hospital, Ottawa, Ontario

Elizabeth Henderson PhD
Peter Lougheed Centre, Calgary, Alberta

Michael John MD
Health Sciences Centre, London, Ontario

Alice Wong MD
Royal University Hospital, Saskatoon, Saskatchewan

Daniel Dalcin MD(c)
Northern Ontario School of Medicine

Syed Zaki Ahmed MD FRCP(C)
Northern Ontario School of Medicine
Department of Internal Medicine, Thunder Bay Regional Health Sciences Centre, Thunder Bay, Ontario

Victoria Bîrlutiu MD PhD
"Lucian Blaga" University Sibiu, Faculty of Medicine Sibiu, Infectious Diseases Clinic, Academic Emergency Hospital Sibiu, Romania

Yuji Hirai MD PhD, Sayaka Asahata-Tago MD, Yusuke Ainoda MD PhD, Takahiro Fujita MD PhD and Ken Kikuchi MD PhD
Department of Infectious Diseases, Tokyo Women's Medical University

Yuji Hirai MD PhD
Department of General Medicine, Faculty of Medicine, Juntendo University, Toyko, Japan

Shalini Desai MD MHSc FRCP(C)
Public Health Agency of Canada, Toronto, Ontario

Shainoor J Ismail MD MSc FRCP(C) and Ian Gemmill MD CCFP
Public Health Agency of Canada, Edmonton, Alberta

Robert Lerch RN BScN MSc
Public Health Agency of Canada, Ottawa

Bryna F Warshawsky MD CCFP
Public Health Ontario, Toronto, Ontario

Melissa Decloe MSc CCPA
Division of Infectious Diseases, Department of Medicine, Toronto East General Hospital, Toronto; Physician Assistant Education Program, McMaster University, Hamilton

Janine McCready MD FRCPC, James Downey MD FRCPC PhD and Jeff Powis MD FRCPC MSc Division of Infectious Diseases, Department of Medicine, Toronto East General Hospital, Toronto
Department of Medicine, University of Toronto, Toronto, Ontario

Cécile Ferrouillet DMV MPH
Groupe de recherche en épidémiologie des zoonoses et santé publique, Faculté de médecine vétérinaire, Université de Montréal, St Hyacinthe
Direction des risques biologiques et de la santé au travail, Institut national de santé publique du Québec, Montréal

François Milord MD MSc
Direction des risques biologiques et de la santé au travail, Institut national de santé publique du Québec, Montréal
Direction de santé publique, Agence de la santé et des services sociaux de la Montérégie, Longueuil

Louise Lambert MD MSc
Direction de santé publique, Agence de la santé et des services sociaux de la Montérégie, Longueuil

Anne Vibien MD FRCP
Service de microbiologie-infectiologie, CSSS Richelieu-Yamaska

André Ravel DMV PhD
Groupe de recherche en épidémiologie des zoonoses et santé publique, Faculté de médecine vétérinaire, Université de Montréal, St Hyacinthe
Département de pathologie et microbiologie, Faculté de médecine vétérinaire, Université de Montréal, St Hyacinthe, Québec

Bruce R Dalton BScPhm PharmD
Department of Pharmacy Services, Alberta Health Services, Calgary
O'Brien Institute of Public Health, Cumming School of Medicine, University of Calgary, Calgary, Alberta

Sandra J MacTavish MSc
Department of Pharmacy Services, Alberta Health Services, Calgary
School of Pharmacy, University of Waterloo, Waterloo, Ontario

Lauren C Bresee BScPharm ACPR MSc PhD
Department of Pharmacy Services, Alberta Health Services, Calgary
School of Pharmacy, University of Waterloo, Waterloo, Ontario
Department of Community Health Sciences, Cumming School of Medicine

Nipunie Rajapakse MD, Otto Vanderkooi MD and Joseph Vayalumkal MD
Department of Pediatrics, Section of Infectious Diseases
Department of Medicine, Cumming School of Medicine, University of Calgary
Alberta Children's Hospital Research Institute, Alberta Health Services

John Conly MD
Alberta Children's Hospital Research Institute, Alberta Health Services
Department of Pathology and Laboratory Medicine, Cumming School of Medicine
Synder Institute for Chronic Diseases
Department of Microbiology, Immunology and Infectious Diseases, Cumming School of Medicine, University of Calgary, Calgary, Alberta

Nelson F Eng PhD, Gustavo Ybazeta PhD, Katrina Chapman BSc, Nya L Fraleigh MSc, Rebecca Letto MSc and Francisco Diaz-Mitoma MD PhD
Advanced Medical Research Institute of Canada, Sudbury

Eleonora Altman PhD
National Research Council of Canada, Ottawa, Ontario

Holly Williscroft MLT
Division of Microbiology, Calgary Laboratory Services, Departments of Pathology & Laboratory Medicine

Deirdre L Church MD PhD, Dylan R Pillai MD and Daniel G Gregson MD
Division of Microbiology, Calgary Laboratory Services, Departments of Pathology & Laboratory Medicine
Division of Medical Microbiology
Medicine, Alberta Health Services and the University of Calgary, Calgary, Alberta, and Department of Pathology & Laboratory Medicine,

Anshula Ambasta MD
Medicine, Alberta Health Services and the University of Calgary, Calgary, Alberta, and Department of Pathology & Laboratory Medicine,

Amanda Wilmer MD
Division of Medical Microbiology

Gordon Ritchie PhD and Sylvie Champagne MD
Division of Medical Microbiology
St Paul's Hospital and the University of British Columbia, Vancouver, British Columbia

Anthony D Bai BHSc
Faculty of Medicine, University of Ottawa, Ottawa

Marilyn Steinberg RN
Mount Sinai Hospital

Lisa Burry PharmD
Mount Sinai Hospital
Leslie Dan Faculty of Pharmacy

George A Tomlinson PhD
Department of Medicine
University Health Network

Adrienne Showler MD
Department of Medicine
Division of Infectious Diseases, University of Toronto, Toronto

Daniel Ricciuto MD
Department of Medicine
Division of Infectious Diseases, University of Toronto, Toronto
Lakeridge Health, Oshawa
Department of Medicine, Queen's University, Kingston

Tania Fernandes PharmD and Anna Chiu BScPhm
Trillium Health Partners, Mississauga

Sumit Raybardhan BScPhm MPH
North York General Hospital

Andrew M Morris MD SM
Mount Sinai Hospital
Department of Medicine
Division of Infectious Diseases, University of Toronto,
Toronto
University Health Network

Chaim M Bell MD PhD
Mount Sinai Hospital
Department of Medicine
University Health Network
Institute for Clinical Evaluative Sciences, Toronto, Ontario

Seyed M Moghadas PhD
Agent-Based Modelling Laboratory, York University,
Toronto, Ontario

**Margaret Haworth-Brockman MSc, Harpa Isfeld-Kiely
MA and Joel Kettner MD**
National Collaborating Centre for Infectious Diseases,
Winnipeg, Manitoba

Madison Dennis MD
Faculty of Medicine, University of Toronto

Mary Jane Salpeter RN BHA
Department of Infection Prevention and Control,
University Health Network;

Susy Hota MSc MD
Faculty of Medicine, University of Toronto;
Department of Infection Prevention and Control,
University Health Network;
Division of Infectious Diseases, Department of Medicine,
University of Toronto, Toronto, Ontario

**Catharine Chambers MSc, Mei Chong MSc and Diana
George MSc**
British Columbia Centre for Disease Control

David M Patrick MD FRCPC MHSc
British Columbia Centre for Disease Control
School of Population and Public Health, University of
British Columbia, Vancouver

Dale Purych MD
LifeLabs Medical Laboratory Services
Fraser Health Authority, Surrey

Fawziah Marra BSc PharmD FCSHP
Faculty of Pharmaceutical Services, University of British
Columbia, Vancouver, British Columbia

Dominique Gagnon MSc and Denis Hamel MSc
Institut national de santé publique du Québec

Nicole Boulianne MSc Bsinf and Eve Dubé PhD
Institut national de santé publique du Québec
Centre de recherche du CHU de Québec
Université Laval, Québec

Sylvie Belley MD and Hélène Gagné Bsinf
Direction de santé publique du Saguenay–Lac-St-Jean,
Chicoutimi

Monique Landry MD
Ministère de la santé et des Services sociaux, Montréal,
Québec

Julie A Bettinger PhD
Vaccine Evaluation Center, BC Children's Hospital,
University of British Columbia, Vancouver, British
Columbia

**Dorothy L Moore, Noni E MacDonald, Canadian
Paediatric Society,**
Infectious Diseases and Immunization Committee
Canadian Paediatric Society, 2305 St Laurent Boulevard,
Ottawa, Ontario K1G 4J8

Davie Wong MD
Internal Medicine, University of Manitoba, Winnipeg,
Manitoba

Julie Carson MD
Section of Microbiology, Department of Pathology and
Laboratory Medicine, University of Calgary
Calgary Laboratory Services

Andrew Johnson MD
Section of Infectious Diseases, Department of Medicine,
University of Calgary, Calgary, Alberta

**Michael A Mitchell MD and Seyed M Hosseini-
Moghaddam MD MPH FRCPC**
Department of Medicine;

Steve Bisch MD and Shannon Arntfield MD FRCSC
Department of Obstetrics and Gynecology, Western
University, London, Ontario, Canada

Xu-Dong Dong PhD
Faculty of Environmental Science and Engineering
Faculty of Life Science and Technology, Kunming
University of Science and Technology, Chenggong
Department of Obstetrics, First People Hospital of
Yunnan Province, Kunming, Yunnan, China

**Xiao-Ran Li PhD, Jian-Jun Luan MM, Xiao-Feng Liu
MS, Yi-Yong Luo PhD and Chen-Jian Liu PhD**
Faculty of Life Science and Technology, Kunming
University of Science and Technology, Chenggong

Juan Peng MS
Department of Obstetrics, First People Hospital of
Yunnan Province, Kunming, Yunnan, China

K Tulloch PharmD
Department of Obstetrics and Gynecology, University of
British Columbia, BC Women's Hospital

I Boucoiran MD MSc, J van Schalkwyk MD and D Money MD
Department of Obstetrics and Gynecology, University of British Columbia, BC Women's Hospital
Women's Health Research Institute, BC Women's Hospital

N Pick MD
Division of Infectious Diseases, University of British Columbia, BC Women's Hospital, Vancouver, British Columbia

F Kakkar MD MPH
Division of Infectious Diseases, Centre hospitalier universitaire Sainte-Justine and Department of Pediatrics, Faculty of Medicine, Université de Montréal
Centre Maternel et Infantile sur le SIDA, Centre hospitalier universitaire Sainte-Justine

M Boucher MD
Centre Maternel et Infantile sur le SIDA, Centre hospitalier universitaire Sainte-Justine
Department of Obstetrics and Gynecology, Université de Montréal, Centre hospitalier universitaire Sainte-Justine, Montreal, Quebec

Safa Edagiz MD
Department of Medical Microbiology, University of Manitoba

Phil Lagace-Wiens MD and James Karlowsky PhD
Department of Medical Microbiology, University of Manitoba
Diagnostic Services Manitoba

Andrew Walkty MD
Department of Medical Microbiology, University of Manitoba
Diagnostic Services Manitoba
Department of Internal Medicine, Section of Infectious Diseases, University of Manitoba, Winnipeg, Manitoba

John Embil MD
Department of Internal Medicine, Section of Infectious Diseases, University of Manitoba, Winnipeg, Manitoba

Philip W Lam BScPhm MD
Department of Medicine, University of Toronto

Andrea V Page BScH MSc MD FRCPC
Division of Infectious Diseases, Mount Sinai Hospital, Toronto, Ontario

Jianhui Xiong PhD and William Chapman MD
Department of Laboratory Medicine

Sigmund Krajden MD and Mark Downing MD
Division of Infectious Diseases
Internal Medicine of St Joseph's Health Centre

John Blondal MD and Urszula Zurawska MD
Internal Medicine of St Joseph's Health Centre

Julianne V Kus PhD and Prasad Rawte MSc
Public Health Ontario

Sigmund Krajden MD and William Chapman MD and V Kus PhD
Department of Laboratory Medicine and Pathobiology, University of Toronto, Toronto, Ontario

George G Zhanel PhD, Andrew J Walkty MD and James A Karlowsky PhD
1Department of Medical Microbiology and Infectious Diseases, College of Medicine, University of Manitoba, Winnipeg, Manitoba

Naheed Rajabali MD
University of Alberta, Edmonton

Thomas Lim MD, Colleen Sokolowski MD, Jason D Prevost MD and Edward Z Lee MD
Red Deer Regional Hospital, Red Deer, Alberta

Eric DR Pond BSc and Sameh El-Bailey MbChb DCP FRCPath
Dalhousie University

Sameh El-Bailey MbChb DCP FRCPath
Microbiology, Saint John Regional Hospital

Duncan Webster MA MD FRCPC
Internal Medicine/Medical Microbiology, Dalhousie University

Stephen Ip MD, Jo-Ann Ford MSN, Kirby Lau BSc, Vladimir Marquez MDCM MSc, Marisa Guan MD, Carolyn Klassen MSN, WC Peter Kwan MD and Eric M Yoshida MD
Department of Medicine, Division of Gastroenterology, University of British Columbia

Jessica Chan MD
United Chinese Community Enrichment Services Society (SUCCESS)

Mel Krajden MD
BC Centre for Disease Control, Vancouver, British Columbia

Raymond SW Tsang MMedSc PhD and Dennis KS Law BA BSc
National Microbiology Laboratory, Public Health Agency of Canada, Winnipeg, Manitoba

Rita R Gad MD DrPH
Communicable Disease Control Unit, Department of Health, Government of New Brunswick, Fredericton, New Brunswick

Tim Mailman MD FRCPC
Department of Pathology and Laboratory Medicine, IWK Health Centre, Halifax, Nova Scotia

Gregory German MD PhD FRCPC
Department of Health, Government of Prince Edward Island, Charlottetown, Prince Edward Island

Robert Needle MSc MLS (ASCP)
Public Health Laboratory and Microbiology, Eastern Health, St John's, Newfoundland and Labrador

Guillaume Mongeau-Martin DCS and Michael Libman MDCM, Momar Ndao DVM PhD, Brian J Ward MSc, MDCM
JD MacLean Tropical Diseases Centre

Gilles Delage MD
Héma-Québec Inc, Ville Saint-Laurent, Quebec

Momar Ndao DVM PhD and Brian J Ward MSc, MDCM
National Reference Centre for Parasitology, Research Institute of the McGill University Health Centre, Montreal

Philippe Guillaume Poliquin MD FRCPC
Section of Paediatric Infectious Diseases, Department of Paediatrics and Child Health

Philippe Lagacé-Wiens MD FRCPC and John M Embil MD FRCPC
Department of Medical Microbiology and Infectious Diseases, University of Manitoba

Philippe Lagacé-Wiens MD FRCPC
Department of Clinical Microbiology, St Boniface General Hospital

Mauro Verrelli MD FRCPC
Section of Nephrology, Department of Internal Medicine, University of Manitoba, and Manitoba Renal Program

David W Allen MD
Section of Cardiology

John M Embil MD FRCPC
Section of Infectious Diseases, Department of Internal Medicine, University of Manitoba, Winnipeg, Manitoba

Derek R MacFadden MD, Wayne L Gold MD, Ibrahim Al-Busaidi MD, Jeffrey D Craig MD, Dan Petrescu MD, Ilana S Saltzman MD and Jerome A Leis MD, MSc
Division of Infectious Diseases, Department of Medicine, University of Toronto;

Jerome A Leis MD, MSc
Centre for Quality Improvement and Patient Safety, University of Toronto, Toronto, Ontario

Abdulaziz Ahmed Hashi MD
Department of Medicine

Johannes Andries Delport MBChB MMed and Sameer Elsayed MD FRCPC FACP
Department of Pathology and Laboratory Medicine

Michael Seth Silverman MD FRCPC FACP and Sameer Elsayed MD FRCPC FACP
Department of Medicine, Division of Infectious Diseases, The University of Western Ontario, London, Ontario

Estelle Ouellet MPA MD(c), Madeleine Durand MD MSc FRCPC, Jason R Guertin MSc PhD(c),
Jacques LeLorier MD PhD FRCPC FISPE and Cécile L Tremblay MD FRCPC
Centre de Recherche du Centre Hospitalier de l'Université de Montréal, Montréal, Québec

Hirotaka Yamashiro MD FRCP C FAAP, Nora Cutcliffe MSc PhD, Simon Dobson MD FRCP C,
David Fisman MD MPH FRCP C and Ronald Gold MD MPH
Pediatrics Section, Ontario Medical Association (PSOMA) and Pediatricians Alliance of Ontario (PAO); 'Pediatricians of Ontario'

Peter Daley MD MSc FRCPC DTM+H, Carla Penney BSc, Susan Wakeham BSc1 and Brendan Barrett MD FRCPC
Memorial University

Glenda Compton MN RN, Aaron McKim MD CCFP and Judy O'Keefe MSW RSW
Long-Term Care, Eastern Health, St John's, Newfoundland and Labrador

Lindsay Nicolle MD FRCPC
University of Manitoba, Winnipeg, Manitoba

Byron M Berenger MD and Sarah E Forgie MD
Department of Medical Microbiology and Immunology, University of Alberta

Byron M Berenger MD
Alberta Provincial Laboratory for Public Health

Shobhana Kulkarni MD
DynaLIFEDx Diagnostic Laboratory Services;
Department of Laboratory Medicine and Pathology;

Brad J Hinz MD
Department of Ophthamology

Sarah E Forgie MD
Department of Pediatrics, University of Alberta, Edmonton, Alberta